MOLECULAR ACTIONS AND TARGETS FOR CANCER CHEMOTHERAPEUTIC AGENTS

BRISTOL-MYERS CANCER SYMPOSIA

Series Editor
MAXWELL GORDON
Bristol Laboratories
Syracuse, New York

1. Harris Busch, Stanley T. Crooke, and Yerach Daskal (Editors). *Effects of Drugs on the Cell Nucleus, 1979.*
2. Alan C. Sartorelli, John S. Lazo, and Joseph R. Bertino (Editors). *Molecular Actions and Targets for Cancer Chemotherapeutic Agents, 1981.*

MOLECULAR ACTIONS AND TARGETS FOR CANCER CHEMOTHERAPEUTIC AGENTS

Edited by

ALAN C. SARTORELLI

JOHN S. LAZO

JOSEPH R. BERTINO

Departments of Pharmacology and Medicine
and
Developmental Therapeutics Program
Comprehensive Cancer Center
Yale University School of Medicine
New Haven, Connecticut

1981

ACADEMIC PRESS

A Subsidiary of Harcourt Brace Jovanovich, Publishers
New York London Toronto Sydney San Francisco

ACADEMIC PRESS, INC.
111 Fifth Avenue, New York, New York 10003

United Kingdom Edition published by
ACADEMIC PRESS, INC. (LONDON) LTD.
24/28 Oval Road, London NW1 7DX

Library of Congress Cataloging in Publication Data
Main entry under title:

Molecular actions and targets for cancer chemotherapeutic agents.

(Bristol-Myers cancer symposia series; v. 2)
Includes bibliographical references and index.
1. Cancer--Chemotherapy--Congresses. 2. Antineoplastic agents--Congresses. 3. Molecular biology--Congresses. I. Sartorelli, Alan Clayton, Date. II. Lazo, John S. III. Bertino, Joseph R. IV. Series: Bristol-Myers cancer symposia; v. 2. [DNLM: 1. Antineoplastic agents--Pharmacodynamics--Congresses. 2. Receptors, Drug--Congresses. 3. Neoplasms--Drug therapy--Congresses. W3 B429 v. 2 1979 / QZ 267 M718 1979]
RC271.C5M64 616.99'4061 80-1683
ISBN 0-12-619280-4

PRINTED IN THE UNITED STATES OF AMERICA

81 82 83 84 9 8 7 6 5 4 3 2 1

Contents

4 Chemotherapeutic Approaches to Cell Populations of Tumors

KATHERINE A. KENNEDY, BEVERLY A. TEICHER, SARA ROCKWELL, and ALAN C. SARTORELLI

5 Suicide Enzyme Inactivators

ROBERT H. ABELES

PART II ANTIBIOTICS

6 DNA Dynamics and Drug Intercalation

HENRY M. SOBELL

7 Molecular Pharmacology of Anthracyclines

STANLEY T. CROOKE, VIRGIL H. DUVERNAY, and SEYMOUR MONG

8 Protein Antibiotics as DNA-Damaging Agents

IRVING H. GOLDBERG, TAKUMI HATAYAMA, LIZZY S. KAPPEN, MARY A. NAPIER, and LAWRENCE F. POVIRK

9 The Action of Bleomycin on DNA in Solution and in Cells

FRANKLIN HUTCHINSON, LAWRENCE F. POVIRK, and KAZUO YAMAMOTO

PART III ANTIMETABOLITES—NUCLEOSIDE ANALOGS

10 Transport of Nucleosides and Nucleoside Analogs by Animal Cells

ALAN R. P. PATERSON

11 Purine Nucleoside Phosphorylase and 5′-Methylthioadenosine Phosphorylase: Targets of Chemotherapy

ROBERT E. PARKS, JR., JOHANNA D. STOECKLER, CAROLYN CAMBOR, TODD M. SAVARESE, GERALD W. CRABTREE, and SHIH-HSI CHU

12 *In Vitro* and *in Vivo* Effects of 5′-Thioadenosine Nucleosides

JAMES K. COWARD

13 Studies on Identifying the Locus of Action of Fluorouracil

FRANK MALEY and GLADYS F. MALEY

14 Inhibition of Thymidylate Synthetase: Mechanism, Methods, and Metabolic Consequences

DANIEL V. SANTI

PART IV ANTIMETABOLITES—FOLATE ANALOGS

15 The Binding of Ligands to Dihydrofolate Reductase

RAYMOND L. BLAKLEY

16 Transport of Folate Compounds in L1210 Cells: Components and Mechanisms

F. M. HUENNEKENS, K. S. VITOLS, M. R. SURESH, and G. B. HENDERSON

17 Membrane Transport and the Molecular Basis for Selective Antitumor Action of Folate Analogs

F. M. SIROTNAK, P. L. CHELLO, J. I. DEGRAW, J. R. PIPER, and J. A. MONTGOMERY

18 Cellular Mechanisms of Resistance to Methotrexate

J. R. BERTINO, B. J. DOLNICK, R. J. BERENSON, D. I. SCHEER, and B. A. KAMEN

PART V RADIATION SENSITIZERS

19 Hypoxia-Dependent Radiation Sensitizers and Chemotherapeutic Agents

G. E. ADAMS and I. J. STRATFORD

20 Mechanistic and Pharmacological Considerations in the Design and Use of Hypoxic Cell Radiosensitizers

J. D. CHAPMAN, J. NGAN-LEE, and B. E. MEEKER

PART VI MEMBRANE TARGETS

21 Plasma Membranes as Targets and Mediators in Tumor Chemotherapy

DONALD F. HOELZL WALLACH, ROSS B. MIKKELSEN, and LESTER KWOCK

22 Altered Plasma Membrane Glycoconjugates of Chinese Hamster Cells with Acquired Resistance to Actinomycin D, Daunorubicin, and Vincristine

JUNE L. BIEDLER and ROBERT H. F. PETERSON

23 Tubulin: A Target for Chemotherapeutic Agents

PETER B. SCHIFF and SUSAN BAND HORWITZ

PART VII ANGIOGENESIS–METASTASIS–ANTICARCINOGENESIS–DIFFERENTIATION

List of Contributors

Numbers in parentheses indicate the pages on which the authors' contributions begin.

ROBERT H. ABELES (103), Graduate Department of Biochemistry, Brandeis University, Waltham, Massachusetts 02254

G. E. ADAMS (401), Division of Physics, Institute of Cancer Research, Royal Cancer Hospital, Sutton, Surrey, SM2 5PX England

R. J. BERENSON (385), Departments of Medicine and Pharmacology, Yale University School of Medicine, New Haven, Connecticut 06510

J. R. BERTINO (385), Departments of Medicine and Pharmacology, Yale University School of Medicine, New Haven, Connecticut 06510

JUNE L. BIEDLER (453), Laboratory of Cellular and Biochemical Genetics, Sloan-Kettering Institute for Cancer Research, Rye, New York 10580

RAYMOND L. BLAKLEY (303), Department of Biochemistry, College of Medicine, The University of Iowa, Iowa City, Iowa 52242

CAROLYN CAMBOR (229), Division of Biology and Medicine, Brown University, Providence, Rhode Island 02912

J. D. CHAPMAN (419), Department of Radiation Oncology, Cross Cancer Institute and Department of Radiology, University of Alberta, Edmonton, Alberta T6G 1Z2 Canada

P. L. CHELLO (349), Laboratory for Molecular Therapeutics, Memorial Sloan-Kettering Cancer Center, New York, New York 10021

SHIH-HSI CHU (229), Division of Biology and Medicine, Brown University, Providence, Rhode Island 02912

JAMES K. COWARD (253), Department of Chemistry, Rensselaer Polytechnic Institute, Troy, New York 12181

GERALD W. CRABTREE (229), Division of Biology and Medicine, Brown University, Providence, Rhode Island 02912

STANLEY T. CROOKE* (137), Research and Development, Bristol Laboratories, Syracuse, New York 13201

JOSEPH E. DE LARCO (541), National Cancer Institute, National Institutes of Health, Bethesda, Maryland, 20205

J. I. DEGRAW (349), SRI International, Menlo Park, California 94025

B. J. DOLNICK (385), Departments of Medicine and Pharmacology, Yale University School of Medicine, New Haven, Connecticut 06510

VIRGIL H. DUVERNAY (137), Department of Pharmacology, Baylor College of Medicine, Houston, Texas 77025

JUDAH FOLKMAN (511), Department of Surgery, Children's Hospital Medical Center, Boston, Massachusetts 02115

ROBERT C. GALLO (555), Laboratory of Tumor Cell Biology, National Cancer Institute, National Institutes of Health, Bethesda, Maryland 20205

IRVING H. GOLDBERG (163), Department of Pharmacology, Harvard Medical School, Boston, Massachusetts 02115

K. R. HARRAP (45), Department of Biochemical Pharmacology, Institute of Cancer Research, Royal Cancer Hospital, Sutton, Surrey SM2 5PX England

TAKUMI HATAYAMA (163), Department of Pharmacology, Harvard Medical School, Boston, Massachusetts 02115

G. B. HENDERSON (333), Department of Biochemistry, Scripps Clinic and Research Foundation, La Jolla, California 92037

SUSAN BAND HORWITZ (483), Department of Cell Biology and Molecular Pharmacology, Albert Einstein College of Medicine, Yeshiva University, Bronx, New York 10461

F. M. HUENNEKENS (333), Department of Biochemistry, Scripps Clinic and Research Foundation, La Jolla, California 92037

FRANKLIN HUTCHINSON (193), Department of Molecular Biophysics and Biochemistry, Yale University, New Haven, Connecticut 06520

A. JENEY (45), Laboratory of Molecular Pathology, Institute of Pathology, Semmelweis Medical University, Budapest, Hungary

*Present address: Research and Development, Smith Kline & French Laboratories, Philadelphia, Pennsylvania 19101.

B. A. KAMEN* (385), Department of Pediatrics and Pharmacology, Yale University School of Medicine, New Haven, Connecticut 06510

LIZZY S. KAPPEN (163), Department of Pharmacology, Harvard Medical School, Boston, Massachusetts 02115

KATHERINE A. KENNEDY (85), Department of Pharmacology and the Developmental Therapeutics Program, Comprehensive Cancer Center, Yale University School of Medicine, New Haven, Connecticut 06510

K. W. KOHN (3), Laboratory of Molecular Pharmacology, Developmental Therapeutics Program, Division of Cancer Treatment, National Cancer Institute, National Institutes of Health, Bethesda, Maryland 20205

LESTER KWOCK (433), Division of Radiobiology, Department of Therapeutic Radiology, New England Medical Center Hospital, Tufts University School of Medicine, Boston, Massachusetts 02111

ROBERT LANGER† (511), Department of Surgery, Children's Hospital Medical Center, Boston, Massachusetts 02115

REUBEN LOTAN‡ (527), Departments of Developmental and Cell Biology and Physiology, College of Medicine, University of California, Irvine, California 92717

FRANK MALEY (265), Division of Laboratories and Research, New York State Department of Health, Albany, New York 12201

GLADYS F. MALEY (265), Division of Laboratories and Research, New York State Department of Health, Albany, New York 12201

B. E. MEEKER (419), Department of Radiation Oncology, Cross Cancer Institute and Department of Radiology, University of Alberta, Edmonton, T6G 1Z2 Canada

ROSS B. MIKKELSEN (433), Division of Radiobiology, Department of Therapeutic Radiology, New England Medical Center Hospital, Tufts University School of Medicine, Boston, Massachusetts 02111

SEYMOUR MONG (137), Department of Pharmacology, Baylor College of Medicine, Houston, Texas 77025

*Present address: Midwest Children's Cancer Center, Department of Pediatrics and Pharmacology, Medical College of Wisconsin and Milwaukee Childrens Hospital, Milwaukee, Wisconsin 53233

†Present address: Department of Nutrition and Food Science, Massachusetts Institute of Technology, Cambridge, Massachusetts.

‡Present address: Department of Biophysics, The Weizmann Institute, Rehovot, Israel

J. A. MONTGOMERY (349), Southern Research Institute, Birmingham, Alabama 35205

MARY A. NAPIER (163), Department of Pharmacology, Harvard Medical School, Boston, Massachusetts 02115

DIANNE L. NEWTON (541), National Cancer Institute, National Institutes of Health, Bethesda, Maryland 20205

J. NGAN-LEE (419), Department of Radiation Oncology, Cross Cancer Institute and Department of Radiology, University of Alberta, Edmonton, Alberta, T6G 1Z2 Canada

GARTH L. NICOLSON* (527), Departments of Developmental and Cell Biology and Physiology, College of Medicine, University of California, Irvine, California 92717

ROBERT E. PARKS, JR. (229), Division of Biology and Medicine, Brown University, Providence, Rhode Island 02912

ALAN R. P. PATERSON (213), Cancer Research Unit, McEachern Laboratory, The University of Alberta, Edmonton, Alberta, T6G 2H7 Canada

ROBERT H. F. PETERSON (453), Laboratory of Cellular and Biochemical Genetics, Sloan-Kettering Institute for Cancer Research, Rye, New York 10580

J. R. PIPER (349), Southern Research Institute, Birmingham, Alabama 35205

LAWRENCE F. POVIRK† (163, 193), Department of Molecular Biophysics and Biochemistry, Yale University, New Haven, Connecticut 06520

P. G. RICHES (45), Protein Reference Unit, Westminster Hospital, London, SW1 England

J. J. ROBERTS (17), Pollards Wood Research Station, Institute of Cancer Research, Royal Cancer Hospital, Chalfont St. Giles, Buckinghamshire HP8 4SP England

ANITA B. ROBERTS (541), National Cancer Institute, National Institutes of Health, Bethesda, Maryland 20205

SARA ROCKWELL (85), Department of Therapeutic Radiology, Yale University School of Medicine, New Haven, Connecticut 06510

*Present address: Department of Tumor Biology, University of Texas System Cancer Center, M.D. Anderson Hospital and Tumor Institute, Houston, Texas 77030

†Present address: Department of Pharmacology, Harvard Medical School, Boston, Massachusetts 02115

Francis W. Ruscetti (555), Laboratory of Tumor Cell Biology, National Cancer Institute, National Institutes of Health, Bethesda, Maryland 20205

Leo Sachs (579), Department of Genetics, The Weizmann Institute of Science, Rehovot, Israel

Daniel V. Santi (285), Department of Biochemistry and Biophysics, and Department of Pharmaceutical Chemistry, University of California, San Francisco, California 94143

Alan C. Sartorelli (85), Department of Pharmacology and the Developmental Therapeutics Program, Comprehensive Cancer Center, Yale University School of Medicine, New Haven, Connecticut 06510

Todd M. Savarese (229), Division of Biology and Medicine, Section of Biochemical Pharmacology, Brown University, Providence, Rhode Island 02912

D. I. Scheer(385),Departments of Medicine and Pharmacology, Yale University School of Medicine, New Haven, Connecticut 06510

Peter B. Schiff (483), Department of Cell Biology and Molecular Pharmacology, Albert Einstein College of Medicine, Yeshiva University, Bronx, New York 10461

F. M. Sirotnak (349), Laboratory for Molecular Therapeutics, Memorial Sloan-Kettering Cancer Center, New York, New York 10021

Henry M. Sobell (119), Department of Radiation Biology and Biophysics, The University of Rochester School of Medicine and Dentistry, Rochester, New York 14627

Michael B. Sporn (541), National Cancer Institute, National Institutes of Health, Bethesda, Maryland 20205

Johanna D. Stoeckler (229), Division of Biology and Medicine, Brown University, Providence, Rhode Island 02912

I. J. Stratford (401), Division of Physics, Institute of Cancer Research, Royal Cancer Hospital, Sutton, Surrey, England

M. R. Suresh (333), Department of Biochemistry, Scripps Clinic and Research Foundation, La Jolla, California 92037

Beverly A. Teicher (85), Department of Pharmacology and the Developmental Therapeutics Program, Comprehensive Cancer Center, Yale University School of Medicine, New Haven, Connecticut 06510

P. J. THRAVES (45), Department of Biochemical Pharmacology, Institute of Cancer Research, Royal Cancer Hospital, Sutton, Surrey, SM2 5PX England

GEORGE J. TODARO (541), Laboratory of Viral Carcinogenesis, National Cancer Institute, National Institutes of Health, Bethesda, Maryland 20205

K. S. VITOLS (333), Department of Biochemistry, Scripps Clinic and Research Foundation, La Jolla, California 92037

DONALD F. HOELZL WALLACH (433), Division of Radiobiology, Department of Therapeutic Radiology, New England Medical Center Hospital, Tufts University School of Medicine, Boston, Massachusetts 02111

R. WILKINSON (45), Department of Biochemical Pharmacology, Institute of Cancer Research, Royal Cancer Hospital, Sutton, Surrey, SM2 5PX England

KAZUO YAMAMOTO (193), Department of Molecular Biophysics and Biochemistry, Yale University, New Haven, Connecticut 06520

Editor's Foreword

The second Bristol-Myers Cancer Symposium was hosted by the Yale University School of Medicine and addressed the subject of Molecular Actions and Targets for Cancer Chemotherapeutic Agents. The range of topics covered was very broad, but a theme was evident throughout the presentations. In a sense, this symposium helped to highlight an evolutionary process that has been gathering momentum for many years and which will now accelerate under the influence of all of the new methodologies in molecular biology and other biomedical sciences.

The historic method of drug discovery has involved, to a large extent, broad screening on a relatively empirical basis. A few of the early cancer drugs, like methotrexate or 5-fluorouracil were designed in the 1940s and 1950s as inhibitors of known essential molecules, following the earlier successes in the 1930s and 1940s in finding the sulfonamides to be useful antagonists of para-aminobenzoic acid. Later, as cell biology became better understood, various enzymes or other *in vitro* systems were enlisted in the screening effort, but the work was still largely empirical.

Today, with the explosive growth of structural and biochemical knowledge about nucleic acids and proteins, people are increasingly making use of this knowledge to improve chemotherapy by studying molecular actions and targets for cancer chemotherapeutic agents. In some cases, the putative drugs are designed based on structural and energetic considerations. In other cases,people continue to screen, but in ever more sophisticated systems. The flowering of research in a variety of natural products, both of microbial origin and from higher life forms, has made much use of the knowledge gained in a dozen disparate disciplines. Agents of microbial origin like doxorubicin, carubicin, aclarubicin, bleomycin, mitomycin C, marcellomycin, and the talisomycins are finding increasing therapeutic use and are contributing immeasurably to our understanding of cancer chemotherapy, nucleic acid inhibition, etc. From the higher plants,the vinca alkaloids, etoposide, teniposide, tripdiolide, bruceantin, etc., form a parade of old and new antitumor molecules. The noble metal derivatives, especially cisplatin, have contributed much to chemotherapy and to a definition of molecular actions and targets. Finally, from mammalian sources,the interferons have opened a new chapter in antitumor and antiviral research. The scientific and financial resources committed to the interferons have telescoped what normally would be decades of research into a few short years. And the new sciences of recombinant DNA and monoclonal antibodies have contributed immeasurably to overall progress. It is all the more remarkable when one considers that the field of recombinant DNA is less than ten years old, and the hybridomas are less than half that age.

Symposia such as that reported in this volume play a key role in the dissemination of new biomedical knowledge, and, even more importantly, in providing another opportunity for creative scientists to meet and inspire each other. We look forward to this continuing voyage of discovery.

Maxwell Gordon
Series Editor

Foreword

In 1978, the first of a series of annual Bristol-Myers Cancer Symposia was organized by Baylor College of Medicine on "Effects of Drugs on the Cell Nucleus." In 1979, Yale University School of Medicine hosted the second symposium on "Molecular Actions and Targets for Cancer Chemotherapeutic Agents," reported in this volume.

The Yale symposium and the previous meeting at Baylor drew scientists from around the world. In a field of such international scope, no one knows where the next forward move in cancer research may occur.

If small gains on numerous, widely separated fronts are to add up to significant progress, the need for extensive worldwide communication is obvious. However, in the scientific community, where the demands and attractions of the laboratory make it difficult to find time for much else, communication can be slow.

The company wants to encourage more rapid interchange by providing, through the Bristol-Myers Cancer Symposia, a means and an excuse for distinguished scientists to break away from their daily routines once a year to assemble. These opportunities for communication will continue as we move into the 1980s.

The 1980 symposium, to be reported in a future volume, was organized by Stanford University School of Medicine on "Advances in Malignant Lymphomas: Etiology, Immunology, Pathology, Treatment." Future symposia are being developed by The Johns Hopkins University School of Medicine and The University of Chicago.

The international thrust of communication on cancer research dates back at least to 1956—a quarter century ago—when Bristol-Myers became involved in anticancer drug research. Even before that, the company had established collaborative research agreements with, among others, the noted Japanese biochemist, Dr. Hamao Umezawa. Our connection with Dr. Umezawa, who discovered the antibiotic bleomycin and saw its promise as a cancer chemotherapeutic agent, was the nucleus from which our subsequent efforts have grown. The company's indebtedness to Dr. Umezawa is great. Today, anticancer drug research holds the top position on the company's research agenda.

The challenges and opportunities in cancer research—including the chances to alleviate the suffering and to improve the lives of untold thousands today and in the future—mean as much to us as they do to cancer scientists. We are proud to play a role in these proceedings.

Richard L. Gelb
Chairman
Bristol-Myers Company

Preface

Chemotherapy has assumed an increasingly important role in the management of patients with cancer. The employment of laboratory and clinical research on the biochemical and pharmacological actions of anticancer drugs should result in new leads that will permit future advances in the chemotherapy of malignancy. This volume represents the proceedings of the Second Annual Bristol-Myers Symposium on Cancer Research hosted by the Department of Pharmacology and the Developmental Therapeutics Program of the Comprehensive Cancer Center of the Yale University School of Medicine. The Symposium and the papers derived therefrom and presented in this volume describe aspects of the biochemical mechanism of action of some of the most important antineoplastic agents in our clinical armamentarium. It is our expectation that such knowledge may assist in the more efficacious clinical use of these agents in refractory cancers. The drug classes considered include alkylating agents, platinum-containing compounds, folate antagonists, purine and pyrimidine nucleoside antimetabolites, and the anthracycline and bleomycin antibiotics. In addition to examining currently employed drugs, a second objective of this volume is to describe possible new biochemical targets and actions for novel therapeutic agents that might lead to the therapies of the future. These include (a) possible membrane targets and radiosensitizers, and (b) noncytotoxic approaches designed to prevent metastases, induce terminal differentiation of malignant cells, inhibit tumor angiogenesis, and suppress carcinogenesis. Such topics were selected for inclusion by the Editors with the conviction that future therapeutic approaches will include noncytotoxic agents. We wish to thank Mrs. Paula A. Wilson and Miss Marion E. Morra for their great assistance in the organization and management of this Symposium, and the Bristol-Myers Company for their support and sponsorship.

Alan C. Sartorelli
John S. Lazo
Joseph R. Bertino

Glossary of Abbreviations

ACM	Aclacinomycin (aclarubicin)
ADA	Adenosine deaminase
ADM	Adriamycin (doxorubicin)
8-AG	8-Aminoguanine
CD	Circular dichroism
CEF	Chick embryo fibroblasts
CH_3B_{12}	Methylcobalamine
CH_2FH_4	5,10-Methylene tetrahydrofolate
CH_3FH_4	5-Methyl tetrahydrofolate
CHIP	*cis*-Dichloro-*trans*-hydroxo-bis-isopropylamine platinum IV
CHO	Chinese hamster ovary
$CHOFH_4$	5-Formyl tetrahydrofolate
CHLZ	Chlorozotocin
CM	Conditioned medium
CMM	Carminomycin (carubicin)
CMNQ	2,3-Dichloromethyl-1,4-naphthoquinone
COMT	Catechol-*O*-methyltransferase
CSA	Colony stimulating activity
5′-dAdo	5′-Deoxyadenosine
d-CMP	2′-Deoxycytidylate
DHF	Dihydrofolate
DHFR	Dihydrofolate reductase
DNM	Daunomycin (daunorubicin)
DSAM	Decarboxylated *S*-adenosylmethionine
EBV	Epstein–Barr Virus
5′-ETFAR	5′-Deoxy-5′-ethylthio-2-fluoroadenosine
F	Folate
FAH_2	Dihydrofolate
FdUMP	5-Fluoro-2′-deoxyuridylate
FH_2	Dihydrofolate
FH_4	Tetrahydrofolate
HEPES	4-(2-Hydroxyethyl)-1-piperazine ethane sulfonic acid
HGPRT	Hypoxanthine-guanine phosphoribosyl transferase
HN_2	2,2′-Dichloro-*N*-methyl diethylamine
HSR	Homogeneously staining region
LAP	Leukocyte alkaline phosphatase

L-PAM	L-Phenylalanine mustard
Ly-CM	Lymphocyte conditioned medium
MAPS	Posttranslational modifications of tubulin
MCD	Magnetic circular dichroism
MCM	Marcellomycin
MGI	Macrophage and granulocyte inducer
MNNG	1-Methyl-3-nitro-1-nitrosoguanidine
MSM	Musettamycin
MTA	Methyl thioadenosine
MTR	5-Deoxy-5-methyl thioribose
MTT	5′-Deoxy-5′-methylthiotubercidin
MTX	Methotrexate
NAC	*N*-Acetyl mercapto ethylamine
NADABA	*N*-Adenosyl-α,γ-diaminobutyric acid
NADP	Nicotinamide adenine dinucleotide phosphate
NBMPR	Nitrobenzylthioinosine
NCS	Neocarzinostatin (zinostatin)
OER	Oxygen enhancement ratio
OPRTase	Orotate phosphoribosyl transferase
PADP	2′-Phospho adenosine-5′-diphosphate
PALA	*N*-Phosphono acetyl aspartic acid
pCMS	*p*-Chloromercuriphenyl sulfonate
PHA	Phytohemagglutinin
PM_2 DNA	Superhelical form of DNA
PNP	Purine nucleoside phosphorylase
PRPP	5-Phosphoribosyl-1-pyrophosphate
PYM	Pyrromycin
QSAR	Quantitative structure–activity relationships
RDM	Rudolfomycin
RSV	Rous sarcoma virus
SAH	*S*-Adenosylhomocysteine
SAM	*S*-Adenosyl-L-methionine
SGF	Sarcoma growth factor
SIBA	*S*-Isobutyl-adenosine
TAF	Tumor angiogenesis factor
TCGF	T-cell growth factor
5-TDG	5-Thio-D-glucose
TMPP	Trimethylphenylphosphonium
TPA	Phorbol myristate acetate
TSCK	Tolylsulfonyl-lysyl chloromethyl ketone
VAB	Vincristine + actinomycin D + bleomycin
VAB III	Vincristine + actinomycin D + bleomycin + cyclophosphamide + adriamycin
WHE-CM	Whole human embryo culture medium
XP	Xeroderma pigmentosum

PART I

Alkylating Agents

1

Molecular Mechanisms of Cross-Linking by Alkylating Agents and Platinum Complexes

K. W. KOHN

Early work on the mechanism of action of alkylating agents evolved the general rule that compounds having a single alkylating group tend to be highly mutagenic and carcinogenic, but that only compounds with two or more alkylating groups are potent cytotoxins and anticancer agents. This led to the hypothesis that the cytotoxic and anticancer activities of these agents are due to cross-linking between macromolecules, especially between DNA molecules (1–5). The double-helical structure of DNA and the finding by Lawley (6) that guanine was susceptible to alkylation at the N-7 position suggested the new possibility of cross-linking between paired DNA strands. Brookes and Lawley (7) reported cross-linkage between two guanines in DNA by nitrogen mustard but could not determine whether the guanines were linked within the same or across opposite strands. Interstrand cross-linking was, however, soon demonstrated accidentally by Geiduschek (8) for nitrogen mustard and again by Iyer and Szybalski (9) in the case of mitomycin. Cross-linking of adjacent bases within the same DNA strand is also possible and is supported in the case of Myleran by the finding of diguanyl products (7) and no interstrand cross-links (10). The possibility of cross-linking between DNA and protein was reported by Rutman *et al.* (11) and Golder *et al.* (12) on the basis of trapping of DNA with precipitated protein from treated cells. It is likely that these cross-linking reactions involving DNA—i.e., interstrand, intrastrand, DNA–protein, or a combination of these linkages—account for the major part of the cytotoxic and antitumor activities of alkylating agents.

MOLECULAR ACTIONS AND TARGETS FOR CANCER CHEMOTHERAPEUTIC AGENTS

ISBN 0-12-619280-4

Although the major inferences from the earlier work have held up, the picture is not quite as simple as was originally thought in that monofunctional alkylating agents have been found to be capable, under some circumstances, of producing cross-links. One possible mechanism of cross-link formation by monofunctional agents is by way of depurination. Alkylated purines may be eliminated from DNA either spontaneously (7) or perhaps enzymatically, leaving a base-free deoxyribose moiety in the DNA backbone. Base-free sites can form interstrand cross-links, possibly by Schiff base formation between the deoxyribose aldehyde group and an amino group on the opposite strand (13). This mechanism may explain the production of interstrand cross-links (14) and possibly also DNA–protein cross-links, by methyl methanesulfonate (15). The ratio of cross-links to monoalkylations, however, is apparently much less than in the case of bifunctional agents.

A more pertinent case is presented by chloroethylnitrosoureas, a group of drugs having extraordinary activity against experimental tumors. These compounds have only one alkylating group, but this single group can produce two alkylations in succession, as demonstrated in the reaction with cytosine moieties (16, 17) (Fig. 1). The nitrosourea molecule initially decomposes to form an active chloroethyldiazohydroxide intermediate (Fig. 2) which is thought to be the alkylating species that transfers chloroethyl groups to nucleophiles. The first alkylation reaction of the nitrosourea is a transfer of the chloroethyl group to either the N-3 or the 4-amino nitrogen of cytosine. A second reaction follows in

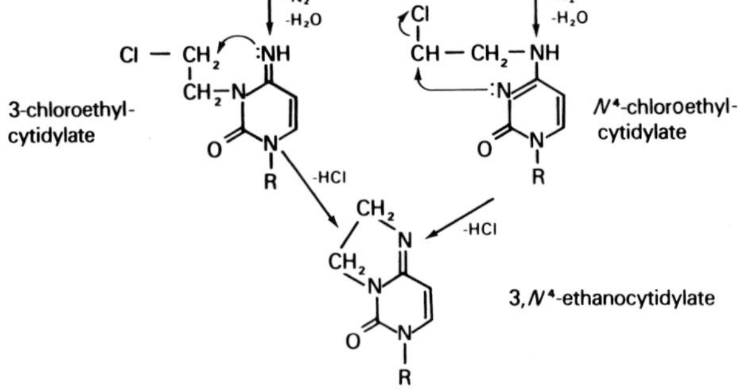

Fig. 1. Successive reactions of a chloroethyl group with a cytosine moiety to form an intramolecular cross-link.

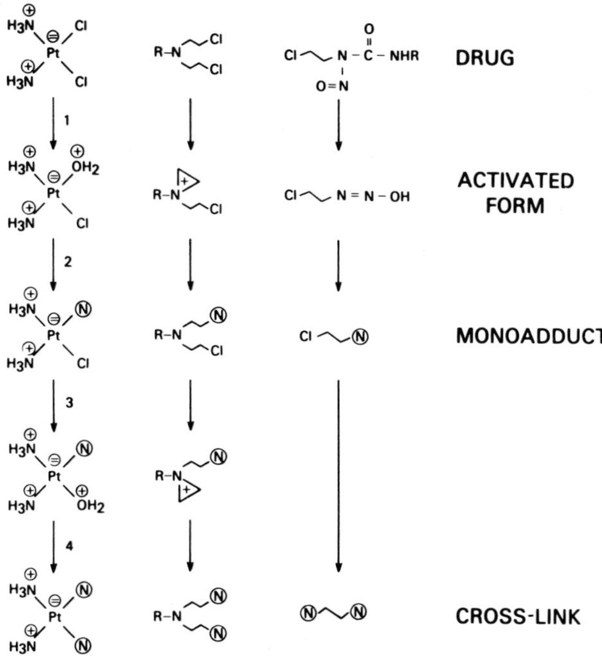

Fig. 2. Reaction steps in the formation of monoadducts and cross-links by Pt(II) complexes, nitrogen mustards, and chloroethylnitrosoureas. Encircled N represents a nucleophilic site on a macromolecule.

which the chloride is displaced and the ethylene chain becomes linked to both nitrogens in the same cytosine residue. When an analogous sequence of reactions occurs between opposite DNA strands, the result is an interstrand cross-link (Fig. 3) (18).

The reaction sequences leading to cross-link formation by three different types of agents are shown in Fig. 2. The classic case of bifunctional nitrogen mustards is shown in the center. (The R group in certain compounds, such as cyclophosphamide, draws electrons away from the nitrogen atom, so that the compound does not undergo any of the reactions shown until a preliminary reaction activates the drug; in Fig. 2, the R group is assumed not to be this type.) The first step leads to a reactive aziridinium intermediate which can alkylate at a nucleophilic site on a macromolecule to form a monoadduct. The process repeats with conver-

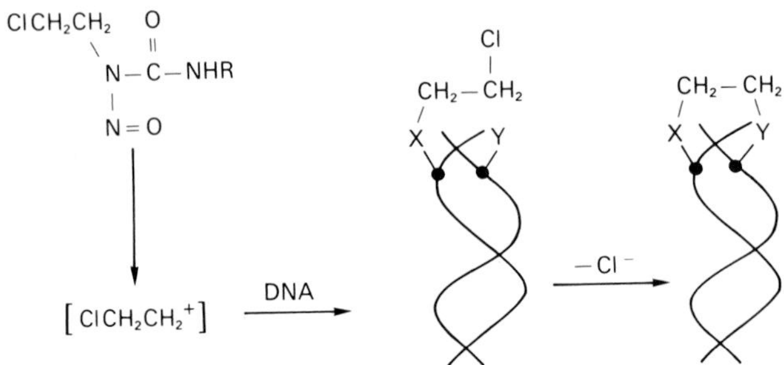

Fig. 3. Scheme for interstrand cross-linking of DNA by chloroethylnitrosoureas. X and Y are nucleophilic sites on opposite DNA strands. [From Kohn (18)].

sion of the second functional group to an aziridinium form which can react with a second nucleophilic site to form a cross-link.

A parallel sequence of reactions occurs in the case of *cis*-diamminedichloroplatinum (II) [*cis*-Pt(II)] complexes (Fig. 2, left). The reactive intermediate in this case is the aquo form, in which a chloride has been replaced by a water molecule. In other respects, the reactions are analogous to those involving nitrogen mustards, although the preferred addition sites on macromolecules may be different.

Chloroethylnitrosoureas (Fig. 2, right) also undergo an initial conversion to a reactive alkylating species. The second alkylation reaction, however, may be direct (but not necessarily rapid), without formation of an intermediate. The essential features of the reaction sequence for the three classes of cross-linking agents are thus qualitatively similar.

In quantitative terms, however, the relative rates of the different reaction steps can differ significantly, even within the same class of agents. A striking example is the difference between two nitrogen mustards: bis(2-chloroethyl)methylamine (HN2) and L-phenylalanine mustard (L-PAM) (Fig.4) (19). The pattern in Fig. 4 applies both to interstrand and to DNA–protein cross-links. In the case of HN2, cross-linking was already near its maximum immediately after a 0.5-hour drug treatment period. Within a few hours, the cross-link level fell significantly, and by 24 hours 90% of the cross-links were gone, in accord with the findings of Yin *et al.* (20). In the case of L-PAM, however, the extent of cross-linking immediately after treatment was low and then rose for 6 hours, after which there was relatively little change over the next 2 hours. The lag in cross-linking by L-PAM, as opposed to HN2, must be due to a slow conversion of monoadducts to cross-links. Although the corresponding delay in the case of HN2 is barely perceptible under these conditions, or in the reaction of HN2 with purified DNA at 37°C, the monoadduct–cross-link reaction has been observed in a purified DNA system at 0°C (21). Both the interstrand and DNA–protein cross-links produced by HN2 in L1210 cells were largely removed over a period of 24 hours (Fig. 4). This removal probably represents repair, since 70% of the cells survive this treatment and form colonies. In the case of L-PAM, however, the cross-links are either not removed as quickly or there is a prolonged steady-state balance between cross-link formation and removal. It should be noted that the delays refered to here are not attributable to time required for preactivation of the drug but rather refer to time required for conversion of monoadducts to cross-links.

The delayed cross-linking pattern exhibted by L-PAM is, in our experience with several types of bifunctional agents, more common than the rapid cross-linking pattern of HN2, although the magnitude of the delay may differ.

The delay in cross-link formation is of interest because it is possible for the monoadducts to be inactivated or to be repaired before they form the presumably

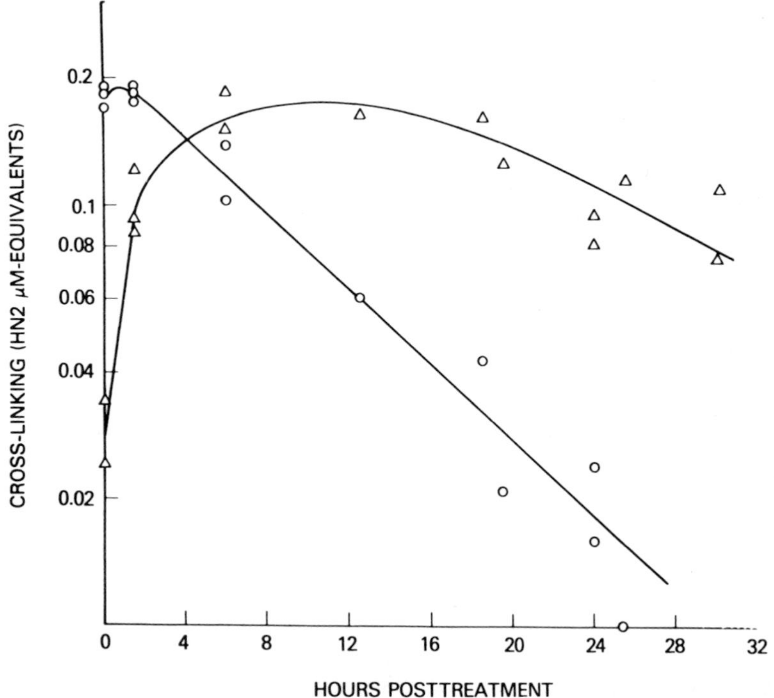

Fig. 4. Kinetics of cross-link formation and removal in mouse leukemia L1210 cells treated with 0.2 μM HN2 (○) or 15 μM L-PAM (△) for 0.5 hour. Cross-linking was assayed by alkaline elution and represents the combined effect of interstrand and DNA–protein cross-links. The results shown are mainly attributable to DNA–protein cross-links. In assays designed to detect only interstrand cross-links, similar kinetics were observed (W. E. Ross, personal communication). The survival of colony-forming ability in the experiment shown was about 70% for HN2 and 30% for L-PAM (but the difference in kinetics is not attributable to the difference in survival). [From Ross *et al.* (19)].

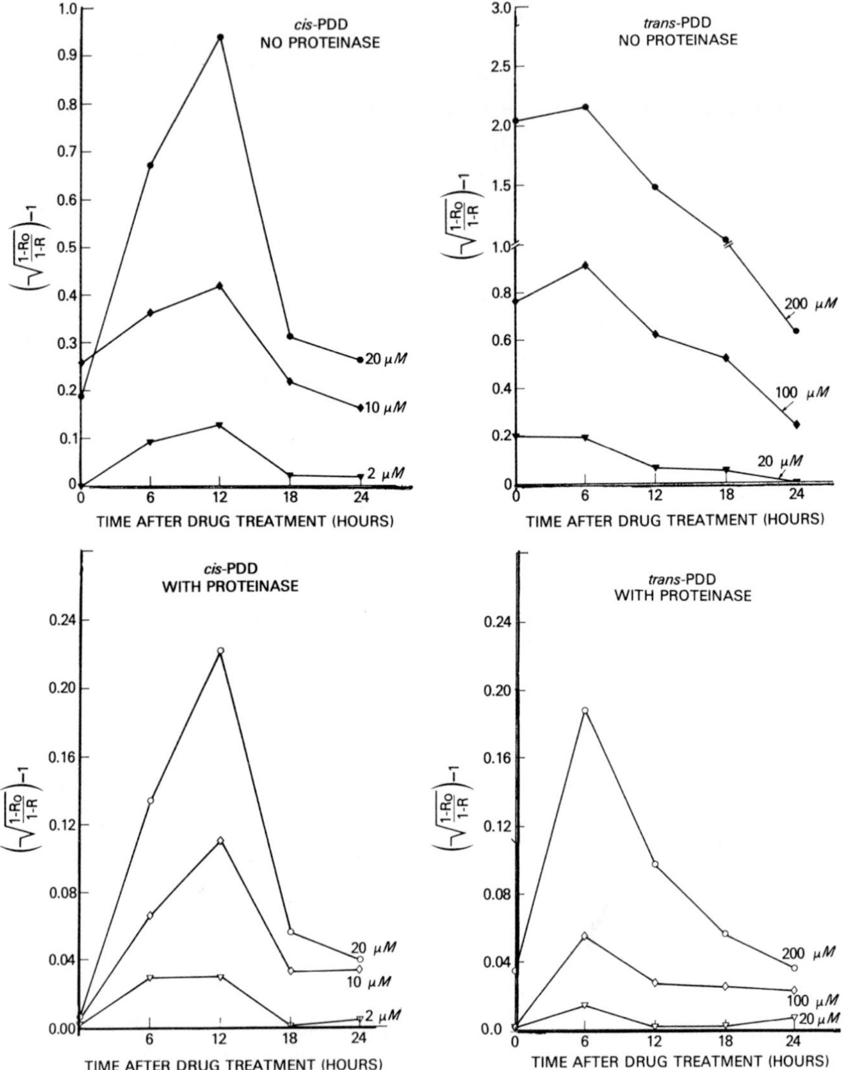

Fig. 5. Formation and removal of cross-links in L1210 cells after treatment with *cis*- or *trans*-Pt(II) (PDD) for 1 hour. Alkaline elution measurements were similar to those illustrated in Fig. 9. The assays without proteinase measure the combined effect of interstrand and DNA–protein cross-links, predominantly the latter, in these experiments. The assays with proteinase measure interstrand cross-links. The ordinate is an empirical measure of cross-link frequency (note differences in scale). [From Zwelling *et al.* (23)].

more lethal cross-links. A possible example of each of these two circumstances will be described.

Compared with L-PAM, the *cis*-Pt(II) complex exhibits even longer delays in cross-link formation and more rapid or more extensive cross-link removal (Fig. 5). Both interstrand and DNA–protein cross-links are formed and repaired. The analogous trans complex has the interesting feature that it produces extensive DNA–protein cross-linking with little interstrand cross-linking (22–24). In this case the repair of DNA–protein cross-links can be clearly studied; the cross-links form rapidly and are removed with a half-time on the order of 20 hours in L1210 cells (Fig. 5). These DNA–protein cross-links are relatively innocuous, since treatment with 100 μM *trans*-Pt(II) (Fig. 5) still permitted approximately 60% survival of colony-forming ability. DNA–protein cross-links produced by different agents may of course involve the linkage of different proteins to different DNA sites with possible unique consequences in each case.

The delay of several hours between the formation of monoadducts and cross-links by *cis*-Pt(II) suggested the possibility that this conversion could be interrupted by an agent that would react relatively quickly with the monoadducts. An agent suitable for this purpose was studied by Filipski *et al.* (25) who found that thiourea, which is known to have an extraordinarily high affinity for platinum, was able to reverse Pt(II)-induced interstrand DNA cross-links in chemical systems. In cell systems, however, the thiourea concentrations necessary to reverse cross-links could not be achieved. Thiourea at subtoxic concentrations was, however, able to prevent the conversion of monoadducts to cross-links (26). According to the hypothesized mechanism (Fig. 6), cross-link formation would be blocked if monoadducts reacted with thiourea more rapidly than with a second DNA site. Figure 7B shows the ability of thiourea to block interstrand cross-link

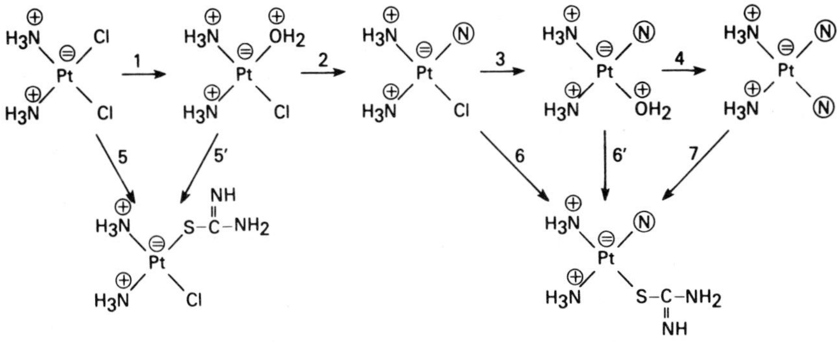

Fig. 6. Scheme for reactions of thiourea with Pt(II) species in the cross-linking sequence. Reactions 5 and 5′ represent reactions of thiourea with free drug; reactions 6 and 6′ represent reactions with monoadducts; reaction 7 represents reversal of cross-links (achieved with purified DNA but not in intact cells). Encircled N represents a nucleophile.

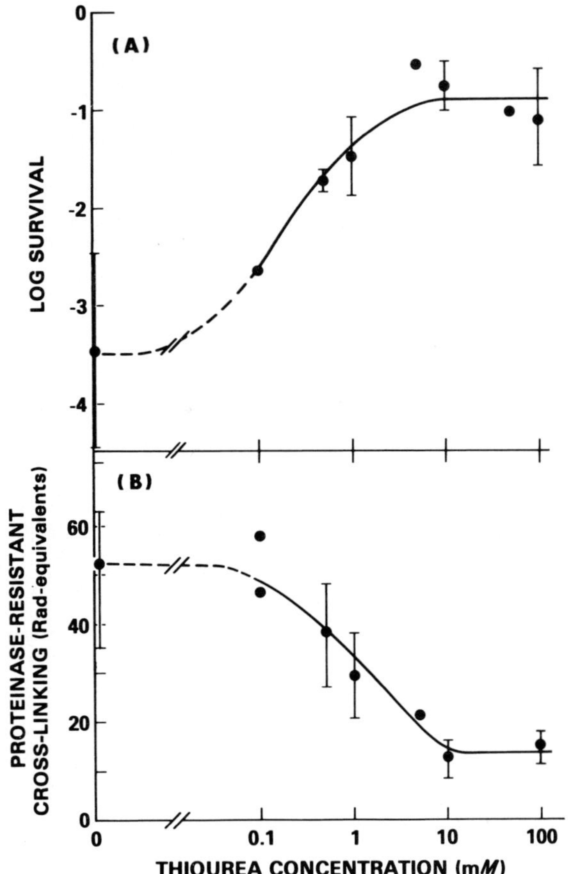

Fig. 7. Prevention of *cis*-Pt(II)-induced cross-linking and cytotoxicity by thiourea. L1210 were treated with 20 μM *cis*-Pt(II) for 1 hour, after which the drug was removed and the cells were exposed to various concentrations of thiourea for 1 hour. Survival was measured by colony formation in soft agar. Interstrand cross-linking was measured 6–12 hours later by proteinase treatment and alkaline elution. [From Zwelling *et al.* 26.]

formation when added after removal of the *cis*-Pt(II). Thiourea concentrations that blocked cross-link formation also enhanced cell survival (Fig. 7A). When thiourea was withheld for 6 hours after *cis*-Pt(II) treatment, the ability to prevent cross-link formation was lost.

Another way in which reactive monoadducts might be removed before conversion to cross-links is through the action of DNA repair mechanisms. The operation of this mechanism is suggested by recent work with chloroethylnitrosoureas, which will be summarized, but some basic aspects of the behavior of these drugs will first be reviewed.

As previously noted, chloroethylnitrosoureas generate a chloroethylating function that can react twice in succession to produce a cross-link (Fig. 2). The two sequential reactions have been resolved both in chemical and in cell systems by measuring delayed cross-link formation occurring after the drug has been removed. When purified DNA is reacted with a chloroethylnitrosourea for a short time, such as 1 hour at 23°C, a small amount of interstrand cross-linking is observed. If the DNA is then separated from the drug and incubated further, the extent of cross-linking continues to increase (18, 27) (Fig. 8). Different chloroethylnitrosoureas differ in the rate of the initial alkylation step, but the kinetics of the second step are the same. This fits the scheme in Fig. 2, since the

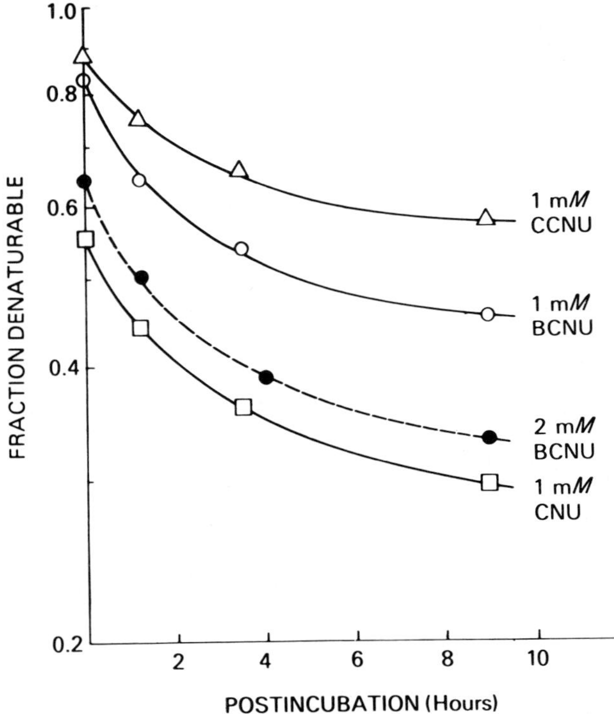

Fig. 8. Kinetics of the delayed step in DNA interstrand cross-linking by chloroethylnitrosoureas. Calf thymus DNA was reacted with drug for 1 hour at 37°C. The DNA was then alcohol-precipitated and redissolved in order to remove the drug. After various times of further incubation at 37°C, interstrand cross-linking was measured by determining the fraction of the DNA irreversibly denatured by exposure to alkali. Cross-linking was evidenced by a reduction in the fraction of DNA that was denaturable. CCNU, 1-(2-Chloroethyl)-1-nitroso-3-cyclohexylnitrosourea; BCNU, bis(2-chloroethyl)nitrosourea; CNU, 1-(2-chloroethyl)-1-nitrosourea. [From Kohn (18)].

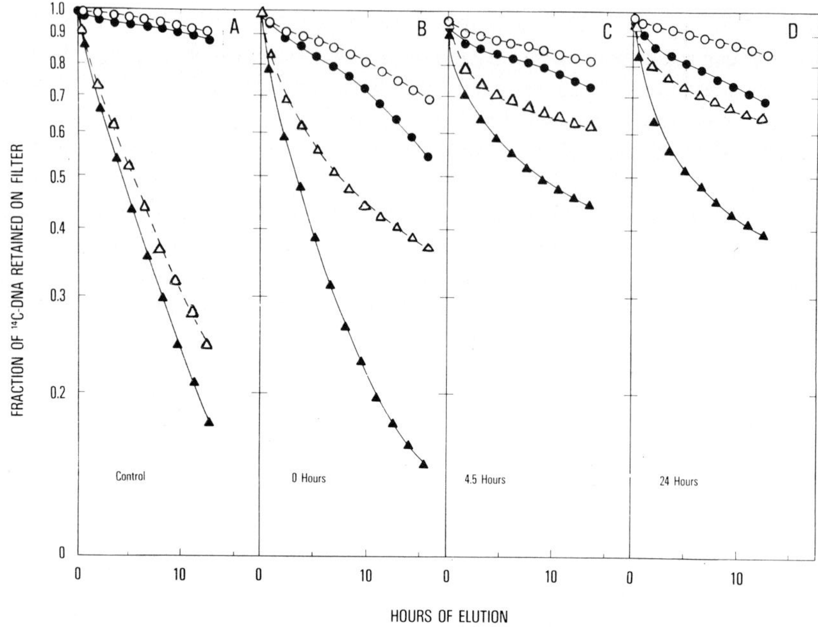

Fig. 9. DNA lesions in L1210 cells at various times after treatment with 50 μ *M* BCNU for 1 hour as measured by alkaline elution. [For details of methodology, see Kohn *et al.* (30, 31)]. The presence of single-strand breaks and/or alkali-labile sites is indicated by an increase in the rate of elution of DNA from filters (●). In order to measure cross-links, the cells were exposed to 300 R of X rays at 0°C to introduce single-strand breaks (△ and ▲). In the direct assay (△), the reduced elution is attributable to a combination of interstrand and DNA–protein cross-links. Interstrand cross-linking per se is exhibited in assays in which proteinase K is used to remove the linked protein (▲). [From Ewig and Kohn (28)]. A, no drug; hours after drug removal: B,0; C,4.5; D,24.

second reaction should involve the same chloroethylated DNA species, regardless of which chloroethylnitrosourea is used.

Delayed interstrand cross-linking by chloroethylnitrosoureas is readily demonstrable in cells by means of alkaline elution methods (Fig. 9, solid triangles) (28, 29). In contrast to interstrand cross-links, however, DNA–protein cross-linking by these drugs shows little or no delay. This may be explained as follows. Proteins are likely to be chloroethylated at amino or sulfhydryl groups. The resulting 2-chloroethylamines or 2-chloroethylsulfides would be potent alkylating groups that could react rapidly with more nucleophilic DNA sites such as the guanine N-7. The formation of interstrand cross-links, on the other hand, could be restricted in the second step by the short distance the ethyl chain can span. Chloride displacement may thereby be restricted to relatively poor nucleophilic DNA sites and therefore may occur relatively slowly.

Interstrand cross-linking by chloroethylnitrosoureas can occur to markedly different extents in different cell types. Interstrand cross-linking by several of these drugs was nearly undetectable in normal human embryo IMR 90 cells, while in the transformed human embryo cell line VA-13 these lesions were quite prominent (32) (Figs. 10 and 11). The difference cannot be attributed to differences in uptake, because it occurred with drugs of widely different chemical

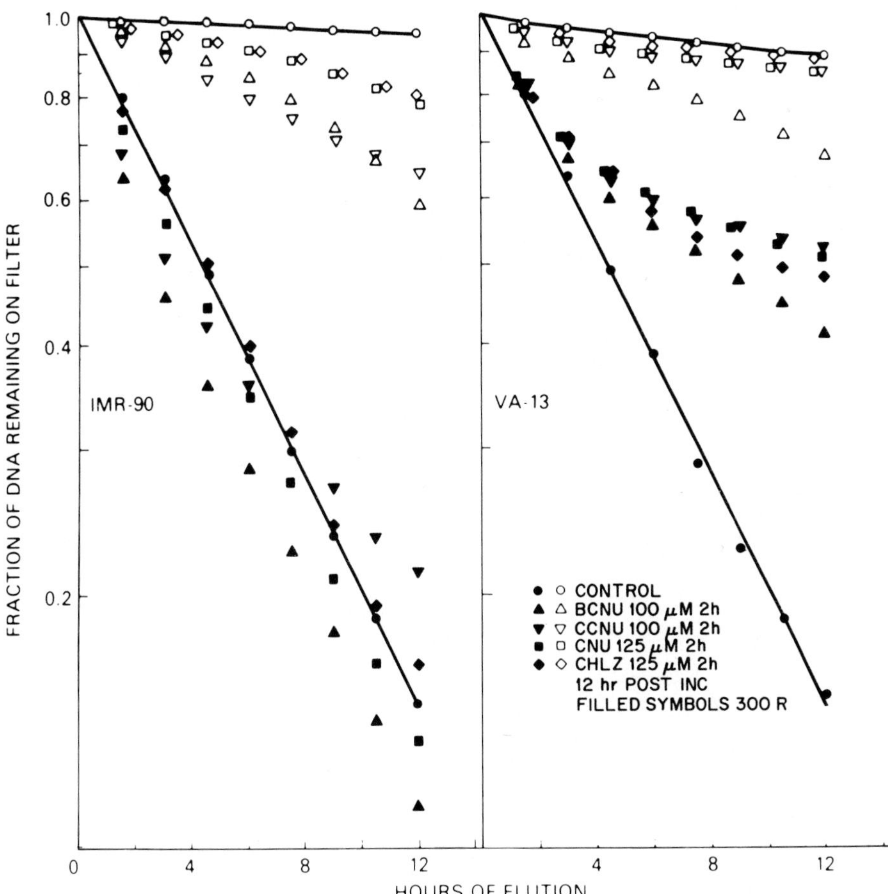

Fig. 10. Interstrand cross-link assays in normal (IMR-90) and transformed (VA-12) human embryo cells treated with various chloroethylnitrosoureas for 1 hour and then incubated for 12 hours to allow the cross-links to develop to their maximum extent. The alkaline elution assays were by the proteinase K method (see Fig. 9). The lines are drawn through the points representing controls not treated with drug. CHLZ, Chlorozotocin. [From Erickson *et al.* (32)].

structures and solubilities, including lipid-soluble compounds not retarded by membrane barriers. Furthermore, the extent of DNA–protein cross-linking in the two cell types was similar (Fig. 12). The normal cells were less sensitive than the transformed line to killing by these drugs. It is possible that the normal cell type is able to remove chloroethyl DNA monoadducts rapidly enough to prevent

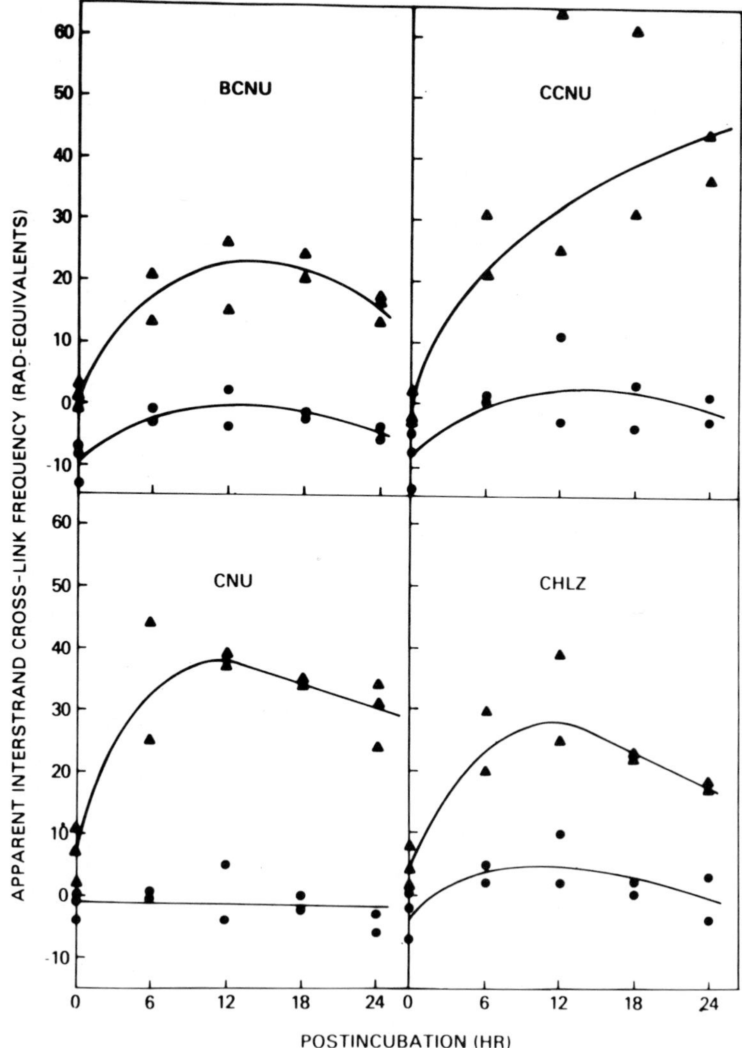

Fig. 11. Interstrand cross-linking as a function of time following 1-hour treatments of IMR-90 (▲) and VA-13 (●) cells with various chloroethylnitrosoureas. [From Erickson *et al.* (32)].

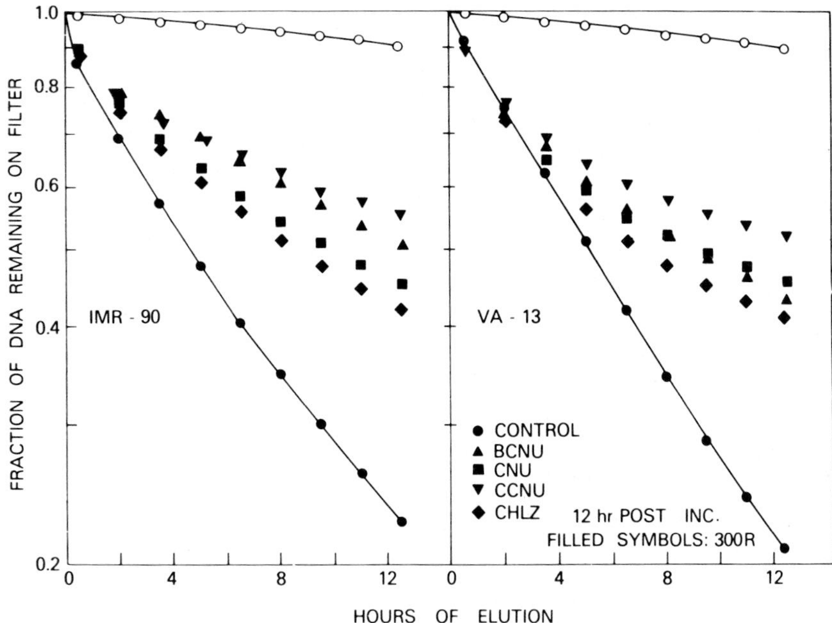

Fig. 12. Total cross-linking in IMR-90 and VA-13 cells treated with various chloroethylnitrosoureas (50 μM) for 1 hour and then incubated for 12 hours. The assays were by alkaline elution without proteinase (see Fig. 9) and show mainly the effect of DNA–protein cross-links [From Erickson *et al.* (32)].

interstrand cross-link formation, while the transformed line lacks this ability. Supporting this idea is the finding of more DNA strand breaks in the normal than in the transformed cell type; these breaks occur transiently following nitrosourea treatment and may reflect a DNA repair process (33).

The hypothesized ability of IMR90 cells to repair chloroethyl monoadducts, however, appears to be specific, since recent experiments by L. C. Erickson and L. A. Zwelling in our laboratory have shown a very different picture with L-PAM and *cis*-Pt(II). Monoadducts formed by these drugs apparently are not rapidly removed by the mechanism that we propose for the removal of chloroethyl monoadducts.

References

1. 1. R. J. Goldacre, A. Loveless, and W. C. J. Ross, *Nature (London)* **163,** 667 (1949).
2. A. Haddow, G. A. R. Kon, and W. C. J. Ross, *Nature (London)* **162,** 824 (1948).
3. A. Loveless and W. C. J. Ross, *Nature (London)* **166,** 1113 (1950).
4. K. A. Stacey, M. Cobb, S. F. Cousens, and P. Alexander, *Ann. N.Y. Acad. Sci.* **68** (3), 682 (1958).

5. P. Alexander and J. T. Lett, *Biochem. Pharmacol.* **4,** 34 (1960).
6. P. D. Lawley, *Proc. Chem. Soc. London* p. 290 (1957).
7. P. Brookes and P. D. Lawley, *Biochem. J.* **80,** 496 (1961).
8. E. P. Geiduschek, *Proc. Natl. Acad. Sci. U.S.A.* **47,** 950 (1961).
9. V. N. Iyer and W. Szybalski, *Proc. Natl. Acad. Sci. U.S.A.* **50,** 355 (1963).
10. K. W. Kohn, C. L. Spears, and P. Doty, *J. Mol. Biol.* **19,** 266 (1966).
11. R. J. Rutman, W. J. Steele, and C. C. Price, *Cancer Res.* **21,** 1134 (1961).
12. R. H. Golder, G. Martin-Guzman, J. Jones, N. O. Goldstein, S. Rotenberg, and R. J. Rutman, *Cancer Res.* **24,** 964 (1964).
13. E. Freese and M. Cashel, *Biochim. Biophys. Acta* **91,** 67 (1964).
14. J. Burnotte and W. G. Verly, *Biochim. Biophys. Acta* **262,** 449 (1972).
15. H. Grunicke, K. W. Bock, H. Becher, V. Gäng, J. Schnierda, and B. Puschendorf, *Cancer Res.* **33,** 1048 (1973).
16. B. S. Kramer, C. C. Fenselau, and D. B. Ludlum, *Biochem. Biophys. Res. Commun.* **56,** 783 (1974).
17. W. J. Lown and L. W. McLaughlin, *Biochem. Pharmacol.* **28,** 2123 (1979).
18. K. W. Kohn, *Cancer Res.* **37,** 1450 (1977).
19. W. E. Ross, R. A. G. Ewig, and K. W. Kohn, *Cancer Res.* **38,** 1502 (1978).
20. L. Yin, E. H. L. Chun, and R. J. Rutman, *Biochim. Biophys. Acta* **324,** 472 (1973).
21. R. J. Rutman, E. H. L. Chun, and J. Jones, *Biochim. Biophys. Acta* **174,** 663 (1969).
22. L. A. Zwelling, K. W. Kohn, W. E. Ross, R. A. G. Ewig, and T. Anderson, *Cancer Res.* **38,** 1762 (1978).
23. L. A. Zwelling, T. Anderson, and K. W. Kohn, *Cancer Res.* **39,** 365 (1979).
24. K. W. Kohn and R. A. G. Ewig, *Biochim. Biophys. Acta* **562,** 32 (1979).
25. J. Filipski, K. W. Kohn, R. Prather, and W. M. Bonner, *Science* **204,** 181 (1979).
26. L. A. Zwelling, J. Filipski, and K. W. Kohn, *Cancer Res.* **39,** 4989 (1979).
27. J. W. Lown, L. W. McLaughlin, and Y.-M. Chang, *Bioorg. Chem.* **7,** 97 (1978).
28. R. A. G. Ewig and K. W. Kohn, *Cancer Res.* **37,** 2114 (1977).
29. R. A. G. Ewig and K. W. Kohn, *Cancer Res.* **38,** 3197 (1978).
30. K. W. Kohn, *Methods Cancer Res.* **16,** 291 (1979).
31. K. W. Kohn, R. A. G. Ewig, L. C. Erickson, and L. A. Zwelling, *In* "DNA Repair: A Laboratory Manual of Research Procedures" (E. Friedberg and P. Hanawalt, eds.), Dekker, New York, 1980.
32. L. C. Erickson, M. O. Bradley, J. M. Ducore, R. A. G. Ewig, and K. W. Kohn, *Proc. Natl. Acad. Sci. U.S.A.* **77,** 467 (1980).
33. L. C. Erickson, M. O. Bradley, and K. W. Kohn, *Cancer Res.* **37,** 3744 (1977).

2

The Mechanism of Action of Antitumor Platinum Coordination Compounds

J. J. ROBERTS

I. Introduction

The initial observation that neutral platinum coordination compounds caused the inhibition of division and the induction of filamentous growth of *Escherichia coli* (1) rapidly led to the recognition of their potential value in the field of cancer chemotherapy (2). *cis*-Diamminedichloroplatinum(II) [*cis*-Pt(II)] and *cis*-

MOLECULAR ACTIONS AND TARGETS FOR CANCER CHEMOTHERAPEUTIC AGENTS

ISBN 0-12-619280-4

diamminetetrachloroplatinum(IV) were shown to have potent antitumor activity against sarcoma 180 and leukemia L1210, whereas the trans geometric isomers of these compounds were ineffective (1,2). After the clear demonstration of activity against a broad range of animal tumors (3–5), clinical trials were initiated by the National Cancer Institute in 1972. These early reports indicated promising anticancer activity, particularly against nonseminomatous testicular tumors, but stressed the limitations imposed by severe toxicity to the kidneys and bone marrow (6). Nausea and vomiting and sometimes audiotoxicity were also severe. However, subsequent studies showed that high doses could be tolerated by means of mannitol diuresis (7). Moreover, with further extended clinical trials of *cis*-Pt(II) there has been confirmation of the early promise of effectiveness against ovarian carcinoma, either when used alone, and not necessarily in high-dose therapy (8–10), or in combination with adriamycin (doxorubicin) and chlorambucil (9). The initially observed extreme sensitivity of testicular tumors to *cis*-Pt(II) (10) has also been confirmed (11,12). Treatment of testicular tumors during the 1960s using several combinations of cytotoxic drugs yielded an overall response rate of 33–71%, with complete remission being rare and not durable. The addition of *cis*-Pt(II) to the previously used combination of vinblastine and adriamycin led to a response rate in 100% of the patients, 74% of whom achieved complete remission (13). Other combinations have included *cis*-Pt(II), vinblastine, actinomycin D, bleomycin, cyclophosphamide, and adriamycin, the so-called VAB III protocol as used by the Memorial Sloan-Kettering Cancer Center (14). A summary of the cumulative response rate compiled by tumor type by Rozencweig *et al.* (15) for a cancer chemotherapy evaluation program notes the lack of effect of *cis*-Pt(II) on all types of leukemias and colorectal tumors. It also notes the encouraging antitumor activity against squamous cell cancer of the head and neck, a tumor that is highly resistant to most chemotherapeutic agents. The non-small-cell lung cancer, again normally resistant to chemotherapy, regressed following platinum combination therapy regardless of histological type (16,17). In a recent extended study on the response of a variety of genitourinary tumors *cis*-Pt(II) was found to be effective not only against testicular tumors but also against prostate carcinomas and bladder carcinomas (12). Some indication of activity against squamous cell carcinomas of the penis and nonfunctioning cortical adrenal carcinomas, but not against renal cell carcinomas, was noted (12). A phase-II trial of *cis*-Pt(II) confirmed some of the early successes and in addition revealed its beneficial action in carcinoma of the uterine cervix (18). Some diminution of the severe nausea and vomiting evoked by *cis*-Pt(II) can be achieved when the drug is given by continuous intravenous infusion (19). For further details of the clinical status of this compound the reader is referred to excellent reviews by Gottlieb and Drewinko (20), Burchenal (21), and Prestayko *et al.* (22).

It is now clear that *cis*-Pt(II) has an established place in cancer chemotherapy, and its use will undoubtedly grow. However, analogues of *cis*-Pt(II) have now been intensively investigated in animal tumors, and some of them have been claimed to have decreased renal toxicity and to offer certain other advantages as compared with *cis*-Pt(II). Some of the most promising compounds are derivatives of 1,2-diaminocyclohexane. The malonato derivative has been shown to produce remissions in acute myeloblastic leukemia (23), as well as regressions in other assorted tumors including some solid tumors. After extensive and promising animal experiments the sulfato derivative has been subjected to a phase-I clinical trial (24), although it is still too early to assess its relative usefulness. The carboxyphthalato derivative has the additional advantage of being appreciably more soluble than the malonato analogue. It is of further interest that studies on the latter compound, on the corresponding malonato derivative, and on 1,2-diaminocycloheptanedichloroplatinum(II) *in vitro* and *in vivo* in mouse leukemias resistant to *cis*-Pt(II) showed no cross-resistance with these three compounds. They were all equally effective, if not more so, than *cis*-Pt(II) against both sensitive and resistant lines of L1210 and P388 (25,26).

It is this encouraging and rapid progress in the clinical development of platinum drugs that has been the main impetus behind studies on their mechanism of action.

The site of the primary lesion in cells that results in toxicity, hence tumor destruction, is now generally agreed to be DNA in preference to other macromolecules such as RNA and protein. Modification of the DNA template results in selective inhibition of DNA synthesis, hence unbalanced growth. The primary biochemical effect in treated cells thus resembles that induced by a number of other cytotoxic and antitumor agents. Therefore the extent to which such agents elicit selective effects on cells may be a reflection of differences in their ability to handle damage to the DNA template. Much effort has therefore been applied in elucidating the nature of the chemical interaction of platinum compounds with DNA and in obtaining evidence for the existence of DNA repair processes which operate on platinum-damaged DNA. It now appears that, not only are platinum-induced lesions in DNA indeed removed by an excision repair process, but also that unexcised damage is circumvented in rodent cells, at least, by some form of replication repair.

I will now consider the biological, chemical, and biochemical evidence that implicates DNA as the principal target molecule for these agents in inducing cytotoxic effects in both cultured cells and cells of tumors and certain organs of rodents.

II. Biological Effects of Platinum Coordination Complexes Indicative of Reactions with DNA

A. Filament Formation in Bacteria

Probably the first observation of an effect of a platinum coordination complex in a biological system, and one which gave a clear indication of its biochemical mode of action, was made during experiments investigating the effect of an electric current on growing bacteria (27). It was noted that, when a low alternating current was passed through platinum electrodes to growing gram-negative bacteria in nutrient media, cell division was inhibited and the bacteria grew into long filaments. Subsequently it was discovered that some of the platinum dissolved under these conditions to give, first, the ionic species ammonium hexachloroplatinate. This compound could itself, at high concentration, inhibit cell division, but aged solutions were found to be far more efficient in producing filaments when exposed to visible light. The photochemical change occurring in a solution of hexachloroplatinate which gave rise to a more active agent was shown to involve replacement of the chloride ligands by NH_3, with the loss of one negative charge per replacement, to give finally a stable neutral species. The new species was shown convincingly to inhibit cell division but not growth, in contrast to the parent ionic species which was a bacteriocide and not a bacteriostat.

Filamentous growth in bacteria is almost certainly indicative of the ability of an agent to react with DNA, leading to selective inhibition of DNA synthesis, with no accompanying effect on other biosynthetic pathways such as those of RNA or protein. A variety of agents, such as UV- and X-irradiation, and cytotoxic alkylating agents, can also elicit this response as a result of their common ability to damage DNA.

B. Induction of Lysogeny

Further important evidence for a direct attack on DNA was provided by the results of Reslova (28), who investigated the ability of platinum compounds to induce the growth of phage from lysogenic strains of *E. coli*. The release of phage DNA to direct synthesis of new phage is normally a rare event. However, agents which can react with DNA can cause phage DNA to be released and phage particles to be synthesized with consequent cell lysis. Reslova (28) has shown that there exists an excellent correlation between the antitumor activity of platinum compounds and their ability to induce lysogenic *E. coli* to enter the lytic cycle.

The important question of whether viruses are similarly induced in mammalian cells by platinum compounds has not been fully resolved. Induction of viruses and subsequent cell lysis have been proposed as a possible explanation for the rapid disappearance of a sarcoma (S180) following administration of *cis*-Pt(II) (29).

C. Mutagenic Properties of Neutral Platinum Complexes

The radiomimetic nature of platinum compounds and the importance of the geometric arrangement of ligands for biological effect also emerge from studies on the mutagenic properties of these agents in a number of prokaryotic and eukaryotic systems (30–34). The cis derivatives were in all cases appreciably more mutagenic than the corresponding trans isomers.

D. Inactivation of Viruses and Transforming DNA

The interactions of platinum compounds with viruses have further indicated the relatively greater importance of reactions with DNA compared to those with protein in producing biological effects. Kutinova *et al.* (35) demonstrated inactivation of the infectious activity of an extracellular papovavirus (SV40) by *cis*-Pt(II). An indication of the mechanism of inactivation was derived by following the capacity of the inactivated virus to induce either tumor or viral antigens. The capacity of the virus to induce the tumor antigen was found to be less sensitive to *cis*-Pt(II) than viral antigen formation or the infectivity of the virus. The slower rate of inactivation of the tumor antigen by *cis*-Pt(II) thus corroborated studies in which SV40 or polyomavirus was inactivated by radiation or hydroxylamine and which revealed that the capacity to induce tumor antigen, thymidine kinase, or transplantation immunity and the transformation activity of the virus were inactivated at a slower rate than the infectivity or the viral antigen-inducing capacity. These findings indicate that viral DNA and not the protein coat is the primary target for both radiation and the platinum compound.

The inactivation of *Bacillus subtilis*-transforming DNA by platinum compounds likewise indicated the effect of these agents on the biological function of DNA (36). Moreover, by examining the changes in transformation frequency of three unlinked genetic markers, the positions of which on the *B. subtilis* chromosome were known, some indication of specificity in the reaction of the platinum complexes with regions of DNA or with individual DNA bases was obtained. The adenine marker, for example, is localized in the region close to the origin of replication and is rich in G-C base pairs in DNA. This was found to be appreciably more sensitive than the methionine marker which is localized at the end of the *B. subtilis* chromosome.

III. Repair of DNA Damage Induced by Platinum Compounds

A. General Comments

Some cells are known to be able to remove or circumvent damage to their DNA, after it has been modified by numerous agents, using various cellular repair processes. This is currently an area of great interest and may well be important in understanding further aspects of drug action. The fact that cells can acquire resistance to drugs is an important limitation to their clinical usefulness. It is now necessary to ask whether tumor cells develop this resistance to platinum compounds by use of a DNA repair mechanism(s). Model studies using prokaryotic and eukaryotic cells *in vitro* indicate that this is indeed a possibility, and these findings strongly support the notion that DNA is indeed the target of these cytotoxic agents.

Investigations of the modifying influence of cellular repair processes on the lethal effects of radiation and chemically induced damage in both microbial and mammalian cells have revealed two basically different repair mechanisms. In one of these, the DNA-bound adducts are recognized and removed by one of two excision processes. If, however, the damage to the DNA is not excised before the DNA is used as a template for DNA replication, it appears that the cell can circumvent the damage either by a mechanism involving recombination or by a process called postreplication repair (or replication repair). Both excision and postreplication repair processes facilitate the recovery of cells from DNA damage introduced by a variety of physical and chemical agents. (See ref. 37 for review).

B. Excision Repair

1. *Bacterial Studies*

The main photoproduct in the DNA of UV-irradiated *E. coli* or mammalian cells is a pyrimidine dimer which is recognized by an excision repair process that removes the dimer attached to an oligonucleotide and resynthesizes the removed section of the DNA. The contribution this excision repair process makes to the ultimate survival of bacterial cells treated with various agents can be assessed by determining the sensitivities of strains of *E. coli* carrying mutations in genes known to code for steps in this repair pathway. It was concluded from such studies that damage introduced into DNA by certain bifunctional agents, such as nitrogen mustard, mitomycin C, and psoralen-plus-visible light, as well as the damage introduced by certain bulky monofunctional carcinogenic agents, such as 4-nitroquinoline-1-oxide and 7-bromomethylbenz(*a*)anthracene, was also eliminated by enzymes encoded by genes known to code for the enzymes required for the repair of UV-induced thymine dimers. From analogous studies on the sensitivities of such DNA repair-deficient *E. coli* mutants to *cis*-Pt(II), it was similarly concluded that the excision repair process(es) contributes only to a small extent to the recovery of strains of *E. coli* from the DNA-damaging effects of this agent (38,39). Some kinds of damage to the DNA of T-odd bacteriophages can be repaired by the enzymatic excision repair system of the host bacterium (host cell repair). The role played by the *hcr* locus is important for the survival of cells after UV irradiation, but not after treatment with 1-methyl-3-nitro-1-nitrosoguanidine (MNNG), and only minimally so after treatment with *cis*-Pt(II). The relatively minor importance of the *hcr* locus in the inactivation of *E. coli* by *cis*-Pt(II) was confirmed by the observation that the bacteriophages T3 and T4 BOL, after treatment with *cis*-Pt(II), gave the same inactivation curves in both *Hcr*$^+$ and *Hcr*$^-$ strains of the indicator bacteria (40). Similarly it was found that platinum-treated transforming DNA did not appear to be more sensitive when assayed in a strain of *Hemophilus influenzae* which carries the *uvrl* mutation, hence lacks the activity of the specific enzymes involved in the repair of UV-irradiated DNA (41).

2. *Mammalian Cell Studies*

Alkaline sucrose gradient sedimentation of prelabeled cellular DNA following treatment of cells with *cis*-Pt(II) did not reveal any accumulation of low-molecular-weight DNA (42). From a knowledge of the extent of reaction of the platinum compound with DNA at the concentration employed, it could be concluded that either lesions were not generally recognized by an endonuclease which inserted nicks into DNA or, alternatively, if the lesions were recognized by an endonuclease, completion of the later stages of the excision repair process(es) led to the rapid restoration of high-molecular-weight DNA. Moreover, since any apurinic sites in DNA would be converted into DNA single-strand breaks under these alkaline conditions, there was no obvious evidence from these studies for the removal of substituted purines by means of a *N*-glycosylase.

On the other hand, the time-dependent changes in the sedimentation profiles of fully labeled DNA observed following a pulse treatment of Chinese hamster cells with *cis*-Pt(II) could be interpreted as being due to the initial formation of DNA interstrand or DNA–protein cross-links that were subsequently removed during several hours, presumably by a DNA excision repair process (42). In these experiments, mammalian cells were lysed under conditions which released labeled DNA sedimenting to positions in an alkaline sucrose gradient corresponding to sedimentation coefficients of 700 S and (in a lesser proportion) 400–650 S. Prior treatment with *cis*-Pt(II) consistently resulted in a dose-dependent increase in the proportion of counts recovered in the 700 S region of the gradient at the expense of the DNA sedimenting in the 400–650 S region of the gradient. Hence treatment of cells with these concentrations of *cis*-Pt(II) hinders the release of DNA from the 700 S "complex."

It is probable that this effect is a consequence of cross-linking of complementary strands of DNA or of cross-linking DNA to protein, which hinders its denaturation under alkaline conditions. This profile was not modified by a 2-hour posttreatment incubation prior to centrifugation. However, by 6 hours a marked change in the profile had occurred, and the DNA sedimented in a narrow band at a position corresponding to 350 S. The latter change could be due to the time-dependent formation of further cross-links in the DNA or between DNA and protein. Twenty-one hours after exposure to the drug, a dose-dependent restitution of the DNA species sedimenting in the 450–650 S range was observed and probably represented enzymatic repair of the platinum-damaged sites in the DNA. While these results cannot be fully interpreted at present because struc-

TABLE I

Relative Sensitivities of Cells to Exposure to *cis*-Pt(II), DNA-Bound Platinum, and Ultraviolet Irradiation[a]

Cell type	D_0 [μM *cis*-Pt(II)]	B_0 (nmoles Pt/gm DNA)	D_0 (J/m^2)
Chinese hamster	15	8.5	
HeLa	4.6	5.5	
Human fetal lung	6.4	7.4	3.1
Xeroderma pigmentosum (XP 12BE)	4.4	1.8	0.55

[a] Data from Refs. 43, 45, 46.

tures with such high *s* values are not fully defined, they do indicate that changes in the molecular weight of DNA or a DNA–protein complex occur under physiological conditions compatible with the concept that platinum-induced damage in DNA can be repaired. More recent studies of the sedimentation properties of DNA from *cis*-Pt(II) treated cells that had a lower, defined molecular weight after alkaline lysis, confirmed this interpretation. (Roberts and Shackleton, unpublished results).

The rare skin condition xeroderma pigmentosum (XP) is characterized by extreme sensitivity to sunlight and a predisposition to skin cancer. Cells taken from persons suffering from this condition are more sensitive to uv irradiation than normal cells and are deficient in excision repair of UV-induced damage. These cells are also sensitive to other DNA-damaging agents such as hydrocarbon epoxides, 4-nitroquinoline-1-oxide, and 7-bromomethylbenz(*a*)anthracene, and sensitivity is again associated with decreased levels of various manifestations of DNA excision repair (for review, see 37). Moreover, these findings were originally thought to indicate that the repair system which excises thymine dimers is also able to excise certain types of chemical damage. It has now been found that these repair-deficient XP cells are also more sensitive than normal fetal lung cells to *cis*-Pt(II) when the lethal effects of the drug are expressed as a function of reaction with DNA rather than as a function of dose of reagent (Table I) (43). It could therefore be reasoned that this increased sensitivity of XP cells is similarly due to their decreased ability to excise *cis*-Pt(II)-induced DNA damage. If this conclusion is correct, then the additional finding that an extract from *Micrococcus luteus* that can incise UV-irradiated DNA does not similarly incise *cis*-Pt(II)-treated DNA indicates that different mechanisms are likely to be involved in repair of the two types of damage.

Loss of platinum from the DNA of mammalian cells, presumably by an enzymatic process, has been unequivocally demonstrated (44). Moreover, the rates of loss of platinum from DNA have been found to correlate with the sensitivities of cells to the platinum-containing drug. Thus Chinese hamster (44) and human fetal lung (45) cells in stationary-phase growth are more sensitive to treatment with *cis*-Pt(II) (when diluted into fresh medium and induced to divide) than either cell type growing exponentially. These differences are not due to greater uptake of the drug by stationary-phase cells. On the other hand, there is a markedly slower rate of loss of platinum from the DNA of stationary-phase cells, which is directly related to their sensitivity, as indicated by values of a DNA-binding index (B_0) for exponentially growing and stationary-phase cells (Table II). (B_0 is defined as the slope of the straight portion of the curve relating log cell survival to binding to DNA.) This relationship lends support to the notion that it is the unexcised lesions in DNA which are responsible for the cellular toxicity of *cis*-Pt(II). This concept was supported by further findings that the recovery of stationary-phase cells from the toxic effects of *cis*-Pt(II) (when these cells were diluted and plated into fresh medium and thus induced to divide) during prolonged holding in the stationary state was accompanied by a loss of platinum-bound adducts from their DNA (44). Moreover, a plot of the amount of platinum bound to DNA against the logarithm of the cell survival accompanying this binding had a slope (B_0) equal to that obtained by plotting the survival of stationary-phase cells treated with a variety of concentrations of *cis*-Pt(II) at zero time against the corresponding levels of DNA-bound platinum (44).

A further indication of the possible role of excision repair in determining the sensitivity of cells in different physiological states to *cis*-Pt(II)-induced damage has come from the observation that cells treated in late G_1 phase are more sensitive to *cis*-Pt(II) than cells treated in mid-S phase (Table III) (46). Replication of the whole genome immediately after platinum-induced modification of the DNA template would be expected to produce more damage (unligated DNA) at the end of the cell cycle compared with mid-S-phase treatment when only part of the DNA is replicated following exposure. Although excision repair is a relatively slow process, involving loss of platinum from exponentially growing cells with a half-life of 28 hours, it is sufficiently rapid for a proportion of the

TABLE II

Relative Sensitivities of Exponentially Growing and Stationary-Phase Cells to DNA-Bound Platinum and Rates of Loss of Platinum from DNA[a]

Cell type	Cell state	B_0 (nmoles Pt/gm DNA)	Loss of platinum from DNA (half-life in hours)
Chinese hamster	Exponentially growing	8.5	28
Chinese hamster	Stationary phase	3.0	96
Human fetal lung	Stationary phase	3.0	108

[a] Data from Refs. 44, 45.

TABLE III

Relative Sensitivities of Cells at Different Stages of the Cell Cycle to Exposure to *cis*-Pt(II) and to DNA-Bound Platinum[a]

Cell type	Cell-cycle phase	D_0 [μM *cis*-Pt(II)]	B_0 (nmoles Pt/gm DNA)
Chinese hamster	G_1	5	3.0
Chinese hamster	S	14	6.5
HeLa	G_1	1.3	4
HeLa	S	4.3	10

[a] Data from Refs. 45, 46.

platinum damage to have been removed before the start of the next round of DNA replication.

C. Postreplication Repair (Replication Repair)

1. *Bacterial Studies*

From the previous discussion, it appears that the majority of DNA–platinum products, involving one strand of a double helix, are chemically stable and are only slowly removed from DNA by an enzymatic process. If this is indeed so, then it could be supposed that persistent lesions in DNA are circumvented during DNA replication by an alternative repair process, one analogous to that which facilitates the survival of excision-defective bacteria after UV irradiation. Evidence has been adduced that gaps are initially left in the daughter DNA opposite thymine dimers in the template strand of DNA; these gaps are subsequently filled by a process involving recombination, which is controlled by *rec* genes and/or *de novo* DNA synthesis, which is probably controlled by the *exr* (*lex*) gene. It was found by Drokník *et al.* (38) that mutation of Exr^+ to Exr^- resulted in a three- to sixfold increase in the sensitivity of *E. coli* to UV irradiation and MNNG, and less than a twofold increase in sensitivity to X-irradiation. On the other hand, the increase in sensitivity of colony-forming ability to *cis*-Pt(II) due to this mutation is 13–23 times. Beck and Brubaker (39) reached a similar conclusion with regard to the important role of this particular repair pathway from a comparison of the effect of treatment with UV light and *cis*-Pt(II) on cell survival and filamentation in recombination repair-deficient mutants of *E. coli* K12. The recombination repair-deficient mutant *recA13* and the double mutant *uvrA6 lexl,* which is known to undergo extensive autodegradation of DNA after treatment with UV irradiation, were particularly sensitive to *cis*-Pt(II).

2. *Mammalian Cell Studies*

It now seems certain that mammalian cells also possess varying capacities to replicate their DNA on a template containing unexcised damage, which may be regarded as indicative of different levels of some form of so-called postreplication repair capacity. It is also apparent, however, that the mechanism of any such repair process differs from that thought to occur in bacteria. Newly synthesized DNA in some UV-irradiated and chemically treated mammalian cells is initially smaller than that in control cells, and it has been proposed that gaps are left in new DNA opposite lesions. The subsequent increase in the molecular weight of nascent DNA during posttreatment incubation of cells (defined operationally as postreplication repair) was, as for bacteria, thought to involve sealing of gaps. However, no evidence for recombinational exchanges was initially forthcoming. Instead it was proposed that so-called gaps were filled by *de novo* DNA synthesis.

On the other hand, other evidence suggests that gaps are not formed in newly synthesized DNA but that there is simply a delay in the rate of synthesis at the site of each lesion. It has further been proposed that the lesion can be circumvented during DNA replication by a mechanism involving strand displacement. However, irrespective of the mechanism involved in synthesizing past radiation or chemically induced lesions in DNA, it has been found that in some cells the process is amenable to inhibition by the trimethylxanthine-caffeine. Thus, it has been shown that the rate of elongation of newly synthesized DNA in UV-irradiated or chemically treated cells is dramatically impaired in the presence of caffeine. As a consequence of this inhibition, many cell lines competent in this replicative bypass repair are rendered extremely sensitive to the lethal effects of these agents by posttreatment incubation in the presence of nontoxic concentrations of caffeine. (For references, see 37).

There is now ample evidence indicating that UV or X-irradiation, or chemically induced cell death is a function of the amount of chromosome damage which can be observed at the first or second mitosis after treatment. Posttreatment incubation in the presence of caffeine enhances dramatically the chromosome-damaging effects of UV irradiation and chemicals in both plant and animal cells.

The various cellular effects of *cis*-Pt(II) and their modification by caffeine suggest that lesions are introduced in DNA by platinum compounds, which are also circumvented by a caffeine-sensitive repair process (47). The potentiating effect of caffeine on *cis*-Pt(II)-induced lethality persists for approximately 24 hours in asynchronously growing Chinese hamster cells and during the first S phase only (i.e., 12 hours) after treatment during the G_1 phase of synchronously growing Chinese hamster cells (48). In this respect therefore the response of *cis*-Pt(II)-treated cells resembles that of UV-irradiated or sulfur mustard-treated cells.

Posttreatment incubation of cells in medium containing 0.75 m*M* caffeine dramatically increases the number of cells with chromosome damage. Caffeine not only increases the number of *cis*-Pt(II)-treated cells containing chromosomal aberrations but also enhances the severity of the damage observed. The most dramatic effect was a marked increase in the number of cells containing shattered chromosomes and those with numerous chromatid deletions and exchanges. The delayed appearance of chromosome abnormalities after *cis*-Pt(II) treatment also suggests that DNA replication is necessary for their formation, and in this respect *cis*-Pt(II) resembles UV irradiation and alkylating agents rather than X-irradiation (47).

The proposal has therefore been made, that inadequate replication of DNA on a DNA-damaged template is responsible for both cell death and chromosome damage and that posttreatment incubation of cells in medium containing caffeine enhances these two effects of DNA damage by inhibiting a process which would permit replication to proceed past lesions. Support for this notion has come from studies on both the rate of DNA synthesis and the size of DNA synthesized in both asynchronous and synchronized populations of *cis*-Pt(II)-treated cells in the presence and absence of caffeine. A study of chromosome damage in Chinese hamster ovary cells treated with another platinum drug has revealed that gaps and breaks are found in the first mitosis after treatment, while chromatid exchanges are present only in cells at the second mitosis (49), a response which is characteristic of compounds that produce lesions repaired by a postreplication repair mechanism.

The dose-dependent depression in the rate of synthesis of DNA in *cis*-Pt(II)-treated, asynchronously growing Chinese hamster cells can be seen as a dose-dependent delay in the peak rate of DNA synthesis (mid-S) in synchronously growing Chinese hamster cells treated in G_1 (48). As a consequence of the dose-dependent extension of the time required for passage through S phase, cells were correspondingly delayed in the time at which they underwent cell division.

It has been found that posttreatment incubation in medium containing a non-toxic concentration of caffeine reverses the *cis*-Pt(II)-induced inhibition of DNA synthesis in asynchronous populations of cells (50), while posttreatment incubation in the presence of caffeine of synchronous cells treated in G_1 leads to a reversal of the *cis*-Pt(II)-induced delay in obtaining the peak rate of DNA synthesis. Under these conditions of *cis*-Pt(II) and caffeine treatment, the peak rate of synthesis approximates in time of appearance that of the control cells (48).

The immediate, dose-dependent, selective, persistent inhibition of DNA synthesis induced in *cis*-Pt(II)-treated Chinese hamster cells as measured by the decreased uptake of [^{3}H]thymidine into DNA, as discussed above, can also be visualized as a dose-dependent decrease in the size of pulse-labeled newly synthesized DNA in treated cells (50). If, however, compensation is made for the reduction in the *rate* of DNA synthesis by increasing the labeling period in *cis*-Pt(II)-treated cells, the alkaline sucrose gradient sedimentation profile of labeled DNA in treated cells is very similar to that of DNA in control untreated cells. It has been concluded from such studies that the replicating machinery is delayed at the site of platinum-induced lesions in the template strand but, given sufficient time, can circumvent the lesions without forming discontinuities (gaps) in the newly synthesized DNA. Alternatively, if gaps are first formed opposite platinum reaction sites in DNA, they must be rapidly filled and will be too transitory for detection. The size of newly synthesized DNA in *cis*-Pt(II)-treated cells may be contrasted with the size of such DNA in cells treated similarly with *cis*-Pt(II) and labeled with [^{3}H]thymidine in the presence of nontoxic concentrations of caffeine. Under these conditions the size of nascent DNA was markedly reduced as compared with that in untreated control cells or cells treated only with *cis*-Pt(II). The decrease in size of DNA was not the result of a decrease in overall rate of DNA synthesis since, as indicated above, the rate of DNA synthesis in *cis*-Pt(II)-treated cells is faster in the presence of caffeine than in its absence. The size of the DNA synthesized during 4 hours in the presence of caffeine in *cis*-Pt(II)-treated cells was dependent on the initial dose of *cis*-Pt(II). It thus appears that caffeine interferes with the mechanism by which the cell replicates its DNA past lesions on the DNA template. Some support for this notion was obtained from a comparison of the distance between platinum-induced lesions on the template strand of DNA and the size of the newly synthesized DNA in cells treated with various doses of *cis*-Pt(II) and postincubated in the presence of caffeine. The distance between platinum atoms on one strand of DNA was calculated from atomic absorption measurements of the platinum bound to DNA isolated from *cis*-Pt(II)-treated cells, and this was found to correspond closely to the size of the newly synthesized DNA. It was concluded therefore that all unexcised platination reactions were normally circumvented during DNA replication by a caffeine-sensitive so-called DNA repair process. A fuller discussion of the effects of platinum compounds on DNA synthesis in various cell systems, and of the arguments favoring the view that this is the result of inactivation of the DNA template, can be found in fuller reviews of the subject (51,52). These various studies have further indicated that enhanced inactivation is produced by a specific type of reaction which occurs in the case of the cis isomers.

IV. Reactions with Cellular DNA Indicative of DNA as the Target Molecule

A. Reactions with Cells in Culture

Additional support for the above notion came from studies on the binding to cellular macromolecules (i.e., DNA, RNA, and protein) with *cis*- and *trans*-Pt(II) at known levels of cell killing (53–55).

To assess the possible importance of DNA, RNA, and protein as primary targets of Pt(II) compounds, these binding data (expressed as moles per gram of macromolecule) were used to construct curves of log survival against the amount

TABLE IV

Extent of Reaction with DNA, RNA, and Protein on a Molar Basis at Concentrations of *cis*-Pt(II) That Reduced Survival of HeLa Cells from *f* to 0.37*f* (B_0 Values)[a]

Molecule	Assumed molecular weight	B_0 (μmoles/gm)	Number of Pt atoms per molecule
DNA	1×10^9	0.0225	22 per DNA
mRNA	4×10^6	0.030	1 per 8 mRNA
rRNA	$0.5\text{–}1 \times 10^6$	0.030	1 per 30 rRNA
tRNA	2.5×10^4	0.030	1 per 1500 tRNA
Protein	1×10^5	0.00675	1 per 1500 protein

[a] Data from Ref. 53.

of drug bound to each type of macromolecule. The resulting graphs were then characterized in a manner similar to those relating log cell survival to dose of drug given to the cells. The shoulder width of the binding curve was given the value B_q and the slope of the straight line portion B_0. For both *cis*- and *trans*-Pt(II), the binding coefficients were higher for RNA than DNA. However, the true significance of these binding coefficients can only be appreciated if account is taken of the molecular weights of the molecules concerned. If one assumes no selectivity in the binding to any particular RNA or protein molecule, then it is possible to calculate the number of platinum molecules bound to each macromolecule at a given toxic dose (53,54). The results of such a calculation performed at the concentration of *cis*-Pt(II) which reduced the surviving fraction from *f* to 0.37*f* (the theoretical concentration required to kill just one cell) shows there are strikingly more molecules bound to DNA than to either RNA or protein, clearly indicating that DNA is the most sensitive cellular target of *cis*-Pt(II) (Table IV).

The binding data further indicate that at this concentration of *cis*-Pt(II) only 1 molecule of protein out of 1500 molecules receives one platination reaction. Unless there is considerable specificity in the reaction of platinum drugs with a particular protein or enzyme molecule, this level of reaction would be too low to inactivate enzyme activity. Moreover, the level of reaction with rRNA, tRNA, or mRNA would not be expected, again in the absence of any selectivity of reaction, to inactivate all such molecules and lead to interference with protein synthesis.

Similar DNA binding and cell survival studies have been carried out with a number of other platinum compounds that have shown encouraging activity against a number of experimental animal tumors (see 51, 52, 56 for discussion of structure–activity relationships). Differences of up to 10-fold were found in the molar concentrations of these agents required to produce equitoxic effects on cells in culture following a 1-hour incubation (D_0 values, Fig. 1). For some

TABLE V

Comparison of the Toxicity of Various Platinum Complexes toward Chinese Hamster V79 379A Cells in Culture and Plasmacytoma ADJ/PC6 Tumor Cells *in Vivo*[a]

	ADJ/PC6A Mouse plasmacytoma				Chinese hamster V79 379 A cells	
Compound[b]	LD_{50} (mg/kg)	ID_{90} (mg/kg)	TI	Solubility (m*M*)	D_0 (μM/1 hour)	B_0 (nmoles/gm)
cis-$Pt(II)Cl_2(NH_3)_2$	13	1.6	8	8.9	15	8.5
cis-$Pt(IV)Cl_2(\textit{iso}\text{-}C_3H_7NH_2)_2(OH)_2$	54	4.2	12.9	44.1	48	2.5
cis-$Pt(II)(1{:}1\text{-CBDCA})(NH_3)_2$[c]	180	14.5	12.4	50	120	3.0
cis-Pt(II)(mal)(1,2-dac)[c]	N.D.[b]	N.D.	N.D.	N.D.	23	2.5
cis-$Pt(II)(SO_4)H_2O$(1,2-dac)[c]	14	0.4	37	36	65	17.5
cis-$Pt(II)Cl_2(C_5H_9NH_2)_2$	480	2.4	200	0.013	120	N.D.

[a] Data from (57, 58).
[b] N.D., Not determined.
[c] CBDCA, Cyclobutanedicarboxylic acid; dac, 1,2-diaminocyclohexane.

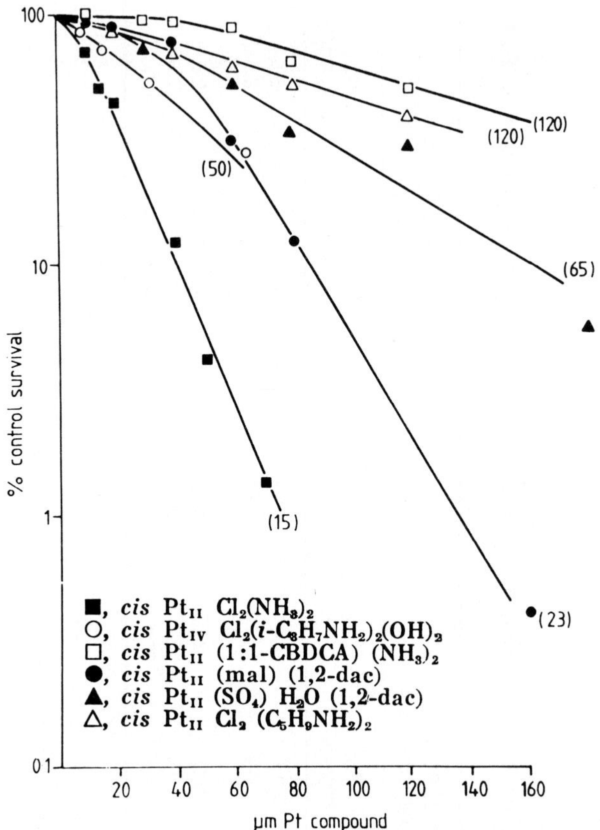

Fig. 1. Effects of different platinum complexes on the survival (colony-forming ability) of Chinese hamster cells. Cells were treated in suspension culture for 1 hour with a number of different concentrations of platinum compounds and then diluted into petri dishes for determination of colony-forming ability. The numbers in parentheses are the calculated slopes of the straight-line portions of the respective survival curves (D_0). CBDCA, Cyclobutane dicarboxylic acid; dac, 1,2-diaminocyclohexane.

agents there is a close relationship between the relative LD_{50} and ID_{90} doses for mice bearing a plasmacytoma and the D_0 dose for hamster cells. The levels of reaction with DNA at equitoxic doses (B_0 values), on the other hand, were of the same order for most compounds and differed by only a few fold (Table V) (57). The lower values of B_0 for diaminocyclohexanemalonatoplatinum(II) and *cis*-dichloro-*trans*-dihydroxobisisopropylamineplatinum(IV) (CHIP) could indicate that nonleaving groups larger than HN_3 are more effective in killing cells. The high value of B_0 for the sulfato compound, compared with its close analogue, the malonato derivative, might conceivably indicate that the former compound gives rise to a different proportion of monofunctional as compared with bifunctional adducts in the DNA than the latter compound.

B. Reactions of Platinum Drugs with DNA *in Vivo*

It is clearly essential, for an understanding of the mechanism of the tumor-inhibitory action of platinum compounds, to establish that the sensitivity of tumor cells is related to the extent of reaction of platinum with their DNA in a manner similar to that for cells treated *in vitro* with these agents. Accordingly, mice bearing a transplanted ADJ/PC6 plasmacytoma were treated with *cis*-Pt(II) and two other active platinum congeners, CHIP and *cis*-diammine(1:1-cyclobutanedicarboxylato)platinum(II) at doses that had an equal inhibitory effects on

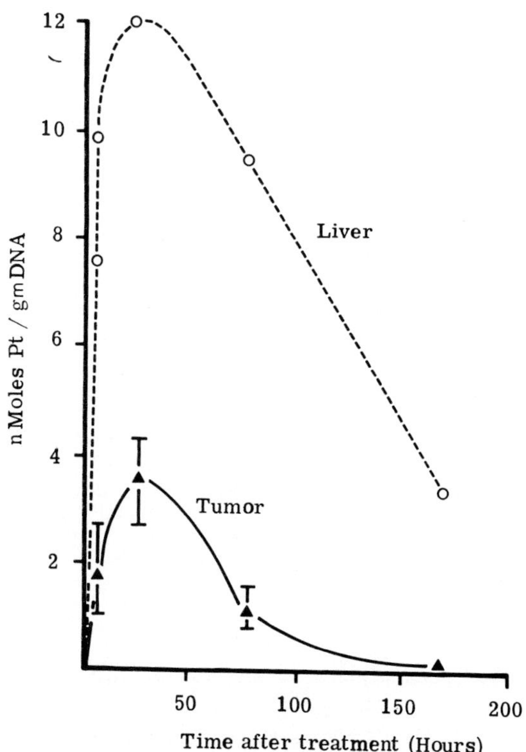

Fig. 2. Time course of binding of *cis*-Pt(II) to the DNA of mouse ADJ/PC6 plasmacytoma and mouse liver. Mice were injected with an ID_{90} dose (58) of *cis*-Pt(II) (1.6 mg/kg), and the DNA isolated and purified and its platinum content determined [all as described in (43)] at the times shown. The values for binding to tumor DNA are the averages of those from not less than three mice, the ranges of which are indicated.

the tumor (ID_{90}; Table VI). Despite the difference in the actual amounts of material adminisied to the mice, the doses did not differ by more than a factor of 2 when expressed in terms of their molar concentrations. Interestingly, the amounts of platinum drugs bound to the tumor DNA at these equitoxic concentrations were all remarkably similar (Figs. 2–4; Table VI) and testify to the essentially similar consequences of binding to the DNA of different types of platinum products. In as much as differences do exist among these three compounds, they are similar to the differences found in the binding of the same agents to the DNA of Chinese hamster cells *in vitro* (Table V). Of more significance, however, is the fact that the actual amounts of the various drugs bound to the DNA of tumor cells at the ID_{90} doses for these agents are of the same order as the previously determined levels of reaction with DNA at approximately equitoxic doses to Chines hamster cells (Table VI). (The ID_{90} doses *in vivo* can be loosely equated to the B_0 doses *in vitro*.). This observation lends considerable support to the notion that it is the interaction of platinum compounds with cellular DNA which is responsible for their cytotoxic action both *in vitro* and *in vivo*.

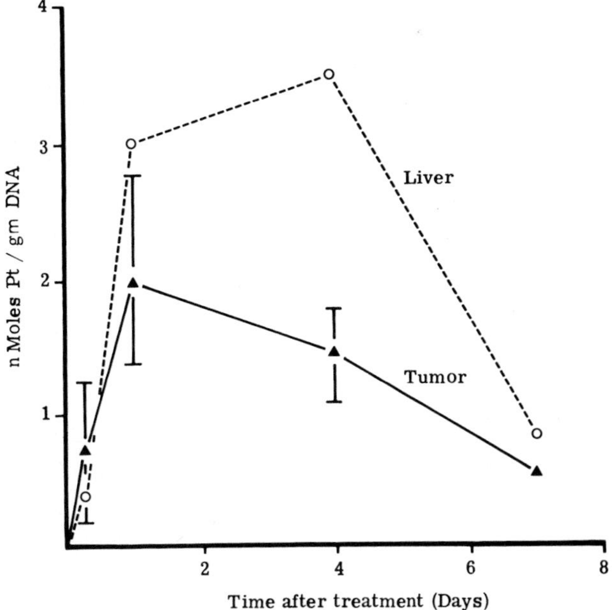

Fig. 3. Time course of binding of CHIP to the DNA of mouse ADJ/PC6 plasmacytoma and mouse liver. Mice were injected with an ID_{90} dose of CHIP [4.2 mg/kg in water (59)], and DNA isolated and purified and its platinum content determined [all as described in (43)] at the times shown. The values for the binding to tumor DNA are the averages of those from not less than three mice, the ranges of which are indicated.

TABLE VI

Comparison of the Binding of Platinum Compounds to the DNA of Tumor Cells *in Vivo* and to the DNA of Chinese Hamster V79 379A Cells *in Vitro*[a]

Compounds	ADJ/PC6 mouse plasmacytoma		Chinese hamster V79 379 A cells	
	ID_{90} (mg/kg)	Binding to tumor DNA (max) (nmoles Pt/gm DNA)	D_0 (μM/1 hour)	nmoles/gm DNA
cis-Pt(II)$Cl_2(NH_3)_2$	1.6	3.5	15	8.5
cis-Pt(IV)Cl_2(*iso*-$C_3H_7NH_2$)$(OH)_2$	4.2	2.0	48	2.5
cis-Pt(II)(1:1-CBDCA)$(NH_3)_2$	14.5	1.8	120	3.0

[a] Data from (57) and J. J. Roberts and H. N. A. Fraval (unpublished results).

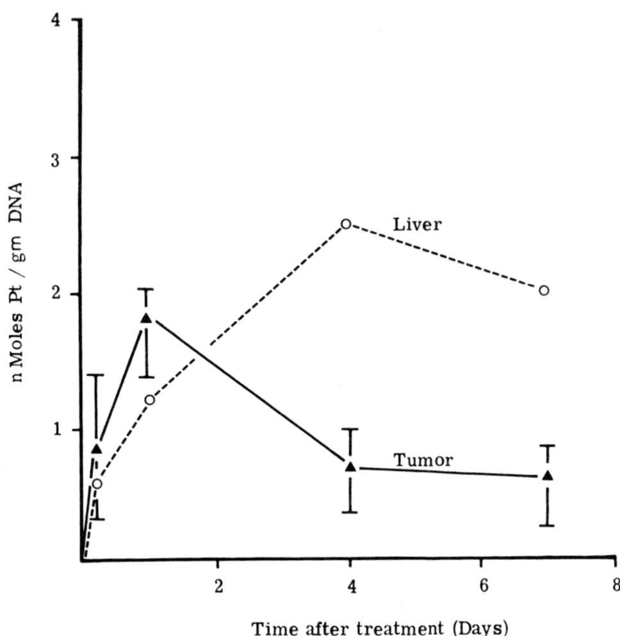

Fig. 4. Time course of binding of diammine(1:1-cyclobutanedicarboxylato)platinum(II) to the DNA of mouse ADJ/PC6 plasmacytoma and mouse liver. Mice were injected with an ID_{90} dose [14.5 mg/kg (59)], and DNA isolated and purified and its platinum content determined [all as described in (43)] at the times shown. The values for the binding to tumor DNA are the averages of those from not less than three mice, the ranges of which are indicated.

The decline, with time, in the amount of platinum bound to the DNA of tumor cells (Figs. 2–4) is probably due to a combination of many factors, including continued DNA synthesis, selective loss of dead cells, and DNA excision repair. On the other hand, the loss of platinum from liver DNA, with a half-life of approximately 2 days in the case of *cis*-Pt(II)- and CHIP-treated animals, is likely to be solely the result of the operation of a DNA excision repair process in this tissue.

The levels of platinum bound to the DNA of liver and tumor tissue when *cis*-Pt(II) was administered to CBA mice bearing a human pancreatic intramuscular tumor xenograft were essentially the same as those in the above similarly treated plasmacytoma-bearing mice. The sensitivity of this tumor to the drug was determined by an *in vitro* plating procedure, and it was found that a dose of 10 mg/kg was required to kill 90% of the cells (D. Courtney-personal communication), and correspondingly more binding occurred with tumor and liver DNA at this higher dose (Figs. 5 and 6). These data might therefore suggest that this particular human tumor is more resistant to *cis*-Pt(II) than the plasmacytoma.

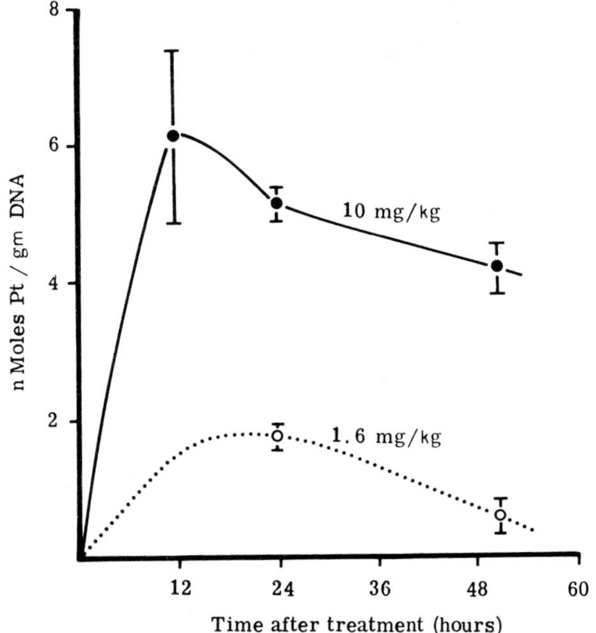

Fig. 5. Time course of binding of *cis*-Pt(II) to the DNA of a human pancreatic tumor xenograft in CBA mice (kindly supplied by D. Courtney). Mice were injected with either 1.6 or 10 mg/kg of *cis*-Pt(II), and the DNA from the tumor isolated and purified and its platinum content determined [as described in (43)] at the times shown. The values shown are the average of those from not less than two mice.

Similar DNA-binding studies with other human tumor xenografts should permit an assessment of the relative inherent sensitivities of other human tumors.

C. Role of Cross-Linking Reactions

The structural requirement for difunctionality and the principal biochemical effects of platinum compounds, as discussed earlier, soon suggested a parallel between platinum drugs and classic bifunctional alkylating agents such as nitrogen mustards. The latter compounds have been thought for some time to produce inhibition of DNA synthesis by their ability to introduce cross-links into the DNA of mammalian cells. It has, however, been a matter of contention as to whether the principal lesion is a cross-link between strands of the DNA helix, cross-links between bases on one strand of DNA or, possibly, even between DNA and protein. In order to estimate cross-links in the DNA, one strand of DNA was given a density and radioactivity label by growing cells in the presence of [^{3}H]bromodeoxyuridine. Cross-linking between a "labeled heavy" strand and a

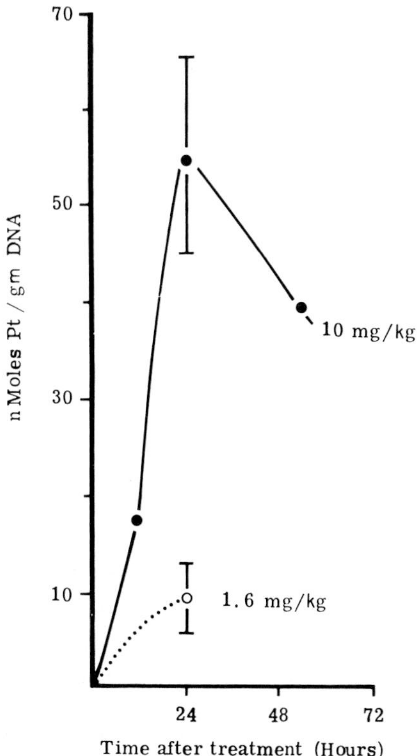

Fig. 6. Time course of binding of *cis*-Pt(II) to the DNA of liver in mice bearing a human pancreatic tumor xenograft. Mice were injected with either 1.6 or 10 mg/kg of *cis*-Pt(II), and the DNA from the liver isolated and purified and its platinum content determined at the times shown. The bars represent the range of the values from two mice.

"light unlabeled" strand produced a "labeled hybrid" species, and this species could be separated in an alkaline $CsCl_2$ gradient (53). Not only was cross-linking of DNA by *cis*-Pt(II) demonstrated by this technique, but also it could be calculated, from a knowledge of the overall extent of platination of DNA at a dose which produced a measured number of cross-links in the DNA of estimated molecular weight, that DNA interstrand cross-linking was, initially at any rate, a relatively rare event.

The possible role of the cross-linking reaction in determining the cytotoxic action of platinum drugs was obtained from a study aimed at answering the question, Does the extent of interstrand cross-linking of DNA correlate with the cytotoxic activity of a range of platinum compounds (54,55)? The relative toxicities of the cis- and trans-isomers of the Pt(II) and Pt(IV) neutral complexes can be defined by the slopes of the survival curves (D_0) obtained by treating HeLa cells in culture (Table VII). Comparison of these two sets of values indicated that

TABLE VII[a]

Concentrations of *cis*- and *trans*-Platinum Compounds Required for Toxicity to HeLa Cells in Culture and to Produce 10% Cross-Linking of DNA *in Vitro* and *in Vivo*

Compound	D_0 (μM)	D_q (μM)	Dose required to produce 10% cross-linking *in vitro* (μM)	Dose required to produce 10% cross-linking *in vivo* (μM)
cis-Pt(II)$(NH_3)_2Cl_2$	3	1	0.5	150
trans-Pt(II)$(NH_3)_2Cl_2$	55	50	1.0	1900
cis-Pt(IV)$(NH_3)_2Cl_4$	1.5	1.0	33.7	420
trans-Pt(IV)$(NH_3)_2Cl_4$	65.0	37.5	67.0	570

[a] Data from (54, 55).

the relative abilities of *cis*- and *trans*-Pt(II) compounds to cross-link DNA *in vivo* (but not *in vitro*) were related to their cytotoxic action. Thus, the relative ability of *cis*- and *trans*-Pt(II) to kill cells, measured either on the basis of dose ($D_0^{trans}/D_0^{cis} = 18$) or DNA binding ($B_0^{trans}/B_0^{cis} = 5.6$) is of the same order as the 12-fold difference in the doses required to produce equal amounts of cross-linking with the two compounds. However, in the case of Pt(IV) compounds, despite an even greater difference in the relative toxicities of the cis and trans compound ($D_0^{trans}/D_0^{cis} = 43$), there was very little difference in their capacities to induce cross-links in DNA either *in vitro* or in whole cells. A reinvestigation of cross-linking of DNA by Pt(II) compounds using a method different from that described above, namely, alkaline elution (60), has confirmed the greater ability of *cis*-Pt(II) as compared with *trans*-(Pt(II) to cross-link cellular DNA. The ability of the method to detect cross-linking of DNA following treatment with concentrations of platinum compounds lower than those required for that used by Roberts and Pascoe (53) permitted a study of the time course of cross-linking. Zwelling *et al.* (60) made the further interesting observation that incubation of treated mouse leukemic L1210 cells in a drug-free medium resulted in an increase in the number of DNA cross-links. Cross-linking effects developed, following treatment with concentrations as low as 1 μM for *cis*-Pt(II) and 5 μM for *trans*-Pt(II), which permitted over 80% survival of colony-forming ability. The maximum cross-linking effect by *cis*-Pt(II) required about a 12-hour posttreatment incubation before it was fully developed, whereas the cross-linking effect of *trans*-Pt(II) was fully developed at the end of 1 hour of drug exposure. The cross-linking effects of both agents were reversed upon further incubation of the cells, presumably as a result of the operation of a DNA excision repair process. More recently, it has been shown that cells can be protected from the toxic effect of *cis*-Pt(II) by preventing the formation of DNA cross-links by incubating cells in the presence of thiourea immediately after treatment (61), a finding which strongly supports a cytotoxic role for DNA interstrand cross-links.

V. Conclusions

This chapter has compiled evidence which clearly indicates that DNA is the principal target molecule of neutral platinum complexes in a variety of biological systems. Currently, the most convincing mechanism for the cytotoxic action of these agents, both on cells in culture and *in vivo,* is that reactions with DNA impair its function as a template for further DNA replication. A variety of reactions with DNA have now been described, but it is not yet known whether all or only some of them are important in inactivating the DNA template. In the case of *cis*-Pt(II), at least, there is good evidence to suggest that DNA interstrand cross-linking is an important cytotoxic reaction. Platinum adducts in DNA seem to be recognized by a DNA excision repair process, and in Chinese hamster cells they are also recognized by a caffeine-sensitive process which facilitates the ability of the replicating machinery to synthesize past them. Inability to synthesize past lesions is associated with mitotic delay, chromosome damage and, eventually, cell death. The similar levels of binding of platinum compounds to the DNA of cells in culture and of tumor cells *in vivo* at equitoxic doses of these agents, as discussed here, indicate that their antitumor action is likely also to result from the same cytotoxic events.

The finding that cells can differ in their response to platinum compounds, either because of a decreased ability to excise lesions (as in the case of xeroderma pigmentosum cells or cells in certain physiological states) or a decreased ability to circumvent lesions during DNA replication by some form of replication repair, as in the case of HeLa cells (62), leaves one hopeful that selective attack on tumor cells is feasible. Although other neutral platinum complexes almost certainly produce their cytotoxic effects by a mechanism similar to that of *cis*-Pt(II), the observed differences in their physiological disposition, as reported here, offer the further hope of finding drugs with selective action against specific tumors and with minimal toxic side effects.

Acknowledgments

I am grateful to the Rustenberg Platinum Mines, Ltd., and the Johnson Matthey Research Centre for financial support over many years and for grants from the Medical Research Council and Cancer Research Campaign. It is with pleasure that I also acknowledge the contributions of my successive collaborators during this period, Drs. J. M. Pascoe, H. W. van den Berg, and H. N. A. Fraval.

References

1. B. Rosenberg, L. Van Camp, J. E. Trosko, and V. H. Mansour, *Nature (London)* **222,** 385 (1969).
2. B. Rosenberg and L. Van Camp, *Cancer Res.* **30,** 1799 (1970).
3. R. W. Talley, *Proc. Am. Assoc. Cancer Res.* **11,** 78 (1970).
4. R. J. Kociba, S. D. Sleight, and B. Rosenberg, *Cancer Chemother. Rep.* **54,** 325 (1970).
5. C. W. Welsh, *J. Natl. Cancer Inst.* **47,** 1071 (1971).
6. M. Rozencweig, D. D. van Hoff, M. Slavik, and F. M. Muggia, *Ann. Intern. Med.* **86,** 803 (1977).
7. D. M. Hayes, E. Cvitkovic, R. Golbey, E. Scheiner, L. Helson, and I. H. Krakoff, *Cancer* **39,** 1371 (1977).
8. H. W. Bruckner, C. C. Cohen, G. Deppe, B. Kabakow, R. C. Wallach, E. M. Greenspan, S. B. Gusberg, and J. F. Holland, *J. Clin. Hematol. Oncol.* **7,** 619 (1977).
9. E. Wiltshaw and T. Kroner, *Cancer Treat. Rep.* **60,** 55 (1976).
10. E. Wiltshaw, *Biochimie* **60,** 925 (1978).
11. D. J. Higby, H. J. Wallace, D. J. Albert, and J. F. Holland, *Cancer* **33,** 1219 (1974).

12. C. E. Merrin, *Biochimie* **60,** 941 (1978).
13. L. H. Einhorn and J. Donahue, *Ann. Intern. Med.* **87,** 293–298 (1977).
14. E. Cvitkovic, E. Cheng, W. F. Whitmore, and R. B. Golbey, *Proc. Am. Soc. Clin. Oncol.* **18,** 324 (1977).
15. M. Rozencweig, D. D. van Hoff, J. S. Penta, and F. M. Muggia, *J. Clin. Hematol. Oncol.* **7,** 672 (1977).
16. R. T. Eagan, J. N. Ingle, S. Frytak, J. Rubin, L. K. Kvols, D. T. Carr, D. T. Coles, and J. R. O'Fallon, *Cancer Treat. Rep.* **61,** 1339 (1977).
17. J. C. Britell, R. T. Eagan, J. N. Ingle, E. R. Creagan, J. Rubin, and S. Frytak, *Cancer Treat. Rep.* **62,** 1207 (1978).
18. M. Hayat, M. Bayssas, G. Brule, P. Cappelaere, A. Cattan, J. Chauvergne, B. Clavel, J. Gouvela, J. Guerrin, J. Lavfer, E. Pommatau, H. Szpirglas, F. Muggia, and G. Mathé, *Biochimie* **60,** 935 (1978).
19. T. L. Loo, S. W. Hall, P. Salem, R. S. Benjamin, and K. Lu, *Biochimie* **60,** 957 (1978).
20. J. A. Gottlieb and B. Drewinko, *Cancer Chemother. Rep.* **59,** 621 (1975).
21. J. H. Burchenal, *Biochimie* **60,** 915 (1978).
22. A. W. Prestayko, J. C. D'Aoust, B. F. Issell, and S. T. Crooke, *Cancer Treat. Rev.* **6,** 17 (1979).
23. J. M. Hill, E. Loeb, A. S. Pardue, A. Khan, N. O. Hill, J. J. King, and R. W. Hill, *J. Clin. Hematol. Oncol.* **7,** 681 (1977).
24. E. Loeb, J. M. Hill, A. S. Pardue, N. O. Hill, A. Khan, and J. J. King, *J. Clin. Hematol. Oncol.* **7,** 701 (1977).
25. J. H. Burchenal, K. Kalaher, K. Drew, L. Lokys, and G. Gale, *Biochimie* **60,** 961 (1978).
26. J. H. Burchenal, K. Kalaher, T. O'Toole, and J. Chisholm, *Cancer Res.* **37,** 3455 (1977).
27. B. Rosenberg, L. van Camp, and T. Krigas, *Nature (London)* **203,** 698 (1965).
28. S. Reslova, *Chem.-Biol Interact.* **4,** 66 (1971–1972).
29. B. Rosenberg, *Cancer Chemother. Rep.* **59,** 589 (1975).
30. D. J. Beck and R. R. Brubaker, *Mutat. Res.* **27,** 181 (1975).
31. C. Monti-Bragadin, M. Tamaro, and E. Banfi, *Chem.-Biol. Interact.* **11,** 469 (1975).
32. P. Lecointe, J.-P. Macquet, J.-L. Butour, and C. Paoletti, *Mutat. Res.* **48,** 139 (1977).
33. J. E. Trosko, *Recent Results Cancer Res.* **48,** 108 (1974).
34. L. A. Zwelling, M. O. Bradley, N. A. Sharkey, T. Anderson, and K. W. Kohn, *Mutat. Res.* **67,** 271 (1979).
35. L. Kutinová, V. Vonka, and J. Drobník, *Neoplasma* **19,** 453 (1972).
36. S. Reslová, M. Srogl, and J. Drobník, *Adv. Antimicrob. Antineoplast. Chemother., Proc. Int. Congr. Chemother., 7th, 1971* Vol. 11, p. 209 (1972).
37. J. J. Roberts, *Adv. Radiat. Biol.* **7,** 211 (1978).
38. J. Drobník, M. Urbánková, and A. Krekulová, *Mutat. Res.* **17,** 13 (1973).
39. D. J. Beck and R. R. Brubaker, *J. Bacteriol.* **116,** 1247 (1973).
40. J. Drobník, A. Blahušková, S. Vasiluková, and A. Krekulová, *Chem.-Biol. Interact.* **11,** 365 (1975).
41. L. L. Munchausen, *Proc. Natl. Acad. Sci. U S A.* **71,** 4519 (1974).
42. H. W. van den Berg and J. J. Roberts, *Chem.-Biol Interact.* **11,** 493 (1975).
43. H. N. A. Fraval, C. J. Rawlings, and J. J. Roberts, *Mutat. Res.* **51,** 121 (1978).
44. H. N. A. Fraval and J. J. Roberts, *Cancer Res.* **39,** 1793 (1979).
45. J. J. Roberts and H. N. A. Fraval (1980). *In* "Cisplatin, Current Status and New Developments." (A. W. Prestayko, S. T. Crooke and S. Carter, eds.), p. 57. Academic Press, New York.
46. H. N. A. Fraval and J. J. Roberts, *Biochem. Pharmacol.* **28,** 1575 (1979).
47. H. W. van den Berg and J. J. Roberts, *Mutat. Res.* **33,** 279 (1975).
48. H. N. A. Fraval and J. J. Roberts, *Chem.-Biol. Interact.* **23,** 99 (1978).
49. I. I. Szumiel and A. H. W. Nias, *Br. J. Cancer* **33,** 450 (1976).

50. H. W. van den Berg and J. J. Roberts, *Chem.-Biol. Interact.* **12,** 375 (1976).
51. J. J. Roberts, *Antibiotics (N.Y.)* **5,** Part 2, 20 (1979).
52. J. J. Roberts and A. J. Thomson, *Prog. Nucleic Acid Res. Mol. Biol.* **22,** 71 (1979).
53. J. J. Roberts and J. M. Pascoe, *Nature (London)* **235,** 282 (1972).
54. J. M. Pascoe and J. J. Roberts, *Biochem. Pharmacol.* **23,** 1345 (1974).
55. J. M. Pascoe and J. J. Roberts, *Biochem. Pharmacol.* **23,** 1359 (1974).
56. M. J. Cleare and J. D. Hoeschele, *Platinum Met. Rev.* **17,** 1 (1973).
57. J. J. Roberts and H. N. A. Fraval, *Biochimie* **60,** 869 (1978).
58. T. A. Connors, M. Jones, W. C. J. Ross, P. D. Braddock, A. R. Khokhar, and M. L. Tobe, *Chem-Biol. Interact.* **5,** 415 (1972).
59. R. Wilkinson, P. J. Cox, M. Jones, and K. R. Harrap, *Biochimie* **60,** 851 (1978).
60. L. A. Zwelling, K. W. Kohn, W. E. Ross, R. A. G. Ewig, and T. Anderson, *Cancer Res.* **38,** 1762 (1978).
61. L. A. Zwelling, J. Filipski, and K. W. Kohn, *Cancer Res.* **9,** 4989 (1979).
62. H. N. A. Fraval and J. J. Roberts, *Chem.-Biol. Interact.* **23,** 111 (1978).

3

Macromolecular Targets and Metabolic Properties of Alkylating Drugs

K. R. HARRAP, A. JENEY, P. J. THRAVES, P. G. RICHES, AND R. WILKINSON

I. General Review

A. Introduction

The initial discovery of the antitumor activity of nitrogen mustard (HN2) (1) prompted the synthesis of a wide range of alkylating agents in a search for more tumor-selective chemicals. Clinically active compounds emerged from studies on congeners of HN2 (chlorambucil); aziridines (triethylene melamine, triethylene thiophosphoramide, Trenimon); alkyl alkanesulfonates (Myleran); and ni-

MOLECULAR ACTIONS AND TARGETS FOR CANCER CHEMOTHERAPEUTIC AGENTS

ISBN 0-12-619280-4

trosoureas [bis(2-chloroethyl)nitrosourea, 1-(2-chloroethyl)nitrosourea]. Attempts were also made to exploit biologically important molecules as carriers of alkylating functions. In this regard, notable successes were the linking of alkylating moieties to amino acids (melphalan), and glucocorticoid hormones [Estracyt (a phenolic *N*-bis(β-chloroethyl)carbamate 17β-phosphate of estradiol) and prednimustine (pregna-1,4-diene-3,20-dione-11,17-dihydroxy-21, 4-*p*-[bis(2-chloroethyl)amino]phenyl butyrate).

Cyclophosphamide, which probably exhibits a wider spectrum of clinical activity than any of the alkylating agents, evolved from attempts to produce a product which would be activated by metabolism. A more recently discovered antineoplastic agent, cisplatin, exhibits features reminiscent of classic alkylating agents in terms of its effects on DNA (2,3). The chemical, biological, biochemical, and pharmacological properties of these compounds have been extensively reviewed (4–15).

B. Macromolecular Targets for Alkylating Agents

1. *Nucleic Acids*

Early recognition of the radiomimetic properties of alkylating agents suggested that DNA might be a major intracellular target (6). The formation of giant cells, resulting from "imbalanced growth" (inhibition of DNA synthesis without major effect on RNA and protein synthesis) endorsed this speculation (16,17). Direct reaction of a bifunctional alkylating agent (sulfur mustard) with tumor cell DNA *in vivo* was first proved by Brookes and Lawley (18), who subsequently demonstrated that the DNA was cross-linked through reaction of the alkylating agent with the N-7 of appropriately disposed guanyl moieties in the double helix (19,20). Similar conclusions emerged from the work of Geiduschek (21) with HN2. These results confirmed the earlier speculations of Goldacre *et al.* (22) that the biological properties of bifunctional alkylating agents might be explained by their cross-linking properties. The formation of both inter- and intrastrand DNA cross-links was subsequently confirmed by several authors (23–28). Investigations with a wide range of mono- and bifunctional alkylating agents have shown that reaction at the N-7 guanine atom in both RNA and DNA is by far the commonest event, less extensive alkylation occurring at the 1- and 3-positions of adenine, the 3-position of cytosine, and the 0-6-position of guanine (7,29,30). It is of interest that only bifunctional alkylating agents exhibit antitumor activity, while both mono- and bifunctional agents are carcinogenic. It appears that the occurrence and persistence of *0*-6-methylguanine correlates well with the carcinogenicity of monofunctional agents (31–33). It has proved difficult to correlate the production of alkylated DNA bases directly with cell death; in particular, 7-methylguanine is rapidly excised and the resultant apurinic site repaired (34–37). The 0-6 alkylation of guanine is less rapidly excised and also causes mispairing if DNA replication occurs on an alkylated template (38,39). In contrast, 7-methylguanine apparently pairs correctly with cytosine (40).

In the case of several newer agents which do not contain a conventional mustard group, DNA has also been shown to be an important target. Thus nitrosoureas alkylate and cross-link DNA (41); in addition, they exhibit carbamoylating activity directed principally at proteins (42). Similarly, cisplatin and other platinum(II) complexes produce DNA interstrand cross-links (43).

DNA excision repair has been implicated by several authors as a major determinant of cellular sensitivity to bifunctional alkylating agents (37,44–47). These findings, which have been exhaustively reviewed recently by Roberts (13), must be regarded as equivocal since as yet, there is no unified consensus that resistance to these agents correlates with enhanced excision repair.

It is generally agreed that DNA is quantitatively the most important intracellular target of alkylating agents. The evidence derives primarily from measurements of the binding (per mole) of either sulfur mustard or *cis*-diamminodichloroplatinum(II) [*cis*-Pt(II)] to DNA, RNA, or protein (13,35,48,49). It is argued that, since the binding to each molecule of DNA is orders of magnitude greater than to RNA or protein, DNA must be the more important target. However, this argument ignores the possible importance of low-level binding to critical regulatory sites in macromolecules. For example, it is known that the chemical alkylation of RNA molecules can destroy or modify their functional integrity, as has been demonstrated for tRNA exposed to dimethyl sulfate (50,51). Furthermore, since the enzymatic methylation of RNA is organ-, tissue-, and species-specific, any additional chemical methylations might disturb this specificity and cause mistranslation (52). For example, the methyl groups on RNA are conserved during maturation and may be necessary for correct processing (52,53). mRNA has a 7-methylguanine at its 5′-end, which is essential for correct translation (54,55), while *0*-6-methyladenines occur in the main body of mRNA (52,56). The insertion of additional 7-methylguanine or *0*-6-methyladenine residues could conceivably modify message integrity. There is ample evidence that such hypermethylation can lead to profound biological disturbance. For example, neoplasia has been associated with both increased and aberrant tRNA methylation (57–60).

After chemical methylation of yeast and rat liver RNA, 7-methylguanine is the major methylated base, although 1-methyladenine and 3-methylcytidine have also been found (61,62). The methylation of tobacco mosaic virus RNA by monofunctional alkylating agents has been described by Singer and Fraenkel-Conrat (63), and intrastrand cross-links in RNA can be produced by bifunctional alkylating agents (23,64–66).

Thus it can be seen that small changes in RNA methylation can modify functional integrity. Low levels of alkylating agent binding to RNA molecules could therefore profoundly alter translational processes and cannot be overlooked.

2. *Protein*

It has been suggested that bifunctional alkylating agents can cross-link DNA to protein. For example, it has been observed that these compounds render DNA resistant to phenol–salt extraction (67–71). Since similar effects are not observed with monofunctional agents, it has been assumed that DNA–protein cross-linking is responsible for the lack of DNA extractability following exposure to bifunctional agents (68,69). Using alkaline elution and treatment with proteinase K, Ewig and Kohn (42) demonstrated the presence of two types of cross-links in cells exposed either to nitrosoureas or to HN2. Proteinase-resistant cross-links were ascribed to DNA–DNA interactions, while proteinase-sensitive cross-links were attributed to DNA–protein binding. The latter formed rapidly, while the former developed more slowly. Repair processes were implicated for both types of lesions. There is also evidence that cisplatin can cross-link DNA to a DNA polymerase (72).

Busch and his co-workers (73–75) were the first to observe that bifunctional alkylating agents may interfere selectively with the synthesis of nonhistone nuclear proteins but not with that of histones or of cytoplasmic proteins. Grunicke and his colleagues (76) showed that Trenimon inhibited histone biosynthesis, while being essentially without effect on the synthesis of nonhistone chromosomal proteins. Subsequently, Grunicke *et al.* (77) found that the effects of Trenimon on histone synthesis in Ehrlich ascites cells were caused by loss of histone mRNA. It is not yet entirely clear whether the effect is due to a specific blockage of histone genes or to an increased degradation of histone mRNA. However, inhibition of histone biosynthesis occurs in the absence of any effect on DNA synthesis (77).

Riches and Harrap (78), in studying the effects of chlorambucil on Yoshida ascites cells *in vivo,* also observed a very rapid inhibition of histone biosynthesis followed 12 hours later by inhibition of nonhistone protein synthesis. These effects occurred prior to inhibition of DNA synthesis. The same authors also noted associated changes in nuclear morphology, predominantly deletion of condensed chromatin and its replacement with diffuse chromatin in cells aspirated from chlorambucil-treated animals. None of these changes occurred in a paired, drug-resistant, cell line. Similar morphological effects were noted subsequently following treatment of animals, carrying sensitive or resistant lines of either the Yoshida or the Walker tumor, with chlorambucil, melphalan, or cyclophosphamide (79). Thus it is apparent that nuclear proteins represent an important target for alkylating agents. The resultant biochemical and morphological changes just described must arise either from direct binding of the drugs to nuclear proteins or from drug-induced changes in their functional organization.

Subcellular binding of chlorambucil was investigated following its administration to rats bearing either drug-sensitive or -resistant lines of the Yoshida tumor (80). Twice as much drug was found associated with the total protein of drug-sensitive cells as compared with that of drug-resistant cells. However, the difference was attributable predominantly to a fivefold excess of binding to the soluble nuclear sap proteins. Binding to nonhistone chromosomal proteins was greater than to histones, the drug being associated with the higher-molecular-weight fractions. Significantly, both covalent and noncovalent binding was observed. Binding to nuclear proteins occurred prior to inhibition of DNA synthesis and tended to persist in sensitive cells, although it was removed much more rapidly in resistant cells. Nuclear proteins from both sensitive and resistant cells appeared closely comparable in amino acid content, polyacrylamide gel electrophoretic patterns and mobilities, and ability to bind [^{3}H]chlorambucil *in vitro* (80–82). These differences in nuclear protein reactivity of chlorambucil in drug-sensitive and -resistant cells were reflected also in differences in the rate of reaction with DNA (83). Cross-links appeared in the DNA of resistant tumors maximally at 6 hours and were "repaired" by 12 hours. In sensitive cells, no DNA reaction was detected at these early times, although extensive binding to, and disaggregation of, chromatin occurred (78,80). Subsequently, progressive and irreversible cross-linking of DNA ensued in drug-sensitive cells. It was suggested that the attendant disaggregation of chromatin in sensitive cells might also be accompanied by impairment of excision repair processes. These findings have been broadly confirmed in two tumor lines (Walker and Yoshida) for three clinically used alkylating agents (chlorambucil, melphalan, and cyclophosphamide) (79,84).

The structural changes induced by alkylating agents in nuclear proteins can also be accompanied by changes in nuclear protein metabolism. In view of the putative role currently proposed for nonhistone chromosomal proteins as gene regulators (85), some attention has been given to the effects of alkylating agents on nuclear protein phosphorylation (82). Again, comparisons have been made of the effects induced by several alkylating drugs following treatment of animals carrying either drug-sensitive or drug-refractory tumors. A consistent finding has been the rapid induction by the alkylating agent of gross nuclear protein phosphorylation in sensitive cells, no such effect being observed in resistant cells (79,82). These phosphorylations are associated predominantly with nuclear sap and nonhistone chromosomal proteins (82).

Glucocorticoids are also known both to stimulate nuclear protein phosphorylation (86) and to modify chromatin structure (87). Prednisolone was found to enhance, reversibly, nuclear protein phosphorylation in both sensitive and resistant tumors following its administration to recipient hosts. Furthermore, in combination with an alkylating agent, prednisolone enhanced nuclear protein phosphorylation in resistant cells to levels comparable to those seen in sensitive tumors following treatment with an alkylating agent alone. This effect was accompanied by morphological changes in the nuclei of drug-refractory tumors, which were highly reminiscent of those seen in sensitive cells responding to an alkylating agent alone (79).

We have proposed a simple model, as a tentative working hypothesis, which may help to account for the effects of alkylating agents and alkylating agent–steroid combinations on chromatin (88). It is suggested that chlorambucil stimulates nuclear protein kinase(s) in drug-sensitive cells, leading to nuclear protein phosphorylation and electrostatic separation of these charged molecules from the DNA. Subsequent alkylation of these charged proteins prevents their reassociation with DNA, thereby rendering DNA more accessible to alkylation. Furthermore, drugs associated noncovalently with the chromatin can provide a depot for continuing DNA reaction. These effects lead to morphological disaggregation of the chromatin and damage to excision repair enzymes. It is suggested that, in cells which have acquired resistance to alkylating agents, the chlorambucil-responsive kinases have either been deleted or impaired; alternatively, these cells may contain abnormally elevated levels of nuclear protein phosphatase(s). In either event, exposure of such resistant cells to an alkylating agent would not produce enhanced nuclear protein phosphorylation and subsequent chromatin disaggregation. However, glucocorticoid hormones are still capable of inducing nuclear protein phosphorylation in these cells, normally a rapidly reversible event, leading to temporary release of the associations of these proteins with DNA. Thus, in resistant cells the steroid should render the DNA accessible to the alkylating agent. Hence the biochemical and morphological events seen in sensitive cells responding to an alkylating agent alone will ensue in resistant cells in the presence of the combination.

It is important that the nuclear reactivities of alkylating drugs be related to current knowledge of chromatin structure. The basic chromatin structural unit, the nucleosome, consists of octomers of histones containing two each of histones H2a, H2b, H3, and H4. This structure is surrounded by approximately 140 bp of helical DNA. The connection between nucleosomes is provided by DNA (40–160 bp), with which the fifth histone, H1, is associated. Nonhistone chromatin proteins are associated with this basic structure in an as yet undefined way (89–95). This same basic structure is present in both transcriptionally active (euchromatin) and inactive (heterochromatin) chromatin (95). However, the former differs from the latter in certain physical properties, rendering feasible the separation of the two structures (96). For example, it has been suggested that the constrained helical configuration of heterochromatin is extended in euchromatin (97). Tew *et al.* (98) have made initial attempts to define further the intrachromatin loci of the action of nitrosoureas on the basis of this model. They have shown that alkylation occurs predominantly with core particle DNA, while carbamoylation is restricted to basic nonhistone proteins.

C. Metabolic and Pharmacokinetic Properties of Alkylating Drugs

Many clinically used alkylating drugs, such as HN2, melphalan, and cisplatin, are apparently metabolically inert and react directly with DNA (see Section

I,B,1). Melphalan was synthesized to exploit the active transport system of its phenylalanine moiety, particularly in multiple myeloma (99,100). In fact, although melphalan exhibits activity against this tumor, it is not actively transported into myeloma cells. However, active transport of melphalan has been described in L5178Y cells (101,102).

The clinically useful alkylating agent cyclophosphamide was synthesized to take advantage of the higher phosphoramidase levels in certain tumors (103). In practice, however, the major determinant of the antitumor activity of this drug is its metabolism in the liver to 4-hydroxycyclophosphamide, which then breaks down chemically to phosphoramide mustard and acrolein, two toxic metabolites (104,105). However, 4-hydroxycyclophosphamide can be detoxified by aldehyde oxidase to yield aldophosphamide in many tissues; the selectivity of the drug is thought to be due to the relative detoxification activities of target tissues (106).

The ability of alkylating agents to bind to serum proteins can also influence their metabolic properties by increasing their half-lives *in vivo*. Hopwood and Stock (107) have shown that the alkylating functions of chlorambucil and melphalan are not impaired as a result of serum protein binding, while the half-lives of these compounds are increased. Protein binding also occurs with the steroidal alkylating agent Prednimustine (108).

Chlorambucil, a nitrogen mustard derivative of phenylbutyric acid, is metabolized *in vivo,* probably via a β-oxidation mechanism (109). The metabolite, phenylacetic mustard, while displaying antitumor activity comparable to that of chlorambucil, is more toxic to the rat (109). Recently, the pharmacological evaluation of chlorambucil has been possible using a high-pressure liquid chromatography (HPLC) method (110). Chlorambucil and phenylacetic mustard can be separated and low plasma concentrations detected, rendering possible a study of their pharmacokinetics in humans without recourse to radiolabeled drugs (110). The half-lives of chlorambucil in humans and rats are 1.7 hours and 45 minutes, respectively. Phenylacetic mustard is a prominent metabolite of chlorambucil in the rat, where it exhibits a half-life of 1.5 hours. However, there is only minor metabolism to phenylacetic mustard in humans (110).

The steroidal alkylating agents Estracyt and Prednimustine were synthesized in an attempt to enhance antitumor selectivity via the transport properties of the steroid carrier (111). Estracyt exhibits useful clinical activity in prostatic cancer (112,113), while Prednimustine has been used in the treatment of leukemias, lymphomas, and carcinomas of the breast and lung (114–119). Prednimustine is considerably less systemically toxic than the parent alkylating agent chlorambucil (120). It is inactive until hydrolyzed to its component molecules, prednisolone and chlorambucil (by nonspecific esterases), in plasma and tissues (108). It is likely therefore that much of the antitumor activity of this compound relates to the nuclear interactions occurring between chlorambucil and prednisolone discussed above (79).

A particularly useful property of prednisolone, when administered in binary combination with chlorambucil, is its ability to potentiate the antitumor activity of the latter while also suppressing its gastrointestinal toxicity (120). Similar effects can be elicited with prednisolone–mustine combinations. However, when the steroid is given with either melphalan or cyclophosphamide, both antitumor activity and host toxicity are enhanced (121).

II. An Experimental Approach

A. Introduction

As outlined above, prednisolone is able both to potentiate the antitumor activity of chlorambucil and to suppress its host toxicity. Significantly, binary combinations of chlorambucil and prednisolone, or prednimustine (the prednisolone ester of chlorambucil), exhibit significant antitumor activity against neoplastic lines which are refractory to treatment with chlorambucil alone. Where tumor cells respond to any of these treatments, extensive morphological changes occur in the chromatin, accompanied by enhanced phosphorylation of nonhistone chromosomal proteins (See Section I,B,2). In view of these findings, the objectives of the present study were as follows.

1. To determine in tumor cells and in several host tissues whether prednisolone modifies the binding of chlorambucil (a) to gross cellular macromolecules and (b) to fractionated chromatin proteins.
2. To locate the binding site of chlorambucil within the chromatin superstructure.
3. To determine whether prednimustine, or combinations of chlorambucil and prednisolone, can produce nuclear protein changes in resistant tumors similar to those seen in drug-sensitive cells responding to chlorambucil alone.
4. To investigate whether the chlorambucil-induced enhancement of nuclear protein phosphorylation may derive from an inhibition of nuclear protein phosphatase activity.
5. In view of the potential clinical utility of prednimustine, to undertake a preliminary evaluation of its pharmacokinetics in the rat.

B. Materials and Methods

1. *Tumor Lines*

The Walker 256 carcinosarcoma and the Yoshida sarcoma were maintained in female Wistar rats as intraperitoneal tumors by transplantation of aliquots of ascitic fluid once a week. Both alkylating agent-sensitive and -resistant lines were used. The resistant Walker tumor was treated with 10 mg/kg of chlorambucil and the resistant Yoshida with 2 mg/kg of melphalan 3 days after each passage to maintain resistance. Experimental animals received a tumor load of 2×10^6 cells, and drug treatments were given subcutaneously in the back of the neck 3 days later, at a tumor load of $3-5 \times 10^7$ cells. Chlorambucil, prednisolone, and prednimustine were administered in dimethyl sulfoxide (DMSO) at 1 ml/kg; control rats received DMSO only.

2. *Macromolecular Binding of Chlorambucil*

[^{3}H]Chlorambucil was prepared by The Radiochemical Centre (Amersham, Bucks, England) by the reductive tritiation of 4,4-bis(2-chloroethyl)amino-2-iodophenyl-3-butyric acid, as previously described by Jarman *et al.* (122). The [^{3}H]chlorambucil was greater than 95% radiochemically pure as measured by HPLC analysis (110) and had a specific activity of 936 mCi/mmole.

[^{3}H]Chlorambucil was administered subcutaneously in DMSO at a dose of 12.4 mg/kg and 38 mCi/kg. Rats receiving [^{3}H]chlorambucil had an ascites tumor load of 5×10^7 cells of either the alkylating agent-sensitive strain of the Walker carcinosarcoma or a paired strain exhibiting acquired resistance to alkylating agent toxicity. In addition, half of the rats also received 10 mg/kg of prednisolone in DMSO 4 hours after the [^{3}H]chlorambucil.

At 6, 24, and 48 hours after [^{3}H]chlorambucil treatment, rats were killed by cervical dislocation. Tumor cells were removed in a 0.9% NaCl solution, as was bone marrow from each femur (at least three rats per point). Cells were centrifuged at 500 g for 3 minutes before being used for the preparation of nuclei (123) and fractionation of DNA, RNA, and protein (124). Livers were also removed, washed in reticulocyte standard buffer (RSB), and chopped, and aliquots were taken for DNA, RNA, and protein fractionation (124) and preparation of nuclei (123). The small intestine was removed and washed in 0.9% NaCl, and the mucosal surface scraped off using a round-ended spatula. The mucosal cells were suspended in 0.9% NaCl, and aliquots were used for DNA, RNA, and protein separation (124) and for preparation of nuclei (123). DNA, RNA, and protein assays were according to the methods of Burton (125), Brown (126), and Lowry *et al.* (127), respectively. Purified nuclei from all tissues were stored at −40°C until required for the fractionation of nuclear proteins.

3. *Fractionation of Nuclear Proteins*

Isolated nuclei were first suspended in 0.14 *M* NaCl–10m*M* Tris–HCl, pH 7.4, extracted twice at 4°C for 20 minutes each in 0.14 *M* NaCl to remove soluble nuclear sap proteins (123). The remaining chromatin was then extracted twice with 0.35 *M* NaCl-10m*M* Tris–HCl, pH 7.4, to remove less tightly bound chromatin proteins, high-mobility-group proteins, and histone H1 (128–130). Extraction with 0.6 M NaCl followed, which released core histones and some nonhistone proteins and DNA (131,132). The residue, containing DNA and associated nonhistone proteins, was solubilized in 5 *M* urea—2*M* NaCl (123). The concentration of [^{3}H]chlorambucil in all these fractions was measured by counting an aliquot in 10 ml of a toluene-based scintillant (Triton X-100, 35%; Butyl PBD, 1%) in an Intertechnique liquid scintillation spectrometer. Nuclear proteins were fractionated from Yoshida sarcoma nuclei on hydroxyapatite, and the fractions characterized by polyacrylamide gel electrophoresis as previously described (80).

4. *Nuclear Protein Phosphorylation*

Whole nuclei were phosphorylated *in vitro* by the method of Rickwood *et al.* (123) both to measure total phosphorylation and prior to assay for nuclear nonhistone protein phosphatase activity. Nuclei (400 μl) were suspended in 0.1 *M* Tris–HC1, pH 8.0, and incubated at 37°C for 5 minutes in 500 μl of 1 *M* sucrose, 200 μl of 1 *M* Tris–HC1, pH 8.0, 200 μl of 0.1 *M* $MgCl_2$, 200 μl of 0.25 *M* NaCl, 30 μl of 1.25 m*M* ATP, 20 μl of [γ^{32}P]ATP (20 Ci/mmole, 250 μCi/ml), and 20 μl of 0.1 *M* phenylmethylsulfonylfluoride in a total reaction volume of 2 ml. Reactions were terminated by cooling on ice and centrifuging at 1000 *g* for 10 minutes. Excess radioactive [γ^{32}P]ATP was removed by washing the pellet in incubation medium containing 12.5 m*M* ATP.

5. *Assay of Nuclear Protein Phosphatase Activity*

Nuclear protein phosphatase activity was determined by the method of Kleinsmith (133).

6. *Micrococcal Nuclease Digestion of Nuclei*

Purified nuclei (123) were incubated for various times at 37°C with 2 units of micrococcal nuclease per 1.0A_{260} unit of nuclei in 50m*M* Tris–HCl, pH 7.5, 25 m*M* KC1, 1 m*M* $MgCl_2$, 10 m*M* $CaCl_2$, and 0.25 *M* sucrose, as previously described (134). Nuclei were then centrifuged at 1000 *g* to remove the reaction mixture, and chromatin was released from the nuclear pellet with 1 m*M* EDTA, pH 8.0. This material was then centrifuged to give the polynucleosome fraction in the supernatant, which was sedimented on a 5–30% sucrose gradient in 1 m*M* EDTA, 0.5 M NaCl, and 1 mM sodium phosphate buffer, pH 7.4. Tubes (6 × 10 ml) were centrifuged in an MSE 65 Superspeed centrifuge at 29,000 rpm for 16 hours (135).

[^{3}H]Chlorambucil binding to chromatin was determined *in vitro*. Walker S cells were removed from the peritoneal cavities of Wistar rats and incubated *in vitro* in RPMI 1640 tissue culture medium supplemented with 10% horse serum (Flow Laboratories, Irvine, Scotland) for 2 hours in the presence of 20 μg/ml of [^{3}H]chlorambucil (61.6 μCi/ml). Nuclei were prepared, and micrococcal nuclease digestion and sucrose gradients performed as described above.

7. *Tissue Culture*

Tissue culture and colony-forming assays on Walker cells were carried out according to Wilkinson *et al.* (108).

8. *Pharmacokinetic Assays of Prednimustine, Chlorambucil, and Phenylacetic Mustard*

These were carried out by HPLC according to the method of Newell *et al.* (110). Radiolabeled prednimustine formulated as previously described (108) was a generous gift from A. B. Leo, Helsingborg, Sweden.

C. Results

1. *Binding of Chlorambucil to Whole Cell Macromolecules*

Figure 1 shows chlorambucil binding to total cellular RNA, which is approximately fivefold greater in the sensitive than in the resistant tumor at 6 hours; in neither case is this modified by prednisolone. Drug amounts at 6 hours in sensitive tumor RNA are approximately comparable to those in liver RNA, while the levels associated with RNA from bone marrow and small intestine are approximately half this value. In normal tissues, as in tumors, prednisolone appears to be without effect on drug–RNA binding. It is notable that, over the 48-hour period of observation, drug is progressively removed from the RNA of all tissues, with the exception of bone marrow where it appears to accumulate.

Binding of chlorambucil to DNA is shown in Fig. 2. The sensitive tumor DNA binds approximately twice as much drug as the resistant tumor. Prednisolone appears to enhance this twofold at 6 hours in the former but not in the latter tumor. Levels of drug associated with liver DNA are considerably greater (approximately 10-fold) than those found in the DNA of other tissues. There is also a suggestion that more drug is present at 6 hours in the DNA of livers taken from animals bearing resistant tumors than from those carrying the drug-sensitive line. Prednisolone does not modify the levels of drug bound to DNA of either the resistant tumor or of normal tissues. As for RNA (Fig. 1), drug is progressively removed from the DNA of all tissues, except for bone marrow, where again accumulation is apparent.

The levels of chlorambucil bound to total cellular proteins were broadly similar in all tissues, as seen in Fig. 3. The steroid did not modify binding to the protein of liver or intestine. In bone marrow, more binding was seen at 24 hours in the presence of prednisolone, while in the sensitive tumor, prednisolone enhanced chlorambucil binding at 6 hours. Binding of chlorambucil was generally greater in sensitive than in resistant cells. The drug was retained, or appeared to accumulate, in proteins from tumor and bone marrow, while the levels progressively decayed in liver and intestine.

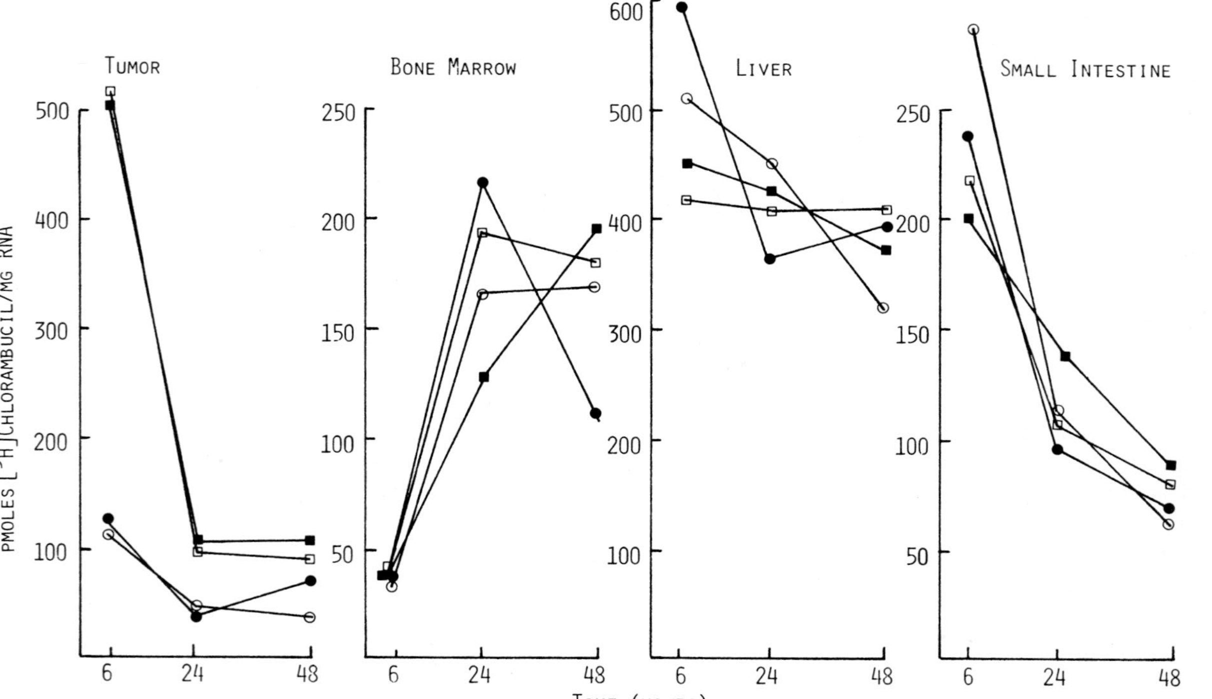

Fig. 1. Binding of [^{3}H]chlorambucil-derived material to total cellular protein. Tumor-bearing rats received 12.4 mg/kg of [^{3}H]chlorambucil (3.08 mCi/mg). Prednisolone-treated animals received 10 mg/kg of the steroid 4 hours later. Tumor and normal tissues were removed and processed as described in Section II,B,2. Points are the mean of duplicate determinations on groups of three (6 and 48 hours) or six (24 hours) rats. ■, Animals bearing drug-sensitive tumors treated with chlorambucil alone; □, animals bearing drug-sensitive tumors treated with chlorambucil followed 4 hours later by prednisolone; ●, animals bearing drug-resistant tumors treated with chlorambucil alone; and ○, animals bearing drug-resistant tumors treated with chlorambucil followed 4 hours later by prednisolone.

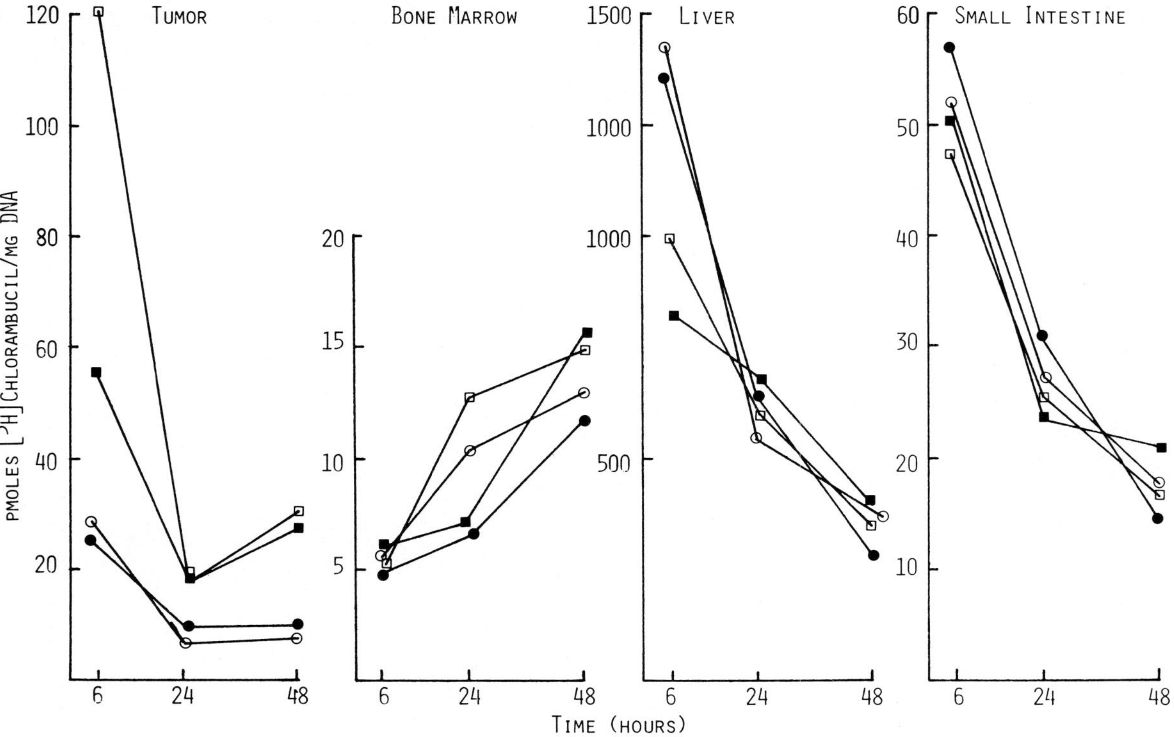

Fig. 2. Binding of [^{3}H]chlorambucil-derived material to total cellular DNA. Tumor-bearing rats received 12.4 mg/kg of [^{3}H]chlorambucil (3.08 mCi/mg). Prednisolone-treated animals received 10 mg/kg of the steroid 4 hours later. Tumor and normal tissues were removed and processed as described in Section II,B,2. Points are the mean of duplicate determinations on groups of three (6 and 48 hours) or six (24 hours) rats. See legend for Fig. 1 for key to symbols.

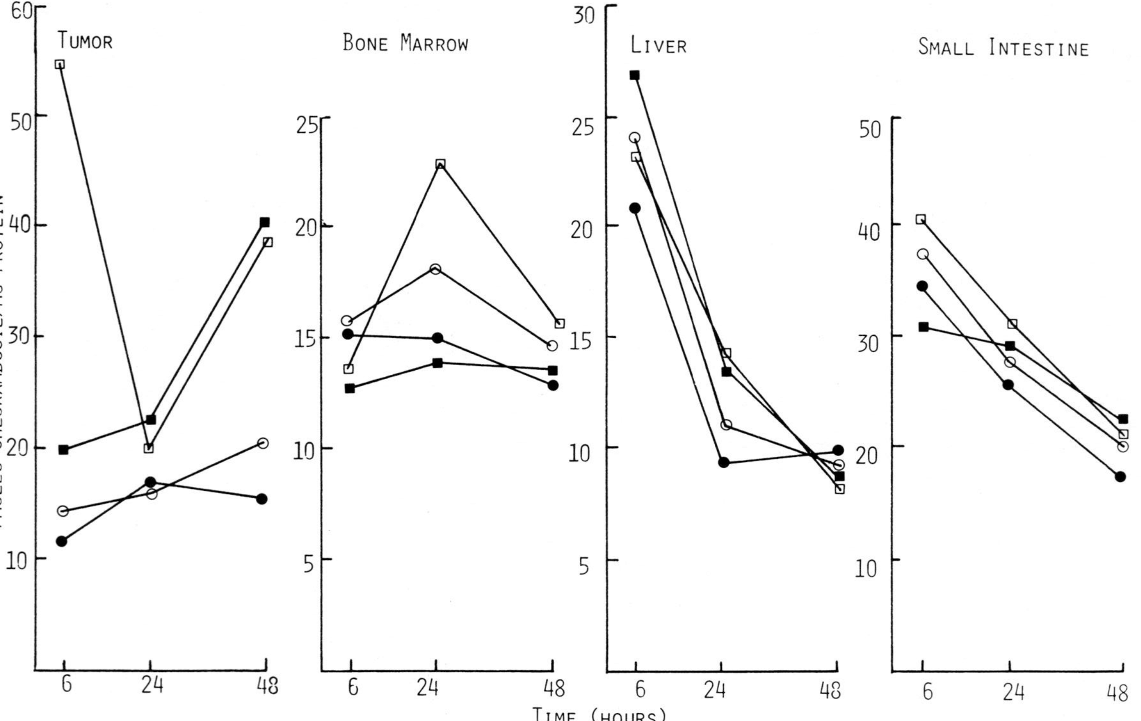

Fig. 3. Binding of [^{3}H]chlorambucil-derived material to total cellular protein. Tumor-bearing rats received 12.4 mg/kg of [^{3}H]chlorambucil (3.08 mCi/mg). Prednisolone-treated animals received 10 mg/kg of the steroid 4 hours later. Tumor and normal tissues were removed and processed as described in Section II,B,2. Points are the mean of duplicate determinations on groups of three (6 and 48 hours) or six (24 hours) rats. See legend for Fig. 1 for key to symbols.

When the molar amounts of chlorambucil associated with unit weights of DNA, RNA, or protein are compared, it is clear that the order of binding for all tissues except liver is RNA > DNA > protein. In liver the order is DNA > RNA > protein. However, when the comparison is made on a molar basis, the order of binding becomes DNA ≫ RNA ≫ protein in all tissues (see Table I). On this basis DNA is apparently the major target for chlorambucil, though it remains possible that low-level binding to other macromolecules may dictate chromatin changes of significance in determining cell death [see above discussion; (79)].

2. *Chromatin Binding of Chlorambucil*

Figure 4 shows the binding of chlorambucil to fractionated chromatin proteins of sensitive and resistant tumors. Consistently, more chlorambucil is associated with fractions of sensitive than resistant tumors, and in both tumors the binding is enhanced by prednisolone treatment, particularly at 6 hours. Steroid enhancement of chlorambucil binding to resistant tumor cells is apparent in the fractionated chromatin proteins, although this difference was not evident in total cell protein.

Figure 5 shows the binding of chlorambucil to chromatin fractions of bone marrow. No consistent changes are apparent. Binding is generally higher in the nuclear sap and salt–urea fractions. It is suppressed by prednisolone in the 0.14 *M* and 0.6 *M* NaCl fractions and enhanced in the 0.35 *M* NaCl and salt–urea fractions. Although the differences observed are small, it is clear that prednisolone does not increase the binding of chlorambucil to bone marrow chromatin, as is the case with tumor chromatin.

The binding of chlorambucil to liver chromatin proteins is not modified by prednisolone, as seen in Fig. 6, and in the small intestine chlorambucil binding is inhibited by prednisolone in all but the 0.6 *M* NaCl fraction (Fig. 7).

With the exception of the nuclear sap fraction in liver, the amounts of drug bound to each fraction from each tissue decayed progressively over the period of study. It is appropriate to draw attention to the striking differences in amounts of drug bound to some tissue fractions and the differential effects of prednisolone on this binding. For example, 6 hours after treatment with chlorambucil alone, the nuclear sap fraction of intestinal cells contains at least 16 times more drug than that found in this fraction from any other tissue. Following treatment with prednisolone, this level of binding is reduced fourfold in intestinal nuclear sap, while conversely the level is expanded fourfold in the corresponding fractions of both tumors. Closely comparable changes are seen in response to prednisolone in the remaining chromatin extracts from intestine and tumor. Thus prednisolone treatment consistently enhances the binding to tumor nucleoproteins, while suppressing binding to intestinal nucleoproteins. Prednisolone is essentially without effect on the chlorambucil levels in chromatin extracts of liver and bone marrow.

In an attempt to locate the site of action of chlorambucil in the chromatin

TABLE I

[^{3}H]Chlorambucil Bound at 6 Hours to Macromolecules[a]

Sample[b]	DNA		RNA		Protein	
	Nmoles/gm	Moles/mole	Nmoles/gm	Moles/mole	Nmoles/gm	Moles/mole
Tumor						
SC	56	56	510	0.51	20	2.0
SC+P	120	120	520	0.52	55	5.5
RC	24	24	120	0.12	11	1.1
RC+P	28	28	110	0.11	14	1.4
Bone marrow						
SC	6.0	6.0	40	0.04	13	1.3
SC+P	5.5	5.5	45	0.05	13.5	1.4
RC	5.0	5.0	50	0.04	15	1.5
RC+P	5.5	5.5	35	0.04	15.5	1.6
Liver						
SC	825	825	450	0.45	27	2.7
SC+P	1000	1000	420	0.42	23	2.3
RC	1300	1300	600	0.60	24	2.4
RC+P	1400	1400	500	0.50	21	2.1
Small intestine						
SC	50	50	200	0.20	31	3.1
SC+P	47	47	220	0.22	40	4.0
RC	57	57	240	0.24	35	3.5
RC+P	52	52	280	0.28	38	3.8

[a] Approximate molecular weights used: DNA, 10^9; RNA, 10^6; protein, 10^5. Data taken from the 6-hour time points in Figs. 1–3.

[b] SC, Animals bearing drug-sensitive tumors treated with chlorambucil alone; SC+P, animals bearing drug-sensitive tumors treated with chlorambucil followed 4 hours later by prednisolone; RC, animals bearing drug-resistant tumors treated with chlorambucil alone; RC+P, animals bearing drug-resistant tumors treated with chlorambucil followed 4 hours later by prednisolone.

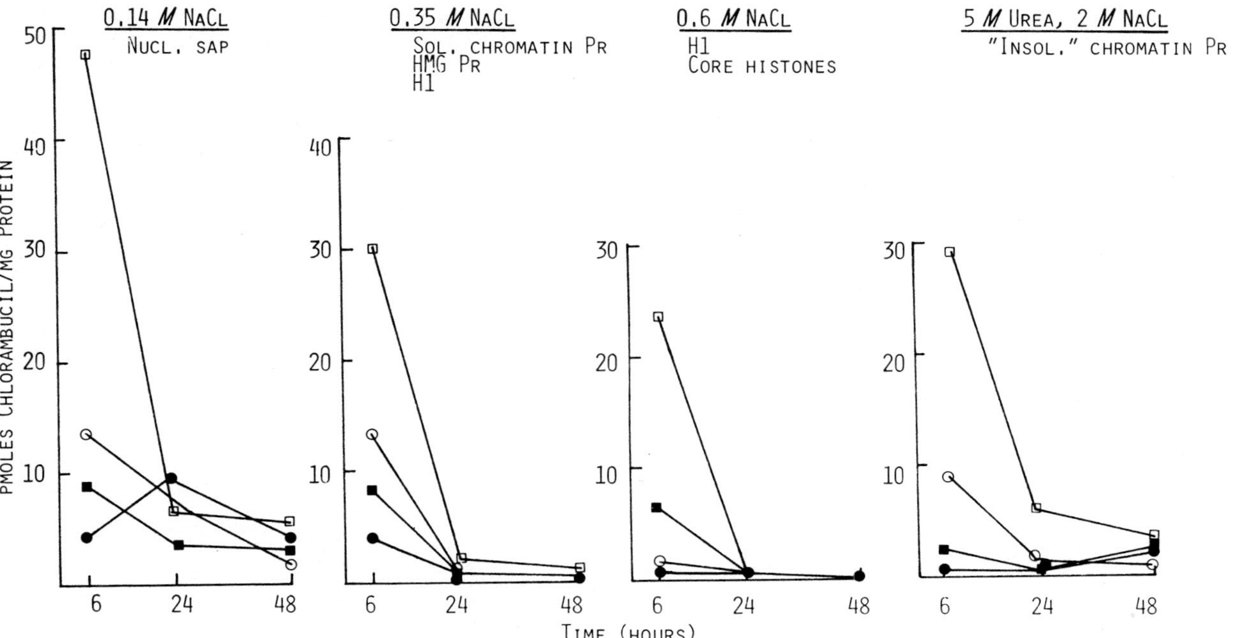

Fig. 4. Binding of [^{3}H]chlorambucil-derived material to chromatin fractions of tumor. Tumor-bearing rats received 12.4 mg/kg of [^{3}H]chlorambucil (3.08 mCi/mg). Prednisolone-treated animals received 10 mg/kg of the steroid 4 hours later. At various times, tissues were removed and nuclei prepared and then fractionated as described in Section II,B,2 and 3. Points are the means of duplicate determinations on groups of three (6 and 48 hours) or six (24 hours) rats. See legend for Fig. 1 for key to symbols.

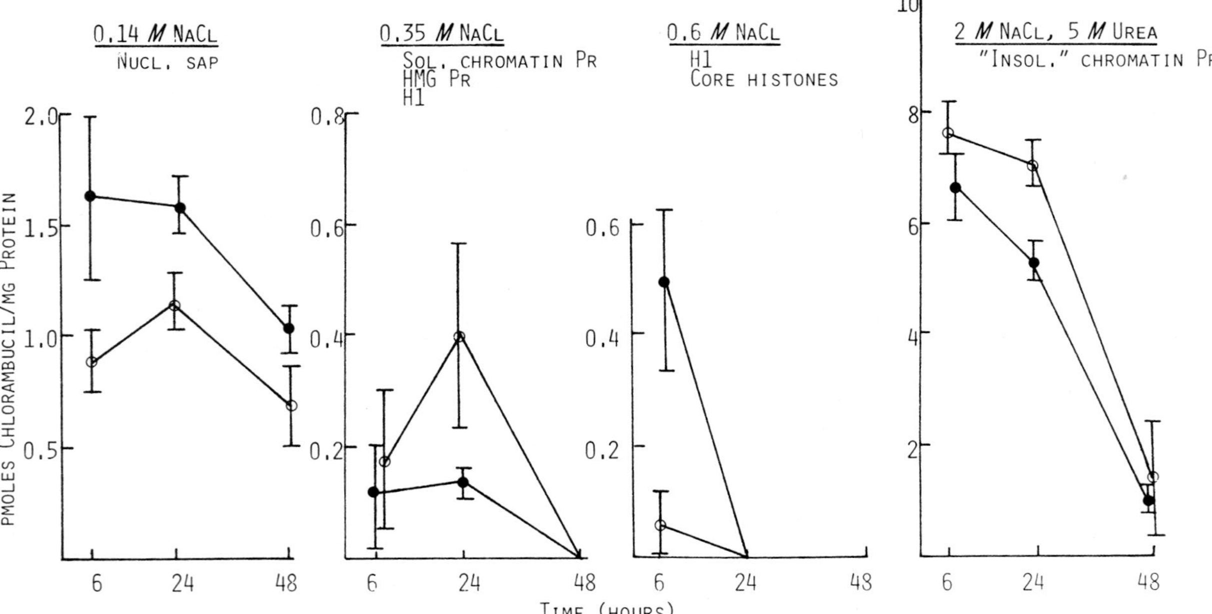

Fig. 5. Binding of [^{3}H]chlorambucil-derived material to chromatin fractions of bone marrow. Tumor-bearing rats received 12.4 mg/kg of [^{3}H]chlorambucil (3.08 mCi/mg). Prednisolone-treated animals received 10 mg/kg of the steroid 4 hours later. At various times, bone marrow was removed and nuclei prepared and then fractionated as described in Section II,B,2 and 3. Points are the means of duplicate determinations in each of two separate experiments. Error bars show the maximum range observed. No differences were apparent between sensitive and resistant tumor-bearing animals in the levels of chlorambucil associated with host bone marrow chromatin fractions. The data have therefore been combined from animals bearing each tumor line. ●, animals treated with chlorambucil alone; ○, animals treated with chlorambucil followed 4 hours later by prednisolone.

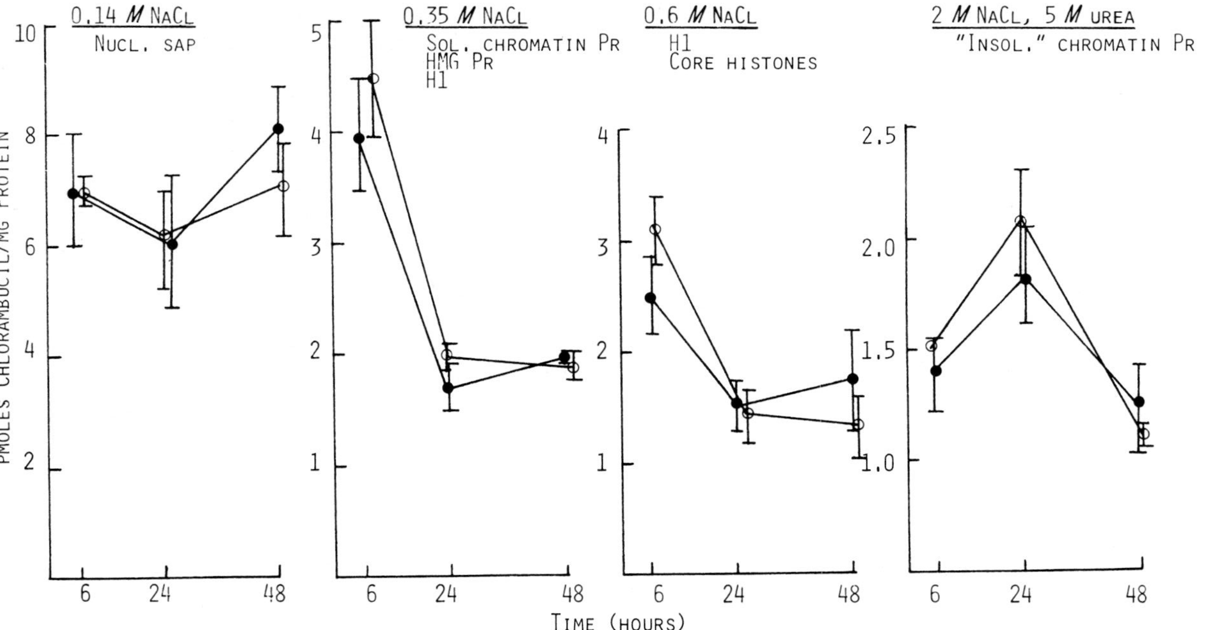

Fig. 6. Binding of [^{3}H]chlorambucil-derived material to chromatin fractions of liver. Tumor-bearing rats received 12.4 mg/kg of [^{3}H]chlorambucil (3.08 mCi/mg). Prednisolone-treated animals received 10 mg/kg of the steroid 4 hours later. At various times, livers were removed and nuclei prepared and then fractionated as described in Section II,B,2 and 3. Points are the means of duplicate determinations in each of two separate experiments. Error bars show the maximum range observed. No differences were apparent between sensitive and resistant tumor-bearing animals in the levels of chlorambucil associated with liver tissue chromatin fractions. The data have therefore been combined from animals bearing each tumor line. See legend for Fig. 5 for key to symbols.

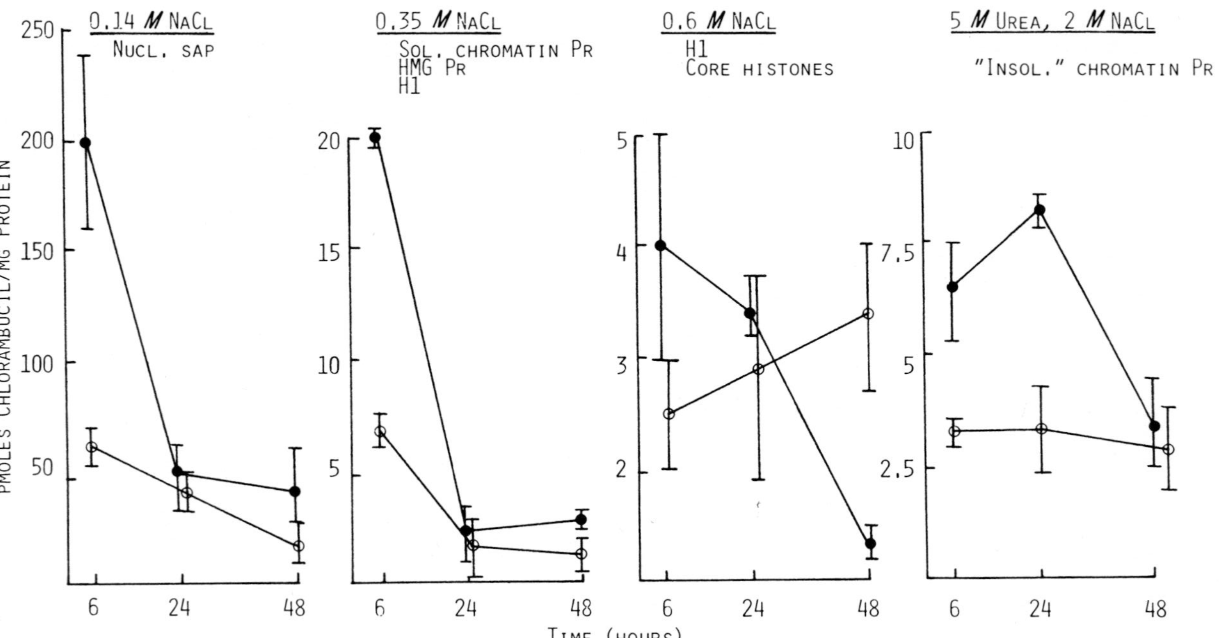

Fig. 7. Binding of [^{3}H]chlorambucil-derived material to chromatin in fractions of small intestine. Tumor-bearing rats received 12.4 mg/kg of [^{3}H]chlorambucil (3.08 mCi/mg). Prednisolone-treated animals received 10 mg/kg of the steroid 4 hours later. At various times, the small intestine was removed and nuclei prepared and then fractionated as described in Section II,B,2 and 3. Points are the means of duplicate determinations in each of two separate experiments. Error bars show the maximum range observed. No differences were apparent between sensitive and resistant tumor-bearing animals in the levels of chlorambucil associated with host tissue chromatin fractions. The data have therefore been combined from animals bearing each tumor line. See legend for Fig. 5 for key to symbols.

superstructure, we have examined its binding to nuclease-digested chromatin. Figure 8 shows the pattern of micrococcal nuclease digestion produced by incubating sensitive Walker tumor nuclei for various times in the presence of micrococcal nuclease. After 2 minutes most of the material is undigested and appears at the bottom of the sucrose gradient (fractions 1–5); after 15 minutes a major band of 8–16 nucleosomes is present (fractions 5–12), and a small mononucleosome peak appears (fractions 14–16); and after 45 minutes most of the material is in the monomer peak (fractions 14–16). By comparison, Fig. 9 shows a 2-minute digestion of nuclei isolated from sensitive cells 6 hours after treatment of the host animals with chlorambucil. It can be seen that chlorambucil treatment enhanced the digestion, and that a band containing 8–16 nucleosomes is produced (fractions 5–12) together with a small mononucleosome peak (fractions 14–16). This is similar to the pattern obtained when control nuclei are incubated with nuclease for 15 minutes, as shown in Fig. 8. Chlorambucil apparently renders chromatin more susceptible to nuclease attack. In an associated *in vitro* experiment, we attempted to identify the site of chlorambucil binding in the chromatin, and Fig. 10 shows a 15-minute digestion with micrococcal nuclease of [^{3}H]chlorambucil-labeled nuclei. The majority of the radioactivity is associated with the top of the gradient (fractions 20–25) and not with the intact mononucleosome region or with the 8–16 nucleosome bands. Although these data are preliminary in nature, they suggest a localization of chlorambucil in specific areas of chromatin rather than a totally random distribution of the drug.

3. *Nuclear Protein Phosphorylation*

We have studied nuclear protein phosphorylation in an attempt to assess the effects of chlorambucil on the functional activity of chromatin. We have shown previously that nuclear protein phosphorylation is enhanced in tumors following treatment with alkylating agents, or with alkylating agent–prednisolone combinations (79,82). Figure 11 summarizes the effects on nuclear protein phosphorylation of various treatments of rats bearing an alkylating agent-resistant strain of the Yoshida ascites sarcoma. In Fig. 11B it can be seen that prednisolone treatment induces a rapidly reversible burst of phosphorylation. In Fig. 11C it is evident that chlorambucil treatment of animals carrying the resistant tumor does not disturb nuclear protein phosphorylation; however, treatment with chlorambucil–prednisolone combinations produces an effect highly reminiscent of that seen in sensitive tumors aspirated from animals treated with chlorambucil alone (82). In Fig. 11A it can be seen that the prednisolone ester of chlorambucil, Prednimustine, enhances phosphorylation in a manner similar to that of the combination.

We have made qualitative investigations of the identity of the phosphorylated products resulting from these treatments. Nuclei were prepared from resistant

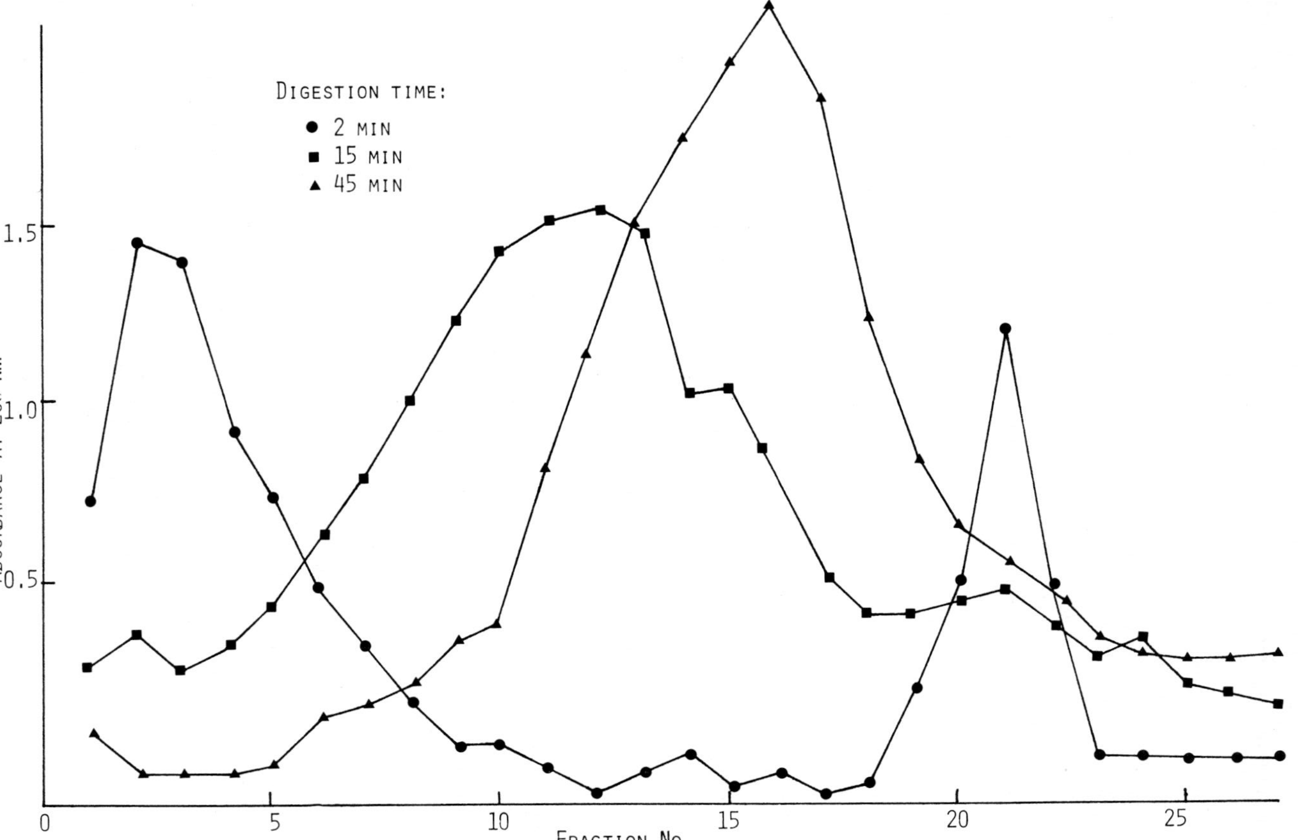

Fig. 8. Sucrose gradient fractionation of Walker(s) chromatin. Sensitive Walker tumor cells were removed from the peritoneal cavities of Wistar rats. Nuclei were prepared and digested at 37°C with micrococcal nuclease, and the digested EDTA-released chromatin was run on 5–30% sucrose gradients as described in Section II,B,6.

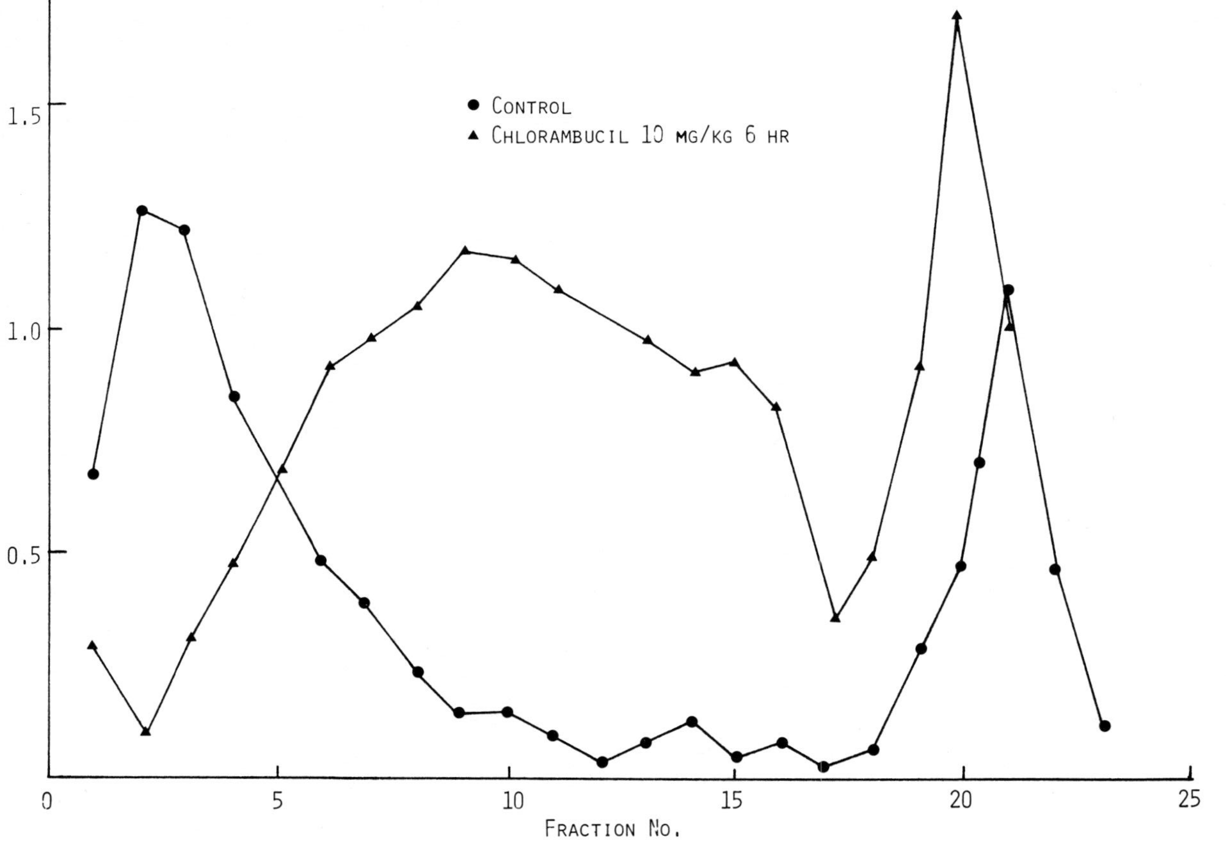

Fig. 9. Sucrose gradient fractionation of Walker(s) chromatin. Sensitive Walker tumor cells were removed from control rats and also from tumor-bearing rats that had received 10 mg/kg of chlorambucil 6 hours earlier. Nuclei were prepared and digested for 2 minutes at 37°C with micrococcal nuclease, and the digested EDTA-released chromatin was run on a 5–30% sucrose gradient.

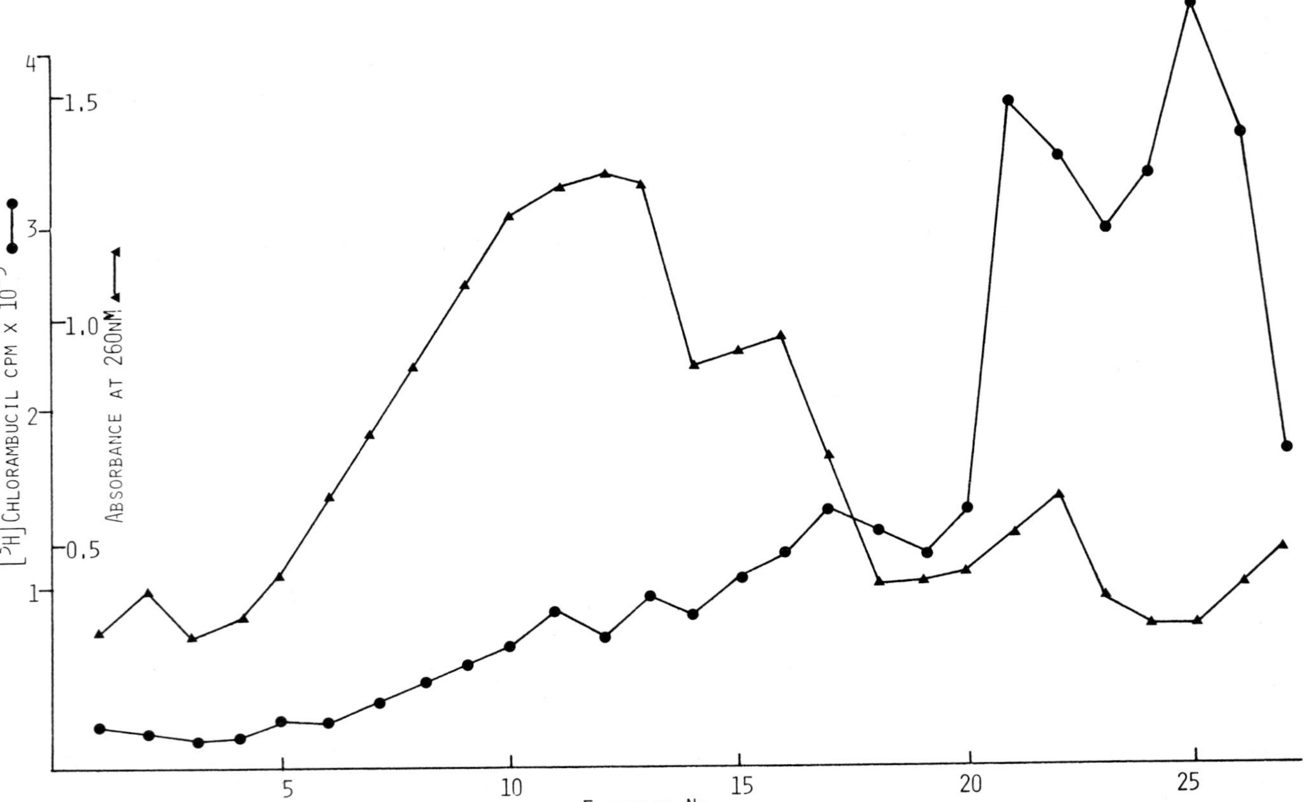

Fig. 10. Sucrose gradient fractionation of Walker(s) chromatin (from chlorambucil-exposed cells). Sensitive Walker tumor cells were removed from the peritoneal cavity and incubated *in vitro* for 2 hours in the presence of 20 μg/ml of [^{3}H]chlorambucil. Nuclei were prepared and digested for 15 minutes at 37°C with micrococcal nuclease as described in Section II,B,6.

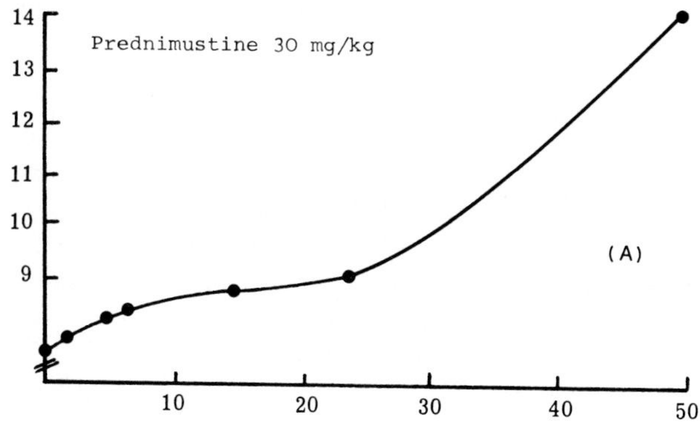

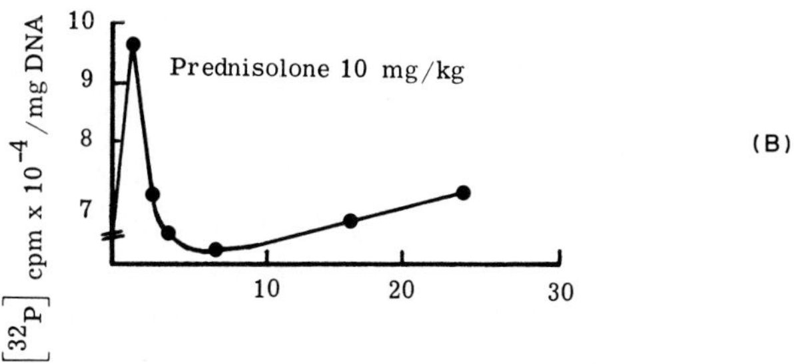

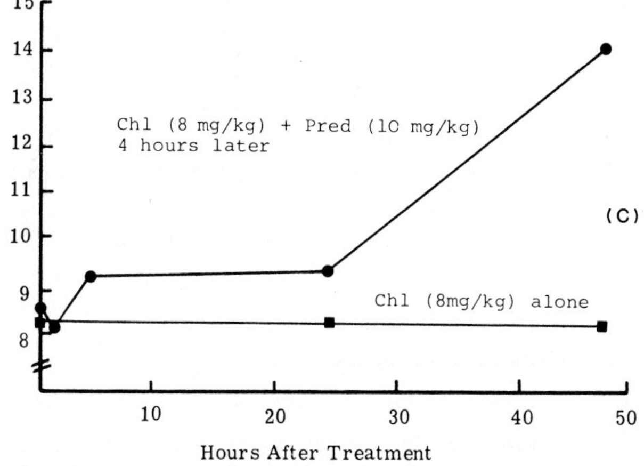

Fig. 11. Total nuclear protein phosphorylation in Yoshida sarcoma cells resistant to alkylating agent toxicity. Tumor-bearing rats received 30 mg/kg of Prednimustine, 10 mg/kg of prednisolone, or 8 mg/kg of chlorambucil followed 4 hours later by 10 mg/kg of prednisolone at time zero. At various times, groups of rats were killed and the tumor cells aspirated; nuclei were prepared, and phosphorylation measured by incubating the nuclei *in vitro* in the presence of [γ-^{32}P]ATP. Total nuclear protein and DNA were isolated, and protein counts expressed per milligram of DNA in the same sample.

Yoshida tumors aspirated from animals previously treated with either prednisolone or Prednimustine. After *in vitro* phosphorylation with [γP^{32}]ATP, nuclear proteins were fractionated on hydroxyapatite and subjected to sodium dodecyl sulfate polyacrylamide gel electrophoresis (see Section II,B,3). No treatment-induced changes were observed in the phosphorylation profile of the histone fraction. It can be seen in Fig. 12 that prednisolone treatment enhanced the phosphorylation level of high-molecular-weight Tris–saline (or nuclear sap) proteins; similar and more extensive enhancement was observed following Prednimustine treatment. In the H2 nonhistone fraction (Fig. 13), both prednisolone and prednimustine produced elevated phosphorylation in the low-molecular-weight region of the gel. Prednimustine appeared to be without effect on the phosphorylation profile of H3 proteins (Fig. 14), although prednisolone treatment led to the appearance of P^{32} label in the high-molecular-weight portion of the gel. It is thus apparent that the phosphorylation enhancement induced by prednisolone and prednimustine in drug-resistant cells is confined to nuclear sap and nonhistone chromatin proteins. Both agents appear to influence closely related proteins in the nuclear sap and H2 fractions. However, only prednisolone exhibits activity in the H3 fractions.

The increased nuclear protein phosphorylation observed following treatment with an alkylating agent or an alkylating agent–steroid combination could be explained either by activation of nuclear protein kinase(s), by inhibition of nuclear protein phosphatases, or by a combination of both effects. Tables II and III show measurements of nuclear protein phosphatase activities in sensitive and resistant strains of the Walker carcinosarcoma. Phosphatase activity was measured both by the loss of [γ-^{32}P]ATP from acid-insoluble material (Table II) and by the appearance of inorganic phosphate in acid-soluble material (Table III). It is apparent that no significant inhibition of phosphatase activity occurred in sensitive cells, nor was phosphatase activity enhanced in resistant cells, following treatment with either chlorambucil alone, prednisolone alone, or a combination of chlorambucil and prednisolone.

From these data, we conclude that modulation of nuclear protein kinase activities is probably responsible for the increased phosphorylation observed. Studies on the separation and characterization of these enzymes are now in progress.

4. *Pharmacokinetics of Prednimustine*

It appears that prednimustine can elicit molecular changes in chromatin comparable to those produced by chlorambucil–prednisolone combinations. This prednisolone ester of chlorambucil is much less toxic systemically than chlorambucil itself (possibly because of its high lipophilicity) and is not cytotoxic *in vitro* until hydrolyzed to its component molecules (108,120). Furthermore, chlorambucil itself undergoes metabolism by β-oxidation to produce phenylacetic mustard, the major metabolite in the rat (109). The data in Fig. 15 demonstrate that

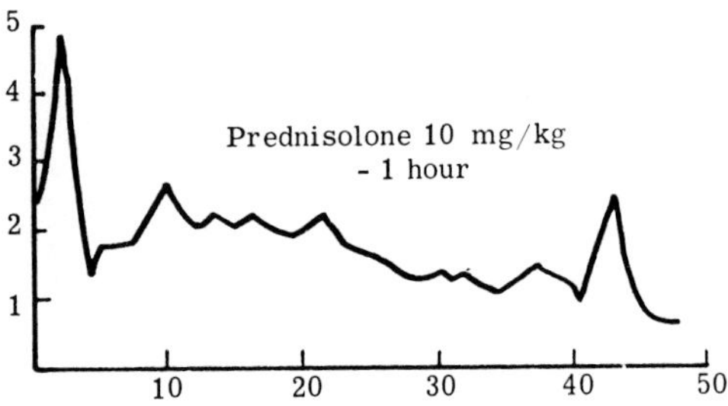

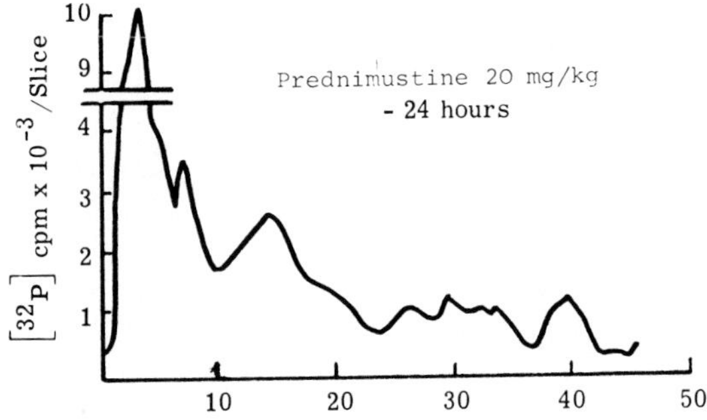

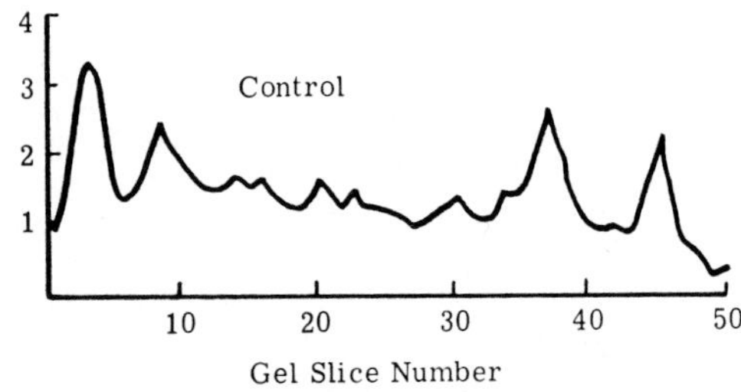

Fig. 12. Polyacrylamide (15%) gel electrophoresis of phosphorylated Tris–saline proteins. Rats bearing the alkylating agent-resistant Yoshida sarcoma received either prednisolone (10 mg/kg) or Prednimustine (20 mg/kg). One hour after prednisolone treatment and 24 hours after Prednimustine treatment, the rats were killed, the tumor aspirated, and nuclei prepared. The purified nuclei were phosphorylated *in vitro* with [γ-^{32}P]ATP and then fractionated. Tris–saline (0.14 *M* NaCl-soluble) proteins were removed, concentrated, and run on 15% polyacrylamide gels. Gels were cut into 2-mm slices, and the radioactivity in each slice counted.

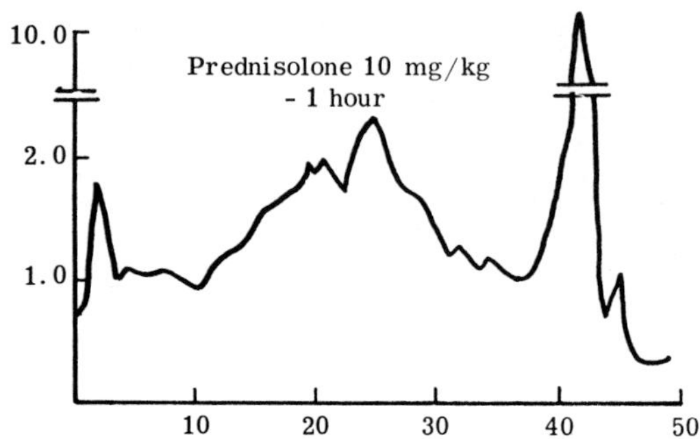

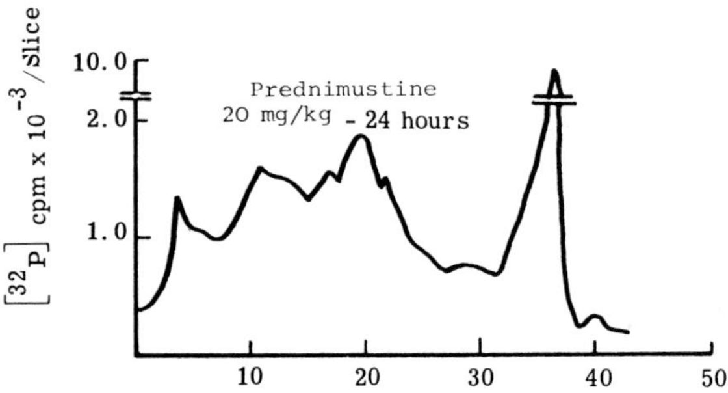

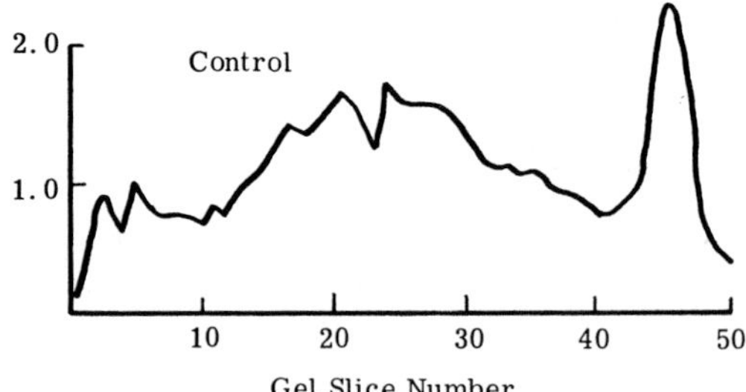

Fig. 13. Polyacrylamide (15%) gel electrophoresis of phosphorylated H2 chromatin proteins. Tumor-bearing rats were treated with prednisolone or prednimustine as described in the legend for Fig. 12. Nuclei were prepared and phosphorylated and, after removal of the Tris–saline (0.14 *M* NaCl-soluble) proteins, the chromatin was further fractionated on a hydroxyapatite column. The H2 fraction was that eluting in 50 m*M* phosphate.

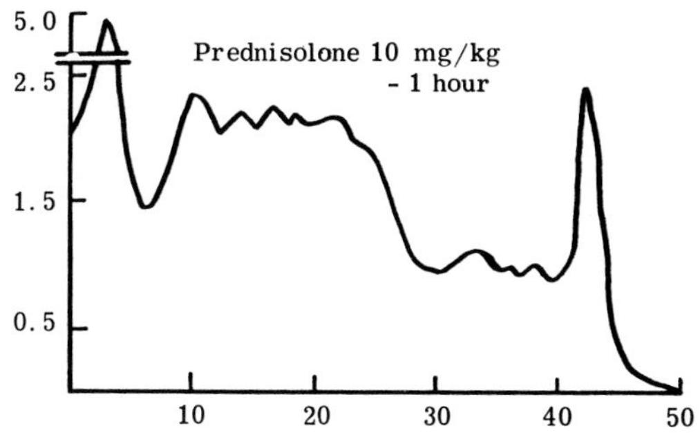

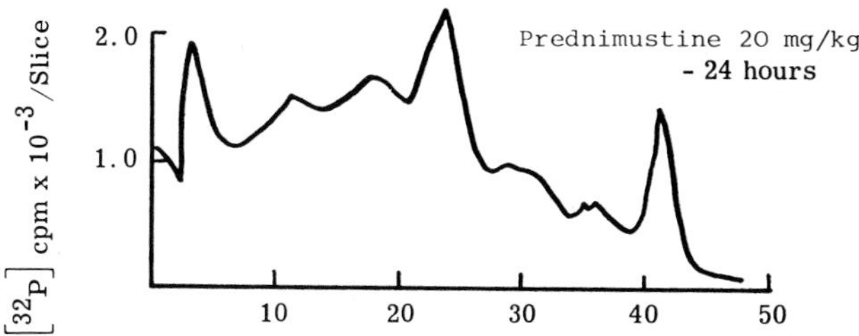

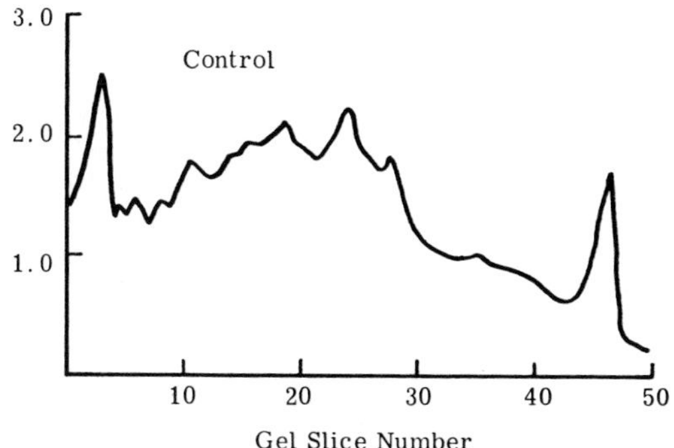

Fig. 14. Polyacrylamide (15%) gel electrophoresis of phosphorylated H3 chromatin proteins. Tumor-bearing rats were treated with prednisolone or prednimustine as described in the legend for Fig. 12. Nuclei were prepared and phosphorylated and, after removal of the Tris–saline (0.14 *M* NaCl-soluble) proteins, the chromatin was fractionated on a hydroxyapatite column. The H3 fraction was that eluting in 200 m*M* phosphate.

TABLE II

Loss of Acid-Precipitable Counts during Incubation of Prelabeled Nuclei[a]

Tumor	Treatment	pmole/min/mg protein		
		6 hours	24 hours	48 hours
Sensitive	None	2.59	3.36	2.98
Walker	Chlor	4.83	4.32	3.40
	Chlor + Pred	6.48	7.49	3.42
	Pred	3.14	5.30	2.60
Resistant	None	1.70	2.72	1.72
Walker	Chlor	2.48	2.39	2.03
	Chlor + Pred	4.63	4.52	4.03
	Pred	N.D.	2.15	2.05

[a] Mean of two separate determinations. Overall scatter not greater than 16%. Rats bearing either the sensitive or resistant Walker tumor received either chlorambucil (Chlor) (10 mg/kg), prednisolone (Pred) (10 mg/kg), or chlorambucil (10 mg/kg), followed 4 hours later by prednisolone (10 mg/kg). Groups of rats were killed at 6, 24, or 48 hours. The tumor was removed, and nuclei were prepared. These were phosphorylated *in vitro* using [γ-^{32}P]ATP, and phosphatase activity measured by following the loss of acid-precipitable counts from total nuclear protein. N.D., Not determined.

phenylacetic mustard is considerably more cytotoxic than chlorambucil. Thus the pharmacological effects produced by prednimustine will be determined by a number of factors including its affinity for various tissues and their respective esterolytic activities; its extent of binding to plasma proteins, which protects it

TABLE III

Release of Inorganic Phosphate during Incubation of Prelabeled Nuclei[a]

Tumor	Treatment	pmoles $^{32}PO_4$/minute/mg protein		
		6 hours	24 hours	48 hours
Sensitive	None	1.72	2.05	2.02
Walker	Chlor	2.87	2.13	2.09
	Chlor + Pred	3.25	2.25	2.26
	Pred	1.11	2.05	2.21
Resistant	None	1.24	1.42	1.06
Walker	Chlor	1.21	1.45	1.53
	Chlor + Pred	1.42	1.50	1.60
	Pred	N.D.	1.30	1.71

[a] Mean of two separate determinations. Overall scatter not greater than 13%. Tumor-bearing rats were treated as described in Table II, footnote *a*, and phosphatase activity measured by the appearance of P^{32}-labeled inorganic phosphate in the acid-soluble fraction of isolated nuclei. N.D., Not determined.

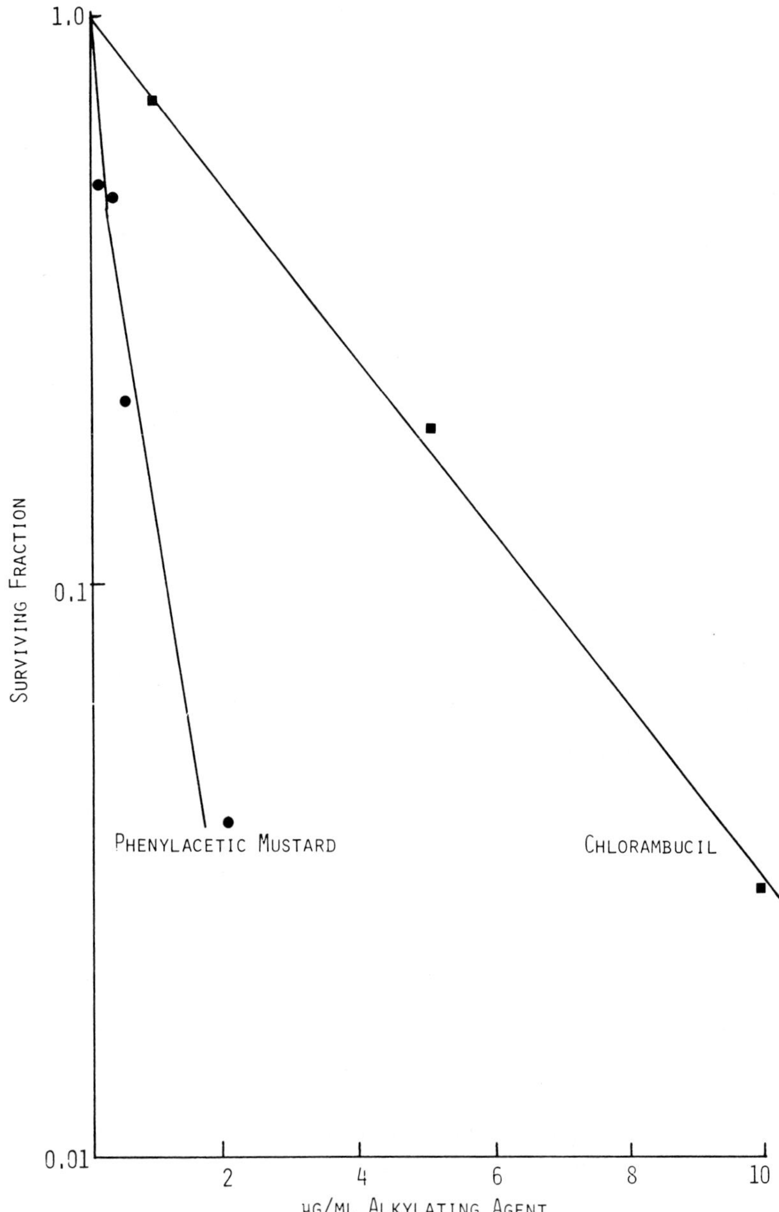

Fig. 15. Survival of colony-forming ability of Walker cells resistant to alkylating agents *in vitro.* Cells in suspension were treated with various doses of chlorambucil or phenylacetic mustard for 60 minutes. Cells were then washed free of excess drug and plated in 0.3% agar at a concentration of 100 cells/ml. Surviving cells were scored as colonies of greater than 32 cells 10 days later.

from hydrolysis (108); the rates with which chlorambucil and phenylacetic mustard are released into the circulation; and the possibility that alkylating moieties released following administration of Prednimustine may possess modified half-lives. In an initial approach to this problem we have compared, in the rat, the pharmacokinetics of Prednimustine, phenylacetic mustard, and chlorambucil. The results are summarized in Fig. 16.

Half-lives of 1.3 hour and 45 minutes may be calculated for the plasma decay of phenylacetic mustard and chlorambucil, respectively, following their intravenous administration. When Prednimustine is given, the resultant circulating levels of chlorambucil and phenylacetic mustard are each $\frac{1}{10}$ of those achieved following administration of equivalent doses of these agents alone. Furthermore, their half-lives are extended. That of chlorambucil is 1.5 hours, while that of phenylacetic mustard is approximately 14 hours. Significantly, no free Prednimustine is detected, and it must be assumed that the compound is rapidly taken up by tissues, whereafter it is slowly hydrolyzed to release chlorambucil, which in turn is metabolized to phenylacetic mustard.

D. Discussion

When the binding of chlorambucil to total cellular macromolecules is considered on a molar basis, it appears that DNA represents a significant target. This finding is in accord with the conclusions of Roberts and colleagues for sulfur mustard, several monofunctional alkylating agents, and cisplatin (136,137). However, as we have pointed out above, such arguments are limited, since they neglect the potential significance of binding to, or metabolic disturbance of, discrete regulatory macromolecules. Prednisolone increased the binding of chlorambucil to total cellular DNA and protein in alkylating agent-sensitive tumor cells but otherwise did not appear to modify binding in any other tissue. However, it was readily apparent that prednisolone modified the binding of this drug to chromatin proteins in a tissue-selective fashion. Prednisolone treatment enhanced the binding of chlorambucil to all nuclear protein fractions from both sensitive and resistant tumors, while conversely suppressing binding to all fractions from intestinal epithelial cells. The steroid was without significant effect on nuclear protein binding in liver and bone marrow.

The increased sensitivity of tumor cell chromatin to micrococcal nuclease digestion after chlorambucil treatment suggests that the drug binds preferentially between clusters or groups of nucleosomes. Renz (138) and Hozier *et al.* (139) described micrococcal nuclease-sensitive sites in chromatin in regions approximately 8–12 nucleosomes apart. In our experiments, micrococcal nuclease digestion of 8–16 nucleosome regions of tumor chromatin was more extensive in chlorambucil-exposed nuclei than in control nuclei. In addition, the drug was associated with chromatin fractions smaller than one nucleosome in size following micrococcal nuclease digestion. Under the salt conditions used for the suc-

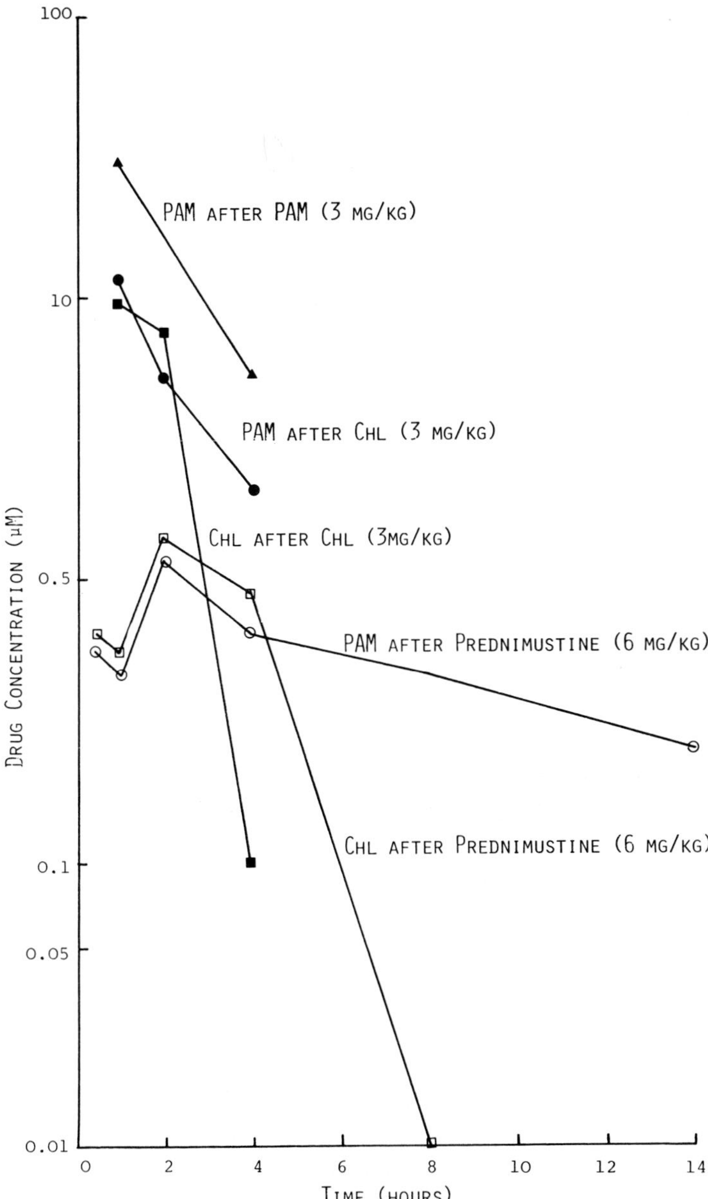

Fig. 16. Non-tumor-bearing female Wistar rats were injected in the tail vein with chlorambucil (Chl) (3 mg/kg) phenylacetic mustard (PAM) (3 mg/kg), or prednimustine (6 mg/kg). All drugs were administered in saline. At various times, thereafter, groups of rats were anesthetized with ether and bled from the heart. Blood collected in heparinized tubes was centrifuged to give a plasma fraction, and drug concentrations in this fraction were assayed by HPLC.

rose gradient (0.5 *M* NaCl), the radioactive peak (fractions 21–22; Fig. 10) could represent [^{3}H]chlorambucil bound to the replicating fork as reported by Schlager and Kripps (135). These authors describe short fragments of nascent DNA which are micrococcal nuclease-resistant and which, in 0.5 *M* NaCl, are released from their nucleosome-like structures and band toward the top of a 5–25% sucrose gradient. The additional peak of radioactive material (fraction 25) probably represents small peaks of linker region DNA released by the EDTA pretreatment. These data suggest that much of the chlorambucil is bound at the replicating fork and is probably associated with the linker region rather than the nucleosome area of chromatin. This is supported by our detection of only low levels of chlorambucil bound to the 0.6 *M* NaCl-soluble fraction of tumor chromatin, which contains the core histones (132).

We have shown previously (79,82) that alkylating agents enhance gross nuclear protein phosphorylation in sensitive but not resistant tumors. However, similar effects can be produced in resistant tumors when the alkylating agent is administered together with prednisolone. The phosphorylation induced by chlorambucil in the chromatin of sensitive tumors appears to be confined to the nuclear sap and a nonhistone (H3) fraction (82). In the present study, we have shown that prednisolone can induce rapid and reversible increases in gross nuclear protein phosphorylation in resistant tumors. When this glucocorticoid is administered together with chlorambucil to rats bearing alkylating agent-resistant tumors, an enhanced phosphorylation of nuclear proteins is obtained which is highly reminiscent of that seen in drug-sensitive tumors responding to alkylating agent alone (82). Furthermore, when chlorambucil and prednisolone are administered in the form of the steroidal ester prednimustine, then the phosphorylation response in resistant tumors appears closely similar to that elicited by the binary combination. Hydroxyapatite fractionation of nuclear proteins from resistant tumors previously exposed to prednisolone or prednimustine has revealed differences in the phosphorylation patterns elicited by the two agents. Prednisolone enhances phosphorylation in low-molecular-weight proteins of the H2 and in high-molecular-weight proteins of the H3 (nonhistone) fractions; there is also a small increase in phosphorylation of high-molecular-weight nuclear sap proteins. On the other hand, prednimustine treatment leads to elevated phosphorylation of high-molecular-weight nuclear sap proteins and low-molecular-weight H2 (nonhistone) proteins. The latter appear not to be identical with those whose phosphorylation is enhanced by prednisolone. Thus it appears that the steroid modulates the pattern of alkylating agent-induced nuclear protein phosphorylation in resistant cells, which is clearly different from that produced in sensitive cells (82).

Nuclear protein phosphatases appear not to be modified by either chlorambucil or prednisolone treatment. These enzymes presumably act in concert with kinases to maintain controlled levels of nuclear protein phosphorylation (140,141). Inhibition of phosphatase activity by alkylating agents might have provided a rationale for the enhanced nuclear protein phosphorylation observed in the present and previous studies (79,82). However, this possibility is eliminated in the present work. The mechanism may relate to alkylating agent-induced changes in kinase specificity, increased synthesis (142), or changes in levels of regulatory effectors such as polyamines (143,144) or cyclic AMP (cAMP) (145–148).

It is possible that cAMP-dependent protein kinases may be involved in the increased nuclear protein phosphorylation observed following alkylating agent treatment. It has been shown that a number of bifunctional alkylating agents, including chlorambucil, can elevate intracellular levels of cAMP, presumably as a result of inhibition of cyclic 3′, 5′-nucleotide phosphodiesterases (149–151). Such effects are not observed in drug-resistant cells (152). This elevation of cAMP levels may be relevant to the enhanced nuclear protein phosphorylations described here and is currently under investigation.

The biochemical properties of alkylating agents outlined here have been derived from experiments on tumor-bearing rats using therapeutically effective doses of the agents concerned. It is apparent that the interesting new agent Prednimustine elicits molecular changes closely comparable to those produced by binary combinations of its components, prednisolone and chlorambucil. However, we have previously shown that prednimustine requires hydrolysis to these componets (by tissue esterases) in order to exhibit cytotoxicity; it is also far more lipophilic than chlorambucil. These considerations have necessitated an examination of the bioavailability of prednimustine and its hydrolysis products in the rat. It is apparent that the drug disappears very rapidly from the peripheral circulation (within 30 minutes). Chlorambucil and phenylacetic mustard are detected at levels approximately $\frac{1}{2}$ of those which would be observed following the administration of equimolar doses of these agents. Furthermore, the resultant half-life of phenylacetic mustard is extended considerably. Phenylacetic mustard is the major circulating metabolite of chlorambucil in the rat (109). It is also more cytotoxic than chlorambucil, as shown here. It is possible that the unique properties of Prednimustine derive from its ability to maintain constant low levels of phenylacetic mustard in the presence of prednisolone. This possibility is currently being evaluated.

III. Summary

The intracellular targets of alkylating drugs have been reviewed in terms of the extents of reaction of these compounds with nucleic acids and proteins. While it is generally concluded that DNA represents their major locus of action, it is emphasized that this assumption overlooks the possibility of critical low-level binding to regulatory macromolecules. Particular emphasis is placed on the role of nonhistone chromosomal proteins, both as targets and determinants of alkylating agent cytotoxicity.

Data have been presented on the tissue-specific modulation of chlorambucil binding by prednisolone which suggest that the interaction of this drug with nuclear proteins correlates better with cytotoxicity (specifically in tumor and intestine) than binding to DNA. Experiments on the internucleosomal location of chlorambucil indicate that this occurs in the DNA linker region. The ability of prednisolone to enhance the antitumor effectiveness of chlorambucil has been discussed in relation to the biochemical effects induced by these agents, and the congener prednimustine, in nonhistone chromatin proteins. The selectivity of this steroidal alkylating agent has been further related to its pharmacokinetic properties.

Acknowledgments

We wish to thank Mrs. F. E. Boxall, Mr. K. G. McGhee, Mr. D. R. Newell, and Miss J. Renshaw for expert technical assistance. The financial support of the Cancer Research Campaign and A. B. Leo, Helsingborg, Sweden, are gratefully acknowledged.

References

1. A. Gilman and F. S. Philips, *Science* **103,** 409 (1946).
2. J. A. Howle and G. R. Gale, *Biochem. Pharmacol.* **19,** 2757 (1970).
3. H. C. Harder and B. Rosenberg, *Int. J. Cancer* **6,** 207 (1970).
4. F. S. Philips, *Pharmacol. Rev.* **2,** 281 (1950).
5. W. C. J. Ross, "Biological Alkylating Agents." Butterworth, London, 1962.
6. L. A. Elson, "Radiation and Radiomimetic Chemicals." Butterworth, London, 1963.
7. P. D. Lawley, *Prog. Nucleic Acid Res. Mol. Biol.* **6,** 89 (1966).
8. A. Loveless, "Genetic and Allied Effects of Alkylating Agents." Pennsylvania State Univ. Press, University Park, 1966.
9. M. Ochoa, Jr. and E. Hirschberg, *in* "Alkylating Agents in Experimental Chemotherapy" (R. J. Schnitzer and F. Hawking, eds.), Vol. 5, p. 1. Academic Press, New York, 1967.
10. J. A. Montgomery, T. P. Johnston, and Y. F. Shealy, *in* "Drugs for Neoplastic Diseases in Medicinal Chemistry" (A. Burger, ed.), 3rd ed., Part I, p.680. Wiley (Interscience), New York, 1970.
11. G. P. Wheeler, *in* "Cancer Medicine" (J. F. Holland and E. Frei, eds.), p.791. Lea & Febiger, Philadelphia, Pennsylvania, 1973.
12. B. Singer, *Prog. Nucleic Acid Res. Mol. Biol.* **15,** 219 (1975).
13. J. J. Roberts, *Adv. Radiat. Biol.* **7,** 211 (1978).
14. K. W. Kohn, *Methods Cancer Res.* **26,** 291 (1979).
15. T. A. Connors, Alkylating Drugs, Nitrosoureas and Dialkyl triazenes in "Cancer Chemotherapy 1979. The EORTC Cancer Chemotherapy Annual 1". Ed H. M. Pinedo. p. 25. Exerpta Med. Amsterdam, Oxford (1979).
16. H. N. Brewer, J. P. Comstock, and L. Aronow, *Biochem. Pharmacol.* **8,** 281 (1961).

17. L. S. Cohen and G. P. Studzinski, *J. Cell. Physiol.* **69,** 331 (1967).
18. P. Brookes and P. D. Lawley, *Biochem. J.* **77,** 478 (1960).
19. P. Brookes and P. D. Lawley, *Biochem. J.* **80,** 496 (1961).
20. P. D. Lawley and P. Brookes, *J. Mol. Biol.* **25,** 143 (1967).
21. E. P. Geiduschek, *Proc. Natl. Acad. Sci. U.S.A.* **47,** 950 (1961).
22. R. J. Goldacre, A. Loveless, and W. C. J. Ross, *Nature (London)* **163,** 667 (1949).
23. P. D. Lawley, J. H. Lethbridge, P. A. Edwards, and K. V. Shooter, *J. Mol Biol.* **39,** 181 (1969).
24. J. G. Walker, *Can. J. Biochem.* **49,** 332 (1971).
25. E. H. L. Chun, L. Gonzales, F. S. Lewis, J. Jones, and R. J. Rutman, *Cancer Res.* **29,** 1184 (1969).
26. K. W. Kohn, C. L. Spears, and P. Doty, *J. Mol. Biol.* **19,** 266 (1966).
27. S. Venitt, *Biochem. Biophys. Res. Commun.* **31,** 355 (1968).
28. W. E. Ross, R. A. G. Ewig, and K. W. Kohn, *Cancer Res.* **38,** 1502 (1978).
29. P. D. Lawley and C. J. Thatcher, *Biochem. J.* **116,** 693 (1970).
30. A. Loveless, *Nature (London)* **223,** 206 (1969).
31. V. M. Craddock, *J. Natl. Cancer Inst.* **47,** 89 (1971).
32. V. M. Craddock, *Nature (London)* **245,** 386 (1973).
33. V. M. Craddock and J. V. Frei, *Br. J. Cancer* **30,** 503 (1974).
34. M. J. Capps, P. J. O'Connor, and A. W. Craig, *Biochim. Biophys. Acta* **331,** 33 (1973).
35. J. J. Roberts, J. M. Pascoe, J. E. Plant, J. E. Sturrock, and A. R. Crathorn, *Chem.-Biol. Interact.* **3,** 29 (1971).
36. J. J. Roberts, J. M. Pascoe, B. A. Smith, and A. R. Crathorn, *Chem.-Biol. Interact.* **3,** 49 (1971).
37. C. R. Ball and J. J. Roberts, *Chem.-Biol. Interact.* **2,** 321 (1970).
38. L. L. Gerchman and D. B. Ludlum, *Proc. Am. Assoc. Cancer Res.* **14,** 13 (1973).
39. P. D. Lawley and P. Brookes, *Biochem. J.* **109,** 433 (1968).
40. R. C. Wilhelm and D. B. Ludlum, *Science* **153,** 1403 (1966).
41. K. W. Kohn, *Cancer Res.* **37,** 1450 (1977).
42. R. A. G. Ewig and K. W. Kohn, *Cancer Res.* **38,** 3197 (1978).
43. L. A. Zwelling, K. W. Kohn, W. E. Ross, R. A. G. Ewig, and T. Anderson, *Cancer Res.* **38,** 1762 (1978).
44. B. D. Reid and I. G. Walker, *Biochim. Biophys. Acta* **179,** 179 (1969).
45. I. G. Walker and B. D. Reid, *Cancer Res.* **31,** 510 (1971).
46. L. Yin, E. H. L. Chun, and R. J. Rutman, *Biochim. Biophys. Acta* **324,** 472 (1973).
47. N. O. Goldstein and R. J. Rutman, *Chem.-Biol. Interact.* **8,** 1 (1974).
48. J. M. Pascoe and J. J. Roberts, *Biochem. Pharmacol.* **23,** 1345 (1974).
49. J. M. Pascoe and J. J. Roberts, *Biochem. Pharmacol.* **23,** 1359 (1974).
50. D. J. Pillinger, J. Hay, and E. Borek, *Biochem. J.* **114,** 429 (1969).
51. J. Hay, D. J. Pillinger, and E. Borek, *Biochem. J.* **119,** 587 (1970).
52. A. E. Pegg, *Adv. Cancer Res.* **25,** 195 (1977).
53. E. K. Wagner, S. Penman, and V. Ingram, *J. Mol. Biol.* **29,** 371 (1967).
54. G. W. Both, A. K. Banerjee, and A. J. Shatkin, *Proc. Natl. Acad. Sci. U.S.A.* **72,** 1189 (1975).
55. S. Muthukrishnan, G. W. Both, Y. Furuichi, and A. J. Shatkin, *Nature (London)* **255,** 33 (1975).
56. R. P. Perry and D. E. Kelley, *Cell* **1,** 37 (1974).
57. E. Borek and S. J. Kerr, *Adv. Cancer Res.* **15,** 163 (1972).
58. S. J. Kerr and E. Borek, *Adv. Enzymol.* **36,** 1 (1972).
59. S. J. Kerr, *Isozymes, Vol. 3 Dev. Biol.* p. 855 (1975). Ed. C. L. Markert, Academic Press, New York, San Francisco, London.

60. J. F. Mushinksi and M. Marini, *Cancer Res.* **39,** 1253 (1979).
61. P. D. Lawley and P. Brookes, *Biochem. J.* **89,** 127 (1963).
62. E. Kriek and P. Emmelot, *Biochemistry* **2,** 700 (1963).
63. B. Singer and H. Fraenkel-Conrat, *Biochemistry* **8,** 3260 and 3266 (1969).
64. K. V. Shooter, P. A. Edwards, and P. D. Lawley, *Biochem. J.* **125,** 829 (1971).
65. W. G. Verly and L. Barkier, *Biochim. Biophys. Acta* **174,** 674 (1969).
66. M. Degré-Couvre and M. D. Mamet-Bratley, *Eur. J. Biochem.* **32,** 292 (1973).
67. R. J. Rutman, W. J. Steel, and C. C. Price, *Cancer Res.* **21,** 1134 (1961).
68. W. J. Steel, *Proc. Am. Assoc. Cancer Res.* **3,** 364 (1962).
69. R. H. Golder, G. Martin-Guzman, J. Jones, N. O. Goldstein, S. Rotenberg, and R. J. Rutman, *Cancer Res.* **24,** 964 (1964).
70. O. Klatt, J. S. Stehlin, Jr., C. McBridge, and A. C. Griffin, *Cancer Res.* **29,** 286 (1969).
71. J. S. Salser and M. E. Balis, *Biochem. Pharmacol.* **19,** 2375 (1970).
72. M. E. Friedman and P. Melius, *J. Clin. Hematol. Oncol.* **7,** 503 (1977).
73. H. Busch and W. I. Steele, *Adv. Cancer Res.* **8,** 41 (1964).
74. H. Busch, S. M. Amer, and W. L. Nyham, *J. Pharmacol. Exp. Ther.* **127,** 195 (1959).
75. H. Busch, D. C. Firszt, A. Lipsey, E. Kohnen, and S. Amer, *Biochem. Pharmacol.* **7,** 123 (1961).
76. H. Wolf, G. Raydt, B. Puschendorf, and H. Grunicke, *FEBS Lett.* **35,** 336 (1973).
77. H. Grunicke, G. Gantner, F. Höldzweber, M. Ihlenfeldt, and B. Puschendorf, *Adv. Enzyme Regul.* **17,** 291 (1979).
78. P. G. Riches and K. R. Harrap, *Cancer Res.* **33,** 389 (1973).
79. R. Wilkinson, M. Birbeck, and K. R. Harrap, *Cancer Res.* **39,** 4256 (1979).
80. P. G. Riches and K. R. Harrap, *Chem.-Biol. Interact.* **11,** 291 (1975).
81. S. M. Sellwood, P. G. Riches, and K. R. Harrap, *Biochem. Soc. Trans.* **3,** 649 (1975).
82. P. G. Riches, S. M. Sellwood, and K. R. Harrap, *Chem.-Biol. Interact.* **18,** 11 (1977).
83. K. R. Harrap and E. W. Gascoigne, *Eur. J. Cancer* **12,** 53 (1976).
84. R. Wilkinson and K. R. Harrap, *Br. J. Cancer* **37,** 470 (1978).
85. G. S. Stein, J. L. Stein, and J. A. Thomson, *Cancer Res.* **38,** 1181 (1978).
86. V. G. Allfrey, C. S. Teng, and C. T. Teng, *in* "Nucleic Acid-Protein Interactions—Nucleic Acid Synthesis in Viral Infection" (D. W. Ribbons, J. F. Woessner, and J. Schultz, eds.), p. 144. North-Holland Publ., Amsterdam, 1971.
87. J. F. Whitfield, A. D. Perris, and T. Youdale, *Exp. Cell Res.* **52,** 349 (1968).
88. K. R. Harrap, P. G. Riches, E. W. Gascoigne, S. M. Sellwood, and C. C. Cashman, *Int. Congr. Ser.—Excerpta Med.* **375,** 106 (1975).
89. R. D. Kornberg, *Science* **184,** 868 (1974).
90. A. L. Olins and D. E. Olins, *Science* **183,** 330 (1974).
91. B. R. Shaw, T. M. Herman, R. T. Kovacic, G. S. Beaudreau, and K. E. Van Holde, *Proc. Natl. Acad. Sci. U.S.A.* **73,** 505 (1976).
92. J. O. Thomas and R. D. Kornberg, *Proc. Natl. Acad. Sci. U.S.A.* **72,** 2626 (1975).
93. A. Worcel and C. Benyajati, *Cell* **12,** 83 (1977).
94. R. D. Kornberg, *Annu. Rev. Biochem.* **46,** 931 (1977).
95. G. Felsenfeld, *Nature (London)* **271,** 115 (1978).
96. R. T. Simpson, *Methods Cell Biol.* **16,** 437 (1977).
97. H. R. Mathews, *Nature (London)* **267,** 203 (1977).
98. K. D. Tew, S. Sudhakar, P. S. Schein, and M. E. Smulson, *Cancer Res.* **38,** 3371 (1978).
99. F. Bergel and J. A. Stock, *Br. Emp. Cancer Campaign, Annu. Rep.* **31,** 6 (1953).
100. R. Alexanian, D. E. Bergsagel, P. J. Migliore, W. K. Vaughn, and C. D. Howe, *Blood* **31,** 1 (1968).
101. G. J. Goldenberg, M. Lee, H. P. Lam, and A. Begleiter, *Cancer Res.* **37,** 755 (1977).

102. A. Begleiter, H. P. Lam, J. Groves, E. Froese, and G. J. Goldenberg, *Cancer Res.* **39,** 353 (1979).
103. G. Gomori, *Proc. Soc. Exp. Biol. Med.* **69,** 407 (1948).
104. P. J. Cox, *Br. J. Cancer* **28,** 81 (1973).
105. T. A. Connors, P. J. Cox, P. B. Farmer, A. B. Foster, and M. Jarman, *Pharmacology* **23,** 115 (1974).
106. P. J. Cox, B. J. Phillips, and P. Thomas, *Cancer Treat. Rep.* **60,** 321 (1976).
107. W. J. Hopwood and J. A. Stock, *Chem.-Biol. Interact.* **4,** 31 (1971/1972).
108. R. Wilkinson, P. O. Gunnarsson, G. Plym-Forshell, J. Renshaw, and K. R. Harrap, "Advances in Tumour Prevention, Detection and Characterisation," Vol. 4, p. 260. Excerpta Med. Int. Congr. Series No. 420 Amsterdam, (1978).
109. A. McLean, D. Newell, and G. Baker, *Biochem. Pharmacol.* **25,** 2331 (1976).
110. D. R. Newell, L. I. Hart, and K. R. Harrap, *J. Chromatogr.* **164,** 114 (1979).
111. I. Konyves and J. Liljekvist, Advances in Tumour Prevention, Detection and Characterisation **3,** 98, Exerpta Med. Int. Congr. Series no. 375 Amsterdam (1975).
112. A. Mittleman, S. K. Shukla, and G. P. Murphy, *J. Urol.* **115,** 409 (1976).
113. R. Nagel and C.-P. Kolln, *Br. J. Urol.* **49,** 73 (1977).
114. L. Brandt, I. Konyves, and T. R. Moller, *Acta Med. scand.* **197,** 317 (1975).
115. J. H. Kaufman, G. L. Hanjura, A. Mittleman, C. W. Aungst, and G. P. Murphy, *Cancer Treat. Rep.* **60,** 277 (1976).
116. Clinical Screening Cooperative Group of E.O.R.T.C., *Biomedicine* **27,** 158 (1977).
117. T. R. Moller, L. Brandt, I. Konyves, and L. G. Lindberg, *Acta Med. scand.* **197,** 323 (1975).
118. I. Konyves, B. Nordenskjold, G. Plym Forshell, A. De Schryver, and H. Westerberg-Larsson, *Eur. J. Cancer* **11,** 841 (1975).
119. H. Catane, R. Catane, H. Takita, J. H. Kaufman, A. Mittleman, and G. P. Murphy, *J. Med. (Basel)* **8,** 115 (1977).
120. K. R. Harrap, P. G. Riches, E. D. Gilby, S. M. Sellwood, R. Wilkinson, and I. Konyves, *Eur. J. Cancer* **13,** 873 (1977).
121. R. Wilkinson and K. R. Harrap, *Br. J. Cancer* **37,** 470 (1978).
122. M. Jarman, L. J. Griggs, and M. J. Tisdale, *J. Med. Chem.* **17,** 194 (1974).
123. D. Rickwood, P. G. Riches, and A. J. MacGillivray, *Biochim. Biophys. Acta* **299,** 162 (1973).
124. H. N. Munro and A. Fleck, *Analyst* **91,** 78 (1966).
125. K. Burton, *Biochem. J.* **62,** 315 (1956).
126. A. H. Brown, *Arch. Biochem. Biophys.* **11,** 269 (1946).
127. O. H. Lowry, N. J. Rosebrough, and A. L. Farr, *J. Biol. Chem.* **193,** 263 (1951).
128. R. A. Montagna and T. Y. Wang, *Cancer Res.* **36,** 3138 (1976).
129. N. C. Kostrava, R. A. Montagna, and T. Y. Wang, *J. Biol. Chem.* **250,** 1548 (1975).
130. D. C. Watson, E. H. Peters, and G. H. Dixon, *Eur. J. Biochem.* **74,** 53 (1977).
131. L. C. Yeoman, J. J. Jordan, R. K. Busch, C. W. Taylor, H. E. Savage, and H. Busch, *Proc. Natl. Acad. Sci. U.S.A.* **73,** 3258 (1976).
132. J. E. Hyde, T. Igo-Kemenes, and H. G. Zachau, *Nucleic Acids Res.* **7,** 31 (1979).
133. L. J. Kleinsmith, *Methods Cell Biol.* **19,** 161 (1979).
134. C. P. Giri, M. H. P. West, M. L. Ramirez, and M. Smulson, *Biochemistry* **17,** 3501 (1978).
135. E. J. Schlaeger and R. Kripps, *Nucleic Acids Res.* **6,** 645 (1979).
136. A. R. Crathorn and J. J. Roberts, *Nature (London)* **211,** 150 (1966).
137. J. J. Roberts and A. J. Thomson, *Prog. Nucleic Acid Res. Mol. Biol.* **22,** 71 (1979).
138. M. Renz, *Nucleic Acid Res.* **6,** 2761 (1979).
139. J. Hozier, M. Renz, and P. Nehls, *Chromosoma* **62,** 301 (1977).
140. H.-C. Li, K.-J. Hsiao, and W. W. S. Chan, *Eur. J. Biochem.* **84,** 215 (1978).
141. L. J. Kleinsmith, J. Stein, and G. Stein, *Proc. Natl. Acad. Sci. U.S.A.* **73,** 1174 (1976).

142. F. Farron-Furstenthal and J. R. Lightholder, *in* "Onco-Developmental Gene Expression" (W. H. Fishman, ed.), p.57. Stewart Sell, New York, San Francisco, London 1976.
143. H. Imai, M. Shimoyama, S. Yamamoto, Y. Tanigawa, and I. Ueda, *Biochem. Biophys. Res. Commun.* **66,** 856 (1975).
144. P. H. Maenpaa, *Biochim. Biophys. Acta* **498,** 294 (1977).
145. E. M. Johnson, J. W. Hadden, A. Inoue, and V. G. Allfrey, *Biochemistry* **14,** 3873 (1975).
146. M. Lasser and V. Daniel, *Biochim. Biophys. Acta* **482,** 41 (1977).
147. U. Eppenberger, K. Talmadge, W. Kung, E. Bechtel, J. Preisz, P. Huber, R. A. Jungmann, and A. Salokangas, *FEBS Lett.* **80,** 229 (1977).
148. A. Datta, C. de Haro, and S. Ochoa, *Proc. Natl. Acad. Sci. U.S.A.* **75,** 1148 (1978).
149. M. J. Tisdale and B. J. Phillips, *Biochem. Pharmacol.* **24,** 1271 (1975).
150. M. J. Tisdale and B. J. Phillips, *Biochem. Pharmacol.* **24,** 205 (1975).
151. M. J. Tisdale and B. J. Phillips, *Biochem. Pharmacol.* **24,** 211 (1975).
152. M. J. Tisdale and B. J. Phillips, *Biochem. Pharmacol.* **25,** 1831 (1976).

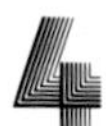

Chemotherapeutic Approaches to Cell Populations of Tumors

KATHERINE A. KENNEDY, BEVERLY A. TEICHER, SARA ROCKWELL, AND ALAN C. SARTORELLI

I. Introduction

Successful therapy of neoplastic disease often involves use of the multiple modalities radiation, surgery, and chemotherapy. Curative therapy requires that all tumor cells capable of indefinite replication be eradicated. These clonogenic cells may exist in several physiological states which confer differing sensitivities to individual agents. By consideration of the various tumor cell subpopulations and the environmental milieu in which each can exist (Fig. 1), therapeutic regimens can be devised to attack specifically each malignant cell type with acceptable host toxicity. This chapter examines the various tumor cell populations, the

MOLECULAR ACTIONS AND TARGETS FOR CANCER CHEMOTHERAPEUTIC AGENTS

ISBN 0-12-619280-4

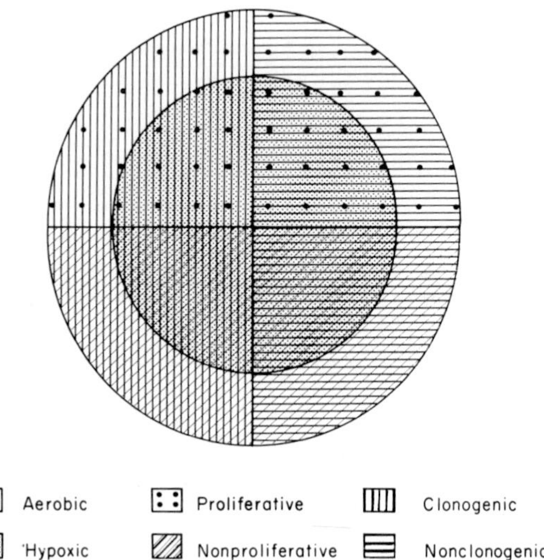

Fig. 1. Diagram of tumor cell subpopulations. The aerobic (unshaded outer rim) and hypoxic (shaded inner circle) tumor cell subpopulations both are composed of proliferating (dots) and nonproliferating or quiescent (slanted lines) cells. In addition, the tumor contains both clonogenic (vertical lines) and nonclonogenic (horizontal lines) cells. Cells can be either aerobic or hypoxic and either proliferating or nonproliferating. These cell populations are not static but dynamic, with cells moving from one population to another.

environmental conditions which exist in tumors, and the design of agents specifically directed against the hypoxic cell subpopulation. The implications of these considerations in the design of rational therapeutic regimens to achieve a concerted attack on the whole tumor are discussed.

II. Characteristics of Tumor Cell Populations

A. Clonogenicity

Cell populations in tumors can be classified according to characteristics such as clonogenicity, proliferative status, and degree of oxygenation (1,2). Clonogenic cells are capable of indefinite proliferation and are therefore responsible for tumor growth and metastatic implantation. Nonclonogenic tumor cells are incapable of sustained proliferation, as a result of differentiation or other factors. Only clonogenic cells must be erradicated in cancer therapy, because only these cells are responsible for tumor progression and metastases.

B. Proliferative Status

Most tumors contain both proliferative cells, which actively progress through the cell cycle, and quiescent cells, which are temporarily or permanently noncycling or slowly cycling because of environmental deficiencies or responses to homeostatic control mechanisms. Quiescent cells, however, may be clonogenic. Many of the common cancer chemotherapeutic agents presently available in our clinical armamentarium, such as arabinosylcytosine, methotrexate, 5-fluorouracil, and vincristine, are toxic only to cells which are actively traversing the cell cycle (3–6). Therefore these agents are directed against proliferating cells and are relatively ineffective against quiescent tumor cells. Chemotherapeutic agents which do not require phase specificity for cytotoxicity, e.g., alkylating agents, often show greater activity toward proliferating cells than toward quiescent cells both *in vitro* and *in vivo* (6), probably as a result of differences in metabolism and in repair capacities of these two cell populations. Chemotherapy may be able to deplete the rapidly proliferating pool of tumor cells, however, the proliferating cell population comprises only a fraction of the neoplastic cells in the tumor. The surviving quiescent tumor cells may resume progression through the cell cycle and reenter the proliferating compartment. As a result, chemotherapy must be extended in an effort to attack quiescent cells as they reenter the proliferative compartment. Prolonged chemotherapy, however, often results in intolerable toxic effects on sensitive normal tissues. Furthermore, quiescent cells may reenter the proliferating pool and cause recurrent tumors to arise years after treatment.

C. Oxygenation Status

Both aerobic and hypoxic cell populations are present in proliferative and nonproliferative compartments of neoplasms. Hypoxia in solid tumors has been of interest to radiotherapists for many years, because hypoxia protects cells from the cytotoxic effects of ionizing radiation. Hypoxic cells have been shown to determine tumor cell survival after large doses of ionizing radiation and to limit the curability of tumors by single-dose radiotherapy (2,7,8). Hypoxic cells occur in virtually all the solid, animal tumors which have been examined and also occur in semisolid or disseminated neoplasms, such as hepatic infiltrates of leukemias and lymphomas (8). In most experimental tumors, a significant proportion of neoplastic cells (often 10–30%) are hypoxic (1,8,9). Furthermore, experimental tumors as small as 1 mm in diameter, as well as large necrotic tumor masses, contain hypoxic cells. Thus most occult metastases, too small to be detected by standard diagnostic techniques, probably contain small or microscopic foci of hypoxic cells.

In addition to being resistant to ionizing radiation, hypoxic cells in solid tumors are probably resistant to chemotherapy. Cytotoxic concentrations of chemotherapeutic agents which have physicochemical properties not conducive to diffusion through tissue or which are unstable or rapidly metabolized to inactive forms may not be achieved in hypoxic cells located in regions of vascular insufficiency. Moreover, the hypoxic cells of solid tumors have abnormal cell proliferation patterns which probably contribute significantly to the ineffectiveness of cell cycle-directed drugs. *In vitro,* the induction of prolonged, severe hypoxia has been shown in some cell lines to result in lengthening of the cell cycle time (10,11). In another cell line, hypoxia produced a block in progression through the G_1 phase of the cell cycle, resulting in a population of G_1-like cells with characteristics similar to those of cells in plateau-phase cultures (12). Furthermore, nutritional and environmental insults to hypoxic cells located in regions of vascular insufficiency may also contribute to the inhibition of cell proliferation. Because the diffusion distance of many nutrients is similar to that of oxygen (13), hypoxic cells may lack necessary energy sources as well as oxygen and, as a consequence, may accumulate lactic acid, CO_2, and other metabolic waste products. A lack of specific nutrients (14,15) or of energy sources such as glucose (15,16), and the exposure to low pH (15,16) or excessive concentrations of lactic acid (16,17), are known to inhibit proliferation in culture by blocking cells in the G_1 phase or by prolonging the cell cycle.

Spheroids, tightly packed balls of cells produced and grown in culture, are used widely as *in vitro* models of solid tumors (18). Very small spheroids grow exponentially, with short, uniform cell cycle times. As spheroids grow, cell proliferation diminishes in the center of the spheroid. Spheroids with radii exceeding about 200 μm have been shown to have central areas of necrosis and radiobiologically hypoxic cells (18). Analyses of mitotic and labeling indexes in these spheroids reveal that hypoxic cells near the edge of necrotic areas are quiescent, while cells on the well-oxygenated periphery are proliferating. Similarly, studies using a corded mouse mammary carcinoma *in vivo* revealed that cells near the blood vessels in the center of the tumor cord were proliferating with a high growth fraction and relatively rapid and uniform cell cycle times (19). As the distance from the blood vessels increased, the proportion of quiescent cells in the tumor cell population increased, and few proliferating cells were present at the edge of the necrotic region. Studies on cell proliferation in EMT6 mouse mammary tumors, which contain small avascular areas of focal necrosis surrounded by well-vascularized tumor tissue, revealed that cells near the edges of the necrotic regions had lower labeling and mitotic indexes than cells in areas with no necrotic features (20). Percent-labeled mitosis curves suggested that cells adjacent to regions of necrosis had slightly longer and more variable cell cycle times. Further analysis of percent-labeled mitoses data and labeling data revealed that the growth fractions are similar in both necrotic and nonnecrotic regions.

These findings suggest that chronically hypoxic cells are probably nonproliferating or proliferate with abnormally long cell cycle times.

In classifying tumor cell populations, it is evident that the various subpopulations described are intersecting rather than exclusive, and that cells may cross from one subpopulation to another (see Fig. 1). For example, most solid rodent neoplasms which have been studied contain more quiescent cells than radiobiologically hypoxic cells, indicating that nonproliferating well-oxygenated cells must exist in these tumors (1,2). Conversely, there is evidence that some radiobiologically hypoxic cells are either cycling or reversibly blocked in the S phase of the cell cycle, rather than being in the G_1-like state generally characteristic of quiescent cells in normal tissues or in cell culture. In KHT sarcomas irradiated with sufficiently large doses of radiation such that only hypoxic cells remained viable, flow microfluorometric analysis combined with cell sorting and cell cloning revealed that some hypoxic cells had DNA contents characteristic of S or G_2 cells rather than the G_1 DNA content generally characteristic of nonproliferating cells (21). Other studies (22,23) have examined the sensitivities of tumor cells to an *in vitro* treatment with hydroxyurea, a drug which selectively kills cells in the S phase of the cell cycle. These experiments, employing EMT6 (22, and S. Rockwell, unpublished observations) and Lewis lung (23) carcinomas, suggest that both of these neoplasms contain radiobiologically hypoxic cells which are sensitive to hydroxyurea, implying that these cells must be in the S phase of the cell cycle. These proliferating hypoxic cells may be derived not only from the tumor cell subpopulation which is chronically hypoxic but also from a subpopulation which is only transiently hypoxic as a result of variations in the blood flow through individual vessels in the tumor. Evidence for the existence of such transiently hypoxic cells in experimental tumors and the therapeutic implications of these cells are discussed in detail elsewhere (24,25). Because clonogenic neoplastic cells probably exist in each of the various subpopulations, multiple therapeutic agents designed to attack each of these subpopulations appear to be required to erradicate the tumor and/or metastases.

III. Tumor Blood Supply and Oxygen Delivery

A. Tumor Blood Supply

Clinically evident tumors are formed only when host tissues provide vessels for the delivery of oxygen and nutrients (26–29). Prevention of neovascularization results in a dormant tumor, as shown by Folkman and co-workers (28,29). Neovascularization of tumor tissue may be a result of the production of factors required for angiogenesis by neoplastic cells (30,31) or by lymphocytes (32,33).

Collapse of portions of the vascular network results in decreased delivery of essential nutrients and oxygen to the neoplasm. There are potentially two causes for the deterioration of tumor vasculature. First, increased interstitial pressure in regions of necrosis may result in the collapse of capillaries, veins, and lymphatics. The hydrostatic pressures generated in tumor tissue can vary from 8 to 30 cm of water (34,35), and such pressures may lead to expansion of interstitial spaces and compression of capillaries, resulting in new areas of necrosis (34,36). Second, many neoplastic cells have doubling times which are shorter than those of capillary endothelial cells (37,38). As a result, the tumor may grow at rates which preclude the formation of adequate vascular beds to support the total neoplastic mass (39,40). Consequently, cells distant from vessels may die following long-term hypoxia and/or nutritional deficiencies. The functional efficiency of the vascular supply decreases as the tumor enlarges (41). Analysis of the vascular spaces of mouse mammary tumors showed that the lengths of tumor capillaries decreased and that the lumen sizes of tumor vessels increased during tumor growth (41). These changes in tumor vasculature result in a decreased surface area for exchange of oxygen and essential nutrients. Other studies of vascular and extravascular spaces have demonstrated a wide heterogeneity in the distribution of these spaces within a tumor, and a decrease in red cell and plasma volume with growth, suggesting the development of central necrosis or relatively avascular areas in the tumors (39,40).

B. Oxygen Delivery

Because oxygen delivery is directly related to the presence of a functional vascular supply, any impairment in microcirculation may result in low oxygen contents in tumor capillaries (34). Other factors which can influence the availability of oxygen to tissues are $p\mathrm{CO_2}$, pH, temperature (all of which influence the shape and position of the oxygen dissociation curve for hemoglobin), and decreased hemoglobin content. It is thought that the most important factor in the development of tumor hypoxia is exhaustion of oxygen supply as a result of insufficient vasculature (34,42,43). This hypothesis has been tested by measuring tumor tissue $p\mathrm{O_2}$ values. As tumors grew larger, mean tumor tissue $p\mathrm{O_2}$ values decreased (42,44,45). Attempts to reverse low tumor $p\mathrm{O_2}$ values with hyperoxia resulted in only slight, insignificant changes in measured $p\mathrm{O_2}$ values (45). These results predicted the demonstration of very low intracapillary hemoglobin–oxygen saturation values, which did not shift significantly during hyperoxia (46). The low hemoglobin–oxygen saturation values were considered evidence for the exhaustion of oxygen supplies to neoplastic cells, resulting in the physiological states of hypoxia and/or anoxia (46). Factors such as maximal oxygen extraction by tumor cells, tissue acidosis, and tissue anemia could contribute to the low hemoglobin–oxygen saturation values in these studies (46,47). Thus the use of hyperoxia in an effort to enhance tumor radiosensitivity actually may provide only a slight increase in tumor oxygen content.

Impaired oxygen delivery may well result in hypoxic or anoxic areas in tumors. Malignant cells may respond to the hypoxic stress by employing glycolytic pathways, resulting in the production of large amounts of lactate (48,49). Because circulation and drainage in tumors are already impaired, metabolic products such as lactate may accumulate and lower the environmental pH. Lowering the extracellular pH, although leading to a further shift in the oxyhemoglobin dissociation curve, will exacerbate the impairment of oxygen delivery.

The processes described above are interconnected and lead to a spiraling production of new areas of hypoxia and necrosis. Treatment with radiation leads to changes in tumor blood flow and oxygenation (8,50,51). The tumor line, the tumor size, and the radiation dose can produce both qualitative and quantitative differences in the tumor blood flow and oxygenation patterns observed after treatment (52–54). One consequence of radiotherapy can be improvement in both blood flow to and reoxygenation of previously hypoxic tumor areas (52), which could result in a changed susceptibility to chemotherapeutic drugs as well as radiation. Changes in tumor blood flow subsequent to therapy must be considered in the design of optimal therapeutic regimens.

IV. Specific Chemotherapeutic Agents for Hypoxic Cells

A. Bioreductive Alkylating Agents

1. *Bioreductive Activation*

During the 1930s it was demonstrated that anaerobic cultures of microbes had a lower half-wave potential (i.e., a greater capacity for reduction) than aerobic cultures. As cultures under either aerobic or anaerobic conditions grew and became more crowded, their redox potentials decreased (55,56). By analogy, this laboratory hypothesized that hypoxic cells in solid tumors probably exist in an environment conducive to reductive processes, which can be exploited by the development of chemotherapeutic agents that become cytotoxic after reductive activation (57). Two classes of agents are presently known which exhibit preferential cytotoxicity toward hypoxic cells through reductive activation: (1) quinone bioreductive alkylating agents, a naturally occurring prototype of which is mitomycin C, and (2) nitroaromatic heterocyclic hypoxic cell radiosensitizing agents.

2. *Quinones*

Bioreductive activation may be important in expression of the cytotoxic activity of several existing antineoplastic agents. It is conceivable that quinones, such as mitomycin C, adriamycin, and daunorubicin, produce reactive species upon

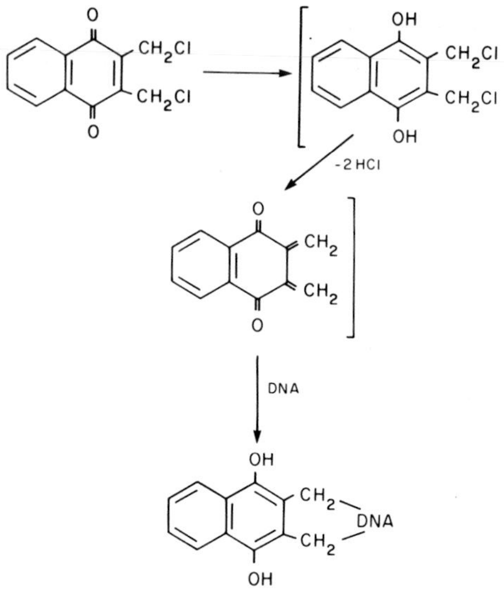

Fig. 2. Activation of 2,3-dichloromethyl-1,4-naphthoquinone to an alkylating species. The proposed activation mechanism for this quinone is characteristic of the steps required for the activation of other quinone bioreductive alkylating agents, e.g., mitomycin C. The first step is a two-electron reduction of the quinone to the hydroquinone followed by spontaneous rearrangement to produce the highly reactive quinone methide which cross-links DNA and/or other biological molecules.

reduction of the quinone moiety (58–64); we have investigated this possibility with mitomycin C.

Early studies demonstrated that mitomycin C and its analogues acted as bifunctional alkylating agents which could form DNA-protein and DNA-DNA cross-links. Reduction of the benzoquinone ring of the mitomycin molecule is a prerequisite for alkylation (62). Studies on the structural requirements of mitomycin molecules for cytotoxic activity suggested that the carbamyl and aziridine moieties were not strictly essential for activation (65,66), and that antineoplastic activity correlated with a low redox potential (67). These studies suggested that simple benzo-, naphtho-, and anthraquinones containing one or two sites capable of generating reactive methides (Fig. 2) after reduction of the quinone moiety might function as bioreductive alkylating agents (58,59,68,69). Several such compounds were synthesized and shown to have significant activity against sarcoma 180 (57,70–76). In addition, the naphthoquinone 2,3-dichloromethyl-1,4-naphthoquinone (Fig. 3) and a variety of anthraquinones are more cytotoxic to hypoxic EMT6 cells than to well-oxygenated cells in culture (77). Studies on the relationship between the oxidation–reduction potential of benzo- and naphthoquinone derivatives and their effectiveness as antitumor agents revealed a good correlation between redox potential and antineoplastic activity (71,76,78); agents having the lowest redox potentials were the most efficacious.

Early studies on the biotransformation of mitomycin C demonstrated that an NADPH-dependent enzyme system was involved in the metabolism of the drug by liver microsomes (60) and was essential for activation of mitomycin C to an alkylating species in bacterial lysates (62). Studies in our laboratory have confirmed and extended these original observations of Schwartz (60) and Iyer and Szybalski (62). We found that mitomycin C was bioactivated under hypoxic conditions in liver microsomes (see Fig. 4) and nuclei by a NADPH-dependent enzyme(s) (79). The enzyme system was inhibited both by oxygen and carbon monoxide. Furthermore, manipulations which inhibited the metabolism of mitomycin C also interfered with the generation of alkylating species as detected with 4-(*p*-nitrobenzyl)pyridine, a trapping agent for activated drug. Using techniques similar to those employed for studying the liver-dependent metabolism of the drug, cell-free systems from the neoplastic cell lines sarcoma 180 and EMT6, were found to activate mitomycin C metabolically to an alkylating agent under hypoxic conditions (Fig. 4); the enzyme system involved appeared to be similar to that in the liver (80).

Although mitomycin C is selectively activated under hypoxic conditions, clinical use of this agent has been limited by severe toxicity to normal tissues, which are presumably well-oxygenated. Toxicity to well-oxygenated tissues is probably the result of a different activation mechanism which involves single-electron

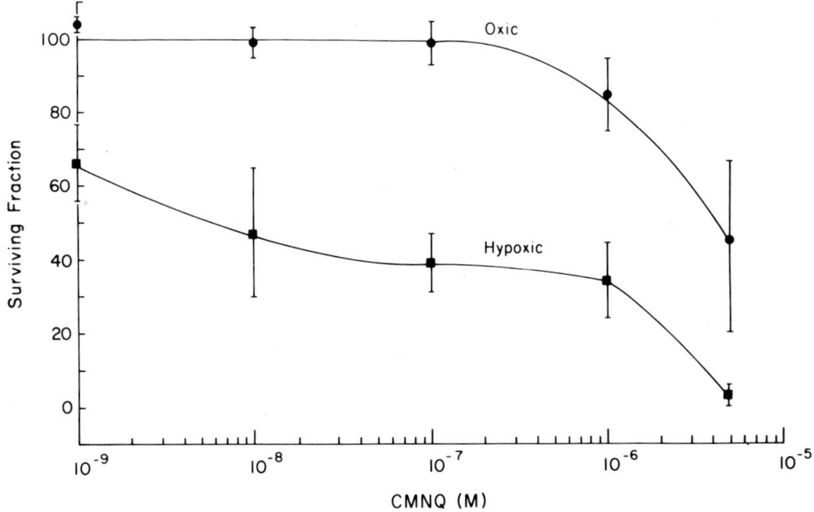

Fig. 3. Cytotoxic activity of 2,3-dichloromethyl-1,4-naphthoquinone (CMNQ) toward aerobic and hypoxic EMT6 cells. EMT6 cells grown in monolayer culture were made hypoxic by exposure to 95% nitrogen–5% CO_2 for 4 hours prior to drug addition. Aerobic cells were maintained under air–5% CO_2 for the same length of time prior to drug exposure. Cell survival was determined by colony formation after 1 hour of drug exposure, as described elsewhere (20, 77, 86).

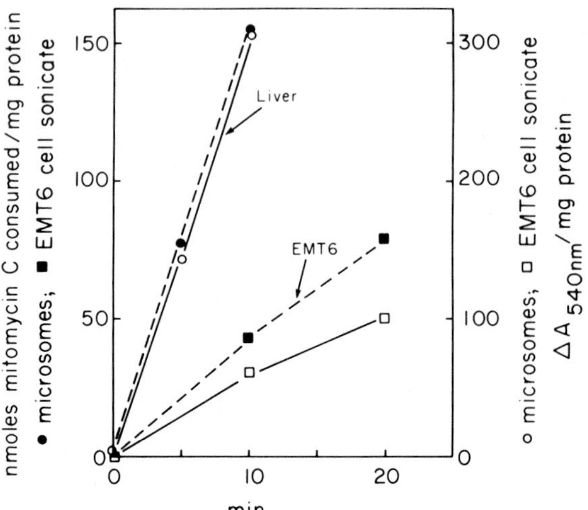

Fig. 4. Metabolism and activation of mitomycin C by liver microsomes and EMT6 cell sonicates. The time dependence of the metabolism of mitomycin C, as measured by substrate disappearance, in liver microsomes and sonicated EMT6 cell preparations is shown. In addition, the formation of activated drug as measured spectroscopically as ΔA_{540} nm by trapping of alkylating species formed during metabolism with 4-(*p*-nitrobenzyl)pyridine, is shown for microsomes and EMT6 cell sonicates.

reduction followed by reoxidation of mitomycin C by oxygen to give the parent compound and the superoxide radical (81–83). The superoxide free radical can dismute, resulting in a variety of extremely reactive species, such as H_2O_2 and hydroxyl radical. The toxicities of these reactive species have been reviewed elsewhere (84,85). Experiments in our laboratory have demonstrated that mitomycin C is more cytotoxic to hypoxic cells than to aerobic cells (80,86). The clinical employment of mitomycin C at maximum tolerated doses does not take advantage of the differential toxicity of this antibiotic for hypoxic cells. However, administration of mitomycin C to cancer patients at low doses might be successfully employed to kill hypoxic tumor cells with minimal oxygen-dependent toxicity. It is also conceivable that compounds could be developed which can be bioactivated by hypoxic cells but which do not support superoxide-generated toxicity in aerobic cells; these agents would be toxic exclusively to hypoxic cells.

B. Nitroaromatic Compounds

Nitroheterocyclic agents, such as metronidazole and misonidazole, increase the sensitivity of hypoxic cells to ionizing radiation (87). In addition, these radiosensitizers have been shown to be toxic to hypoxic cells *in vitro,* whereas well-oxygenated cells were insensitive to nitroimidazoles (88,89). The susceptibility of cells to misonidazole-induced cytotoxicity is determined by the severity of the hypoxia (88). Relatively large amounts of *N*-hydroxy and amine metabolites were produced in hypoxic cells, indicating that reduction of the nitro group occurred (88–90), whereas few metabolites were found in aerobic cells (89). The selective toxicity of misonidazole to hypoxic cells appeared to be related to the generation and retention of metabolites (89–92), implying that tumor cells can metabolize this compound by pathways which are dependent on the state of cellular oxygenation. Studies employing chemically reduced nitroimidazoles supported the concept that reduction of the nitro group could lead to reactive species capable of interacting with macromolecules such as DNA (93,94). Furthermore, incubation of $CH2B_2$ cells with metronidazole or misonidazole under hypoxic conditions resulted in substantial time-dependent damage to DNA, measured as alkali-labile lesions, which were interpreted as single-strand breaks (95).

Although the enzymatic systems responsible for the reduction of nitroimidazoles in mammalian tumor cells have not been well characterized, nitroreductase activity in hepatic microsomes is known to be dependent upon either NADH or NADPH, inhibited by oxygen, and stimulated by flavins (96–98). Complete reduction of the nitro group involves a six-electron transfer from pyridine nucleotides and results in the formation of a primary amine (97). Because microsomal flavins and cytochromes are almost invariably one-electron donors, the first step in the reduction would be formation of the nitro radical anion (99). Many aromatic and aliphatic nitro compounds form complexes (most likely as nitroso derivatives) with hemoproteins presenting an access to the heme pocket, such as cytochrome P-450, cytochrome P-420, hemoglobin, and myoglobin (100). Further reduction of the nitroso and hydroxylamine compounds can also occur. Studies on the reduction of *N*-hydroxyphentermine have shown that this material is reduced by at least two enzyme systems, one of which is inducible by phenobarbital, requires NADPH, and is sensitive to carbon monoxide (101). Similar enzyme systems may exist in tumor cells and allow reductive activation of nitroimidazoles to cytotoxic compounds.

Although the electron-affinic radiosensitizers are selectively cytotoxic to hypoxic cells in the absence of radiation, this cytotoxicity requires prolonged contact times (several hours) and relatively high drug concentrations (e.g., 1–5 m*M* misonidazole) (90, 102–105). Consequently, the selective action of these agents on hypoxic cells may not be exploitable in the treatment of human cancer. Incorporation of a nitroaromatic moiety into a molecule specifically designed to be activated to a highly reactive alkylating species under the reducing conditions present in hypoxic neoplastic cells should result in agents which are selectively toxic to hypoxic cells. To test this hypothesis, *o*- and *p*-nitrobenzyl halides and carbamates were prepared as prototypes of nitroreductase-catalyzed bioreductive alkylating agents. As shown in Table I, the first half-wave potentials of these nitrobenzyl compounds are quite similar to those of metronidazole, with misonidazole being slightly more electron-affinic.

The survivals of hypoxic EMT6 tumor cells exposed to *o*-nitrobenzyl alcohols, halides, and carbamates were significantly lower than those of aerobic cells treated with these agents. In contrast, no significant differences in cytotoxicity toward aerobic and hypoxic cells were observed with corresponding *p*-nitrobenzyl halides and carbamates, *o*- or *p*-nitrobenzyl alcohols, nitrotoluenes, benzyl halides, and benzyl carbamates. These data suggest that the presence of the nitro group in an ortho orientation to the halomethylene or carbamylmethylene group is necessary for selective toxicity to hypoxic cells. The selective cytotoxicity of these compounds is thought to involve bioreduction of the nitro substituent to produce a highly nucleophilic amino group adjacent to the methylene moiety bearing a good leaving group (Fig. 5). The participation of the

TABLE I

Half-wave Reduction Potentials and Aerobic versus Hypoxic Kill Ratios of *o*- and *p*-Nitrobenzyl Alcohols, Halides, and Carbamates

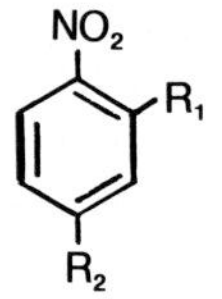

R_1	R_2	$E_{1/2}$ (V)[a]	Aerobic/hypoxic ratio[b]
H	CH_2OH	−0.84	2.8
H	CH_2Br	−0.75	2.0
H	CH_2Cl	−0.72	1.4
H	$CH_2OCONHCH_3$	−0.82	1.4
H	$CH_2OCONHC_2H_5Cl$	−0.77	3.0
CH_2OH	H	−0.83	2.0
CH_2Br	H	−0.75	26.7
CH_2Cl	H	−0.72	12.8
$CH_2OCONHCH_3$	H	−0.79	800.0
$CH_2OCONHC_2H_5Cl$	H	−0.76	1000.0
Misonidazole		−0.68	
Metronidazole		−0.74	

[a] First half-wave reduction potentials were measured in 0.05 *M* potassium phosphate buffer prepared in water-ethanol (1:1, v/v), pH 7.0, by differential pulse polarography (PAR 174A polarographic analyzer). The values were obtained in volts versus a saturated calomel reference electrode using 0.1 *M* KCl as the supporting electrolyte.

[b] The ratio of drug concentration necessary to decrease the surviving fraction of aerobic cells 50% to the drug concentration required to decrease the surviving fraction of hypoxic cells by the same percentage.

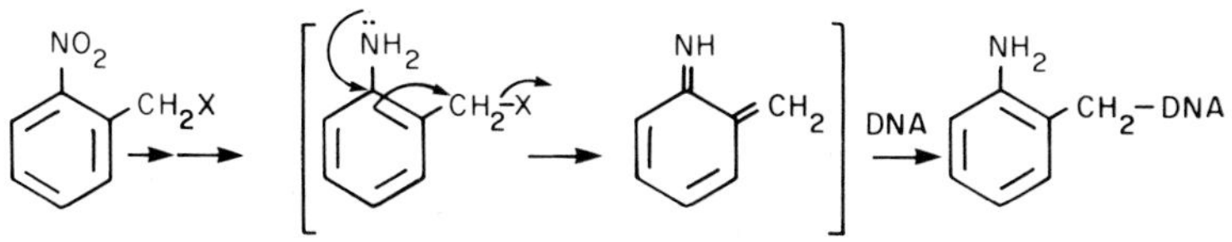

Fig. 5. Activation scheme for *o*-nitrobenzyl compounds. The proposed activation scheme for *o*-nitrobenzyl halides, alcohols, and carbamates requires nitro group reduction to the amine followed by intramolecular rearrangement to produce the anilinium methide-containing compound which can react with cellular macromolecules such as DNA.

amino function in forming the postulated reactive methide intermediate is necessary to overcome energy barriers associated with the aromaticity of the benzene ring, with intramolecular rearrangement leading to the anilinium ion and the highly reactive methide. Upon reaction of the methide with an available cellular nucleophile, such as nucleic acid or protein, the aromaticity of the system is restored.

Nitrobenzyl halides and carbamates are clearly more cytotoxic to hypoxic cells than misonidazole and metronidazole. One log of cell kill could be achieved with *o*-nitrobenzyl halides and carbamates when cells were exposed to a concentration of 10 μM drug for 1 hour. In contrast, misonidazole required concentrations of 1–5 m*M* and incubation times of 2–5 hours to produce a comparable kill of hypoxic cells (90,102–105). Moreover, the selective toxicity of *o*-nitrobenzyl halides and carbamates for hypoxic cells was evident at concentrations as low as 0.01 μM. Although *o*-nitrobenzyl halides, especially *o*-nitrobenzyl bromide, were toxic to mice when administered intraperitoneally in saline suspensions, *o*-nitrobenzyl-*N*-substituted carbamates were well-tolerated by animals given daily doses as large as 500 mg/kg (106,107).

V. The Design of Chemotherapeutic Regimens for Solid Tumors

A consideration of the physiological status of the tumor cell subpopulations (Fig. 1) suggests that a rational approach to cancer therapy requires a combination of agents and/or modalities directed toward each of the cell types in the tumor, including the cycling and noncycling populations of both the aerobic and hypoxic compartments. Based on these concepts, the combinations of drugs (or other treatment modalities) selected for therapy should include the following.

1. A bioreductive alkylating agent designed to attack the hypoxic cell compartment by exploiting the capacity of these cells for reductive activation: Mitomycin C appears to be the most efficacious agent of this class presently available for clinical use. To maximize the differential cytotoxicity of this compound, it should be administered in relatively low doses for a prolonged period.

Concurrent administration of mitomycin C with an agent selected for its ability to kill aerobic cells should minimize any loss of effectiveness of the mitomycin due to reoxygenation of hypoxic cells.

2. An agent or modality to attack specifically any nonproliferating aerobic cells present in the tumor (i.e., plateau phase-like cells): Bleomycin, *cis*-diamminedichloroplatinum(II), and nitrosoureas such as 1-(2-chloroethyl)-3-cyclohexylnitrosourea and 1,3-bis(2-chloroethyl)nitrosourea which appear to be more toxic to nonproliferative plateau-phase cells than to exponentially growing cells (108–113), are clinically used agents which could be employed to attack the quiescent cell subpopulation present in tumors.

3. Agents or a treatment modality with specificity for well-oxygenated proliferating cells: Agents for this purpose include arabinosylcytosine, methotrexate, vincristine, and actinomycin D. Each of these drugs is most effective against rapidly proliferating cells.

Agents such as bleomycin, procarbazine, and streptonigrin may be useful in the attack of cells in categories 2 and 3, because these drugs appear to require oxygen for the full expression of antineoplastic activity. Similarly, radiation could be used to kill both proliferative and quiescent well-oxygenated cells. It is apparent that the combination of modalities and agents employed to attack the tumor must cause biochemical lesions resulting in cell death in all subpopulations without inflicting unacceptable toxicity to normal host tissues. By careful selection and employment of agents, it may be possible to cure neoplastic diseases currently considered to have a poor prognosis.

Acknowledgments

This work was supported in part by U.S. Public Health Service Grants CA-02817, CA-16359, and CA-06519 from the National Cancer Institute; a grant from the Bristol-Myers Company; and National Institutes of Health Postdoctoral Fellowships CA-06177 (K.A.K.) and CA-06365 (B.A.T.).

References

1. G. G. Steel, "Growth Kinetics of Tumors." Oxford Univ. Press (Clarendon), London and New York, 1977.
2. R. F. Kallman and S. Rockwell, *in* "Cancer: A Comprehensive Treatise" (F. F. Becker, ed.), Vol. 6, p.225. Plenum, New York, 1977.
3. M. L. Mendelsohn, *Cancer* **29,** 2390 (1969).
4. G. G. Steel and L. F. Lamerton, *Natl. Cancer Inst., Monogr.* **30,** 29 (1969).
5. I. F. Tannock, *Cancer Treat. Rep.* **62,** 8 (1978).
6. F. Valeriote and L. van Putten, *Cancer Res.* **35,** 2619 (1975).
7. K. A. Kennedy, B. A. Teicher, S. Rockwell, and A. C. Sartorelli, *Biochem. Pharmacol.* **29,** 1 (1980).

8. R. F. Kallman, *Radiology* **105,** 135 (1972).
9. J. F. Fowler and J. Denekamp, *Pharmacol. Ther.* **7,** 413 (1979).
10. J. S. Bedford and J. B. Mitchell, *Br. J. Radiol.* **47,** 687 (1974).
11. R. Born, O. Hug, and H.-R. Trott, *Int. J. Radiat. Oncol., Biol. Phys.* **1,** 687 (1976).
12. C. J. Koch, J. Kruuv, H. E. Frey, and R. A. Snyder, *Int. J. Radiat. Biol. Relat. Stud. Phys., Chem. Med.* **23,** 67 (1973).
13. I. F. Tannock, *Br. J. Radiol.* **45,** 515 (1972).
14. K. D. Ley and R. A. Takey, *J. Cell Biol.* **47,** 453 (1970).
15. J. R. Gautschi, R. Schinder, and C. Hürni, *J. Cell Biol.* **51,** 653 (1971).
16. C. Cerrarini and H. Eagle, *Nature (London), New Biol.* **233,** 271 (1971).
17. D. W. Fodge and H. Rubin, *J. Cell. Physiol.* **85,** 635 (1975).
18. R. M. Sutherland, *Pharmacol. Ther.* **8,** 105 (1980).
19. I. F. Tannock, *Br. J. Cancer* **22,** 258 (1972).
20. S. Rockwell, R. F. Kallman, and L. F. Fajardo, *J. Natl. Cancer Inst.* **49,** 735 (1972).
21. M. G. Pallavicini, M. E. Lalande, R. G. Miller, and R. P. Hill, *Cancer Res.* **39,** 1891 (1979).
22. S. Rockwell, E. Frindel, A. J. Valleron, and M. Tubiana, *Cell Tissue Kinet.* **11,** 279 (1978).
23. A. E. Bateman and G. G. Steel, *Cell Tissue Kinet.* **11,** 445 (1978).
24. R. M. Sutherland and A. J. Franko, *Int. J. Radiat. Oncol., Biol. Phys.* **6,** 117 (1980).
25. J. M. Brown, *Br. J. Radiol.* **52,** 650 (1979).
26. P. M. Gullino, *J. Natl. Cancer Inst.* **61,** 639 (1978).
27. J. Folkman, *Adv. Cancer Res.* **19,** 331 (1974).
28. M. A. Gimbrone, Jr., S. B. Leapman, R. S. Cotran, and J. Folkman, *J. Exp. Med.* **136,** 261 (1972).
29. J. Folkman, *N. Engl. J. Med.* **285,** 1182 (1971).
30. M. Greenblatt and P. Shubek, *J. Natl. Cancer Inst.* **41,** 111 (1968).
31. P. M. Gullino, *Methods Cancer Res.* **5,** 45 (1970).
32. Y. A. Sidky and R. Auerbach, *J. Exp. Med.* **141,** 1084 (1975).
33. R. Auerbach, L. Kubai, and Y. Sidky, *Cancer Res.* **36,** 3435 (1976).
34. R. H. Thomlinson, *J. Clin. Pathol.* **30,** Suppl. 11, 105 (1977).
35. T. P. Butler and P. M. Gullino, *Cancer Res.* **35,** 3084 (1975).
36. R. J. Goldacre and B. Sylvén, *Br. J. Cancer* **16,** 306 (1962).
37. I. F. Tannock, *Cancer Res.* **30,** 2470 (1970).
38. I. F. Tannock and S. Hayashi, *Cancer Res.* **32,** 77 (1972).
39. L. Karlsson, M. Alpsten, K. L. Appelgren, and H. I. Peterson, *Microvasc. Res.* **19,** 71 (1980).
40. H. I. Peterson, *in* "Tumor Blood Circulation: Angiogenesis, Vascular Morphology and Blood Flow of Experimental and Human Tumors" (H. I. Peterson, ed.), p. 103. CRC Press, Boca Raton, Florida, 1979.
41. A. W. Vogel, *J. Natl. Cancer Inst.* **34,** 571 (1965).
42. P. Vaupel, *Microvasc. Res.* **13,** 399 (1977).
43. H. S. Reinhold, *in* "Tumor Blood Circulation: Angiogenesis, Morphology and Blood Flow of Experimental and Human Tumors" (H. I. Peterson, ed.), p. 115. CRC Press, Inc., Boca Raton, Florida, 1979.
44. P. Vaupel and G. Thews, *Oncology* **30,** 475 (1974).
45. P. Vaupel, *Bibl. Anat.* **15,** 288 (1977).
46. P. Vaupel, R. Manz, W. Müller-Klieser, and W. A. Grunewald, *Microvasc. Res.* **17,** 181 (1979).
47. P. Vaupel, *in* "Tumor Blood Circulation: Angiogenesis, Morphology and Blood Flow of Experimental and Human Tumors" (H. I. Peterson, ed.), p. 143. CRC Press Inc., Boca Raton, Florida, 1979.
48. P. M. Gullino, *in* "Cancer: A Comprehensive Treatise" (F. F. Becker, ed.), Vol. 3, p. 327. Plenum, New York, 1975.

49. K. G. M. M. Alberti, *J. Clin. Pathol.* **30,** Suppl. 11, 14 (1977).
50. H. S. Reinhold, B. Blachiewicz, and A. Berg-Blok, *Eur. J. Cancer* **15,** 481 (1979).
51. H. S. Reinhold, *Eur. J. Cancer* **15,** 481 (1979).
52. D. E. Hilmas and E. L. Gillette, *Radiat. Res.* **61,** 128 (1975).
53. M. Mäntylä, J. Kuikka, and A. Rekonen, *Br. J. Radiol.* **49,** 335 (1976).
54. C. W. Song, J. T. Payne, and S. H. Levitt, *Radiology* **104,** 693 (1972).
55. L. F. Hewitt, "Oxidation Reduction Potentials in Bacteriology and Biochemistry," 4th ed., p. 19. London County Council, London, 1936.
56. J. R. Porter, "Bacterial Chemistry and Physiology," p. 56. Wiley, New York, 1946.
57. A. J. Lin, L. A. Cosby, C. W. Shansky, and A. C. Sartorelli, *J. Med. Chem.* **15,** 1247 (1972).
58. J. S. Driscoll, G. F. Hazard, H. B. Wood, Jr., and A. Goldin, *Cancer Chemother. Rep., Part 2* **4**(2), 1 (1974).
59. H. W. Moore, *Science* **197,** 527 (1977).
60. H. S. Schwartz, *J. Pharmacol. Exp. Ther.* **136,** 250 (1962).
61. H. S. Schwartz, J. E. Sodergren, and F. S. Philips, *Science* **142,** 1181 (1963).
62. Y. N. Iyer and W. Szybalski, *Science* **145,** 55 (1964).
63. W. Szybalski and V. G. Arneson, *Mol. Pharmacol.* **1,** 202 (1965).
64. H. Murakami, *J. Theor. Biol.* **10,** 236 (1966).
65. S. Kinoshita, K. Uzu, K. Nakano, M. Shimizu, T. Takahashi, and M. Matsui, *J. Med. Chem.* **14,** 103 (1971).
66. S. Kinoshita, K. Uzu, K. Nakano, and T. Takahashi, *J. Med. Chem.* **14,** 109 (1971).
67. S. T. Crooke and W. T. Bradner, *Cancer Treat. Rev.* **3,** 121 (1976).
68. A. J. Lin, L. A. Cosby, and A. C. Sartorelli, *Cancer Chemother. Rep., Part 2* **4**(4), 23 (1974).
69. L. A. Cosby, R. S. Pardini, R. E. Biagini, T. L. Lambert, A. J. Lin, Y. M. Huang, K. M. Hwang, and A. C. Sartorelli, *Cancer Res.* **36,** 4023 (1976).
70. A. J. Lin, R. S. Pardini, L. A. Cosby, B. J. Lillis, C. W. Shansky, and A. C. Sartorelli, *J. Med. Chem.* **16,** 1268 (1973).
71. A. J. Lin and A. C. Sartorelli, *J. Org. Chem.* **38,** 813 (1973).
72. A. J. Lin, C. W. Shansky, and A. C. Sartorelli, *J. Med. Chem.* **17,** 558 (1974).
73. A. J. Lin, B. J. Lillis, and A. C. Sartorelli, *J. Med. Chem.* **18,** 917 (1975).
74. A. J. Lin and A. C. Sartorelli, *J. Med. Chem.* **19,** 1336 (1976).
75. A. J. Lin, R. S. Pardini, B. J. Lillis, and A. C. Sartorelli, *J. Med. Chem.* **17,** 668 (1974).
76. A. J. Lin and A. C. Sartorelli, *Biochem. Pharmacol.* **25,** 206 (1976).
77. T. S. Lin, B. A. Teicher, and A. C. Sartorelli, *Abst. Pap., 179th Natl. Meet., Am. Chem. Soc.* MEDI 62 (1980).
78. G. Prakash and E. M. Hodnett, *J. Med. Chem.* **21,** 369 (1978).
79. K. A. Kennedy and A. C. Sartorelli, *Fed. Proc., Fed. Am. Soc. Exp. Biol.* **38,** 443 (1979).
80. K. A. Kennedy, S. Rockwell, and A. C. Sartorelli, *Cancer Res.* **40,** 2356 (1980).
81. K. Handa and S. Sato, *Gann* **66,** 43 (1975).
82. N. Bachur, S. Gordon, and M. V. Gee, *Cancer Res.* **38,** 1745 (1978).
83. N. Bachur, S. Gordon, M. V. Gee, and K. Hon, *Proc. Natl. Acad. Sci. U.S.A.* **76,** 954 (1979).
84. I. Fridovich, *Acc. Chem. Res.* **5,** 321 (1972).
85. W. A. Pryor, *Photochem. Photobiol.* **28,** 787 (1978).
86. S. Rockwell and K. A. Kennedy, *Int. J. Radiat. Oncol., Biol. Phys.* **5,** 1673 (1979).
87. R. L. Wilson, W. A. Cramp, and R. M. J. Ings, *Int. J. Radiat. Biol. Relat. Stud. Phys., Chem. Med.* **26,** 557 (1974).
88. J. K. Mohindra and A. M. Rauth, *Cancer Res.* **36,** 930(1976).
89. Y. C. Taylor and A. M. Rauth, *Cancer Res.* **38,** 2745 (1978).
90. T. W. Wong, G. F. Whitmore, and S. Gulyas, *Radiat. Res.* **75,** 541 (1978).
91. I. J. Stratford, *Br. J. Cancer* **38,** 130 (1978).

92. I. J. Stratford and G. E. Adams, *Br. J. Radiol.* **51,** 745 (1978).
93. N. F. La Russo, M. Tomasz, and M. M. Müller, *Gastroenterology* **71,** 917 (1976).
94. N. F. La Russo, M. Tomasz, M. M. Müller, and R. Lipman, *Mol. Pharmacol.* **13,** 872 (1977).
95. F. Hohman, B. Palcic, and L. D. Skarsgard, *Radiat. Res.* **67,** 529 (1976).
96. J. A. Fouts and B. B. Brodie, *J. Pharmacol. Exp. Ther.* **119,** 197 (1957).
97. J. R. Gillette, J. J. Kamm, and H. A. Sasame, *Mol. Pharmacol.* **4,** 541 (1968).
98. L. A. Poirier and J. H. Weisburger, *Biochem. Pharmacol.* **23,** 661 (1974).
99. R. P. Mason and J. L. Holtzman, *Biochemistry* **14,** 1626 (1975).
100. P. Mansuy, P. Gans, J. C. Chottard, and J. F. Bartoli, *Eur. J. Biochem.* **76,** 607 (1977).
101. C. Y. Sum and A. K. Cho, *Drug Metab. Dispos.* **4,** 436 (1976).
102. I. Wodinsky, R. K. Johnson, and J. J. Clement, *Proc. Am. Assoc. Cancer Res.* **20,** 230 (1979).
103. B. A. Moore, B. Palcic, and L. D. Skarsgard, *Radiat. Res.* **67,** 459 (1976).
104. J. L. Foster, *Int. J. Radiat. Oncol., Biol. Phys.* **4,** 153 (1978).
105. C. R. Geard, S. F. Povlas, M. B. Astoy, and E. J. Hall, *Cancer Res.* **38,** 644 (1978).
106. B. A. Teicher and A. C. Sartorelli, *Abstr. Pap., 178th Natl. Meet. Am. Chem. Soc.* MEDI 67 (1979).
107. B. A. Teicher and A. C. Sartorelli, *J. Med. Chem.* **23,** 955 (1980).
108. S. C. Barranco and J. K. Novak, *Cancer Res.* **34,** 1616 (1974).
109. S. C. Barranco, J. K. Novak, and R. M. Humphrey, *Cancer Res.* **33,** 691 (1973).
110. B. K. Bhuyan, T. J. Fraser, and K. J. Day, *Cancer Res.* **37,** 1057 (1977).
111. G. M. Hahn, L. F. Gordon, and D. A. Kurkjian, *Cancer Res.* **34,** 2373 (1974).
112. R. M. Sutherland, *Cancer Res.* **34,** 3501 (1974).
113. J. J. Roberts, this volume, Chapter 2.

5

Suicide Enzyme Inactivators*

ROBERT H. ABELES

It is frequently desirable, in physiological studies or for pharmacological purposes, to inhibit specific enzymes. This is generally achieved in one of two ways: (1) through molecules which bind to the target enzyme reversibly and thereby prevent catalysis or reduce the rate of catalysis; competitive inhibitors and transition-state analogues fall into this category; and (2) through molecules which inactivate the enzyme irreversibly by forming a covalent bond with it. The type of inactivator I shall discuss falls into the second category. Well-known examples of irreversible enzyme inactivators are active site-directed inactivators, for example, tolylsulfonyl-lysyl chloromethyl ketone (TPCK) (1). The TPCK molecule incorporates two important features:

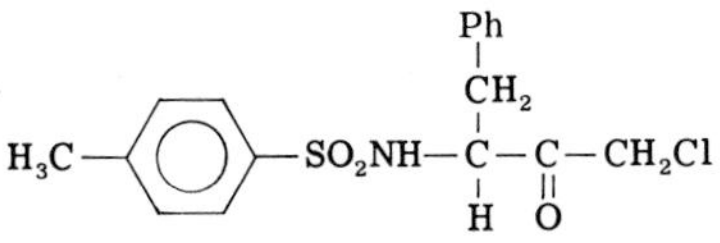

$$H_3C-C_6H_4-SO_2NH-\underset{H}{\overset{\overset{Ph}{|}}{\overset{CH_2}{\overset{|}{C}}}}-\underset{\|}{\overset{}{C}}\underset{O}{}-CH_2Cl$$

TPCK

It resembles a normal chymotrypsin substrate and is therefore bound to the active site of this enzyme. The molecule also contains a chloro ketone ($-\underset{O}{\overset{C}{\|}}-CH_2Cl$), which is a reactive alkylating agent and can therefore interact with a nucleophile at the active site. This compound labels a histidine residue. Inactivators of this type have been extremely useful in identifying active site residues. A disadvantage to the use of these inhibitors is that, because they are intrinsically reactive molecules, they can react with molecules other than the target enzymes. The latter event could be particularly undesirable when one uses these inhibitors *in vivo*.

*In this chapter I shall deal primarily with inactivators which were studied at Brandeis University, as well as with some inactivators developed by others which are related to those we have studied. Several comprehensive reviews on the subject of suicide inactivators or mechanism-based inactivators have been published (21–26).

MOLECULAR ACTIONS AND TARGETS FOR CANCER CHEMOTHERAPEUTIC AGENTS

ISBN 0-12-619280-4

Another category of enzyme inactivators are suicide enzyme inactivators. These inactivators have also been called mechanism-based inactivators, K_{cat} inactivators, and Trojan horse inactivators. Suicide enzyme inactivators also form a covalent bond with the enzyme, but the principle underlying their mode of action is different from that of active site-directed inactivators. Suicide enzyme inactivators are relatively unreactive molecules which structurally resemble the substrate and therefore bind to the active site of the enzyme. Once bound to the active site, the enzyme acts on them as it does on the normal substrate. For instance, the enzyme might abstract a proton. This action triggers a chemical change in the inactivator, which leads to the formation of a highly reactive species at the active site. This reactive species then reacts with a functional group on the enzyme to cause inactivation of the enzyme. The characteristic feature of a suicide inactivator is that the active form of the inactivating compound is generated at the active site through the catalytic capability of the enzyme. The specificity of these inactivators not only lies in their structural similarity to the substrate but is also dependent on the mechanism of action of the target enzyme.

The concept underlying suicide enzyme inactivators was suggested to us by the work of Bloch (2) and Morisaki and Bloch (3) on the mechanism of action of β-hydroxydecanoyl dehydrase. β-Hydroxydecanoyl dehydrase catalyzes the following reaction:

$$CH_3(CH_2)_6CHOHCH_2CONAC \rightleftharpoons CH_3(CH_2)_6CH{=}CHCONAC \rightleftharpoons CH_3(CH_2)_5CH{=}CHCH_2CONAC \quad (1)$$

$NAC = SCH_2CH_2NHCOCH_3$

It has been found that $H_3C(CH_2)_5C{\equiv}CCH_2COSCH_2CH_2NHCOCH_3$ inactivates the enzyme and becomes covalently attached to an histidine residue at the active site. The following mechanism has been proposed for the inactivation:

$$CH_3(CH_2)_5C{\equiv}CCH_2CONAC \underset{}{\overset{\text{enzyme-catalyzed}}{\rightleftharpoons}} CH_3(CH_2)_5CH{=}C{=}CHCONAC \xrightarrow{\text{His—enzyme}} CH_3(CH_2)_5CH{=}\underset{\text{His—enzyme}}{\underset{|}{C}}CH_2CONAC \quad (2)$$

(or perhaps the α, β isomer)

In this case, the acetylene is not actually an inactivator. Inactivation occurs through the allene generated at the active site through the catalytic capabilities of the enzyme. The normal catalytic process most probably involves the following events: (1) protonation and deprotonation of the α position, (2) protonation of the β-hydroxy group to facilitate its elimination, and (3) protonation and deprotonation of the γ position. Appropriate functional groups must be present to serve as acids or bases. The same catalytic events and functional groups are probably involved in conversion of the acetylene to the allene. To bring about this conversion, a proton must be abstracted from the α position of the acetylene and a proton must be added to the γ position. Furthermore, addition of the histidine to the allene again requires protonation of the α position. The mammalian enzyme crotonase, which carries out a similar dehydration but does not catalyze the $\alpha,\beta \rightleftharpoons \beta,\gamma$ conversion, is not inactivated by the acetylenic substrate analogue. Since the enzyme does not carry out the isomerization, it probably does not have a functional group which interacts with the γ position of the substrate and therefore may not be able to catalyze conversion of the acetylene to the allene.

The work of Bloch suggested to us that any enzyme which catalyzed proton abstraction from the substrate should be subject to inactivation by acetylenic substrate analogues. Therefore our first attempts to synthesize suicide inactivators involved acetylenic substrate analogues.

Before discussing specific examples of suicide inactivators, I shall briefly consider the experimental criteria by which these inactivators can be recognized. The most definitive method requires complete characterization of the enzyme inhibitor adduct, i.e., identification of the functional group on the enzyme which is labeled and identification of the structural changes the inhibitor has undergone. Such an investigation is time-consuming and frequently very difficult, because of the limited amounts of enzymes generally available. However, relatively simple kinetic experiments can give useful information. In examining a potential suicide inhibition, one should first establish the kinetics of inhibition. For suicide inactivators, a time-dependent loss of enzyme activity is expected. Time dependence provides good but not definitive evidence that covalent modification has taken place. Demonstration that the loss of enzyme activity, at constant inactivator concentration, is first-order, provides evidence that inactivation occurs before the inactivator is released from the enzyme, a fundamental property of suicide inhibition. This distinguishes the inactivation process from cases in which the enzyme converts a substrate to a reactive species which is released and later reacts with the enzyme from solution.

At the time we started this work, we were investigating the mechanism of action of plasma amine oxidase (a Cu^{2+} protein) and several flavoprotein oxidases, i.e., lactic oxidase and mitochondrial amine oxidase. Our studies led to the conclusion that these reactions were initiated by proton abstractions. These enzymes are therefore ideal candidates for inactivation by acetylenic compounds. These enzymes should also catalyze the abstraction of a proton from an acetylenic substrate analogue, and this should then lead to conversion of the acetylene to an allene. A nucleophile on the enzyme can then attack the allene,

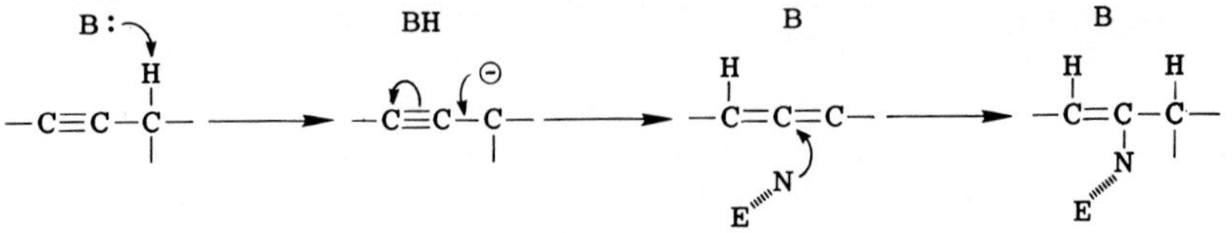

$$-C\equiv C-\overset{|}{\underset{|}{C}}H- \longrightarrow -C\equiv C-\overset{\ominus}{C}- \longrightarrow -\overset{H}{C}=C=C- \longrightarrow -\overset{H}{C}=\underset{N-E}{C}-\overset{H}{C}- \quad (3)$$

and a covalent bond is formed with the inactivator. In other words, these enzymes should be subject to the same principle of inactivation as that described for β-hydroxydecanoyl dehydrase. It was already known that mitochondrial amine oxidase was inhibited by pargyline and propynylamine. We found that propynylamine also inactivated plasma amine oxidase (4). Lactic oxidase, a flavoprotein, is inactivated by the substrate analogue 2-hydroxybutynoic acid (5,6).

$CH\equiv C-CH_2NH_2$	$\phi-CH_2-N(CH_3)-CH_2-C\equiv CH$	$CH\equiv C-CH(OH)-COO^-$
Propynylamine	Pargyline	2-Hydroxybutynoic acid

Thus our expectations were born out. Acetylenic substrate analogues proved to be effective inhibitors of these enzymes. Is the mechanism of inactivation as expected? In each case the inactivators meet the criteria for suicide inactivators outlined above. We have little information beyond this for plasma amine oxidase. The spectrum of inactivated mitochondrial amine oxidase shows that, in the course of inactivation, the enzyme-bound flavin is modified. The structure of the modified flavin is shown in Fig. 1 (7). Inactivation of lactic oxidase by 2-hydroxybutynoic acid also leads to modification of the flavin. Figure 2 represents the structure of the adduct formed (5,6).

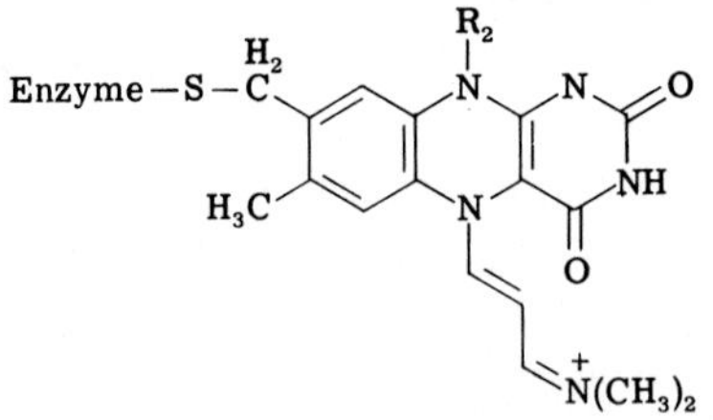

Fig. 1. Flavin adduct from mitochondrial amine oxidase inactivated with $CH\equiv C-CH_2NH_3$.

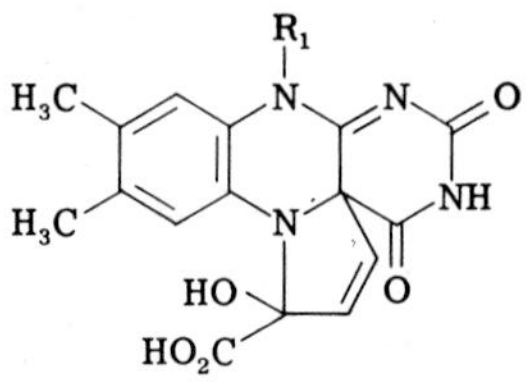

Fig. 2. Flavin adduct from lactic oxidase inactivated with $CH\equiv C-CHOHCOO^-$.

Adduct formation is not as expected; i.e., covalent bond formation does not occur alpha to the carbon from which the proton is abstracted. What is the reason for this? The allene formed from hydroxybutynoic acid and propargylamine is not analogous to the allene formed in the inactivation of β-hydroxydecanoyl dehydrase. These allenes, if formed, have electron-releasing substituents, and it is difficult to predict how they will react with a nucleophile. A number of

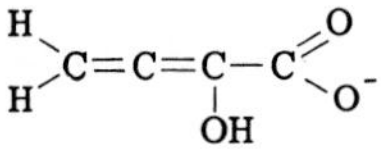

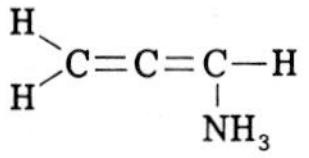

$$H_2C{=}C{=}C(OH){-}COO^- \qquad H_2C{=}C{=}C(NH_3){-}H$$

alternative mechanisms for inactivation have also been considered. We shall show these for lactic oxidase, but similar mechanisms could apply to mitochondrial amine oxidase; (1) An allenic anion could be formed, which then adds to the flavin:

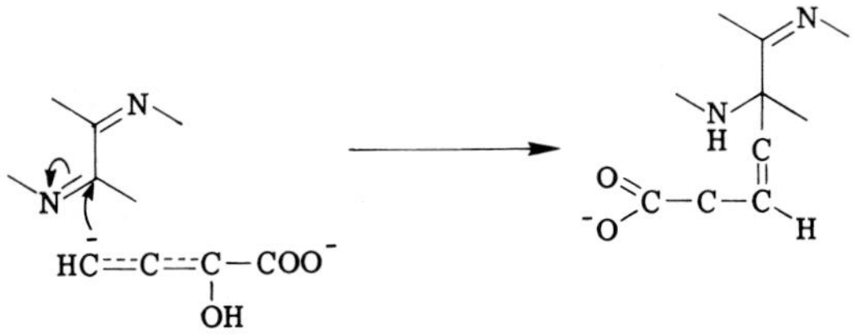

(4)

(2) The inhibitor could be oxidized and the reduced flavin could add to the oxidized inactivator through a Michael-type addition:

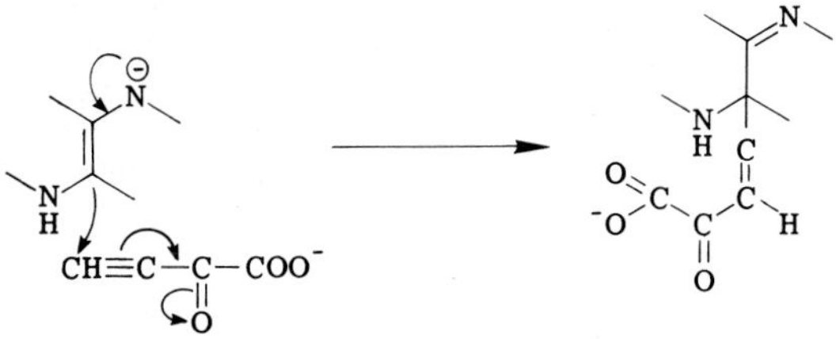

(5)

At this time, we have no way of deciding which of these mechanisms, if either, applies.

Recently, we have found another type of inhibition of flavoproteins by an acetylenic substrate. Butynoylpantotheine appears to be a suicide inactivator of butyryl-CoA dehydrogenase and of glutaryl-CoA dehydrogenase (8). With these enzymes the inactivator does not react with the flavin, since the spectrum of the flavin in the inactivated enzyme is unchanged; i.e., the inactivated enzyme shows a normal oxidized flavin spectrum. The inactivation obtained with butynoyl pantotheine may be a case in which a nucleophile at the active site adds to an allenic intermediate.

The results obtained with the various flavoproteins indicate that acetylenic inactivators may be more versatile than we had originally anticipated. It now appears that acetylenic substrate analogues can inactivate through at least three different mechanisms:

1. Through allene formation followed by nucleophilic attack of a base on the allene:

$$-C{\equiv}C-\overset{H}{\underset{|}{C}}- \longrightarrow -\underset{H}{C}{=}C{=}C- \;(\text{N attacks central C}) \longrightarrow -C{=}\underset{N}{C}-\overset{H}{C}- \qquad (6)$$

2. Formation of the allenic anion followed by addition of this anion to an electrophile at the active site:

$$-C{\equiv}\overset{H}{C}-C- \longrightarrow -\overset{-}{C}{=}C{=}C- \;(\text{attacks } X{=}Y) \longrightarrow -\underset{X-YH}{C}{=}C{=}C- \qquad (7)$$

3. Oxidation of the inactivator to produce a compound containing an acetylynic group alpha-beta to a carbonyl group; the nucleophile then adds through a Michael-type addition:

$$-C{\equiv}C-\underset{X}{C}- \xrightarrow{[O]} -C{\equiv}C-\underset{\underset{X}{\|}}{C}- \;(\text{N attacks}) \longrightarrow -\underset{N}{C}{=}\overset{H}{C}-\underset{\underset{X}{\|}}{C}- \qquad (8)$$

The inactivation of γ-cystathionase by propargylglycine (I) has been studied in some detail (9). In this inactivation it appears reasonably certain that an intermediate allene is involved. γ-Cystathionase catalyzes the following reaction:

$$H_2O + XCH_2CH_2\underset{NH_3^+}{CH}COO^- \longrightarrow HX + CH_3CH_2\underset{\underset{O}{\|}}{C}COO^- + NH_4^- \qquad (9)$$

$$X = -SCH_2\underset{NH_3^+}{CH}COO^-;\ -OH$$

This enzyme probably operates as illustrated in Eq. (10). The enzyme has the ability to catalyze the abstraction of both the α and β hydrogens of the substrate and probably also facilitates the leaving of group X by protonation. A mechanism for the inactivation by propargylglycine (I) is shown by Eq. (11).

$$HC{\equiv}CCH_2\underset{^+NH_3}{CH}CO_2^- \qquad\qquad CH_2{=}\overset{Cl}{C}CH_2\underset{^+NH_3}{CH}CO_2^-$$

I II

The inactivation is based on the ability of the enzyme to abstract a β hydrogen and probably also its ability to deliver a proton near the terminal end of the molecule. Both of these capabilities are utilized in the normal catalytic process.

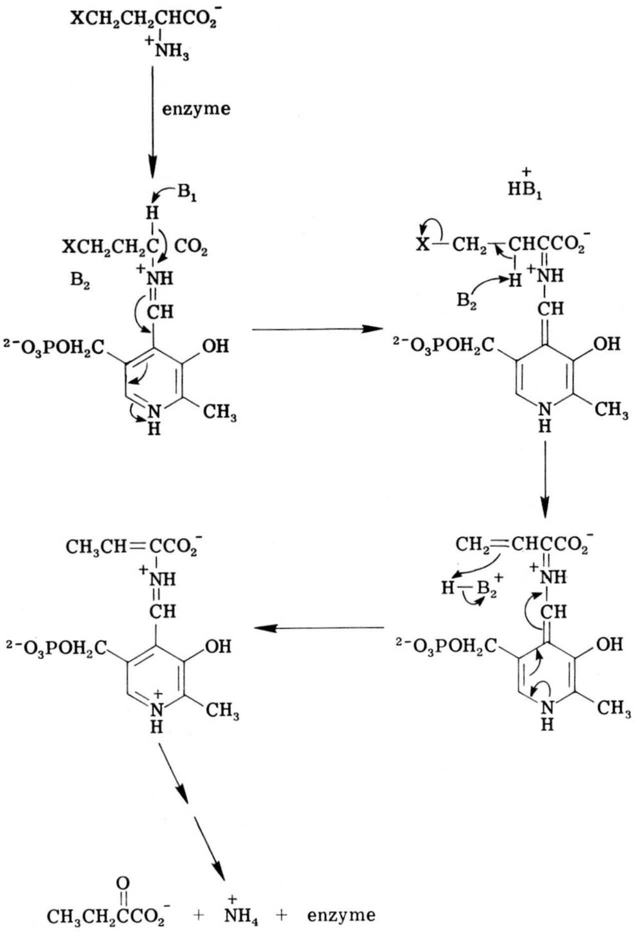

$XCH_2CH_2CHCO_2^-$ ($^+NH_3$)

enzyme

$$\text{XCH}_2\text{CH}_2\text{C(H)(CO}_2\text{)}{=}\overset{+}{\text{N}}\text{H}{=}\text{CH–Py} \;\longrightarrow\; \text{X–CH}_2\text{–CH–CCO}_2^-{=}\overset{+}{\text{N}}\text{H–CH}{=}\text{Py} \;\longrightarrow\; \text{CH}_2{=}\text{CHCCO}_2^-{=}\overset{+}{\text{N}}\text{H–CH}{=}\text{Py} \;\longrightarrow\; \text{CH}_3\text{CH}{=}\text{CCO}_2^-{=}\overset{+}{\text{N}}\text{H}{=}\text{CH–Py}$$

(10)

$$CH_3CH_2\overset{O}{\overset{\|}{C}}CO_2^- + \overset{+}{N}H_4 + \text{enzyme}$$

(B_1 and B_2 are nucleophilic groups of the enzyme)

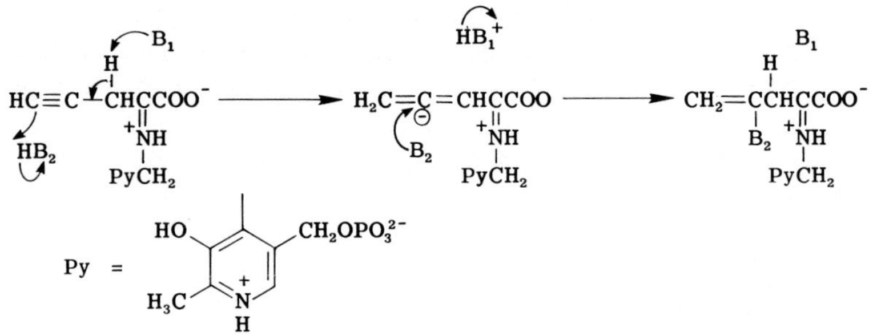

$$HC{\equiv}C{-}CHCCOO^-(=\overset{+}{N}H{-}PyCH_2) \longrightarrow H_2C{=}\overset{\ominus}{C}{=}CHCCOO(=\overset{+}{N}H{-}PyCH_2) \longrightarrow CH_2{=}C(B_2)CHCCOO^-(=\overset{+}{N}H{-}PyCH_2) \quad (11)$$

Py = 3-hydroxy-2-methyl-5-($CH_2OPO_3^{2-}$)pyridinium-4-yl (HO, H_3C, $\overset{+}{N}H$)

$$H_2C{=}C(Cl){-}CHCCOO^-(=\overset{+}{N}H{-}PyCH_2) \longrightarrow H_2C{=}C{=}CHCCOO^-(=\overset{+}{N}H{-}PyCH_2) \longrightarrow CH_2{=}C(B)CHCCOO^-(=\overset{+}{N}H{-}PyCH_2) \quad (12)$$

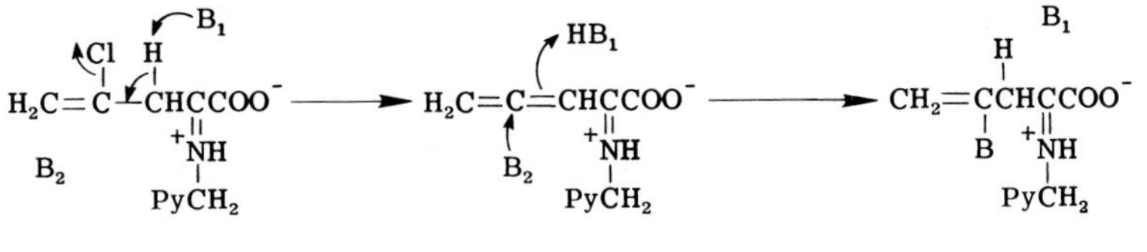

Compound II also inactivates the enzyme, probably through the mechanism shown in Eq. (12). Here the intermediate allene can be formed by the elimination of HC1 rather than through rearrangement of an acetylenic bond. This inactivation is based on the ability of the enzyme to catalyze the abstraction of a substrate β proton.

Through the efforts of several laboratories, acetylenic inactivators for many enzymes have now been developed. Some examples of enzymes which have been inactivated by acetylenic inactivators are:

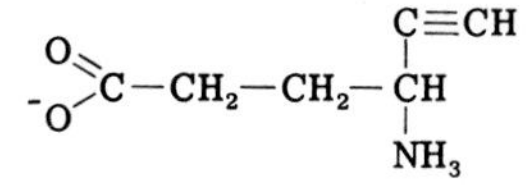

$$^{-}O(O=)C-CH_2-CH_2-CH(C\equiv CH)-NH_3$$

γ-Aminobutyric acid (GABA) transaminase (10) and glutamate decarboxylase

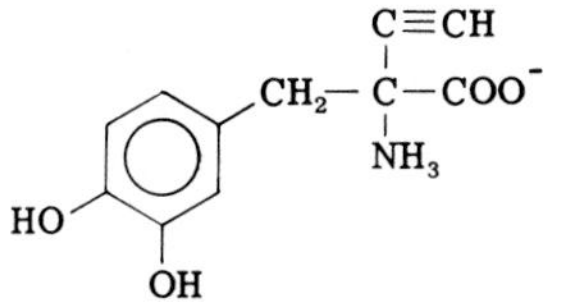

$$(3,4\text{-}HO)_2C_6H_3-CH_2-C(C\equiv CH)(NH_3)-COO^-$$

Dopa decarboxylase (11)

$$NH_2-CH(C\equiv CH)-(CH_2)_2-CH_2-NH_2$$

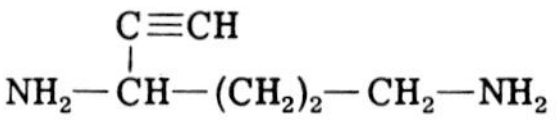

Ornithine decarboxylase (12)

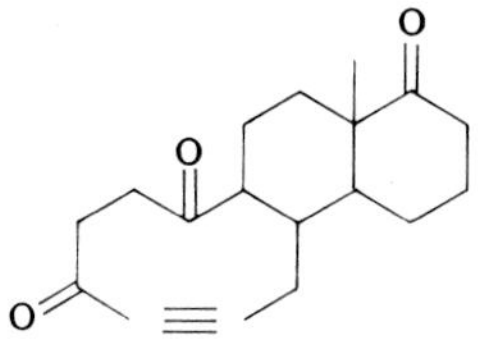

Δ^5-3-Ketosteroid isomerase (13,14)

It is unlikely that inactivators of decarboxylases operate through an allene mechanism. It is more probable that they operate through oxidation of the inactivator to produce a compound containing an acetylynic group alpha-beta to a carbonyl group followed by addition of the nucleophile through a Michael-type reaction.

There are a number of pyridoxal phosphate-dependent enzymes which catalyze β-elimination reactions:

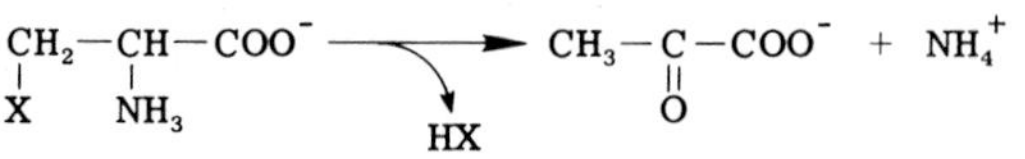

$$CH_2(X)-CH(NH_3)-COO^- \xrightarrow{-HX} CH_3-C(=O)-COO^- + NH_4^+ \qquad (13)$$

These reactions involve the following intermediate:

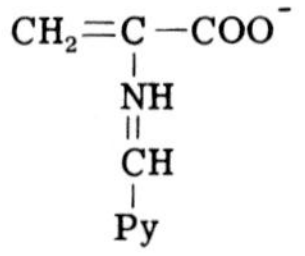

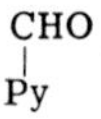

$$CH_2=C(COO^-)-NH=CH-Py \qquad\qquad Py-CHO = \text{pyridoxal phosphate}$$

This intermediate seems to be a reasonably reactive Michael acceptor and could therefore react with a nucleophile at the active site. However, these enzymes do not become inactive during catalysis, and therefore the intermediate is not a sufficiently reactive Michael acceptor, or no nucleophile is in the vicinity of the intermediate. We therefore undertook to modify the substrate so that the intermediate would become more susceptible to nucleophilic attack. Attachment of halogens to the β carbon should enhance the susceptibility to nucleophilic attack. Thus if these enzymes are allowed to act on β,β-dichloroalanine or β,β,β-trifluoroalanine, the following intermediates will be formed:

$$CHCl{=}C(NH{=}CH{-}Py){-}COO^- \qquad CF_2{=}C(NH{=}CH{-}Py){-}COO^-$$

These intermediates should then be subject to nucleophilic attack. We do not know at this stage whether our reasoning is correct, but polyhaloalanines inactivate a number of enzymes which catalyze β-elimination reactions (15,16).

The following mechanism was established for the inactivation of γ-cystathionase by trifluoroalanine:

$$F_3C{-}CH(NH_3^+){-}{}^{14}COO^- + CHO{-}Pyr \rightleftharpoons F_2C(F){-}CH(NH^+{=}CH{-}Pyr){-}{}^{14}COO^- \;(B:) \rightleftharpoons F_2C{=}C(NH^+{=}CH{-}Pyr){-}{}^{14}COO^- + F^- \;(B:)$$

$$\rightleftharpoons B{-}F_2C{-}C^{-}(NH^+{=}CH{-}Pyr){-}{}^{14}COO^- \xrightarrow[-2F^-]{H_2O} B{-}C(=O){-}C(=NH^+{-}CH^{-}{-}Pyr){-}{}^{14}COO^- \underset{}{\overset{H_3O^+}{\rightleftharpoons}} B{-}C(=O){-}CH(NH^+{=}CH{-}Pyr){-}{}^{14}COO^- \xrightarrow{-{}^{14}CO_2} B{-}C(=O){-}CH_2{-}NH^+{=}CH{-}Pyr \quad (14)$$

The inactivation is somewhat more complex than we had originally anticipated. The three fluorine atoms are lost, and the trifluoromethyl group is converted to an acyl group. This is probably advantageous, since it leads to the formation of a more stable bond than that which would be formed had the nucleophile simply added to the double bond formed through the elimination of the first fluoride. This mechanism is very similar to that proposed for the inactivation of thymidylate synthetase by trifluorothymidylic acid (17,18).

The following properties of the trifluoromethyl group make it a useful component of inactivators: (1) Fluorine is a relatively small atom and does not cause steric problems; in this respect, it is superior to chlorine which is large, and because of this chlorine-containing inactivators appear to bind poorly. (2) Elimination of fluoride alpha to a carbanion occurs relatively readily. (3) Hydrolysis can occur after addition of the nucleophile, so that an acyl group is finally formed and a relatively irreversible adduct is formed between inactivator and enzyme.

Although trifluoromethyl groups have proved useful in the inactivation of a number of enzymes, there are several examples where these compounds are ineffective. For instance, trifluoroalanine does not inactivate cystathionine synthase, although it is generally believed that the mechanism of action of this enzyme is very similar to that of other enzymes which catalyze β-eliminations and which are inactivated by trifluoroalanine. Similarly, neither GABA transaminase nor glutamate decarboxylase is inactivated by trifluoromethyl GABA, although on mechanistic grounds one might expect this compound to inactivate.

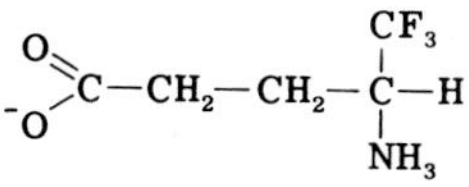

$$\begin{array}{c} O \\[-2pt] ^-O \end{array}\!\!>\!C-CH_2-CH_2-\overset{\displaystyle CF_3}{\underset{\displaystyle NH_3}{\overset{|}{\underset{|}{C}}}}-H$$

In spite of the fact that some compounds containing trifluoromethyl groups failed to inactivate as expected, it is very likely that many additional compounds can be synthesized which contain trifluoro and difluoromethyl groups which will be effective enzyme inactivators.

The inactivators discussed so far are based on enzyme mechanisms involving carbanionic intermediates. I would like to discuss one additional group of inactivators which are not dependent upon carbanion formation. These are inactivators based on cyclopropanone. We became aware of these inactivators through our studies on the mushroom toxin coprine (19). Coprine causes severe illness after ingestion of alcohol, probably as a result of the inhibition of aldehyde dehydrogenase. *In vitro,* coprine does not inhibit aldehyde dehydrogenase. *In vivo,* the compound is hydrolyzed to 1-hydroxy-1-aminocyclopropane and probably also to 1,1-dihydroxycyclopropane. Both of these compounds inhibit aldehyde dehydrogenase *in vitro*. Most of our studies were carried out with the dihydroxy compound. Before discussing a probable mechanism of inactivation, it will be useful to indicate the mechanism of action of aldehyde dehydrogenase.

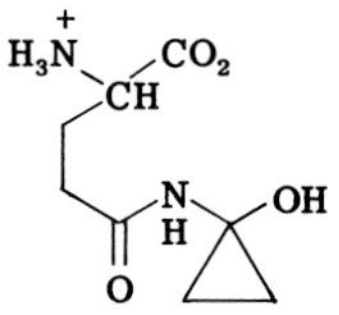

Coprine

Aldehyde oxidation is believed to involve initial interaction between a sulfhydryl group at the enzyme site and the aldehyde. The resulting thiohemiacetal is then oxidized:

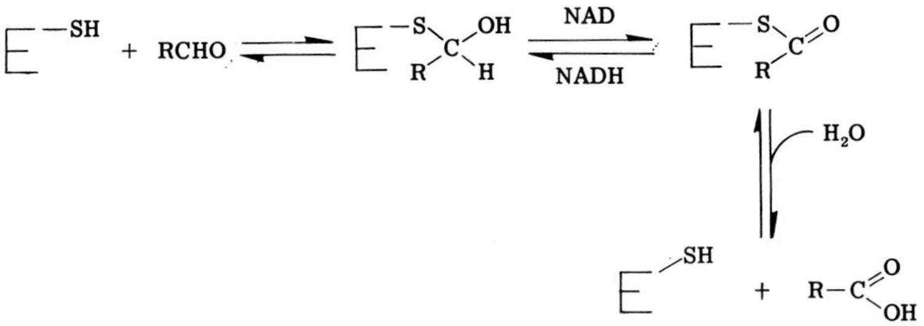

$$E{-}SH + RCHO \rightleftharpoons E{-}S{-}CH(OH)R \underset{NADH}{\overset{NAD}{\rightleftharpoons}} E{-}S{-}C(=O)R \overset{H_2O}{\rightleftharpoons} E{-}SH + R{-}C(=O)OH \quad (15)$$

The inactivation mechanism proposed for cyclopropane hydrate is very similar to the normal oxidation process: This type of inactivation may not, strictly speaking, involve suicide inactivation, since a nonenzyme-catalyzed conversion of cyclopropanone hydrate to cyclopropanone occurs. These compounds therefore also inactivate other sulfhydryl enzymes; i.e., there is lack of specificity. In addition, the inactivation is reversible with a $t_{1/2}$ of 4–5 days. It should also be pointed out that cyclopropane hydrate is effective *in vivo* and reduces the rate of acetaldehyde metabolism.

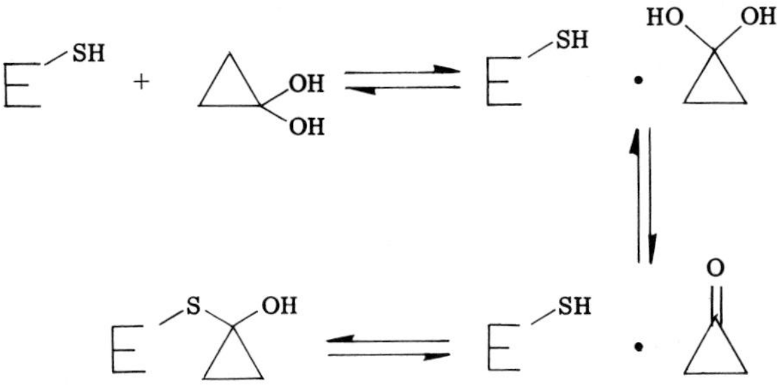

(16)

The mechanism established for the inactivation of aldehyde dehydrogenase may be applicable to the inactivation of other enzymes. Cyclopropylamine is known to inhibit monoamine oxidase and plasma amine oxidase. The mechanism of inactivation of these enzymes is unknown. The mechanism of inactivation of plasma amine oxidase is currently under investigation in our laboratory, and that of mitochondrial amine oxidase is being studied by Richard Silverman (Department of Chemistry, Northwestern University, Chicago, Illinois). Based on the evidence we have at this time, we postulate the following mechanism of inactivation for plasma amine oxidase:

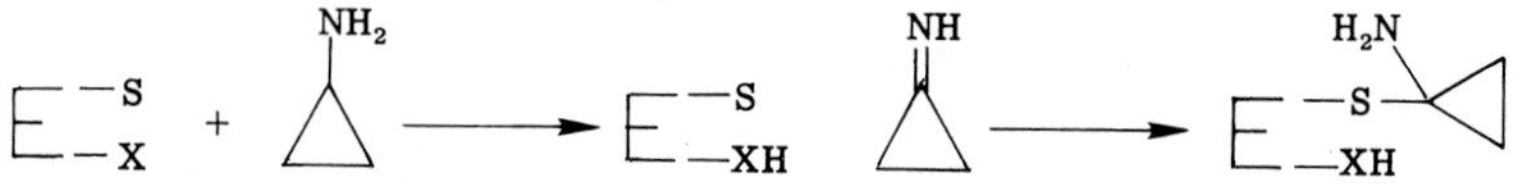

(17)

An early step in the inactivation is believed to be the oxidation of cyclopropylamine to cyclopropylimine. Evidence for this oxidation is provided by the occurrence of an isotope effect on the rate of inactivation by [1-^{2}H]cyclopropylamine. Inactivation occurs then by addition of a nucleophile to the imine.

Since cyclopropanone forms a stable adduct with nucleophiles, it seems that it should be useful as an inactivator for other enzymes. Peptides containing aldehyde analogues of amino acids are effective inhibitors (not inactivators) of proteolytic enzymes. For instance, Ac-Leu-Leu-phenylalaninale strongly inhibits chymotrypsin (20). It would be of interest to test analogous peptides containing a cyclopropanone hydrate moiety. These peptides may have two advantages over the aldehydic inhibitor: (1) They might bind more tightly; and (2) unlike the aldehydic peptides, they are not subject to oxidation and would therefore be more useful *in vivo*.

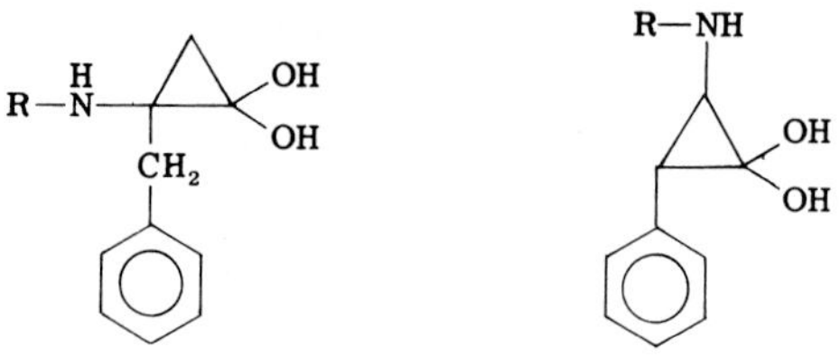

Analogues containing the cyclopropane hydrate structure

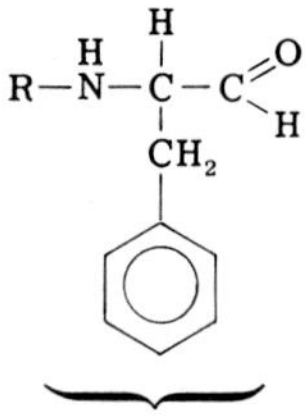

Ac-Leu-Leu-phenylalaninale

References

1. E. Shaw, *in* "The Enzymes" (P. D. Boyer, ed.), 3rd ed., Vol. 1, p. 91. Academic Press, New York, 1970.
2. K. Bloch, *in* "The Enzymes" (P. D. Boyer, ed.), 3rd ed., Vol. 5, p. 441. Academic Press, New York, 1971.

3. M. Morisaki and K. Bloch, *Biochemistry* **11,** 309 (1972).
4. R. C. Hevey, J. Babson, A. L. Maycock, and R. H. Abeles, *J. Am. Chem. Soc.* **95,** 6125 (1973).
5. S. Ghisla, H. Ogata, V. Massey, A. Schonbrunn, and R. H. Abeles, *Biochemistry* **15,** 1791 (1976).
6. A. Schonbrunn, R. H. Abeles, C. T. Walsh, S. Ghisla, H. Ogata, and V. Massey, *Biochemistry* **15,** 1798 (1976).
7. A. L. Maycock, R. H. Abeles, J. I. Salach, and T. P. Singer, *Biochemistry* **15,** 114 (1976).
8. B. Gomes and R. H. Abeles, unpublished.
9. W. Washtein and R. H. Abeles, *Biochemistry* **16,** 2485 (1977).
10. M. J. Jung and B. W. Metcalf, *Biochem. Biophys. Res. Commun.* **67,** 301 (1975).
11. A. Maycock, S. D. Aster, and A. A. Patchett, *in* "Drug Design: Mechanism-Based Enzyme Inhibitors" (T. I. Kalman, ed.), p. 115. Am. Elsevier, New York, 1979.
12. B. W. Metcalf and P. Casara, *Tetrahedron Lett.* p. 3337 (1975).
13. F. H. Batzold and C. H. Robinson, *J. Am. Chem. Soc.* **97,** 2576 (1975).
14. F. H. Batzold and C. H. Robinson, *J. Org. Chem.* **41,** 313 (1976).
15. R. B. Silverman and R. H. Abeles, *Biochemistry* **16,** 5515 (1977).
16. R. B. Silverman and R. H. Abeles, *Biochemistry* **15,** 4718 (1976).
17. T. T. Sakai and D. V. Santi, *J. Med. Chem.* **16,** 1079 (1973).
18. D. V. Santi and T. T. Sakai, *Biochemistry* **10,** 3598 (1971).
19. J. S. Wiseman and R. H. Abeles, *Biochemistry* **18,** 427 (1979).
20. A. Ito, K. Tokawa, and B. Shimizu, *Biochem. Biophys. Res. Commun.* **49,** 343 (1972).
21. R. R. Rando, *Science* **185,** 320–324 (1974).
22. R. R. Rando, *Acc. Chem. Res.* **8,** 281–288 (1975).
23. R. R. Rando, *Biochem. Pharmacol.* **24,** 1153–1160 (1975).
24. C. T. Walsh, *Horiz. in Biochem. and Biophys.* **3,** 36–81 (1977).
25. N. Seiler, M. J. Jung, and J. Koch-Weser (eds.). "Enzyme-Activated Irreversible Inhibitors," Elsevier North Holland. Biomedical Press (1978).
26. R. H. Abeles and A. L. Maycock, *Acc. Chem. Res.* **9,** 313–319 (1976).

PART II

Antibiotics

6

DNA Dynamics and Drug Intercalation

HENRY M. SOBELL

I. Introduction

What is the dynamic nature of DNA (and double-helical RNA) structure that gives rise to drug intercalation? How does this same dynamic structure give rise to DNA breathing—the transient disruption of hydrogen bonding between base pairs at temperatures well below the melting temperature [as evidenced, for example, by tritium exchange (1,2), formaldehyde reactivity (3,4), and polarographic studies (5,6)]—and how are these premelting changes related to melting at elevated temperatures?

More generally, how is the subject of DNA premelting related to understand-

MOLECULAR ACTIONS AND TARGETS FOR CANCER CHEMOTHERAPEUTIC AGENTS

ISBN 0-12-619280-4

ing protein–DNA interactions? For example, what is the nature of the promoter and how does the RNA polymerase recognize and bind to the promoter? What about single-strand-specific DNA-binding proteins—Do their interactions with DNA involve intercalation and if so why? What do nucleases "see" when they cleave DNA and, related to this, why—in eukaryotic chromatin—are active genes about five times more nuclease-sensitive than inactive genes? Is DNA in active genes, ribosomal genes in particular, held by histones in a conformation *different* from the Watson–Crick structure? Does this give rise to the differential nuclease sensitivity and to the selective inhibition of RNA synthesis by actinomycin and echinomycin?

Here we describe our theory for understanding the dynamic nature of DNA and RNA structure in solution. Although primarily a structural theory designed to provide insight into the mechanism of drug intercalation and DNA breathing, phenomena collectively known as premelting phenomena, the theory makes important additional predictions concerning the nonuniformity in the magnitude of energy fluctuations in different regions of DNA—this reflects the presence of acoustic phonons in its structure and the heterogeneity in DNA flexibility associated with different stacking energies that stabilize various combinations of nucleotide sequences. We will review the physical nature of this effect and its biological implications here.

We begin by envisioning DNA in solution to be continuously bombarded by solvent molecules along its length. Although the vast majority of these solvent collisions transfer energy into the polymer to give rise to anharmonic motions in its structure that eventually dissipate energy back into solution as a result of viscous damping, occasionally solvent molecules with the appropriate momentum (i.e., having their directions oriented along the dyad axes in DNA) collide with DNA, and this gives rise to harmonic motion in the polymer.

By harmonic motion we mean specific normal mode oscillations in DNA structure that either remain localized to a site (to produce a conformational change) or travel along the helix at the speed of sound in the form of normal mode waves. At low amplitudes, these harmonic motions cause DNA to oscillate between B DNA and a right-handed superhelical variant of B DNA that contains approximately 10 bp per turn and has a pitch of about 34 Å. Such structures balance the unwinding in the helix with right-handed superhelical writhe to keep the linkage invariant, a feature that creates minimal perturbation in DNA structure. Higher-amplitude harmonic motions give rise to similar structures, except that these contain somewhat more than 10 bp per turn and have base pairs inclined more acutely to the helix axis. Their presence could contribute to the apparent net unwinding of DNA and the altered tilt of base pairs relative to the helix axis—features observed for DNA in solution (7,8). At small amplitudes of oscillation, DNA behaves as an elastic body that accumulates strain energy in its structure through small changes in torsional angles that define the geometry of the sugar–phosphate backbone. These changes are localized primarily in the furanose rings of alternate deoxyribose sugar residues (normally, the puckering of the furanose ring in B DNA is C-2′ *endo;* however, the effect of introducing strain energy into the helix is to alter the magnitude and direction of this puckering). At larger amplitudes of oscillation, the enhanced strain energy in the sugar–phosphate chains begins to flatten out the furanose ring. Finally, at some critical oscillation amplitude, alternate sugars "snap" into a C-3′ *endo* sugar conformation with a concomitant partial unstacking of base pairs. This structure (denoted β-kinked DNA) corresponds to an inelastic distortion in DNA structure and arises from a transient high-energy normal mode oscillation in the helix localized at a specific site. Such a structure is hyperflexible and therefore experiences enhanced energy fluctuations during its lifetime—this reflects the presence of acoustic phonons associated with traveling normal mode waves in DNA. The energy from these fluctuations can be used to further separate base pairs (so as to allow drugs and dyes to intercalate into DNA) and to rupture hydrogen bonds connecting base pairs (as occurs in DNA breathing). We have qualitatively described structural aspects of these processes elsewhere (9–11).

Here we document these conformational changes in greater detail. Using a linked-atom least squares approach for building and refining nucleic acid structures with defined stereochemistry (12,13), we are able to follow the structural intermediates involved in drug intercalation and DNA breathing. An important related question concerns the structural nature of the B $\rightleftharpoons$ A transition in DNA, which we now describe.

II. The B $\rightleftharpoons$ A Transition in DNA

It has been known for many years that a variety of naturally occurring and synthetic DNA polymers can exist in two major families of double-helical structures, the A and B families (14,15). Although considerable variation exists within each family, members of the B family of helices all contain C-2′ *endo* sugar residues in the high anti conformation, while members of the A family all contain C-3′ *endo* sugar residues in the low anti conformation. The B $\rightleftharpoons$ A transition occurs in all naturally occurring DNA preparations and in most synthetic DNA polymers. First detected in oriented fibers of Na DNA at 75% relative humidity by X-ray diffraction (16), the transition has also been observed in 70–80% ethanol–water mixtures with a variety of other physical techniques (15,17–20). The transition occurs over a narrow range of humidity and ethanol–water concentrations and is highly cooperative. Cross-linking DNA by photodimerization inhibits the B $\rightleftharpoons$ A transition, as do a variety of intercalative drugs and dyes.

What is the structural nature of the B $\rightleftharpoons$ A transition? Here we show that it is

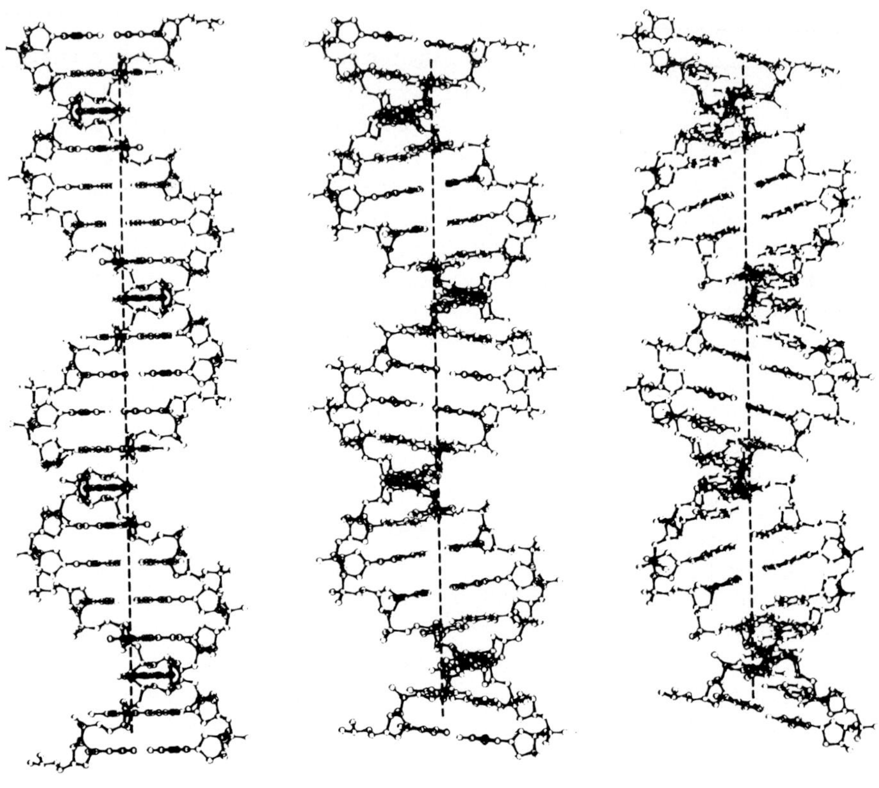

A

Fig. 1A. Conformational intermediates in the B ⇌ A transition as computed by linked-atom least squares energy minimization methods. The key structural intermediate in the B ⇌ A transition is β-kinked DNA; this structure (shown on the far right) has a dinucleotide with a mixed C-3′ endo (3′–5′) C-2′ endo sugar puckering as the asymmetric unit and has helical parameters that lie midway between B and A DNA. The transition from B DNA to β-kinked DNA shown here corresponds to a low-frequency normal mode oscillation in B DNA structure. See text for further discussion.

possible to deform B DNA to A DNA continuously along a minimum energy pathway by changing the dihedral angles that define the geometry of the sugar–phosphate backbone. These changes primarily occur in the furanose rings of *alternate* deoxyribose sugar residues. Levitt and Warshel (21) have shown that both ribose and deoxyribose sugar rings are extremely flexible, having stable energy minima at C-2′ *endo* and C-3′ *endo* sugar conformations. The barrier separating these conformations is about 0.5 kcal/mole, a value well below the normal C—C single-bond energy barrier (i.e., 2–3 kcal/mole, in most cases)

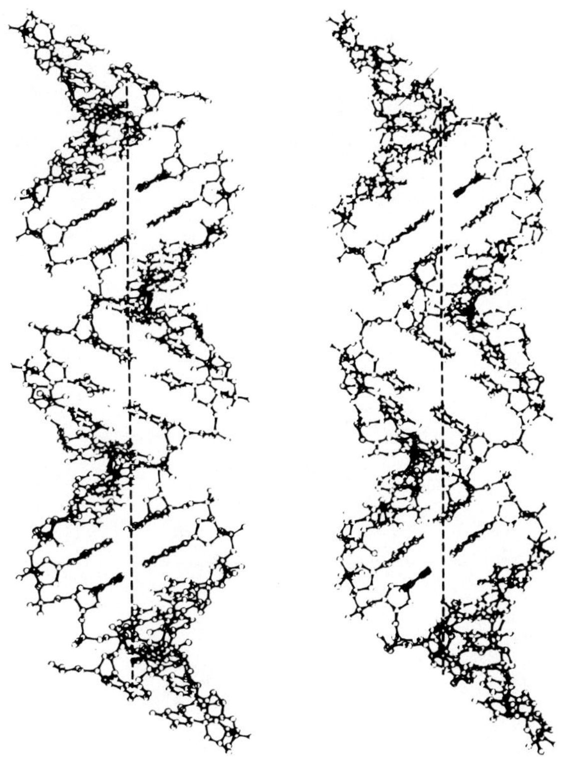

Fig. 1A. (*continued*)

and, for this reason, conformational changes in both DNA and RNA are expected to involve alterations in sugar puckering as well as in torsional angles describing the phosphodiester region of the sugar–phosphate backbone.

Figure 1 shows the conformational intermediates calculated for the B $\rightleftharpoons$ A transition using linked-atom least squares energy minimization methods. A key structural intermediate in the B $\rightleftharpoons$ A transition is β-kinked DNA; this structure has a dinucleotide with the mixed C-3′ *endo* (3′−5′) C-2′ *endo* sugar puckering as an asymmetric unit and has helical parameters that lie midway between B and A DNA. Preliminary calculations suggest its energy to be intermediate between that of B and A structures and to fall in a local minimum—β-kinked DNA therefore could be a metastable intermediate in the B $\rightleftharpoons$ A transition pathway. (It is important to note, however, that these calculations involve the poly(dA-dT)$_n$ polymer sequence kinked at pTpA; we are expanding our calculations to include other DNA sequences and will report on these at a later time.) Although the B $\rightleftharpoons$ A transition has been calculated as a uniform transition simultaneously involving the entire polymer length (20 bp of which are shown in Fig. 1), we envision a

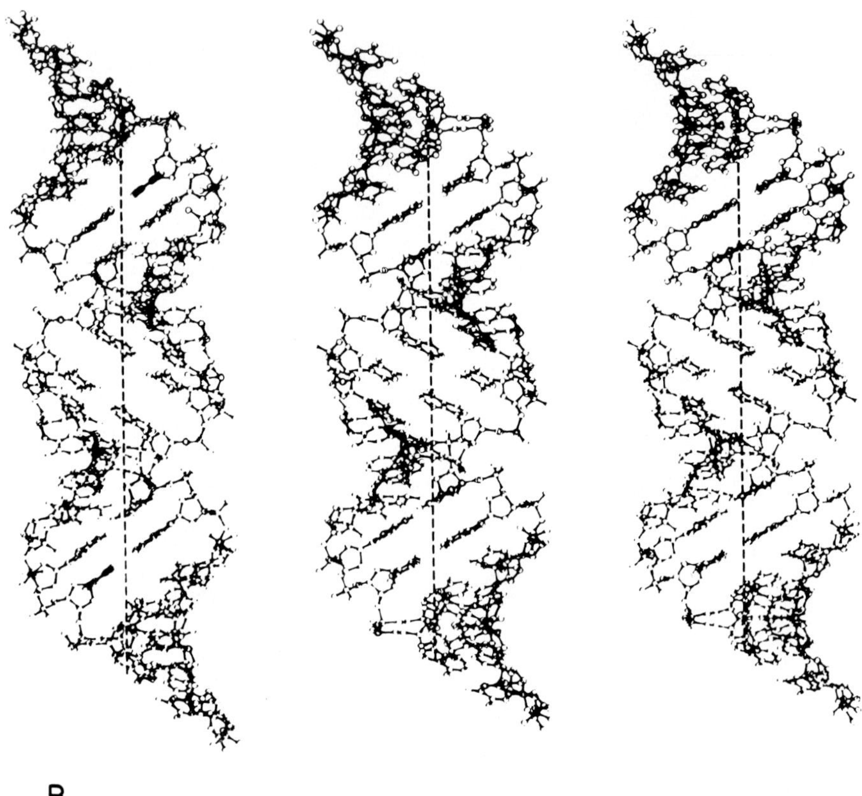

B

Fig. 1B. Transition from β-kinked DNA to A DNA conformation as computed by linked-atom least squares energy minimization methods. This series of conformational changes forms as the result of a low-frequency normal mode oscillation in A DNA structure. Double-stranded RNA may possess a similar low-frequency normal mode oscillation in its structure that gives rise to a conformational change from A (or A′) RNA to β-kinked RNA; this would subsequently allow double-helical RNA to undergo drug intercalation into its structure.

gradation of structures connecting B DNA with A DNA to serve as dynamic interfaces connecting the two. A moving structure such as this could leave behind either B or A DNA, depending on the relative stabilities of these forms under given conditions.

The pathway from B DNA to β-kinked DNA (and the pathway from A DNA to β-kinked DNA) shown in Fig. 1 reflects a specific low-frequency normal mode oscillation in B DNA (and A DNA) structure that is excited by thermal fluctuations. Double-stranded RNA may possess a similar low-frequency normal mode oscillation in its structure that gives rise to a conformational change from A (or A′) RNA to β-kinked RNA—this would subsequently allow double-helical RNA

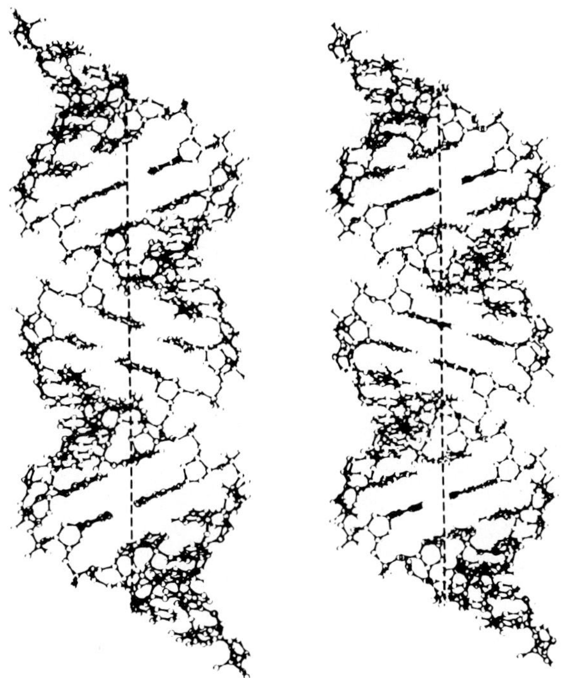

Fig. 1B. (*continued*)

to undergo drug intercalation into its structure (see Sections III and IV). The conversion of β-kinked RNA to the B structure may not be possible for steric reasons. We are therefore computing the A (or A′) $\rightleftharpoons$ B transition for double-helical RNA as well and will describe the results of these calculations elsewhere.

III. β-Kinked DNA $\rightleftharpoons$ β-Intercalated DNA Conformational Changes

A key property of the β-kinked DNA structure is its flexibility; this readily allows it to undergo further lengthening and unwinding to form the β-intercalated structure (see Fig. 2). These changes primarily involve alterations in the glycosidic torsional angles of the nucleotides, although a series of other minor changes occur in the torsional angles defining the phosphodiester region of the sugar–phosphate backbone. The β-kinked DNA $\rightleftharpoons$ β-intercalated DNA transition is accompanied by a monotonic rise in energy without any intervening energy minimum and corresponds to a second low-frequency (i.e., acoustic) normal mode oscillation in DNA structure that can be excited by thermal energies.

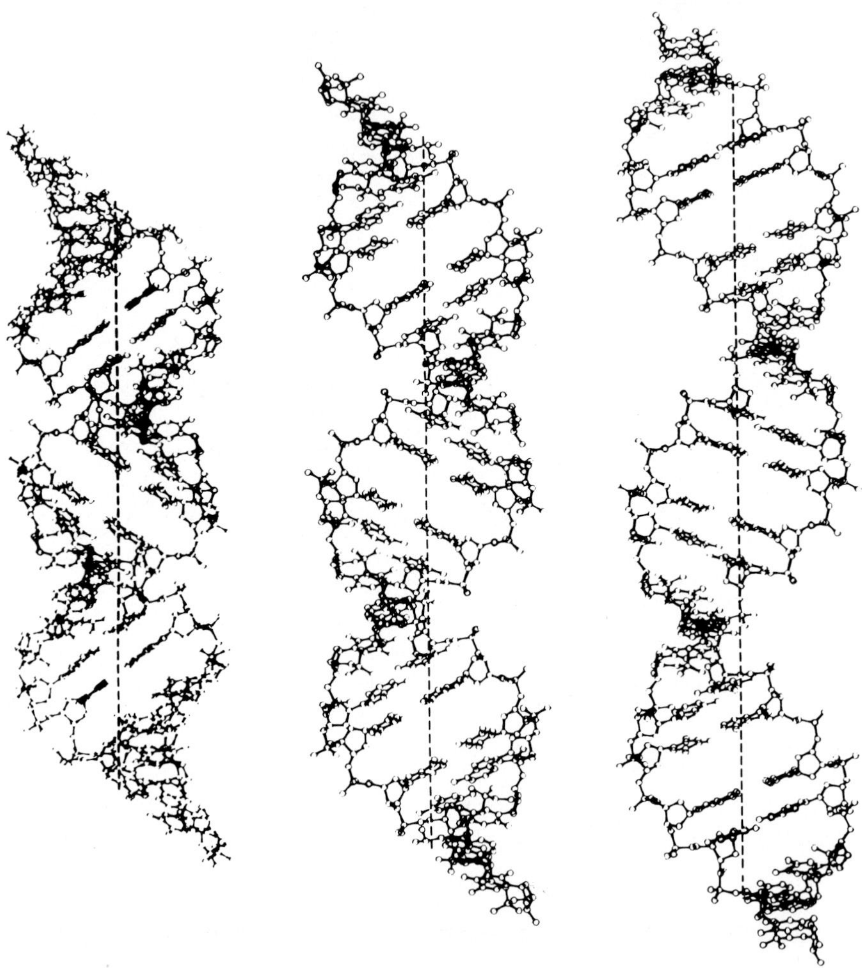

Fig. 2. Conformational intermediates in the β-kinked DNA$\rightleftharpoons$-intercalated DNA transition as computed by linked atom least squares energy minimization methods. These intermediate structures correspond to a specific low-frequency normal mode oscillation in the β-kinked DNA structure.

IV. Compound Normal Mode Oscillations in DNA Structure That Give Rise to Mono- and Bifunctional Drug Intercalation

The information described above has allowed us to compute the compound normal mode oscillations in DNA structure that give rise to the stereochemistries necessary for drug intercalation (both mono- and bifunctional) and DNA breath-

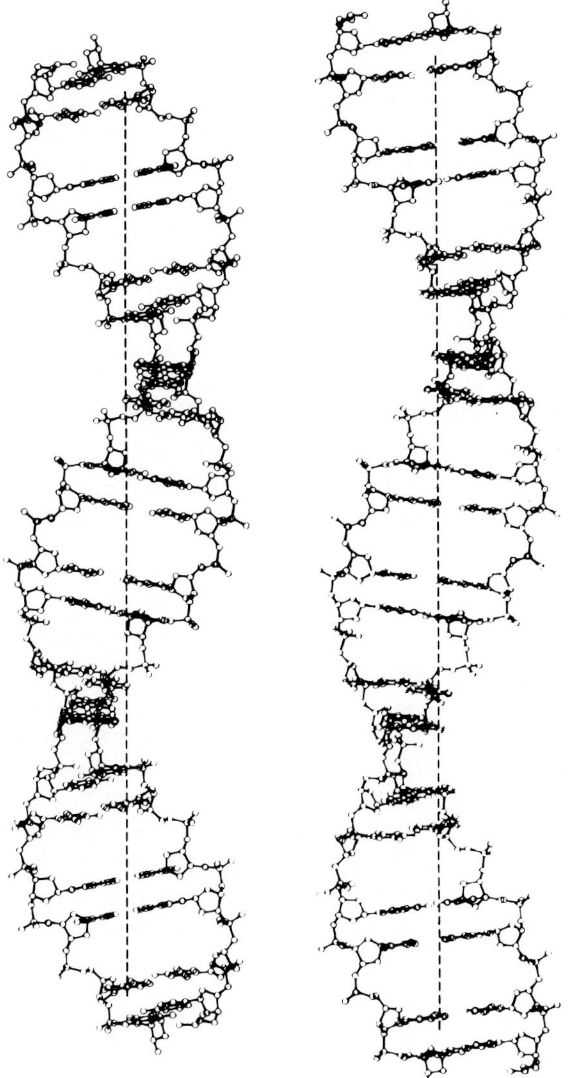

Fig. 2. *(continued)*

ing. These calculations are in progress, and we cannot yet describe them in detail. However, one can obtain considerable insight into this by considering an analogous problem in mechanics in the macroscopic domain.

Let us consider the example of an aluminum rod that is hit by a hammer perpendicular to its long axis at some initial time. If the momentum transferred by the hammer to the rod does not exceed its elastic limit, the rod undergoes (elastic) deformation at the point of impact, and this gives rise to a series of elastic traveling waves having different frequencies. If the rod is finite in length, these elastic traveling waves rebound from the ends and undergo subsequent constructive and destructive interference events. As time proceeds, a standing wave having a defined frequency emerges (i.e., the rod "rings"), and this vibration (along with its overtones) corresponds to a specific normal mode excited in this system.

If, however, the rod in this example is infinite in length, no such normal modes will appear; the elastic traveling waves created by the impact of the hammer on the rod will simply continue to travel along the rod to infinity. This second example is more relevant to DNA. Here elastic traveling waves take the form of normal mode waves that continuously appear as a result of fluctuations (as explained earlier, these appear because of a specific class of solvent collisions with DNA—collisions that strike DNA down its dyad axis). These normal mode waves are associated with the presence of acoustic phonons that travel along the polymer at the speed of sound, eventually undergoing viscous damping. For this reason, DNA is not expected to undergo normal modes (as defined in the classic sense) in aqueous solution.

What happens if the momentum transferred by the hammer to the rod exceeds some elastic limit? The rod bends, that is, undergoes a structural change at the point of impact—an event known as inelastic deformation. If the structural defect associated with this bend creates a hyperflexible joint (i.e., crack), elastic energy that exists on either side of the defect will migrate into this hyperflexible region and snap the rod—an event known as a recoil phenomenon. With DNA, an occasional "hot" solvent collision could excite a normal mode oscillation in the B helix whose amplitude exceeds the elastic limit of the polymer (in Section V, however, we describe how multiple fluctuations can transiently concentrate energy at flexible regions of DNA because of the presence of acoustic phonons to effect a conformational change, and we consider this to be the more probable explanation); this gives rise to either the single- or double-kinked (that is, β-kinked) DNA structures. Both structures contain hyperflexible joints (i.e., kinks) into which elastic energy can migrate; this elastic energy partially arises from the initial "hot" solvent collison with DNA (i.e., the recoil phenomenon) and from energies from other fluctuations that occur along the polymer at different times and arrive in the form of acoustic phonons. This additional (elastic) energy can be used to further separate base pairs (to allow drugs and dyes to intercalate into DNA) and to rupture hydrogen bonds connecting base pairs (as occurs in DNA breathing)—motions that characterize the normal mode oscillation in the β-kinked DNA structure (see Section III). Both types of normal mode oscillations (i.e., B DNA $\rightleftharpoons$ β-kinked DNA and β-kinked DNA $\rightleftharpoons$ β-intercalated DNA) act to produce the series of conformational changes necessary for mono- and bifunctional drug intercalation; we therefore refer to these as compound normal mode oscillations in DNA structure that give rise to drug intercalation and DNA breathing.

In the rod analogy, the term "inelastic deformation" has been used to describe a permanent structural deformation associated with net work done on the system. Of course, for DNA in solution, fluctuations produce only transient work on the polymer; DNA kinking is a reversible process having forward and backward rate constants. The reversibility of this process reflects the small energies involved in this conformational change and—related to this—maintenance of the covalent integrity of the sugar–phosphate backbone.

Computations describing the compound normal mode oscillations in DNA structure involve combining a gradation of structural information from the B DNA $\rightleftharpoons$ β-kinked DNA and the β-kinked DNA $\rightleftharpoons$ β-intercalated DNA transitions. Similar calculations are being carried out to understand the dynamic nature of double-helical RNA structure. We will describe the results of these computations elsewhere.

V. The Influence of Acoustic Phonons on the Magnitude of Energy Fluctuations in DNA

An important consequence of the presence of acoustic phonons in DNA structure is the altered nature of energy fluctuations along the helix at equilibrium. This is because, when calculating the magnitude of energy fluctuations at specific places on DNA, one has to take into account not only fluctuations that arise locally at this site but in addition fluctuations that occur at a distance and then travel to this site in the form of acoustic phonons. Since DNA is a heterogeneous polymer—having variable flexibility as a result of different stacking energies between base pairs in different sequences—it follows (see below), that the probability that a specific region will experience a fluctuation with a given energy depends on the elasticity of this region and of neighboring regions. Generally, more flexible DNA regions experience larger energy fluctuations; the magnitude of these enhanced fluctuations increases the probability that transient DNA conformational change can occur (i.e., B DNA $\rightleftharpoons$ β-kinked DNA) and that, once formed, this conformationally altered DNA structure will experience still larger energy fluctuations (i.e., β-kinked DNA $\rightleftharpoons$ β-intercalated DNA).

We have already described the physical nature of this effect and its biological importance in several previous publications (22,23). We describe one of our more recent treatments of this effect here (24).

The general expression for fluctuations in condensed matter is

$$\Delta w^2 = -[kT(\partial P/\partial T)_V - P]^2 kT(\partial V/\partial P)_T + C_V(kT)^2$$

where Δw^2 is the mean squared energy fluctuation, T is the absolute temperature, P is the pressure, V is the volume, k is Boltzmann's constant and C_V is the heat capacity (25).

To calculate Δw^2, we will need to calculate the free energy, which is given by

$$F = N\epsilon_0 + kT\sum_{\alpha} \ln (1 - e^{-\hbar\omega_\alpha kT})$$

where N is the number of base pairs, ϵ_0 is the interaction energy per base pair at equilibrium, and ω_α are characteristic frequencies of longitudinal lattice oscilations.

For a linear polymer, the number of eigenvalue oscillations in the interval of wave vector dk is equal to

$$Na(dk/2\pi) = Na\ (d\omega/2\pi u)$$

where a is the lattice constant (i.e., for DNA, this corresponds to 3.4 Å) and u is the velocity of longitudinal phonons ($u = \omega/k$).

For temperatures well below the Debye temperature, low frequencies (i.e., acoustic phonons) play a predominant role in determining the free energy. In this approximation, we obtain

$$F = N\epsilon_0 + kT(Na/2\pi u) \int_0^\infty \ln (1 - e^{-\hbar\omega\, kT}) d\omega = N\epsilon_0 - Na\ (\pi(kT)^2/12\hbar u)$$

and therefore

$$C_V = (\partial/\partial T)[F - kT(\partial F/\partial T)] = Na(\pi(kT)^2/12\hbar u)$$

For qualitative estimates, we can consider the volume of DNA to be constant. Then

$$\Delta w^2 = Na\ \pi(kT)^3/6\hbar u$$

In DNA, the velocity of longitudinal phonons is given by $u = \sqrt{E/\rho}$, where E is Young's modulus and ρ is the linear density of DNA. Although ρ is approximately constant along the polymer, E is not, because of different stacking energies for A-T and G-C base pairs (26). For this reason, phonons travel along the DNA molecule with nonuniform velocities. This gives rise to larger magnitude energy fluctuations in the regions of the polymer having greatest flexibility.

VI. Does DNA Have Two Structures That Coexist at Equilibrium?

What is the structure of DNA in solution at equilibrium? Is it only B DNA? We have proposed that DNA has *two* discrete structures in dynamical equilibrium—B DNA and β-kinked DNA (22, 23). Drugs and dyes intercalate into the β-kinked

DNA structure. In addition to the transient formation of β-kinked DNA at different points along the polymer, specific regions of DNA could become permanently β-kinked—this being a function of temperature. Here, β-kinked DNA corresponds to a second-order phase transition in the polymer—different regions of DNA undergoing this transition at different temperatures. Because of their enhanced flexibility, these regions could be particularly prone to undergo DNA breathing motions (i.e., further base unstacking and hydrogen bond breakage). The energies for these breathing motions arise from both local fluctuations and fluctuations originating in neighboring regions that propagate energy in the form of acoustic phonons along DNA.

Regions of second-order phase transition such as these could serve to nucleate DNA melting at higher temperatures. They may also have an important biological function—they may serve as binding sites for a variety of protein–DNA interactions. We will now describe these and other related concepts.

VII. Protein-DNA Interactions

A. RNA Polymerase-Promoter Recognition

What is the nature of the promoter and how does the RNA polymerase recognize and bind to it?

We propose that the promoter is in fact a region of DNA that has undergone a second-order phase transition in its structure (i.e., β-kinked DNA, as described above) and that the recognition and attachment of RNA polymerase for promoter regions reflects this. Thus RNA polymerase may bind to the promoter by intercalating—either partially or completely—aromatic side chains into DNA and, in addition, by interacting with specific nucleotide bases and sugar–phosphate groups through hydrogen bonds, van der Waals interactions, and electrostatic interactions as it forms the tight binding complex.

An important feature of our model is the prediction that DNA exists in an altered premelted form at the promoter. Another key prediction is that this same structure accompanies RNA polymerase as it moves along the DNA template synthesizing RNA chains (i.e., this corresponds to the "bubble" often shown in schematic illustrations of RNA polymerization). Our model predicts therefore that intercalative drugs and dyes interfere with RNA synthesis in at least two ways: first, by binding to the promoter to interfere with the initiation of new RNA chains, and second, by binding to the β-kinked DNA structure traveling with the RNA polymerase enzyme to interfere with the elongation of growing RNA chains. Evidence that ethidium does in fact interfere with both the initiation and the elongation of RNA chains has already appeared (27).

B. Single-Strand-Specific DNA-Binding Proteins

How do the single-strand-specific DNA binding proteins (i.e., T4 gene *32* protein, fd gene *5* protein) bind to DNA? Do their interactions with single-stranded DNA involve intercalation and if so why? What is the structure of single-stranded DNA when it interacts with these DNA-binding proteins?

Our model predicts that single-stranded DNA assumes a premelted structure during DNA unwinding with the following structural characteristics: a perfectly alternating pattern of sugar puckering down the polynucleotide backbone (i.e., C-3′ *endo* (3′ − 5′) C-2′ *endo* (3′ − 5′) C-3′ *endo*, and so on), with (potential) intercalating spaces between every other nucleotide base. This being the case, single-strand-specific DNA-binding proteins will almost certainly intercalate (either partially or completely) aromatic amino acid side chains between the bases when binding to DNA. In addition, other interactions will utilize hydrogen bonding, van der Waals interactions, and electrostatic interactions—interactions all centered on recognizing structural features of the premelted single-stranded DNA structure we have postulated.

C. Nuclease Specificity and the Organization of DNA in Chromatin

What do nucleases "see" when they cleave DNA and, related to this, why, in eukaryotic chromatin, are active genes some five times more nuclease-sensitive than inactive genes? Is DNA in active genes, ribosomal genes in particular, held by histones in a conformation *different* from the Watson–Crick structure, and does this give rise to the differential nuclease sensitivity and to the selective inhibition of ribosomal RNA synthesis by actinomycin and echinomycin?

Transcriptionally active chromatin has been shown to be particularly sensitive to pancreatic DNase digestion—active genes being digested between four and five times faster than inactive genes (28–30). DNA in active genes appears to remain bound to histones, as evidenced by staphylococcal nuclease limit digest studies (31) and measurements of the thickness of chromatin fibers actively undergoing RNA transcription (about 70 Å wide) (32). There is no evidence for a beaded structure in (ribosomal) transcriptionally active chromatin—rather, the structure appears to be an extended one in which the DNA exists in some state particularly sensitive to pancreatic DNase.

We have wondered whether this state is β-kinked DNA. If pancreatic DNase recognizes kinks in DNA (see below), then it would digest this structure approximately five times faster than κ-kinked DNA (a time-averaged structure we postulate to exist in inactive chromatin). Since β-kinked DNA has an axial repeat length similar to that of B DNA, the chromatin fiber could be extended about the same length as that predicted assuming B DNA in these regions. Finally, gene activation could be achieved along the lines originally suggested by Weintraub *et al.* (33), in which the histone–DNA complex exists as a linear structure (active chromatin) or a helical structure (inactive chromatin). The flip-flop interconversion of these forms could convert the left-handed superhelical writhe in the κ helix into unwinding in the β helix, this unwinding being localized at the kinks. Such a mechanism could allow control of premelting changes in DNA necessary for RNA transcription.

Inactive chromatin is now established to consist of a beaded structure in which DNA is complexed to each of four histones (H2a, H2b, H3, H4). Each bead is an octamer of histones complexed to 140 bp, most likely, as a left-handed superhelix around the periphery of the histone core (34). An important observation concerns the pancreatic DNase digestion patterns observed from inactive chromatin—this demonstrates periodicities of approximate integral multiples of 10 nucleotide bases (i.e., fragments 10, 20, 30, . . . up to 300 have been observed), suggesting the presence of nuclease-sensitive sites periodically located every 10 bp. In more recent experiments, Lutter (35) has demonstrated this repeat to be somewhat variable but centered at 10.4 bp on the average.

We have postulated these sites to be kinks. The kink could serve as a substrate for both pancreatic DNase and splenic acid DNase II (these nucleases could partially intercalate into DNA, positioning these enzymes along the dyad axis of the kink to effect staggered cleavage about this symmetry axis). A kink placed every 10 bp in DNA gives rise to a left-handed superhelical structure with approximately the same dimensions as the nucleosome. We have postulated this structure (denoted κ-kinked DNA) or, more precisely, a time-averaged structure of this type, to exist in the organization of DNA in inactive chromatin.

VIII. Conclusion

The subject of drug intercalation is a multidimensional one, concerned with understanding the dynamic structure of DNA in solution and the molecular basis of its flexibility. Our X-ray crystallographic studies of drug intercalation have allowed us to propose unifying structural models to understand a large number of drug–DNA (and drug–RNA) interactions; these models have led us to formulate further dynamic concepts of DNA structure that give rise to drug intercalation. The phenomenon of drug intercalation is more broadly related to DNA breathing (or DNA premelting) and involves a second DNA structure that arises because of fluctuations that exist at equilibrium. This DNA structure (β-kinked DNA) is a hyperflexible DNA region that undergoes enhanced energy fluctuations during its lifetime as a result of the presence of acoustic phonon energy in DNA. These fluctuations give rise to further base unstacking (so as to follow for drug intercalation) and hydrogen bond breakage (to allow DNA breathing).

More generally, we have asked whether DNA could have two discrete structures that coexist at equilibrium at a given temperature—B DNA and β-kinked DNA. Here, β-kinked DNA corresponds to a second-order phase transition in the polymer, different regions of DNA undergoing this transition at different temperatures. Such (permanently) premelted regions could nucleate DNA melting at higher temperatures. They could also serve an important biological function. They may be binding sites for a variety of protein–DNA interactions.

Thus promoters could be permanently β-kinked DNA regions recognized in part by the RNA polymerase through partial or complete intercalation of its aromatic side chains into DNA. Such a structure could migrate along with the enzyme to form the activated complex in the polymerization reaction. Histones may have evolved to control this DNA activation process through a flip-flop mechanism in which inactive DNA (κ-kinked DNA) is converted into active DNA (β-kinked DNA) through the use of topological constraints. Nucleases may have evolved to "see" kinks in DNA by partially intercalating aromatic amino acid side chains into DNA.

We can expect major advances in future years in our understanding of how proteins bind to DNA and recognize specific structural features of its base sequence. Almost certainly, these advances will be provided by X-ray crystallography, the most powerful tool we now have to understand the structure of biological macromolecules. It will then be possible to evaluate the relevance of dynamic DNA structure—and the phenomenon of drug intercalation—to understand protein–DNA interactions.

Acknowledgments

This work has been supported in part by the American Cancer Society and the National Institutes of Health. Additional partial support has been obtained from the Department of Energy, and this paper has been assigned report no. UR-3490-1819 at the DOE, the University of Rochester.

References

1. J. D. McGhee and P. H. von Hippel, *Biochemistry* **14,** 1281 and 1297 (1975).
2. H. Teitelbaum and S. W. Englander, *J. Mol. Biol.* **92,** 55 and 79 (1975).
3. J. D. McGhee and P. H. von Hippel, *Biochemistry* **16,** 3267 (1977).
4. J. D. McGhee and P. H. von Hippel, *Biochemistry* **16,** 3276 (1977).
5. E. Palecek, *In* "Methods in Enzymology" (L. Grossman and K. Moldave, eds.), Vol. 21, p. 3. Academic Press, New York, 1971.
6. E. Palecek, *Prog. Nucleic Acid. Res. Mol. Biol.* **18,** 151 (1976).
7. M. Hogan, N. Dattagupta, and D. M. Crothers, *Proc. Natl. Acad. Sci. U.S.A.* **75,** 195 (1978).
8. J. C. Wang, *Cold Spring Harbor Symp. Quant. Biol.* **43,** 29 (1978).
9. H. M. Sobell, C.-C. Tsai, S. C. Jain, and S. C. Gilbert, *J. Mol. Biol.* **114,** 333 (1977).
10. H. M. Sobell, B. S. Reddy, K. K. Bhandary, S. C. Jain, T. D. Sakore, and T. P. Seshadri, *Cold Spring Harbor Symp. Quant. Biol.* **42,** 87 (1977).

11. H. M. Sobell, *in* "Effects of Drugs on the Cell Nucleus" (H. Busch, ed.), Vol. 1, pp. 145–160. Academic Press, New York (1979).
12. P. J. Smith and S. Arnott, *Acta Crystallogr. Sect. A* **34,** 3 (1978).
13. A. Banerjee, R. Ramani, E. D. Lozansky, and H. M. Sobell, unpublished observations.
14. V. I. Ivanov, L. E. Minchenkova, A. K. Schyolkina, and A. I. Poletayev, *Biopolymers* **12,** 89 (1973).
15. V. I. Ivanov, L. E. Minchenkova, E. E. Minyat, M. D. Frank-Kamentskii, and A. K. Schyolkina, *J. Mol. Biol.* **87,** 817 (1974).
16. R. E. Franklin and R. G. Gosling, *Acta Crystallogr.* **6,** 673 (1953).
17. J. Brahms and W. F. H. M. Mommaerts, *J. Mol. Biol.* **10,** 73 (1964).
18. J. C. Girod, W. C. Johnson, Jr., S. K. Huntington and M. F. Maestre, *Biochemistry* **12,** 5092 (1973).
19. R. Herbeck, T.-J. Yu, and W. L. Peticolas, *Biochemistry* **15,** 2656 (1976).
20. S. C. Erfurth and W. L. Peticolas, *Biopolymers* **14,** 247 (1975).
21. M. Levitt and A. Warshel, *J. Am. Chem. Soc.* **100,** 2607 (1978).
22. E. D. Lozansky, H. M. Sobell and M. Lessen, *in* "Stereodynamics of Molecular Systems" (Ramaswamy H. Sarma, ed.), p. 265. Pergamon, Oxford, (1979).
23. H. M. Sobell, E. D. Lozansky, and M. Lessen, *Cold Spring Harbor Symp. Quant. Biol.* **43,** 11 (1978).
24. E. D. Lozansky, and H. M. Sobell, *Proc. Nat. Acad. Sci.* submitted.
25. L. D. Landau and E. M. Lifshitz, "Statistical Physics," p. 353. Addison-Wesley, Reading, Massachusetts, 1969.
26. V. A. Bloomfield, D. M. Crothers, and I. Tinoco, Jr., "Physical Chemistry of Nucleic Acids." Harper, New York, 1974.
27. J. P. Richardson, *J. Mol. Biol.* **78,** 703 (1973).
28. H. Weintraub, and M. Groudine, *Science* **193,** 848 (1976).
29. A. Garel and R. Axel, *Cold Spring Harbor Symp. Quant. Biol.* **42,** 701 (1977).
30. S. J. Flint and H. M. Weintraub, *Cell* **12,** 783 (1977).
31. R. D. Camerini-Otero, B. Sollner-Webb, R. H. Simon, P. Williamson, M. Zasloff, and G. Felsenfeld, *Cold Spring Harbor Symp. Quant. Biol.* **42,** 43 (1977).
32. V. E. Foe, L. E. Wilkinson and C. D. Laird, *Cell* **9,** 131 (1976).
33. H. Weintraub, A. Worcel and B. Alberts, *Cell* **9,** 409 (1976).
34. See, for example, "Chromatin," *Cold Spring Harbor Symp. Quant. Biol.* **42** (1977).
35. L. Lutter, *Nucleic Acids Res.* **6,** 41 (1979).

7

Molecular Pharmacology of Anthracyclines

STANLEY T. CROOKE, VIRGIL H. DUVERNAY, AND SEYMOUR MONG

I. Introduction

Anthracyclines represent a major class of antineoplastic drugs, and their importance has increased significantly since the discovery of adriamycin (ADM) and daunomycin (DNM) (1,2). Clearly, ADM is the most important single anticancer drug available because of its relatively broad spectrum of activity, and DNM is an important agent in the treatment of leukemias (3). Equally clearly, ADM and DNM possess significant toxic liabilities, the most important of which are myelosuppression and cardiotoxicity (3).

A measure of the importance of anthracyclines is the number of programs

MOLECULAR ACTIONS AND TARGETS FOR CANCER CHEMOTHERAPEUTIC AGENTS

ISBN 0-12-619280-4

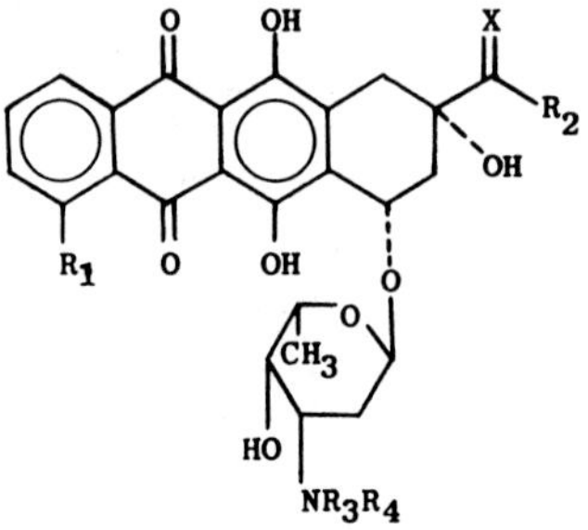

Compound	R_1	R_2	R_3	R_4	X
ADRIAMYCIN	OCH_3	CH_2OH	H	H	O
DAUNOMYCIN	OCH_3	CH_3	H	H	O
CARMINOMYCIN	OH	CH_3	H	H	O
RUBIDAZONE	OCH_3	CH_3	H	H	$NNHCOC_6H_5$
AD-32	OCH_3	$CH_2OCOC_4H_9$	H	$COCF_3$	O
AD-41	OCH_3	CH_2OH	H	$COCF_3$	O

Fig. 1. The general structure and structural modifications of the ADM-DNM class of anthracyclines.

directed toward the development of improved compounds of this class. Emanating from these programs have been numerous analogues which promise clinically significant improvements in therapeutic index in the future and which have provided a great deal of information that permits a better understanding of the molecular pharmacology and the structure–activity relationships of anthracyclines. These analogues may be divided chemically into two groups. Figure 1 shows the general structure of the ADM-DNM class of anthracyclines, and Fig. 2 shows the general structure of the aclacinomycin (ACM)–cinerubin A class of anthracyclines (4). This group differs chemically from the former group in that the compounds have a carbomethoxy substitution at C-10, they lack a carbonyl function at C-13 and, with the exception of pyrromycin (PYM), all the compounds are di- or trisaccharides.

In this chapter, the molecular pharmacologic characteristics of anthracyclines and known structure–activity relationships will be briefly discussed. In addition, the evidence that anthracyclines should be divided into multiple mechanistic classes will also be discussed.

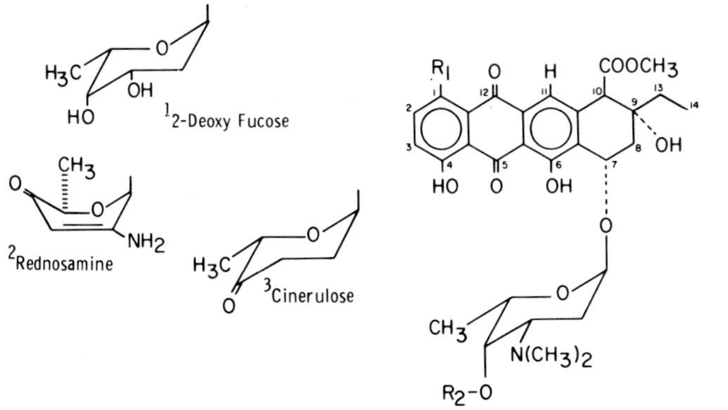

ANTHRACYCLINE	R_1	R_2
PYRROMYCIN	OH	H
MUSETTAMYCIN	OH	2-DEOXYFUCOSE[1]
RUDOLFOMYCIN	OH	2-DEOXYFUCOSE - REDNOSAMINE[2]
ACLACINOMYCIN	H	2-DEOXYFUCOSE - CINERULOSE[3]
MARCELLOMYCIN	OH	2-DEOXYFUCOSE - 2-DEOXYFUCOSE
CINERUBIN A	OH	2-DEOXYFUCOSE - CINERULOSE

Fig. 2. Structures and structural modifications of the ACM-cinerubin A class of anthracyclines.

II. The Interaction of Anthracyclines with Isolated DNA

A. Binding to Linear DNA

Most anthracyclines have been shown to bind to DNA derived from multiple sources. The binding is thought to be due to intercalation of the planar ring structure and to ionic interactions between the sugar(s) and the sugar–phosphate backbone of DNA (5–10). Moreover, studies from several laboratories have shown that the biological activities of many anthracyclines are related to their ability to bind to DNA (4,11–15).

In our laboratory, we have explored the interaction of several anthracyclines with DNA using a number of techniques, one of which is fluorescence quenching. Since all anthracyclines have fluorescent properties, and the fluorescence is quenched when they bind to DNA, this technique has proven to be of value. Figure 3 shows the fluorescence spectrum PYM, the fluorescence quenching by DNA, and that no peak shifts were induced by its interaction with DNA. Based on the information obtained from such studies, binding constants can be determined for each drug and each type of DNA.

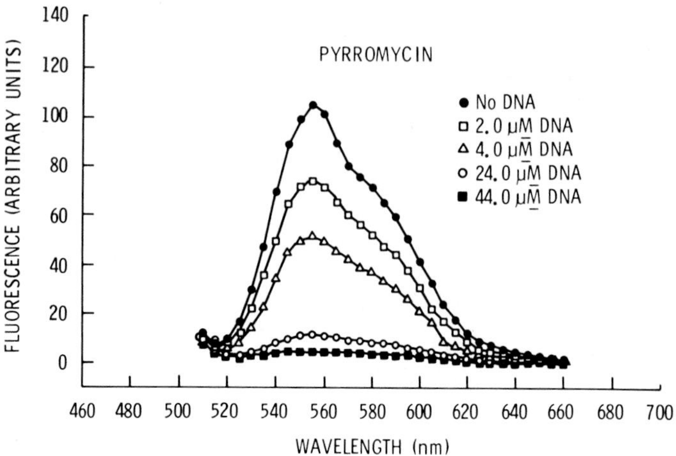

Fig. 3. Fluorescence spectrum of PYM, and the fluorescence spectral changes which occur upon interaction with salmon sperm DNA. Spectra were obtained using 5 μM anthracycline.

To explore the variations induced in DNA binding of anthracyclines by variations in the base composition of DNA, we employed four naturally occurring DNA species and two synthetic polynucleotides. Figure 4 shows a typical Scatchard analysis of the interaction of three anthracyclines with three DNA species, and Fig. 5 shows Scatchard analyses of PYM and ACM with poly(dA-dT)–poly(dA-dt) and poly(dG-dC)–poly(dG-dC), Tables I (see ref. 16) and II provide a quantitative review of data on a variety of anthracyclines and demonstrate that ADM behaved in a manner quite different from pyrromycinone-based anthracyclines in that it clearly showed an absolute requirement for G-C for binding to DNA. This is graphically illustrated in Fig. 6. Clearly, pyrromycinone-based anthracyclines exhibited no G-C content specificity, and in fact bound with more avidity to poly(dA-dT)–poly(dA-dT) than any other polynucleotide, differing qualitatively from ADM.

To explore structure–activity relationships affecting DNA interactions, we have studied a series of pyrromycinone-based analogues. Figure 7 shows the structures of marcellomycin (MCM), rudolfomycin (RDM), and their 10-decarbomethoxy analogues. In addition, we studied the 10-carbomethoxy epimers of MCM and musettamycin (MSM), shown in Fig. 8. Table III shows the DNA-binding parameters observed for MCM and RDM and their decarbomethoxy analogues. Clearly, removal of the carbomethoxy group resulted in a significant decrease in affinity for the DNA species studied. Furthermore, the results shown in Table IV demonstrated that the interaction was highly stereospecific in that the epimers bound to DNA with less avidity than even the decarbomethoxy analogues.

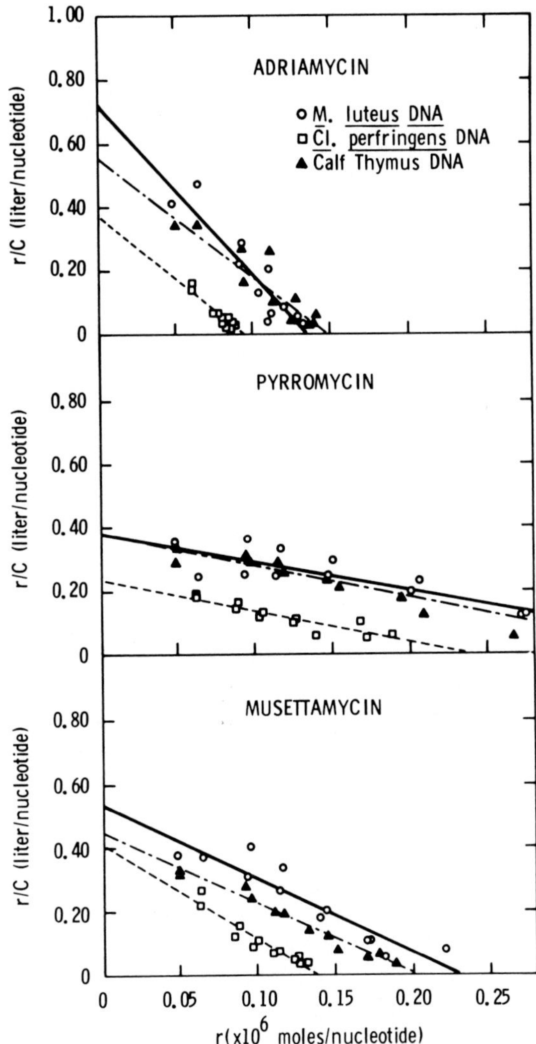

Fig. 4. Scatchard plots of the binding data for the interaction of anthracyclines with calf thymus DNA, *Clostridium perfringens* DNA, and *Micrococcus luteus* DNA.

Similar studies demonstrated the importance of the glycosidic chain length and the affinity for DNA. For example, Fig. 9 shows a comparison of the three pyrromycinone-based anthracyclines which differ only in glycosidic chain length, and Table V shows that increasing chain length resulted in greater affinity for DNA. Furthermore, the terminal sugar 2-deoxyfucose appeared to confer a DNA binding advantage over other terminal sugars. Thus the binding of

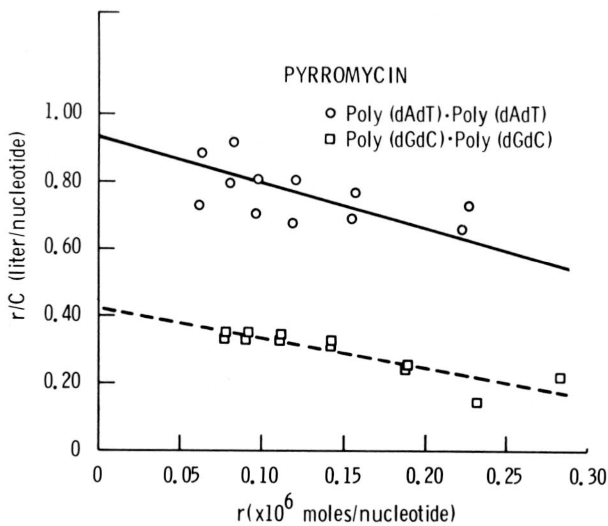

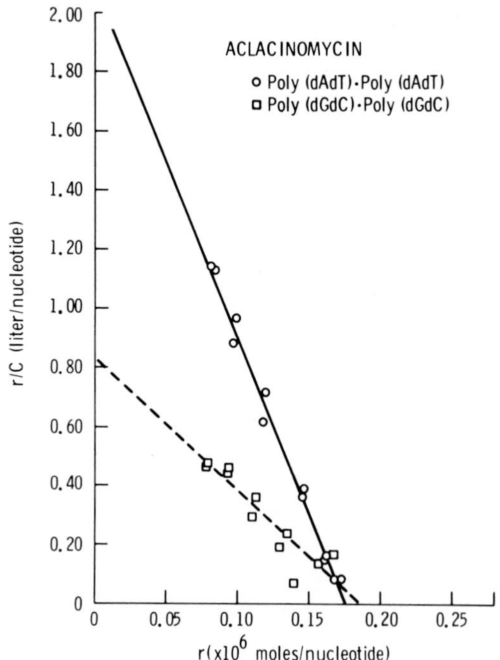

Fig. 5. Scatchard plots of the binding data for the interaction of PYM and ACM with poly(dA-dT)–poly(dA-dT) and poly(dG-dC)–poly(dG-dC).

TABLE I

Calf Thymus DNA-, *Micrococcus luteus* DNA-, and *Clostridium perfringens* DNA-Binding Parameters of Anthracyclines[a,b]

	Calf thymus DNA, 43% G-C		*Micrococcus luteus* DNA, 72% G-C		*Clostridium perfringens* DNA, 28% G-C	
Anthracycline	K_{app} ($\times 10^6\ M^{-1}$)[c]	n_{app}[d]	K_{app} ($\times 10^6\ M^{-1}$)[c]	n_{app}[d]	K_{app} ($\times 10^6\ M^{-1}$)[c]	n_{app}[d]
Adriamycin	3.67 ± 0.42	0.15 ± 0.05	5.46 ± 0.76	0.14 ± 0.08	3.97 ± 0.55	0.10 ± 0.04
Pyrromycin	0.98 ± 0.13	0.38 ± 0.02	0.87 ± 0.18	0.43 ± 0.03	1.01 ± 0.13	0.24 ± 0.02
Musettamycin	2.21 ± 0.13	0.20 ± 0.02	2.32 ± 0.30	0.23 ± 0.04	2.96 ± 0.28	0.14 ± 0.03
Rudolfomycin	1.98 ± 0.16	0.22 ± 0.02	2.02 ± 0.35	0.29 ± 0.05	2.44 ± 0.34	0.16 ± 0.04
Aclacinomycin	2.48 ± 0.16	0.18 ± 0.02	2.37 ± 0.34	0.19 ± 0.04	1.75 ± 0.29	0.11 ± 0.02
Marcellomycin	5.03 ± 0.23	0.19 ± 0.03	5.25 ± 0.46	0.23 ± 0.07	6.05 ± 1.23	0.13 ± 0.13

[a] All p values were determined from tables of significance limits for correlation coefficients (56); as such, p values were all <0.001. The number of averaged values used to construct composite Scatchard curves was no less than 10 and usually 12.

[b] Standard deviations of slopes (K_{app}) and x intercepts (n_{app}) were calculated from linear regression analyses (16).

[c] Values were obtained by linear regression analyses of composite Scatchard curves obtained from two or more separate experiments, each of which contained duplicate or triplicate values at each DNA concentration.

[d] Apparent number of binding sites per nucleotide. Values were obtained as for K_{app}.

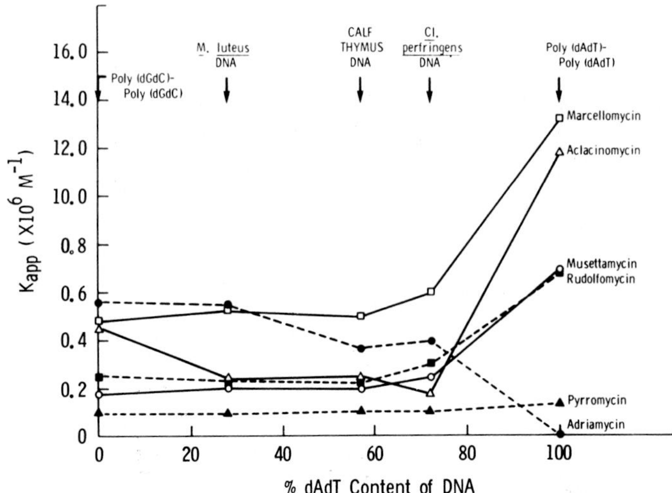

Fig. 6. The effect of varying DNA base compositions on the apparent association constants of anthracyclines. Results were obtained from Tables I and II. Percentage of dA-dT sequences varied depending upon the DNAs studied: poly(dG-dC)–poly(dG-dC), 0%; *M. luteus* DNA, 28%; calf thymus DNA, 57%; *C. perfringens* DNA, 72%; poly(dA-dT)–poly(dA-dT), 100%.

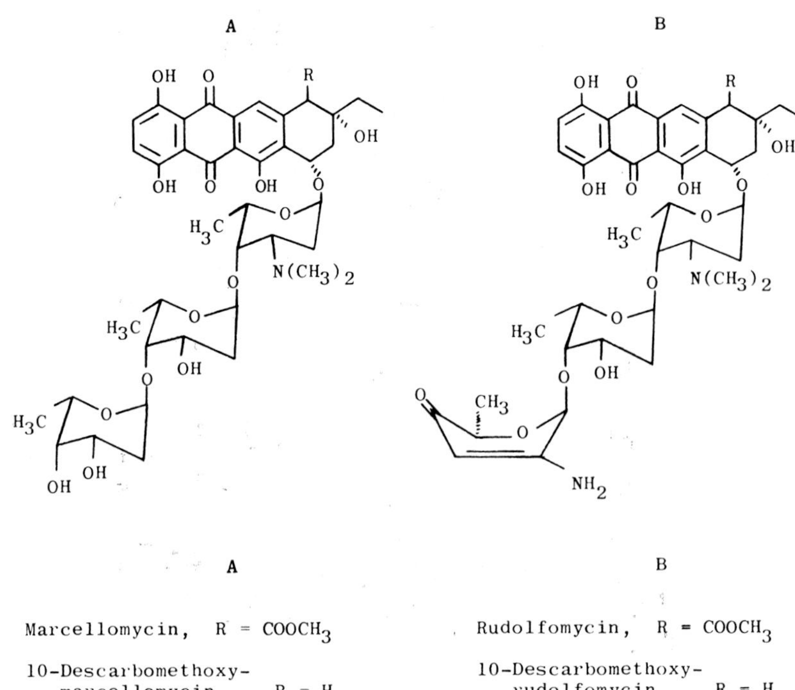

Marcellomycin, R = $COOCH_3$

10-Descarbomethoxy-marcellomycin, R = H

Rudolfomycin, R = $COOCH_3$

10-Descarbomethoxy-rudolfomycin R = H

Fig. 7. Structures of MCM, 10-descarbomethoxymarcellomycin, RDM, and 10-descarbomethoxyrudolfomycin.

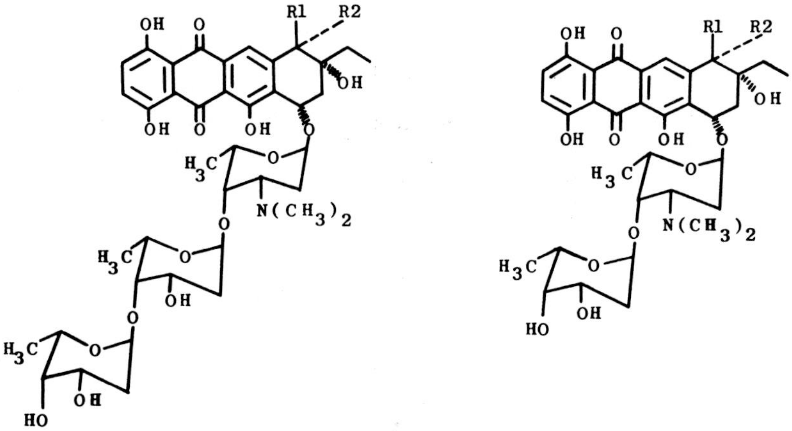

	R1	R2
MARCELLOMYCIN	$COOCH_3$	H
MIMIMYCIN	H	$COOCH_3$

	R1	R2
MUSETTAMYCIN	$COOCH_3$	H
COLLINEMYCIN	H	$COOCH_3$

Fig. 8. Structures of MCM, MSM, and their C-10 epimers, mimimycin and collinemycin, respectively.

TABLE II

Poly(dA-dT)-Poly(dA-dT) and Poly(dG-dC)-Poly(dG-dC) DNA-Binding Parameters of Anthracyclines[a,b]

Anthracycline	Poly(dA-dT)-poly(dA-dT) K_{app} ($\times 10^6\ M^{-1}$)[c]	Poly(dA-dT)-poly(dA-dT) n_{app}[d]	Poly(dG-dC)-poly(dG-dC) K_{app} ($\times 10^6\ M^{-1}$)[c]	Poly(dG-dC)-poly(dG-dC) n_{app}[d]
Adriamycin	No detectable binding	No detectable binding	5.54 ± 0.61	0.16 ± 0.06
Pyrromycin	1.33 ± 0.21	0.70 ± 0.04	0.88 ± 0.14	0.48 ± 0.02
Musettamycin	6.79 ± 0.57	0.28 ± 0.10	2.46 ± 0.23	0.30 ± 0.04
Rudolfomycin	6.88 ± 0.72	0.31 ± 0.13	1.74 ± 0.33	0.35 ± 0.05
Aclacinomycin	11.81 ± 0.37	0.18 ± 0.05	4.48 ± 0.68	0.18 ± 0.08
Marcellomycin	16.13 ± 1.78	0.20 ± 0.25	4.75 ± 0.50	0.25 ± 0.08

[a] All p values were <0.001 (see Table I). The number of averaged values used to construct composite Scatchard curves was no less than 11 and usually 12.

[b] See Table I, footnote *b*.

[c] See Table I, footnote *c*.

[d] See Table I, footnote *d*.

TABLE III

Structure–Activity Relationships of Class II Anthracyclines: The Carbomethoxy Group at Position 10 of the Aglycone

Anthracycline	K_{app} ($\times 10^6\ M^{-1}$)				IC_{50} NoRNA synthesis (μM)	IC_{50} cell survival (μM)	*In vivo* antitumor activity (mg/kg/dose)
	M. luteus DNA	Calf thymus DNA	Salmon sperm DNA	*C. perfringens* DNA			
Marcellomycin	5.25	5.03	9.51	6.05	0.01	0.75	0.20
Descarbomethoxy-marcellomycin	1.21	2.14	1.28	1.26	2.56	3.80	4.0
Rudolfomycin	2.02	1.98	3.11	2.44	0.29	0.31	0.20
Descarbomethoxy-rudolfomycin	0.42	1.42	1.54	0.96	9.13	>5.0	16.0

TABLE IV

Binding Parameters of Marcellomycin, Musettamycin, Mimimycin, and Collinemycin for Salmon Sperm DNA and Calf Thymus DNA

	Salmon sperm DNA, 41% G-C		Calf thymus DNA, 43% G-C	
Anthracycline	K_{app}[a]	n_{app}[b]	K_{app}[a]	n_{app}[b]
Marcellomycin	9.51	0.17	5.03	0.19
Mimimycin	0.32	0.28	0.33	0.28
Musettamycin	1.99	0.26	2.21	0.20
Collinemycin	0.59	0.23	0.42	0.26

[a] See Table I, footnote *c*.
[b] See Table I, footnote *d*.

pyrromycinone-based anthracyclines to DNA is clearly dependent on the carbomethoxy group at C-10 and the glycosidic chain length. Moreover, as will be discussed in subsequent sections, a reduction in DNA affinity was correlated with a decrease in nucleolar RNA (NoRNA) synthesis inhibitory potency, cytotoxicity and *in vivo* antitumor activity for these compounds.

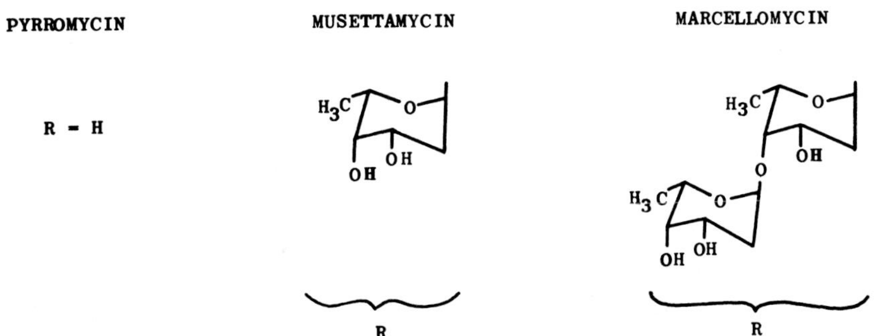

Fig. 9. Structural comparison of PYM, MSM, and MCM.

TABLE V

Structure–Activity Relationships of Class II Anthracyclines: The Length of the Glycosidic Side Chain

Anthracycline	Number of sugar groups	K^{*}_{app} ($\times 10^6$ M^{-1})[a]					IC_{50} NoRNA synthesis (μM)[b]
		Poly(dG-dC)-poly(dG-dC)	*M. luteus* DNA	Calf thymus DNA	*C. perfringens* DNA	Poly(dA-dT)-poly(dA-dT)	
Pyrromycin	1	0.88	0.87	0.98	1.01	1.33	6.15
Musettamycin	2	2.46	2.32	2.21	2.96	6.79	0.014
Marcellomycin	3	4.75	5.25	5.03	6.05	13.23	0.009

[a] Obtained from Tables I and II.
[b] Obtained from Table VII.

B. Binding to Superhelical DNA

The interaction of intercalating agents with superhelical DNA has been shown to induce marked conformational changes. Agarose gel electrophoresis of superhelical (form I) PM2 DNA treated with intercalating agents has demonstrated unwinding–rewinding of the DNA (5,17–20). This is a sensitive method for determining binding of anthracyclines and is useful complement to fluorescence quenching techniques because it measures effects on the macromolecule rather than relying on effects on the ligand. We have employed this technique to explore additional aspects of the interaction of anthracyclines with DNA.

Figure 10 shows the effects of several anthracyclines on the electrophoretic mobility of form I PM2 DNA. Each anthracycline induced a concentration-dependent diffuse electrophoretic pattern typical of intercalative agents. Posttreatment of anthracycline-treated DNA with bleomycin resulted in typical bleomycin fragmentation of the DNA, demonstrating that the patterns observed were not due to degradation of the DNA. From such studies, the relative affinities for DNA of each of the anthracyclines were determined and were found to be equivalent to the relative affinities determined using fluorescence quenching techniques.

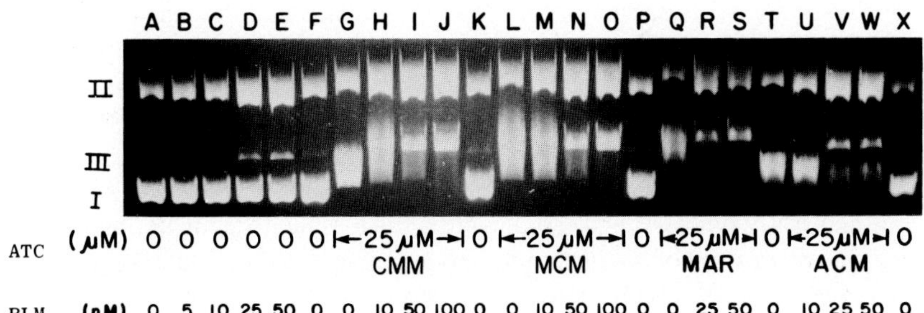

Fig. 10 Effects of anthracycline (ATC) pretreatment of PM2 DNA on degradation induced by bleomycin A_2 (BLM). Results obtained from Mong *et al.* (19). ccc-PM2 DNA was incubated with various anthracyclines (25 μM) in the presence of 20 mM 2-mercaptoethanol for 30 minutes, as described previously (19), and then incubated with increasing concentrations of bleomycin A_2. The products of the reactions were separated by agarose gel electrophoresis. (A) Control PM2 DNA; (B) 5 nM bleomycin A_2; (C) 10 nM bleomycin A_2; (D) 25 nM bleomycin A_2; (E) 50 nM bleomycin A_2; (F) control PM2 DNA, (G–J) PM2 DNA treated with 25 μM CMM posttreated with 0, 10, 50, and 100 nM of bleomycin A_2; (K) control PM2 DNA; (L–O) PM2 DNA treated with 25 μM ADM posttreated with 0, 10, 50, and 100 nM of bleomycin A_2; (P) control PM2 DNA; (Q–S) PM2 DNA treated with MCM and then posttreated with 0, 25, and 50 nM bleomycin A_2; (T) control PM2 DNA; (U–W) PM2 DNA treated with 25μM ACM and then posttreated with 10, 25, and 50 nM bleomycin A_2; (X) control PM2 DNA.

C. Degradation of Purified DNA

Studies demonstrating extensive chromosomal damage in cells treated with ADM have been reported (21,22). More recently, the degradation of purified form I PM2 DNA by ADM has been reported (23,24). However, these studies have employed high concentrations of ADM (0.2 or 0.4 m*M*), a high temperature, and high concentrations of reducing agents. In our laboratory, we have confirmed that anthracyclines can degrade purified PM2 DNA under the reported conditions; however, at lower concentrations and under less harsh conditions anthracyclines induced conformational alterations in PM2 DNA without evidence of degradation (Fig. 10). Thus the effects which appear to be more important mechanistically are the conformational alterations induced in DNA.

III. Effects of Anthracyclines on Nucleic Acid Synthesis

Most of the anthracyclines studied (see Section VIII for discussion of anthracyclines that may not rely on DNA interactions or nucleic acid synthesis inhibition for cytotoxicity) have been shown to inhibit synthesis of both DNA and RNA rapidly and effectively (4,25–30). It has also been reported that ADM and DNM inhibit DNA polymerase α selectively (31). Table VI shows the concentrations necessary to inhibit DNA and RNA synthesis in L1210 leukemia cells *in vitro*. As can be seen, ADM and DNM and most other anthracyclines inhibit DNA and RNA synthesis at approximately equivalent concentrations. In contrast, several of the anthracyclines noted in Table I have been reported to inhibit whole-cell RNA synthesis more effectively than DNA synthesis (32,33). As a consequence of the report on ACM, we undertook a detailed examination of the effects of several anthracyclines on nucleic acid synthesis.

In our laboratory we have studied the effects of anthracyclines on whole-cell DNA and RNA synthesis and, employing a double-label technique, on the synthesis and processing of nucleolar pre-rRNA. Table VII shows that the anthracyclines studied can be divided into two classes on the basis of their relative specificities for inhibition of NoRNA synthesis. Class I anthracyclines (ADM, carminomycin (CMM), and PYM) inhibited NoRNA synthesis at concentrations equal to those required to inhibit DNA synthesis. Class II anthracyclines (MSM, RDM, ACM, and MCM) inhibited NoRNA synthesis at concentrations approximately 200- to 1300-fold lower than those required to inhibit DNA synthesis. Moreover, removal of the 10-carbomethoxy group of the pyrromycinone-based anthracyclines reduced the NoRNA synthesis selectivity of the class II anthracyclines. Other studies showed that none of the anthracyclines studied had discernible effects on the processing of NoRNA.

The structure–activity relationships responsible for NoRNA synthesis inhibition selectivity are summarized in Fig. 11. To be nucleolus-selective, anthracyclines must have a carbomethoxy group at position 10, and data not shown demonstrate that the carbomethoxy group must be in the proper attitude, as the

TABLE VI

Inhibition of RNA and DNA Synthesis in Cultured Mouse L1210 Cells by Anthracycline Antibiotics[a]

	IC_{50} values (μM)		
Anthracycline	DNA synthesis	RNA synthesis	IC_{50} DNA/IC_{50} RNA ratio
Adriamycin	0.80	0.90	0.89
Daunorubicin	0.30	0.30	1.00
Rhodomycin B	2.10	0.10	21.0
Nogalamycin	4.00	0.40	10.0
Cinerubin A	0.30	0.03	10.0
Cinerubin B	1.50	0.20	7.5
Aclacinomycin A	1.20	0.12	10.0

[a] Determined by assaying drug effect on the incorporation of [^{3}H]thymidine and [^{3}H]uridine into DNA and RNA, respectively (32).

epimers at C-10 of MCM and MSM are much less selective toward NoRNA synthesis. In addition, the compound must be at least a disaccharide, as PYM is not NoRNA-selective even though it has the proper aglycone. Table VIII shows that NoRNA synthesis inhibition is essential for the activity of class II anthracyclines, in that structural changes which induced changes only in NoRNA synthesis inhibitory activity resulted in marked reductions in cytotoxicity and *in vivo* antitumor activities. Furthermore, the effects on NoRNA synthesis were correlated with DNA binding affinity as shown in Table IX.

TABLE VII

Inhibition by Anthracyclines of Nucleolar RNA Synthesis Relative to Whole-Cell DNA Synthesis

Anthracycline	IC_{50} NoRNA synthesis (μM)	$\frac{IC_{50}\text{ DNA synthesis}}{IC_{50}\text{ NoRNA synthesis}}$ ratio
Adriamycin	6.00	1.02
Carminomycin	13.06	1.12
Pyrromycin	6.15	0.93
Musettamycin	0.014	714
Rudolfomycin	0.290	240
Aclacinomycin	0.037	170
Marcellomycin	0.009	1256
Descarbomethoxy-marcellomycin	2.56	7.42
Descarbomethoxy-rudolfomycin	9.13	2.01

CLASS I ANTHRACYCLINES

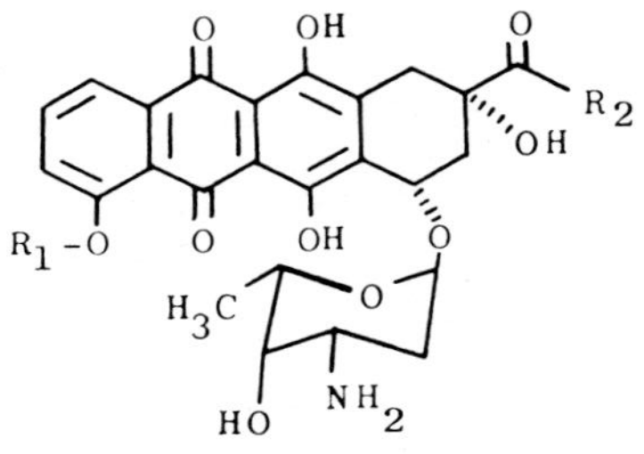

	R_1	R_2
ADRIAMYCIN	CH_3	CH_2OH
CARMINOMYCIN	OH	CH_3

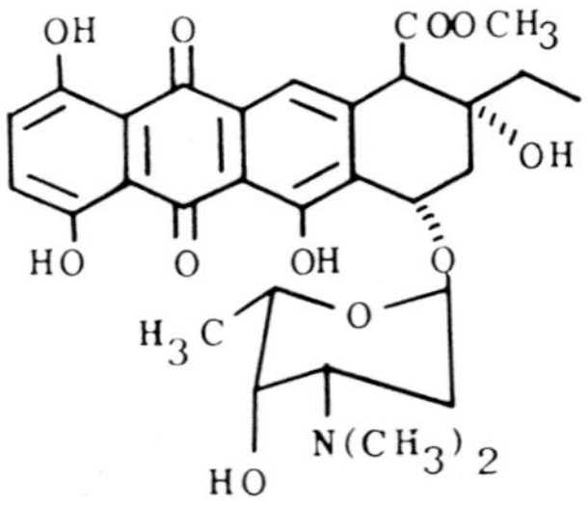

PYRROMYCIN

CLASS II ANTHRACYCLINES

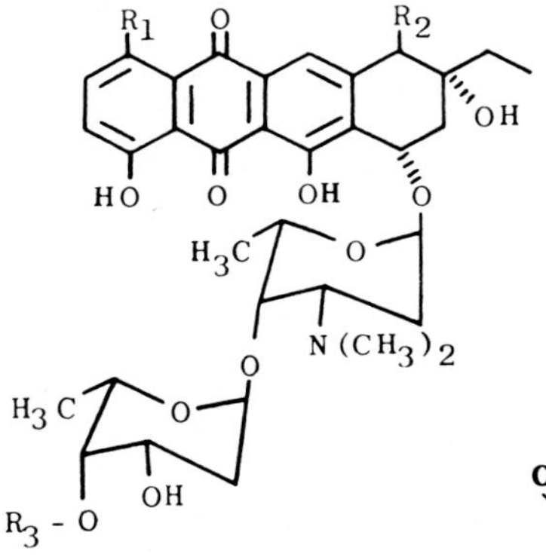

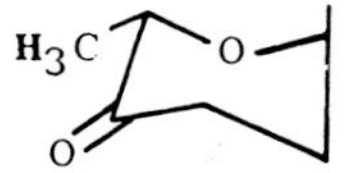

CINERULOSE

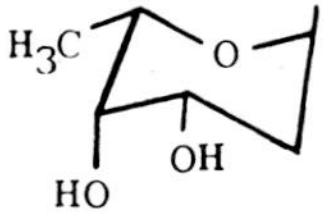

2-DEOXYFUCOSE

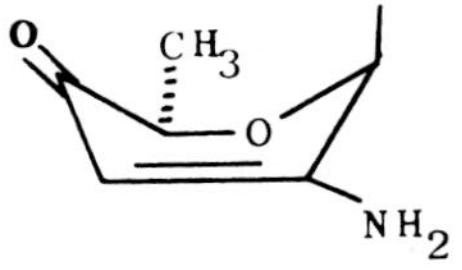

REDNOSAMINE

ANTHRACYCLINE	R_1	R_2	R_3
MUSETTAMYCIN	OH	$COOCH_3$	H
RUDOLFOMYCIN	OH	$COOCH_3$	REDNOSAMINE
ACLACINOMYCIN	H	$COOCH_3$	CINERULOSE
MARCELLOMYCIN	OH	$COOCH_3$	2-DEOXYFUCOSE
DESCARBOMETHOXY-MARCELLOMYCIN	OH	H	2-DEOXYFUCOSE
DESCARBOMETHOXY-RUDOLFOMYCIN	OH	H	REDNOSAMINE

Fig. 11. Structures of class I and class II anthracyclines and the 10-descarbomethoxy analogues of MCM and RDM.

TABLE VIII

Inhibition of DNA, RNA, and NoRNA Synthesis and Cell Viability by Class II Anthracyclines in Comparison with *in Vivo* Antitumor Data

	In vitro IC_{50} values (μM)				
	DNA synthesis	RNA synthesis	NoRNA synthesis	Cell viability	*In vivo* antitumor activity in L1210 leukemia (mg/kg/dose)
Marcellomycin (MCM)	13.52	3.03	0.014	0.75	0.20
10-Decarbomethoxy-marcellomycin (D-MCM)	18.99	4.07	2.56	3.80	4.0
D-MCM/MCM ratio	1.40	1.34	183	5.10	20
Rudolfomycin (RDM)	69.70	3.65	0.29	0.31	0.20
10-Decarbomethoxy-rudolfomycin (D-RDM)	18.37	7.24	9.13	>5.0	16.0
D-RDM/RDM ratio	0.264	1.98	31	>16	80

TABLE IX

Structure–Activity Relationships of Class II Anthracyclines: The Carbomethoxy Group at Position 10 of the Aglycone

Anthracycline	K_{app} ($\times 10^6\ M^{-1}$)						
	M. luteus DNA	Calf thymus DNA	Salmon sperm DNA	*C. perfringens* DNA	IC_{50} NoRNA synthesis (μM)	IC_{50} cell survival (μM)	*In vivo* antitumor activity (mg/kg/dose)
Marcellomycin	5.25	5.03	9.51	6.05	0.01	0.75	0.20
Decarbomethoxy-marcellomycin	1.21	2.14	1.28	1.26	2.56	3.80	4.0
Rudolfomycin	2.02	1.98	3.11	2.44	0.29	0.31	0.20
Decarbomethoxy-rudolfomycin	0.42	1.42	1.54	0.96	9.13	>5.0	16.0

IV. Effects on Protein Synthesis

Cellular protein synthesis appears to be much less sensitive than other metabolic processes to the action of anthracyclines (4,34,35). The inhibition that occurs appears to be secondary to other cellular effects such as inhibition of RNA synthesis. However, no studies have as yet been reported on the effects of anthracyclines on the synthesis of specific proteins or classes of proteins.

V. Antimitotic Effects of Anthracyclines

Silvestrini *et al.* (36) reported evidence for antimitotic effects of DNM in cultured mouse cells at drug concentrations which affect nuclei acid synthesis. The antimitotic effect was rapid in onset, occurring even when DNM was administered within minutes prior to prophase. Kitaura *et al.* (34) demonstrated similar effects for ADM. Furthermore, more recently, ACM has been reported to bind to tubulin and to inhibit mitosis (37). Thus anthracyclines may have significant effects on the mitotic apparatus, and much remains to be elucidated.

VI. Effects of Anthracyclines on Mitochondrial Function

Studies have shown that ADM affects mitochondria in a number of ways, including superoxide generation (38), perturbation of the electron transport system (39–41), and inhibition of the synthesis of cytochromes a and a_3 (42). Gosalvez *et al.* (43) demonstrated significant inhibition of respiration of mitochondria isolated from normal and tumor cells. Similarly, Iwamoto *et al.* (44) demonstrated that ADM, CMM, DNM, and adriamycin-14-O-octanoate inhibited the respiratory chain enzymes succinooxidase and NADH oxidase, which require the cofactor coenzyme Q_{10}. Comparatively high drug levels were required to elicit these effects in both studies. Kishi *et al.* (39) have demonstrated that ADM inhibits beef heart mitochondrial succinooxidase and NADH oxidase and that this inhibition can be prevented by the addition of several forms of coenzyme Q. It was further shown that daunomycinone was significantly less inhibitory than adriamycinone, indicating that the hydroxyl group of the latter may be important for receptor binding. The role of lipid peroxidation in cardiac toxicity has been reported (45), and its amelioration by α-tocopherol has been suggested (46). A similar observation has been reported for coenzyme Q_{10} (39,40,45). Thus the effects of anthracyclines on mitochondrial function may be responsible in part for the antitumor actions of these drugs; in addition it is possible that the cardiotoxicity of ADM may be largely due to the inhibition of

CoQ_{10}-mediated enzymes which are present in high concentrations in cardiac tissue.

VII. Effects of Anthracyclines on Membrane Synthesis and Function

Studies on the effects of ADM on sarcoma 180 cells demonstrated that cytotoxicity correlated better with changes in the rate of cellular agglutination by concanavalin A than with alteration of nucleic acid synthesis, and that ADM-induced membrane changes occurred at very low concentrations (47). Additional studies further suggested direct interactions with membranes and the cellular cytoskeleton (48–52).

In our laboratory, we have examined the effects of pyrromycinone-based anthracyclines on membrane synthesis as determined by fucose or glucosamine incorporation into acid-insoluble components. Figures 12 and 13 show typical kinetic studies on the effects of ADM and MCM on $[^3H]$fucose and $[^{14}C]$-glucosamine incorporation into acid-insoluble material. None of the anthracyclines studies had demonstrable effects on membrane synthesis at any of the concentrations studied. Effects on membrane function remain to be investigated.

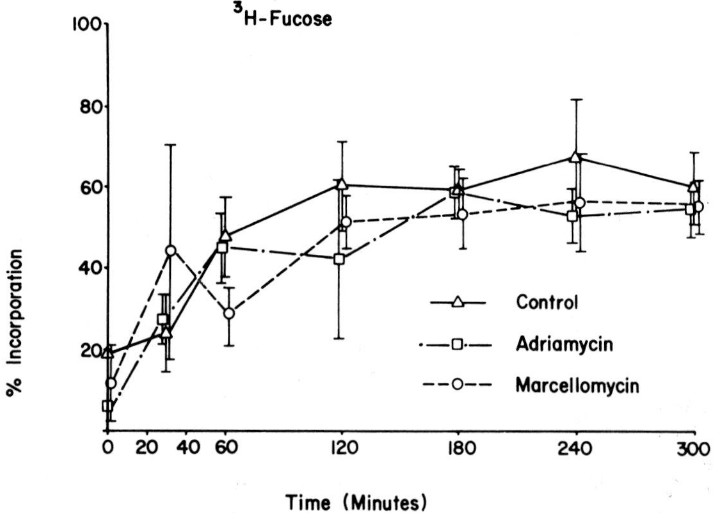

Fig. 12. Time course of the effects of MCM and ADM on the incorporation of $[^3H]$ fucose into membrane components. Cultured NHAC were treated with drugs and labeled with precursor, and aliquots were assayed at the appropriate times. The data are presented as the percentage of cell-associated radioactivity incorporated into trichloroacetic acid-insoluble radioactivity. Means of a minimum of triplicate determinations are shown, and the curves represent typical results of duplicate experiments.

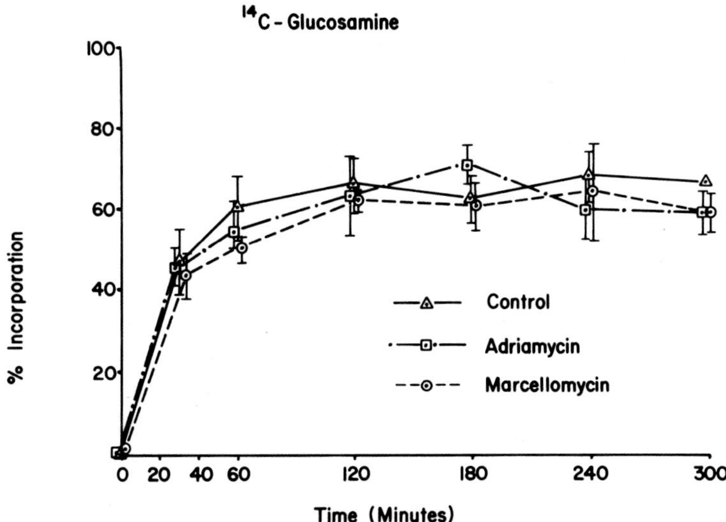

Fig. 13. Time course of the effects of MCM and ADM on the incorporation of [C] glucosamine into membrane components. The data presented were obtained as indicated in the legend for Fig. 12, and the time courses represent typical results of duplicate experiments.

VIII. Anthracyclines Which May Not Depend on DNA Interactions for Cytotoxicity

AD-32, the structure of which is shown in Fig. 1, exhibited antitumor activity against P388 and L1210 leukemias (53). However, AD-32 has been reported not to bind to DNA and to localize to the cytoplasm rather than the nucleus (54,55). Thus it has been suggested that AD-32 induces cytotoxicity by mechanisms involving cellular components other than DNA.

Studies in our laboratory on CMM and its 11-methyl ether (CMM-OMe) have suggested that these two compounds may be cytotoxic primarily as a result of mechanisms other than DNA binding. Both compounds are close structural analogues of ADM (Fig. 14).

Table X shows binding parameters of the three agents to calf thymus and salmon sperm DNA and demonstrates that CMM and CMM-OMe bind with much less avidity than ADM. Studies using PM2 DNA confirmed the results obtained with fluorescence quenching techniques (Fig. 15). Moreover, although CMM is approximately 10-fold more potent as a cytoxic agent than ADM, and CMM-OMe is approximately equipotent, they were relatively ineffective in inhibiting the synthesis of nucleic acids. Clearly, therefore, inhibition of DNA synthesis cannot account for the cytotoxicity of CMM or CMM-OMe. Nor can

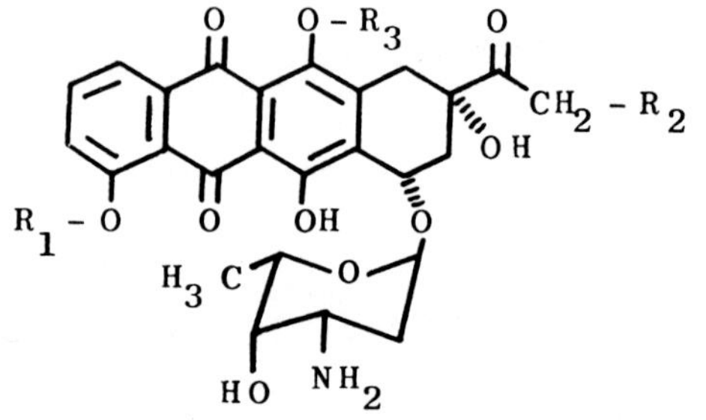

	R_1	R_2	R_3
Adriamycin	CH_3	OH	H
Carminomycin	H	H	H
Carminomycin-11-methyl ether	H	H	CH_3

Fig. 14. Structures of ADM, CMM, and carminomycin-11-methyl ether.

TABLE X

DNA-Binding Parameters of Adriamycin, Carminomycin, and Carminomycin-11-Methyl Ether[a]

	Calf thymus DNA		Salmon sperm DNA	
Anthracycline	K_{app} ($\times 10^6$ M^{-1})[b]	n_{app}[c]	K_{app} ($\times 10^6$ M^{-1})[b]	n_{app}[c]
Adriamycin	3.67	0.15	11.68	0.12
Carminomycin	0.26	0.50	0.15	0.65
Carminomycin 11-methyl ether	N.D.		N.D.	

[a] All p values were determined from tables of significance limits for correlation coefficients. Most p values were <0.01 with the exception of CMM salmon sperm DNA, which was $p < 0.05$. The number of averaged values used to construct composite Scatchard curves was no less than 8 and usually 12. Values are derived from the results of duplicate or triplicate experiments.

[b] See Table I, footnote *c*. N.D., Not detectable.

[c] See Table I, footnote *d*.

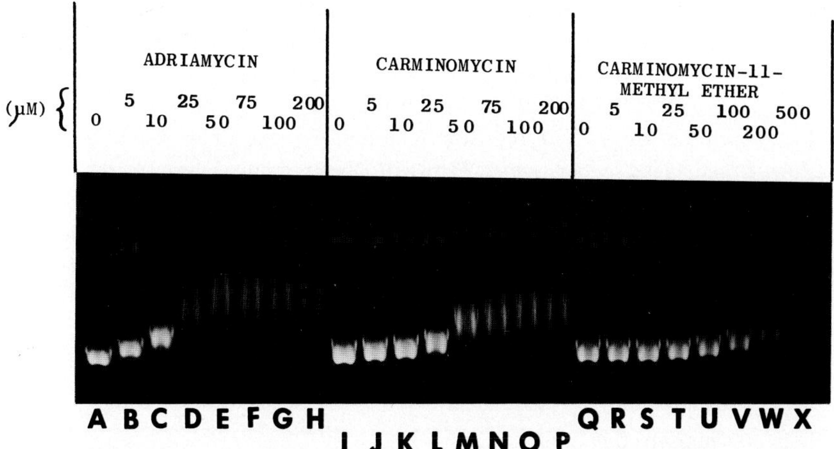

Fig. 15. Agarose gel electrophoretic separations of anthracycline-PM2 DNA reaction products. Reactions were performed, and agarose gel electrophoresis conducted as previously reported (19). Direction of electrophoresis is from top to bottom; the fastest migrating band was the superhelical ccc-PM2 DNA and the slowest migrating band (faintly visible) was the relaxed form of DNA. Lanes A through H correspond to increasing concentrations of ADM of 0, 5, 10, 25, 50, 75, 100, and 200 μM, respectively. Lanes I through P correspond to identical concentrations of CMM. Lanes Q through X correspond to increasing concentrations of carminomycin-11-methyl ether of 0, 5, 10, 25, 50, 100, 200, and 500 μM, respectively. Electrophoresis was at 5 V/cm for 10 hours at room temperature. Gels were stained with 0.5 μg/ml of ethidium bromide.

inhibition of RNA or NoRNA synthesis. Moreover, studies on membrane biosynthesis as described above have failed to demonstrate significant inhibitory activity. Thus the mechanism of action of these agents has not been defined. It is possible that microsomal activation and free-radical formation play a role in their activities as previously suggested (56).

IX. Conclusions

That minor structural modifications result in significant changes in the molecular pharmacological action of anthracyclines has become increasingly evident, suggesting that there may be multiple mechanistic classes of these agents. The studies presented here suggest that CMM and CMM-OMe may form a separate class of anthracyclines. The dissimilarity between pyrromycinone-based anthracyclines and ADM, based on DNA-binding characteristics, suggests that ADM may fall into a class of its own. Thus the results presented suggest the existence of five mechanistic classes of anthracyclines. The two classes of anthracyclines obtained, based on selectivity for the inhibition of NoRNA synthesis, can each be further subdivided. When comparing the affinity constants for binding to DNA, class I anthracyclines can be subdivided into CMM (low K_{app} values) versus PYM and ADM (intermediate to high K_{app} values). Also, ADM is clearly different from PYM and from the other pyrromycinone-based anthracyclines, based on the sequence specificities of DNA binding. Furthermore, ADM is different from CMM and CMM-OMe, based on DNA-binding characteristics, nucleic acid synthesis inhibitory activities, and antitumor activities. In addition, the class II anthracyclines MCM, RDM, MSM, and ACM are distinct from decarbomethoxymarcellomycin, decarbomethoxyrudolfomycin, clacinomycin, and mimimycin on the basis of DNA-binding characteristics and biological activities. Therefore, five mechanistic classes of anthracyclines can be defined based on the present results:

Nucleolar nonselective anthracyclines
- Adriamycin
- Carminomycin and carminomycin-11-methyl ether
- Pyrromycin

Nucleolus-selective anthracyclines
- Marcellomycin, aclacinomycin, mussettamycin, and rudolfomycin
- 10-Decarbomethoxymarcellomycin, 10-descarbomethoxyrudolfomycin, mimimycin, and collinemycin

Acknowledgments

The authors wish to express their appreciation to Dr. A. W. Prestayko for his review of the manuscript for this chapter and also to Ms. Julie Durantini and Ms. Carol Boyd for assistance in typing.

References

1. F. Arcamone, G. Cassinelli, G. Fantini, A. Grein, P. Orezzi, C. Pol, and C. Spalla, Adriamycin, 14-Hydroxy-daunomycin, a new antitumor antibiotic from *S. peucetius var. caesius* (1969). *Cancer Treat. Rep.* **53,** 842–848.
2. A. DiMarco, V. Gaetani, P. Orezzi, B. Scarpinato, R. Silvestrini, M. Soldati, T. Dasdia, and L. Valenti, *Nature (London)* **201,** 706 (1964).
3. R. H. Blum and S. K. Carter, *Ann. Intern. Med.* **80,** 249 (1974).
4. S. T. Crooke, V. H. DuVernay, L. Galvan, and A. Prestayko, *Mol. Pharmacol.* **14,** 290 (1978).
5. M. Waring, *J. Mol. Biol.* **54,** 247 (1970).
6. W. J. Pigram, W. Fuller, and L. D. Hamilton, *Nature (London) New Biol.* **235,** 17 (1972).
7. D. C. Ward, E. Reich, and I. H. Goldberg, *Science* **149,** 1259 (1965).
8. A. DiMarco, F. Arcamone, and F. Zunino, *Antibiotics (N.Y.)* **3,** (1975).
9. K. C. Tsou and K. F. Yip, *Cancer Res.* **36,** 3367 (1976).

10. T. Facchinetti, A. Montovani, L. Cantoni, R. Cantoni, and M. Salmona, *Chem.-Biol. Interact.* **20,** 97 (1978).
11. E. J. Gabbay, D. Grier, R. Fingele, R. Reiner, S. W. Pearce, and W. D. Wilson, *Biochemistry* **15,** 2062 (1976).
12. F. Zunio, R. Gambetta, A. DiMarco, A. Zaccara, and G. A. Luoni, *Cancer Res.* **35,** 754 (1975).
13. V. H. DuVernay, J. M. Essery, T. W. Doyle, W. T. Bradner, and S. T. Crooke, *Mol. Pharmacol.* **15,** 341 (1979).
14. V. H. DuVernay, J. A. Pachter, and S. T. Crooke, *Mol. Pharmacol.* (in press).
15. V. H. DuVernay, J. A. Pachter, and S. T. Crooke, *Biochemistry* **18,** 4024 (1979).
16. K. Diem and C. Lentner, eds., "Scientific Tables," 7th ed. Ciba-Geigy, Basel, 1970.
17. B. M. J. Revet, M. Schmir, and J. Vinograd, *Nature (London) New Biol.* **229,** 10 (1971).
18. R. T. Esperjo and J. Lebowitz, *Ann. Biochem.* **72,** 95 (1976).
19. S. Mong, J. E. Strong, V. H. DuVernay, and S. T. Crooke, *Mol. Pharmacol.* (in press).
20. S. Mong, J. E. Strong, J. A. Bush, and S. T. Crooke, *Antimicrob. Agents & Chemother.* (in press).
21. H. S. Schwartz, *Res. Commun. Chem. Pathol. Pharmacol.* **10,** 51 (1975).
22. W. N. Hittleman and P. N. Ras, *Cancer Res.* **35,** 3027 (1975).
23. J. W. Lown, S. K. Sim, K. C. Majundar, and R. Y. Chang, *Biochem. Biophys. Res. Commun.* **76,** 705 (1977).
24. A. Someya and N. Tanaka, *J. Antibiot.* **8,** 839 (1979).
25. A. DiMarco, R. Silvestrini, S. DiMarco, and T. Dasdia, *J. Cell Biol.* **27,** 545 (1965).
26. A. Theologides, J. W. Yarbo, and B. J. Kennedy, *Cancer* **21,** 16 (1968).
27. A. Rusconi and A. DiMarco, *Cancer Res.* **29,** 1507 (1969).
28. K. Danø, S. Frederiksen, and P. Hellung-Larsen, *Cancer Res.* **32,** 1307 (1972).
29. L. E. Crook, K. R. Rees, and A. Cohen, *Biochem. Pharmacol.* **21,** 281 (1972).
30. W. D. Meriwether and N. R. Bachur, *Cancer Res.* **32,** 1137 (1972).
31. G. P. Sartiano, W. E. Lynch, and W. D. Bullington, *J. Antibiot.* **32,** 1038 (1979).
32. D. W. Henry, *ACS Symp. Ser.* **30,** 15 (1976).
33. T. Oki, Y. Matsuzawa, A. Yoshimoto, K. Numata, I. Kitamura, S. Hori, A. Takamutsu, H. Umezawa, M. Ishizuka, H. Naganawa, H. Suda, M. Hamada, and T. Takeuchi, *J. Antibiot.* **28,** 830 (1975).
34. K. Kitaura, R. Imai, Y. Ishihara, H. Yanai, and H. Takahira, *J. Antibiot.* **25,** 509 (1972).
35. J. J. Wang, D. S. Chervinshy, and J. M. Rosen, *Cancer Res.* **32,** 511 (1972).
36. R. Silvestrini, A. DiMarco, and T. Dasdia, *Cancer Res.* **30,** 966 (1970).
37. M. Misumi, H. Yamaki, T. Akiyama, and N. Tanaka, *J. Antibiot.* **31** (1), 48 (1979).
38. W. S. Thayer, *Chem.-Biol. Interact.* **19,** 265 (1977).
39. T. Kishi, T. Watanabe, and K. Folkers, *Proc. Natl. Acad. Sci. U.S.A.* **73,** 4653 (1976).
40. C. Bertazzoli and H. Ghione, *Pharmacol. Res. Commun.* **9,** 235 (1977).
41. C. Bertazzoli, L. Sala, L. Ballerini, T. Watanabe, and K. Folkers, *Res. Commun. Chem. Pathol. Pharmacol.* **15,** 797 (1976).
42. G. Andreini, C. M. Beretta, and O. Sonzogni, *Pharmacol. Res. Commun.* **9,** 155 (1977).
43. M. Gosalvez, M. Blanco, J. Hunter, M. Miko, and B. Chance, *Eur. J. Cancer* **10,** 567 (1974).
44. Y. Iwamoto, I. L. Hansen, T. H. Porter, and K. Folkers, *Biochem. Biophys. Res. Commun.* **58,** 633 (1974).
45. C. E. Myers, W. P. McGuire, R. H. Liss, I. Iffim, K. Grotzinger, and R. C. Young, *Science* **197,** 165 (1977).
46. C. E. Myers, W. McGuire, and R. Young, *Cancer Treat. Rep.* **60,** 961 (1976).
47. S. A. Murphee, L. S. Cunningham, K. M. Hwang, and A. C. Sartorelli, *Biochem. Pharmacol.* **25,** 1227 (1976).

48. T. R. Tritton, S. A. Murphee, and A. C. Sartorelli, *Biochem. Biophys. Res. Commun.* **84,** 802 (1978).
49. S. A. Murphee, T. R. Tritton, and A. C. Sartorelli, *Fed. Proc. Fed. Am. Soc. Exp. Biol.* **36,** 303 (1977).
50. G. Schioppocassi and H. S. Schwartz, *Res. Commun. Chem. Pathol. Pharmacol.* **18,** 519 (1979).
51. R. Goldman, T. Faccinetti, D. Bach, A. Raz, and M. Shinitzky, *Biochim. Biophys. Acta* **512,** 254 (1978).
52. C. Na and S. N. Timasheff, *Arch. Biochem. Biophys.* **182,** 147 (1977).
53. M. Israel, E. J. Modest, and E. Frei, III, *Cancer Res.* **35,** 1365 (1975).
54. S. K. Sengupta, R. Seshadri, E. J. Modest, and M. Israel, *Proc. Am. Assoc. Cancer Res.* **17,** 109 (1976).
55. A. Krishan, R. N. Ganpathi, and M. Israel, *Cancer Res.* **38,** 3656 (1978).
56. N. R. Bachur, S. L. Gordon, and M. J. Gee, *Cancer Res.* **38,** 1745 (1978).

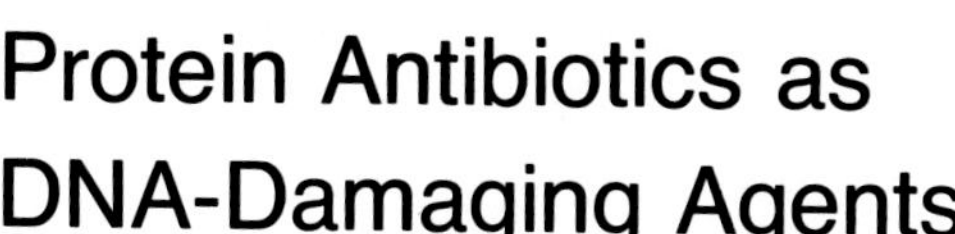

Protein Antibiotics as DNA-Damaging Agents

IRVING H. GOLDBERG, TAKUMI HATAYAMA, LIZZY S. KAPPEN, MARY A. NAPIER, AND LAWRENCE F. POVIRK

I. Introduction

In recent years a number of macromolecular (>10,000-dalton) antitumor antibiotics have been obtained from culture filtrates of *Streptomyces*. The agents

MOLECULAR ACTIONS AND TARGETS FOR CANCER CHEMOTHERAPEUTIC AGENTS

ISBN 0-12-619280-4.

that have been best characterized with regard to their chemical and biological properties are the protein antibiotics neocarzinostatin (NCS) (1), auromomycin (2) [and macromomycin (3)], and actinoxanthin (4). Interestingly, these three distinct agents contain regions of amino acid sequence homologous with one another (5–7) and, at least in the case of the first two agents, have some similarities in their biological effects. In this chapter we shall focus on work from our laboratory on the molecular basis of the action of NCS. Where possible, we shall compare the information available on the action of NCS with that emerging on auromomycin (and macromomycin).

II. Molecular Basis of Action of Protein Antitumor Antibiotics

A. Relation of Structure of Neocarzinostatin to Biological Activity

The antitumor antibiotic NCS, isolated from culture filtrates of *Streptomyces carzinostaticus* variant F-41 (1), is an acidic single-chain polypeptide with a molecular weight of 10,700 (5). The protein has been purified to homogeneity, and its amino acid sequence (Fig. 1) (5,8–10) and physical properties (11,12) have been determined. A preliminary X-ray diffraction study of NCS has been reported (13). The 20 amino acids at the NH_2-terminus are not required for full biological activity (14). This compound exists in a tight, proteolysis-resistant conformation with an antiparallel, β-pleated sheet structure (15). It possesses two reduction-resistant disulfide bridges and lacks methionine and histidine. The positions of the disulfides have not yet been unambiguously assigned. In NCS two tryptophan residues occur at positions 46 (buried) and 79, and one buried tyrosine residue at position 32. Oxidation of tryptophan 79 does not result in loss of biological activity (15). Similarly, acylation of the amino groups (alanine 1 and lysine 20) does not affect the activity of NCS (16,17). On the other hand, modification of the carboxyl groups results in loss of activity (17). Furthermore, spontaneous deamidation of asparagine 83 at a weakly acidic pH has been reported to generate a material which lacks biological activity (18). The chemically deamidated compound is thought to be the same as the biosynthetic precursor preneocarzinostatin (pre-NCS), isolated from culture filtrates, that antagonizes NCS activity (19).

B. Spectroscopic Characterization of a Nonprotein Chromophore in Neocarzinostatin

Optically active absorption bands have been reported for NCS above 300 nm (15,20), and inactivation of NCS by irradiation with 300 to 400-nm light has been found (21–23). Since these spectral characteristics are unusual for a purified

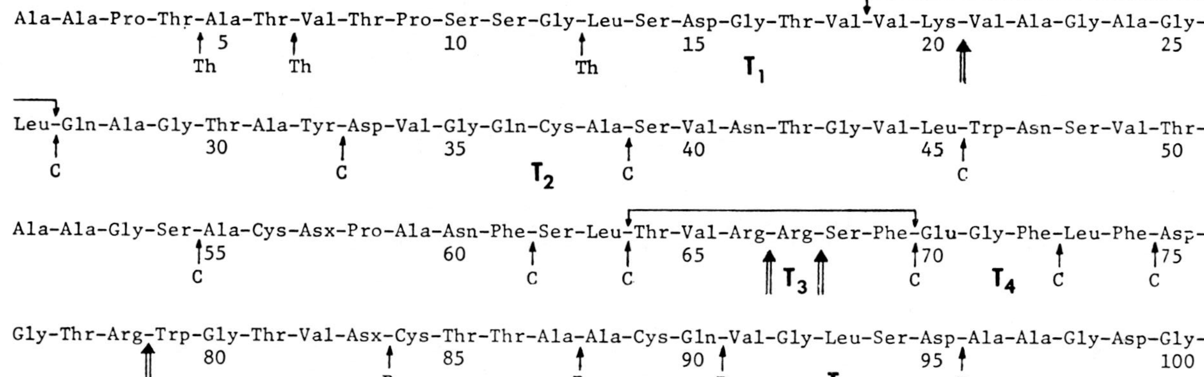

Fig. 1. Structure of NCS. Double arrows indicate tryptic cleavage; small arrows show some of the subsequent cleavages by thermolysin (Th), chymotrypsin (C), and pepsin (P). Overlap peptides are indicated by a bridged arrow. From Meienhofer *et al.* (5).

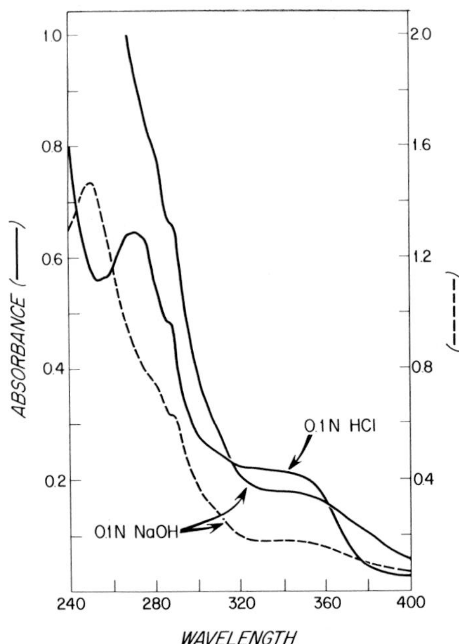

Fig. 2. The UV and visible light absorption spectra of NCS (2.7×10^{-5} *M*) in 0.1 *N* HCl and NCS (2.8×10^{-5} *M*) in 0.1 *N* NaOH.

protein, we further characterized native NCS spectroscopically and separated a highly fluorescent chromophore from the protein (20). As shown in Fig. 2, at an acid pH, NCS exhibits a broad absorption maximum at about 270 nm with an abnormally high extinction coefficient (ϵ 23,000) and a broad shoulder between 300 and 360 nm, with tailing between 360 and 400 nm (ϵ_{340} ~8000). Furthermore, strong optical activity is found above 300 nm with extremes in the magnetic circular dichroism (MCD) at 320 and 365 nm corresponding to the circular dichroism (CD) minima at these wavelengths (Fig. 3) (20). In alkaline solution an absorption maximum is seen at 250 nm; there is hypochromicity between 320 and 360 nm and a more gradual tailing that extends beyond 400 nm (Fig. 2).

The fluorescence spectrum of NCS has major excitation maxima at 285, 340, and 380 nm, with emission maxima at 345, 420, and 490 nm, respectively (20). The 345 nm emission band is attributable to tryptophan residues, but the intensity is low for the two tryptophans present, 45% of the intensity of an equivalent concentration of *N*-acetyltryptophanamide. The tryptophan emission is enhanced by treatment with reducing or denaturing agents. In the presence of 0.01 *M* 2-mercaptoethanol or 4 *M* guanidine–HCl, in 0.05 *M* Tris–HCl, pH 8.0, for 24 hours, the 345-nm emission is increased 1.4- and 2.0-fold, respectively. *S*-Carboxymethylated NCS, which has virtually no absorption or fluorescence excitation above 300 nm, exhibits normal tryptophan emission. Guanidine–HCl-treated NCS has increased absorption below 270 nm and a broad maximum at 380 nm. The fluorescence emission intensity is increased 1.4-fold at 420 nm and 8-fold at 490 nm. When treated with 2-mercaptoethanol (or $NaBH_4$), NCS exhibits some small changes in absorption above 300 nm. The intensity of the 420- and 490-nm emission bands, however, is increased 2.4- and 1.3-fold, respectively. The reduced tryptophan fluorescence emission of native NCS might be due to quenching resulting from its tightly folded structure which is relaxed by these treatments, as measured by CD (12,23). It is more likely that the altered emission is due to dissociation of a nonprotein chromophore, which quenches the tryptophan emission by competitively absorbing excitation energy and by serving as an energy acceptor. It is of interest that the 89-amino-acid tryptic fragment lacking the 20 amino acids at the NH_2-terminus possesses the same absorption and fluorescence spectroscopic properties as native NCS (14).

Separation of a nonprotein uv or visible light-absorbing material from the NCS protein is possible by several procedures (20). Sephadex G-50 chromatography of guanidine-treated, of 2-mercaptoethanol-treated, or of base-treated (0.1 *N* NaOH), but not of acid-treated (0.1 *N* HCl) NCS, separates the protein and nonprotein components. We have also found that chromatography of NCS on Amberlite XAD-7 and elution with distilled water leads to the recovery of a protein essentially free of chromophore as judged by uv and fluorescence measurements (23,24). The most convenient separation procedure for study of the chromophore, however, is methanol extraction of the lyophilized drug. The methanol fraction (A) (Fig. 4), free of common amino acids, has two broad absorption shoulders near 270 and 340 nm, CD and MCD activity above and below 300 nm, and fluorescence emission at 420 and 490 nm (20). The methanol-insoluble fraction (B), with an amino acid composition identical to that of NCS, exhibits typical protein absorbance (Fig. 4), with λ_{max} at 277 nm (ϵ

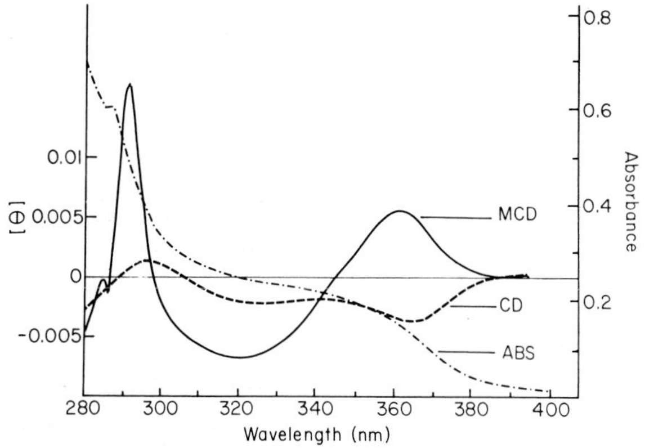

Fig. 3. The MCD, CD, and absorption (ABS) spectra of NCS (3.5×10^{-4} *M*, 0.015 *M* sodium acetate, pH 4.5). From Napier *et al.* (20).

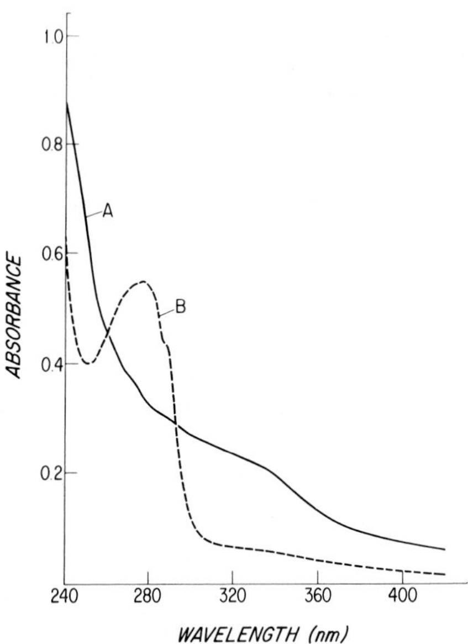

Fig. 4. Methanol extraction of NCS. Absorption spectra of methanol-soluble fraction A in methanol and methanol-insoluble fraction B in water. The fractions were diluted to a volume approximately equivalent to 1 mg/ml NCS. From Napier *et al.* (20).

14,000). The absorption at 250 nm, seen for NCS, is reduced. Absorption and optical activity above 300 nm are virtually absent. Also, there are no changes in the tryptophan residues as determined by MCD. The major fluorescence remaining is the tryptophan emission at 345 nm. The spectral properties of fraction B are similar to those found for *S*-carboxymethylated NCS which has lost the nonprotein chromophore probably as a result of the reduction and methanol extraction procedures used in its preparation (9). Thus NCS purified by chromatography is an acid-stable complex of a protein and a nonprotein chromophore which can be dissociated and separated by a number of procedures. It is of interest that carzinostatin, an uncharacterized antibiotic isolated from the parent strain of *S. carzinostaticus,* has been described as a complex consisting of a methanol-soluble fraction and a methanol-insoluble, water-soluble fraction (25). Neither fraction has significant biological activity alone, but recombination restores activity. The biological properties of NCS, a more stable antibiotic isolated from variant 41 of *S. carzinostatin,* are similar to those of carzinostatin.

C. Cellular DNA as a Target in the Action of Neocarzinostatin

There is considerable evidence that DNA is an important target in the action of NCS. Thus low levels of NCS selectively inhibit DNA synthesis in sensitive bacteria and mammalian cells (26–30), induce degradation of existing DNA in bacteria (26,31), and produce breaks in the DNA of mammalian cells (28–30,32–35). A correlation exists between the ability of NCS to induce breakage of cellular DNA in HeLa cells and its inhibition of DNA replication and cell growth (29,35). In fact, in common with other agents causing DNA strand breaks, such as X-irradiation and photolysis of bromodeoxyuridine-substituted DNA, NCS selectively inhibits initiation of DNA synthesis in replicons in mammalian cells (L. F. Povirk and I. H. Goldberg, unpublished data) and differs from uv radiation which selectively inhibits DNA chain elongation. Single-strand breaks induced in HeLa cells by NCS can be repaired to a considerable extent, but repair of double-strand breaks is less efficient (30), and the latter may account for the cell-killing activity of the antibiotic. We estimate that there are about 55–60 double-strand breaks per cell at the mean lethal dose (at which there is 37% survival of cells) of 0.01 μg/ml NCS (30). Thus it appears that a small number of such breaks in a critical region of the genome may be the lethal event. Furthermore, the so-called DNA complex consisting of DNA, lipid, and protein is disrupted by NCS treatment of HeLa cells, and this is accompanied by release within the cell of free DNA (30). DNA repair synthesis is activated by NCS-induced DNA damage, as revealed by the induction of unscheduled DNA synthesis in treated lymphocytes (36) and by the marked stimulation of thymidine incorporation into parental (but not newly made replicative) DNA in HeLa cells and isolated nuclei (37). Furthermore, low levels of NCS cause a block in the G_2 phase of the cell cycle (38,39) and chromosomal abberrations in mammalian cells (39,40).

Strong evidence for the involvement of DNA in NCS action comes from experiments showing that NCS is a mutagen for *Escherichia coli* and that mutagenicity and cell killing are affected in inverse ways by a *recA* mutation (41). We have also found NCS to be mutagenic for *Salmonella typhimurium,* especially in strains bearing the plasmid pKM101 which has been implicated in error-prone repair (42,43). Finally, the lethal effect of NCS on L1210 cells has been found to be potentiated by caffeine, an inhibitor of postreplication repair (44,45).

D. Properties of Auromomycin and Macromomycin

Macromomycin, produced by *Streptomyces macromomyceticus* (3), is a weakly acidic protein (pI 5.4) with a molecular weight of about 12,500 (2,46–48) that is active in cell cultures (49,50) and against several experimental murine tumors (51). Macromomycin inhibits DNA synthesis selectively (47,49,52–55) and induces DNA strand scissions *in vivo* (52–56). It has only recently been appreciated that macromomycin preparations are often contaminated with the more cytotoxic auromomycin (2), and it seems likely that this accounts for its biological activity (23). Auromomycin is the same as macromomycin but contains a chromophore absorbing at 357 nm (2). Auromomycin also selectively inhibits DNA synthesis and induces DNA strand scission in bacterial and mammalian cells (55,57,58). We have also found that auromomycin is mutagenic for bacteria. (E. Eisenstadt and I. H. Goldberg, unpublished data).

E. Requirements for *in Vitro* DNA Strand Scission by Protein Antibiotics

Single-strand nicks in superhelical and linear duplex DNA are caused by NCS *in vitro* (Fig. 5), and this reaction is stimulated at least 1000-fold by the presence of a mercaptan (32,33,35,55,59–64). At higher doses of NCS, double-strand breaks are produced, presumably as a result of the random placement of single-strand breaks within a small number of base pairs of one another. Auromomycin has also been found to induce DNA strand cleavage *in vitro* in linear duplex and superhelical DNA, and this reaction is little affected by 2-mercaptoethanol (Fig. 5) (55,58,65). Double-strand breaks produced as single events appear to be

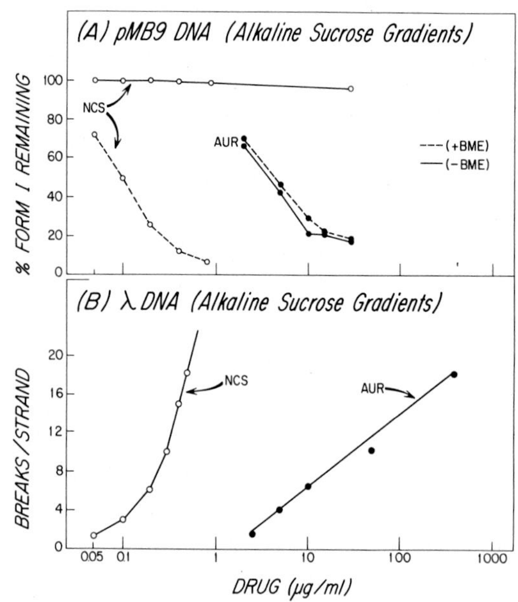

Fig. 5. Strand breakage in pMB9 and λ DNA by NCS and auromomycin (AUR). (A) Standard reactions (0.1 ml) contained 0.94 μg (1.8×10^4 cpm) of superhelical pMB9 DNA and varying amounts of the drugs in the presence and absence of 10 m*M* 2-mercaptoethanol. The data have been adjusted as though there was 100% form I at the start of the reaction. (B) λ DNA (0.4 μg, 2.4×10^4 cpm) was incubated with the drugs in a final volume of 0.1 ml. 2-Mercaptoethanol (BME) was added only to the samples containing NCS. After incubation for 30 minutes, the reaction mixtures were analyzed on alkaline sucrose gradients. From Kappen *et al.* (55).

caused by this agent (55). In contrast, macromomycin caused very slight scission of linear or circular duplex DNA even at levels of 500 μg/ml, with or without 2-mercaptoethanol (52,54,55,65), although Sawyer *et al.* (48) reported that supercoiled PM2 DNA was cleaved by this antibiotic in the absence of reducing compounds. On the other hand, Suzuki *et al.* (65) have found that, in the presence of $NaBH_4$ or dithiothreitol, macromomycin caused DNA breakage *in vitro*. The significance of this finding remains to be determined, although it seems highly likely that the degree of auromomycin contamination determines the extent of biological activity (23). Similar to the apparent lack of association between the *in vivo* and *in vitro* effects of macromomycin on DNA strand scission, Vandré and Montgomery (56) found that an acetylated form of macromomycin lost almost all of its ability to break DNA strands in KB cells but retained a significant portion of its DNA synthesis-inhibitory action. We have also found that auromomycin-induced scission of DNA *in vitro* is inhibited by intercalating drugs such as ethidium bromide, daunorubicin, proflavin, and actinomycin D at low concentrations, while concentrations at least 10 times higher are required for inhibition of the NCS reaction (55).

In contrast to the results with macromomycin, with NCS the changes in cytotoxicity are always accompanied by like changes in DNA scission activity *in vivo* and *in vitro* (14,24,35). It should also be noted, as shown in Fig. 5 that about 40 times or more auromomycin is required to produce the same degree of DNA strand scission as NCS (with 2-mercaptoethanol), even though in cells auromomycin is at least as cytotoxic (55).

F. Template Properties of Neocarzinostatin-Treated DNA

DNA treated by NCS is a much poorer primer for *E. coli* DNA polymerase I than untreated DNA (61,66), and this enzyme has been shown to bind to the site of DNA damage in a nonfunctional form (61). The degree of inhibition of DNA synthesis by NCS depends on the concentrations of NCS and 2-mercaptoethanol during pretreatment and is related to the number of single-strand breaks produced in the DNA. That NCS-induced strand breakage generates inactive binding sites for DNA polymerase I is shown in experiments in which either untreated DNA or excess enzyme is able to overcome the inhibition in a competitive way. Furthermore, [^{203}Hg]DNA polymerase I binds to NCS-treated DNA, and binding correlates with the extent of nicking (61). It appears that one molecule of enzvme binds to each break introduced by NCS.

G. DNA Base Specificity in Neocarzinostatin Action

The breaks possess both 3′- and 5′-phosphoryl termini, indicative of the existence of a gap of one or more nucleotides (60,67). As expected, generation of a 3′-hydroxyl group by treatment of NCS-nicked DNA with alkaline phosphatase converts the DNA into a much better primer for DNA polymerase I than DNA unexposed to the antibiotic. DNA strand cleavage is also accompanied by release of the bases thymine (59,60) and adenine (60). Only about 15% as much adenine is released as thymine. The requirement for thymidylic and deoxyadenylic acids in the scission reaction was also revealed by experiments in which various synthetic and natural DNAs of different base composition were tested for their ability to protect against the cutting of radioactive λ virus DNA (60). Furthermore, using the DNA sequencing technique of Maxam and Gilbert (68), NCS was shown to cleave double-stranded φX174 DNA restriction fragments in the presence of 2-mercaptoethanol almost exclusively at deoxythymidylic and deoxyadenylic acid residues (69,70). Overall, deoxythymidylic acid residues are attacked much more frequently than deoxyadenylic acid residues (Fig. 6), although there is variability in the attack rate for both nucleotides at different locations in the DNA molecule. While all deoxythymidylic acid residues are sites of scission, not all deoxyadenylic acid residues are cleavage sites, but there appears to be no clear-cut nucleotide sequence specificity in determining cleavage frequency. In agreement with the protection experiments, single-stranded DNA is a very poor substrate for NCS-induced scission. It is of interest that both members of a base pair, deoxythymidylic and deoxyadenylic acids, are the main targets of NCS, for the chances of producing double-strand breaks in A-T-poor or homopolymeric regions is significantly increased over that caused by the otherwise random placement of single-stranded scissions. Since double- and not single-strand breaks are considered lethal events (71,72), this action of NCS may be important in determining its cytotoxicity. Furthermore, these results on base specificity are in agreement with the earlier finding with DNA polymerase I that DNA synthesis directed by poly[d(A-T)] is much more sensitive to NCS than that directed by poly[d(G-C)] (61).

H. Evidence for Direct Sugar Damage in Neocarzinostatin Action

Evidence has been obtained that the drug-induced gaps in DNA are not caused by simple splitting of the phosphodiester bond. We have found that sugar damage plays an important role in the NCS-induced DNA strand scission reaction (73). The release of [^{3}H]-labeled compounds, mainly as formic acid and water, from [5′-^{3}H] thymidine-λDNA, accounts for 50–80% of the thymine released without or with post-incubation alkaline treatment, respectively. The release of these labeled sugar degradation products correlates well with the increase in both thymine release and 5′-phosphate ends due to post-incubation alkaline treatments. In addition, a malonaldehyde-like substance (characterized by its reaction with thiobarbituric acid and its chromatographic properties), containing label derived from the 1′,2′-carbons of the deoxyribose moiety of thymidylate in DNA, is produced in a bound form concomitantly with the strand breaks and

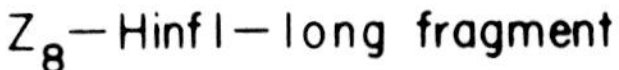

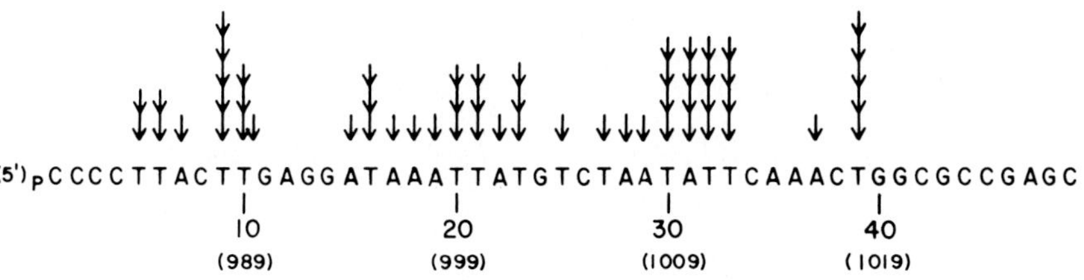

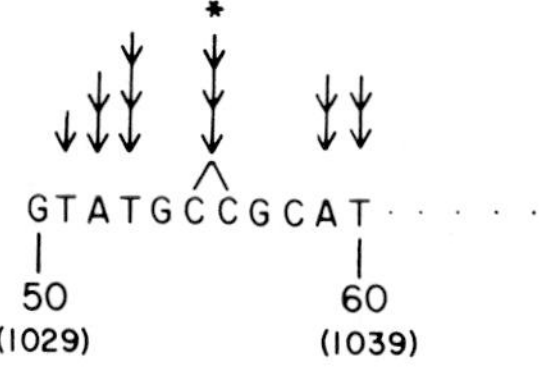

Z_8—Hinf I—short fragment

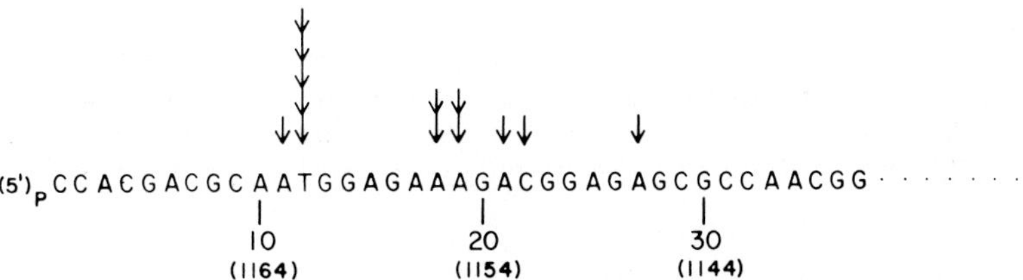

Fig. 6. Cleavage sites of NCS in two restriction enzyme fragments of duplex ϕX174 DNA as determined by the DNA-sequencing technique of Maxam and Gilbert [68]. The number of arrows indicates the relative intensity of the bands on the autoradiograms. Very faint bands deserving significantly less than one arrow are not shown. The asterisk indicates the position attacked by NCS in the single-stranded fragment. The nucleotide position on the Sanger map is indicated in parentheses. The sequence of the short fragment is the complement of that on the Sanger map. From Hatayama *et al.* (69).

thymine release; its production is dependent on the presence of mercaptans and oxygen, is stimulated by isopropanol, and is inhibited by α-tocopherol. Labeled malonaldehyde-like material and water are released from DNA only after alkaline treatment and account for about 40% of the corresponding thymine released.

Thymine release is significantly increased by post-incubation alkaline treatment. The number of thymines released by various post-incubation treatments is

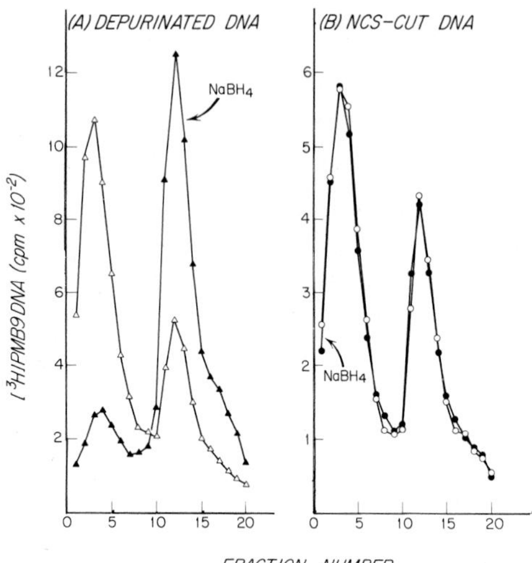

Fig. 7. Effect of $NaBH_4$ reduction on depurinated DNA (A) and NCS-cut DNA (B) as analyzed on alkaline sucrose gradients. Supercoiled pMB9 DNA was partially depurinated at 50°C in 0.05 *M* sodium citrate, pH 3.5, for 3 minutes. DNA (34 μg/ml, 1.9×10^4 cpm/μg) was cut with NCS (0.5 μg/ml) under standard conditions as in Fig. 5. Reduction by $NaBH_4$ (22 °C, 90 minutes) was carried out in 200 μl of reaction mixture containing 50 m*M* potassium phosphate, pH 6.5, and treated DNA (1.4 μg NCS-treated DNA and 2.5 μg depurinated DNA). At 15-minute intervals $NaBH_4$ was added in aliquots to a final concentration of 0.5 *M*. Portions (85 μl) of the reaction mixture were then analyzed on 5–20% alkaline sucrose gradients. Sedimentation is from left to right. The faster and slower sedimenting peaks represent forms I and II of pMB9 DNA, respectively. Open symbols are without $NaBH_4$ treatment.

consistent with the number of 5′-phosphate ends generated at the DNA gaps as determined by the combined use of alkaline phosphatase and polynucleotide kinase; and after alkaline treatment (0.3 *N* NaOH, 37°C, 30 min) both values are in good agreement with the number of single-strand breaks, as estimated by alkaline sucrose gradients. Taken together these data indicate that NCS generates damage in the DNA that requires alkali for its full expression as measured by thymine release and the generation of 5′-phosphate ends. In addition to true single-strand breaks, NCS can produce up to half alkali-labile breaks (67, unpublished data), but these seem not to be due to simple aldehydic apurinic–apyrimidinic sites since treatment with $NaBH_4$ of drug-treated DNA fails to decrease the number of breaks observed on alkaline sucrose gradients (Fig. 7). Also, we have found that base substitution, such as occurs upon alkylation of DNA by methyl methanesulfonate or nitrogen mustard, does not occur with NCS treatment since, unlike the effect of these agents, the glycosidic bond is not cleaved by heating at 54°C at neutral pH to generate alkali-labile breaks (L. S. Kappen and I. H. Goldberg, unpublished data).

I. Evidence for Formation of an Active, Labile Form of Neocarzinostatin

While NCS-induced cutting of DNA *in vitro* is markedly stimulated by the presence of a mercaptan, high levels of the mercaptan inhibit the reaction (Fig. 8) (62). This effect is seen especially clearly with the radiation protector (and free-radical scavenger) *S*,2-aminoethylisothiuronium bromide–HBr (AET).

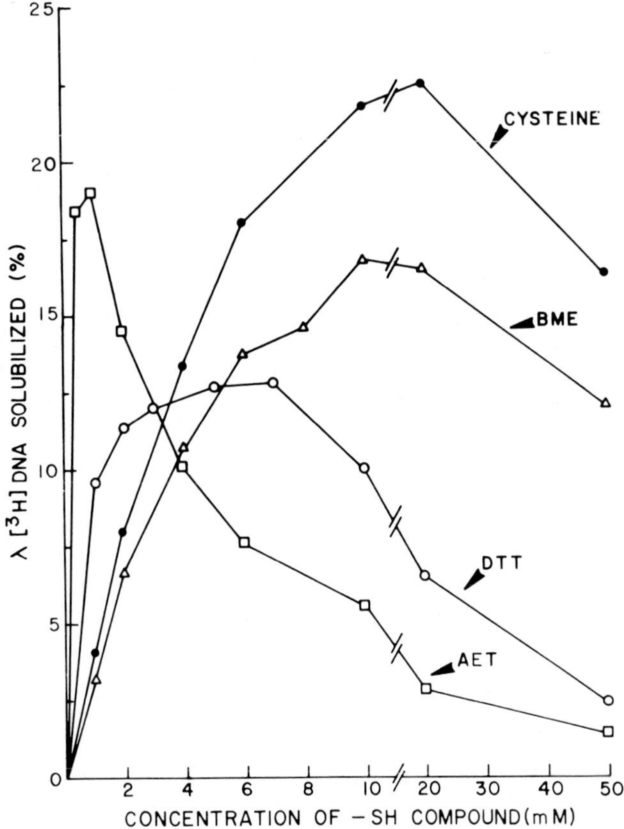

Fig. 8. Effect of different sulfhydryl compounds on the activity of NCS (100 μg/ml). The concentrations of the sulfhydryl agents [cysteine, 2-mercaptoethanol (BME), dithiothreitol (DTT), AET] were varied as indicated. The trichloroacetic acid solubility of λ [^{3}H]DNA was measured at 20 minutes. From Kappen and Goldberg (62).

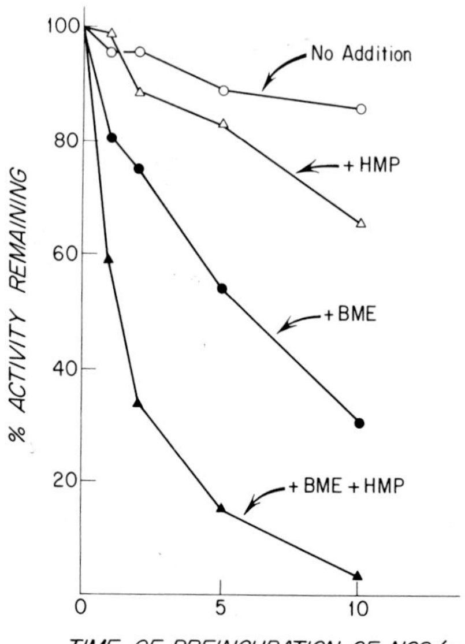

Fig. 9. Rate of inactivation of NCS in the presence of a sulfhydryl compound and hexamethylphosphoramide (HMP). NCS (125 μg/ml) was preincubated in 62.5 m*M* Tris-MCl buffer, pH 8.0, alone or with 0.5 *M* hexamethylphosphoramide in the presence and absence of 5 m*M* 2-mercaptoethanol (BME). At the various times shown, 80-μl aliquots were removed and added to tubes containing λ DNA (0.8 μg, 3.6×10^4 cpm). The complete reaction mixture had 100 μg/ml of NCS and 10 m*M* 2-mercaptoethanol. After 30 minutes of incubation, the amount of trichloroacetic acid-solubilized radioactivity was determined. Without preincubation the percentage of the DNA made acid-soluble was 8.2 and 31% without and with hexamethylphosphoramide, respectively. From Kappen and Goldberg (24).

Since AET rearranges rapidly when neutralized to form 2-mercaptoethylguanidine, it is likely that the latter is the active form. While less active than a mercaptan, we have found that $NaBH_4$ can also activate the reaction. In addition, preincubation of NCS with a mercaptan results in its rapid inactivation (Fig. 9) (62,64), and this inactivation is not prevented by the absence of oxygen or the presence of EDTA or catalase. Support for the possible involvement of a radical mechanism comes from the requirement for oxygen in the DNA scission reaction (22,62,63) and its inhibition by low concentrations of the potent peroxyl free-radical scavenger α-tocopherol (62). Acid-solubilization of DNA by NCS was blocked 50% at 50 μM α-tocopherol. The effect of α-tocopherol on NCS-induced cleavage of supercoiled pMB9 DNA is shown in Fig. 10. We have also found that α-tocopherol blocks the auromomycin scission of DNA (55). On the other hand, exogenous metals have yet to be implicated in either reaction, since various metal chelators (e.g., EDTA, 8-hydroxyquinoline, deferoxamine,

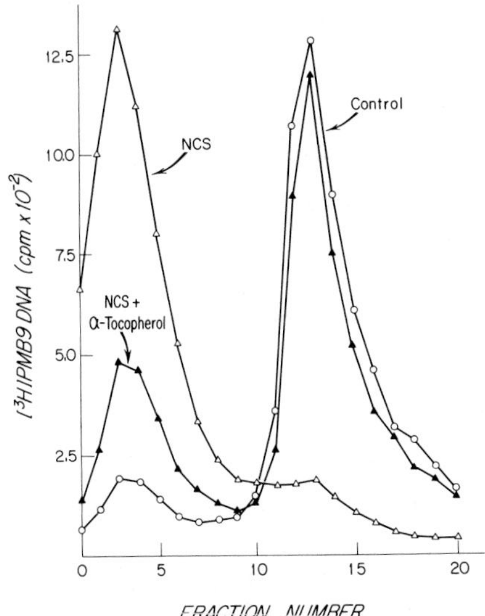

Fig. 10. Inhibition of NCS cutting of pMB9 DNA by α-tocopherol. Supercoiled pMB9 DNA (0.6 μg, 7×10^3 cpm/μg) was treated with NCS (0.5 μg/ml) under standard conditions (10 mM 2-mercaptoethanol) in the presence or absence of 0.5 mM α-tocopherol. The reaction mixture was analyzed on 5–20% alkaline sucrose gradients. Addition of 0.5 mM α-tocopherol to control DNA did not affect its sedimentation profile (not shown). Sedimentation is from left to right.

diethyldithiocarbamate, neocuproine, cuprizone) do not block the reaction (62, and unpublished data). Furthermore, we have found the clinical form of NCS (after dialysis against water) to be free of iron, zinc, cobalt, and copper. Similarly, superoxide dismutase and catalase do not inhibit the reaction.

Unexpectedly, various alcohols, organic solvents, and other agents, such as urea, that affect protein conformation have been found to stimulate the mercaptan-dependent reaction significantly (24,62) (Fig. 11). Hexamethylphosphoramide was the most potent of the stimulators tested. Kinetic analysis of NCS-induced DNA scission in the presence of isopropanol showed that the solvent effect was on the initial rate of the reaction (Fig. 12) and that the V_{max} and not the K_m was affected (24). In contrast, guanidine-HCl at subdenaturing levels strongly inhibited the reaction (50% inhibition at 0.05 M). It is of interest that, like the mercaptans, the organic solvents inactivate NCS in a preincubation (Fig. 9). It seemed possible that the organic solvents, in both activation and inactivation, facilitate the release and generation of an active, labile form of the antibiotic by unfolding the protein (24). As described in a subsequent section (II,M), this prediction has been found to be the correct one.

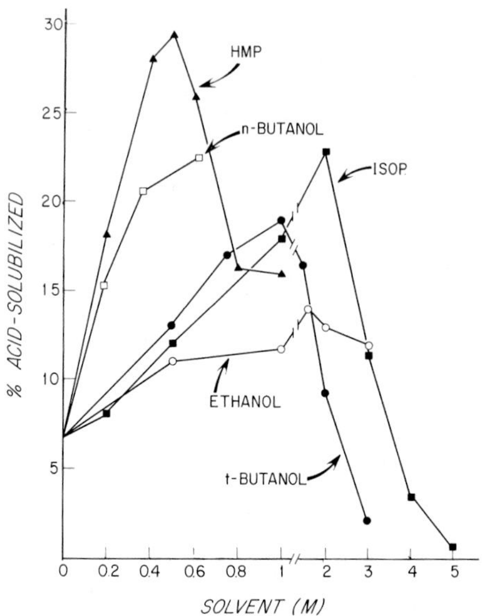

Fig. 11. Effect of organic solvents on NCS activity. Standard reaction mixtures (100 μl) contained 0.8 μg of λ DNA (2.4×10^4 cpm), 100 μg/ml of NCS, and varying amounts of solvents. After incubation for 30 minutes, the amount of trichloroacetic acid-soluble radioactivity was determined. HMP, Hexamethylphosphoramide; ISOP, isopropanol. From Kappen and Goldberg (24).

J. Effect of Chromophore Removal on Neocarzinostatin Activity

The nonprotein chromophore of NCS can be removed or destroyed by any of several different procedures (20) (Section II,K). In an effort to remove the chromophore as gently as possible, so as to be able to determine the effect of chromophore loss alone on the activity of the drug, we have employed Amberlite XAD-7 chromatography in a manner similar to that described for the preparation of macromomycin (2), except that protein was eluted with distilled water before elution with 30% ethanol (23,24). The water-eluted protein and the 30% ethanol-eluted protein constituted 65 and 24%, respectively, of the total protein placed on the column. Absorbance and fluorescence spectroscopy revealed that both fractions were severely depleted in material absorbing above 300 nm, with water-eluted material being more chromophore-free than the fraction eluting with 30% ethanol (Fig. 13). Both materials possessed the amino acid composition of the original NCS. Biological activity as determined by DNA synthesis inhibition in HeLa cells and DNA scission activity *in vitro* was markedly decreased in the two chromatography fractions, with the water-eluted material having about 0.5% and the 30% ethanol-eluted fraction having about 5% of the original activity in both assays. These data suggest a correlation between the extent of chromophore

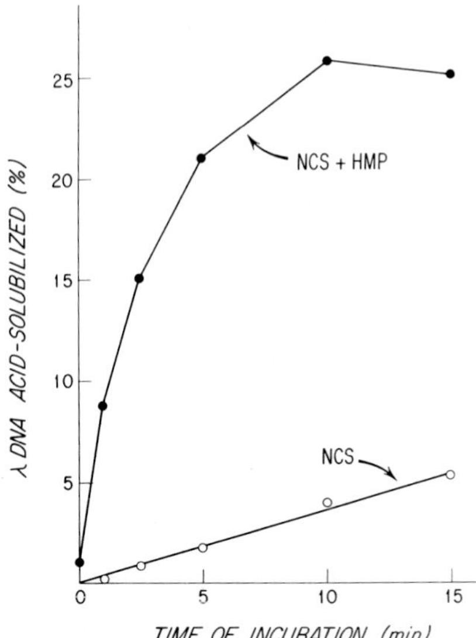

Fig. 12. Time course of stimulation of NCS activity by hexamethylphosphoramide (HMP). Incubations (1 ml) were as in Fig. 11. Portions of 100-ml were withdrawn at the indicated times for the determination of acid-solubilized radioactivity. From Kappen and Goldberg (24).

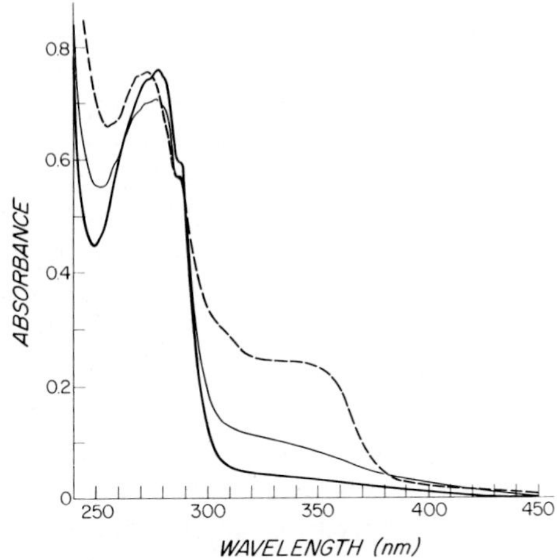

Fig. 13. The UV and visible light absorption spectra of proteins eluted from Amberlite XAD-7 chromatography of NCS. Heavy solid line, Water-eluted protein (5.3×10^{-5} *M,* 0.57 mg/ml, in water, ϵ 14,000); light solid line, 30% ethanol-eluted protein (5×10^{-5} *M,* 0.55 mg/ml, in water, assuming ϵ 14,000); dashed line, native NCS (3.2×10^{-5} *M,* 0.34 mg/ml, in 0.01 M sodium acetate, pH 5.0). From Nupier *et al.* (23).

removal and the amount of activity remaining. We have also carried out Amberlite XAD-7 chromatography on "purified" macromomycin and have found that the material eluted by distilled water has only about 10% of the DNA synthesis inhibition activity of the starting material, raising the likelihood that the activity attributed to macromomycin is due to contaminating auromomycin. These data suggested that the nonprotein chromophore is responsible for antibiotic activity.

K. Inhibition of DNA Interaction by Inactivated Antibiotics

Although evidence had been presented that active drug enters mammalian cells (29,74,75), there was no direct evidence that the drug forms a stable complex with DNA. Commonly employed methods involving chromatography and centrifugation techniques with a radioactive form of the drug had failed to give evidence for direct binding of NCS to DNA (74, L. S. Kappen and I. H. Goldberg, unpublished data). We have used an indirect method, involving the ability of NCS rendered inactive by denaturing agents or other treatments, to block the activity of native NCS (24). Acid solubilization of λ DNA by native NCS was measured in the presence of increasing amounts of inactivated NCS. Both heat-denatured and 2-mercaptoethanol-inactivated NCS block the activity of native NCS; 50% inhibition was obtained at about equimolar levels with native drug (24). Inhibition is less at higher DNA/native drug ratios. In order to establish the specificity of this assay we have compared the effects of NCS treated by different agents to those of other acidic proteins and the protein antibiotics macromomycin and auromomycin (Table I). It can be seen that NCS inactivated by different methods inhibits the activity of native NCS. It is interesting to note that arginine-blocked NCS, which is not active *in vitro* or *in vivo* (14), does not inhibit the reaction of NCS with or without heat treatment. On the other hand, the 89-amino-acid peptide derivative of NCS, which is as active as NCS *in vitro* and *in vivo* (14), inhibits NCS activity after heat inactivation. Little (<1%) if any *in vitro* or *in vivo* biological activity is retained by NCS from which the chromophore has been removed by methanol extraction (23) and, as seen in Table I, this is a potent inhibitor of native drug in cell-free DNA scission. Similar results were obtained with the water-eluted chromophore-free NCS prepared by Amberlite XAD-7 chromatography (Fig. 14). Auromomycin, macromomycin (data not shown), bovine serum albumin, and pepsinogen (all with or without heat denaturation) do not have any effect on the activity of NCS. These results were confirmed in experiments in which DNA strand breakage was followed on alkaline and neutral sucrose gradients, although because of the relatively high ratio of DNA to native NCS, larger amounts of inactive drug were required for comparable inhibition. Similarly, we have found that *in vitro* DNA strand scission by auromomycin is blocked specifically by heated auromomycin or by macromomycin (Fig. 15), heated or unheated, in a dose-dependent way (23). On the other hand, an inactivated form of actinoxanthin (gift of Y. A.

TABLE I

Effect of Inactivated Neocarzinostatin and Other Proteins on the Activity of Native Neocarzinostatin[a] (24)

Addition (μg/ml)[b]	Inhibition (%)
None	
Heat-inactivated NCS (200)	70
UV-inactivated NCS[c] (180)	63
6 *M* Guanidine-treated NCS (80)	59
Methanol-extracted NCS (100)	75
Arginine-blocked NCS (200)	None
Arginine-blocked NCS after heat treatment (200)	None
Heat-inactivated 89-amino-acid peptide of NCS (50)	53
Heat-inactivated auromomycin (200)	None
Bovine serum albumin (500)	None
Ovalbumin (500)	None
Pepsinogen (500)	None

[a] The effect of addition of the proteins listed to incubations containing native NCS and λ [^{3}H]DNA was determined by measuring the amount of trichloroacetic acid-soluble radioactivity; 8.7 % of the DNA was made acid-soluble by NCS (100 μg/ml) without addition of other proteins.

[b] Details of the various treatments are described in Kappen and Goldberg (23).

[c] Exposure to long-wavelength UV light (Mineralight Lamp, Model UVSL-58, 366 nm) for 45 minutes at 15 cm.

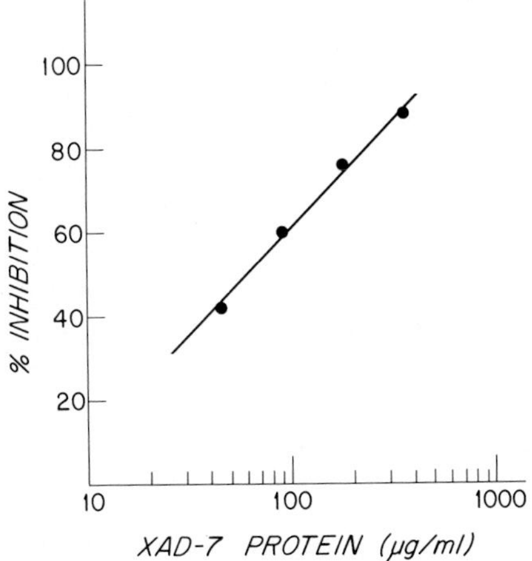

Fig. 14. Inhibition of NCS activity by water-eluted protein from Amberlite XAD-7 chromatography of NCS. Reaction mixtures (100 μl) contained 100 m*M* Tris–HCl, pH 8.0, 10 m*M* 2-mercaptoethanol, 0.4 μg λ DNA (1.8 × 10^4 cpm), 95 μg/ml active NCS, and varying amounts of protein obtained by Amberlite XAD-7 chromatography of NCS. After 30 minutes of incubation at 37°C, the amount of trichloroacetic acid-solubilized radioactivity was determined. With NCS alone, 86 cpm was made acid-soluble. From Napier *et al.* (23).

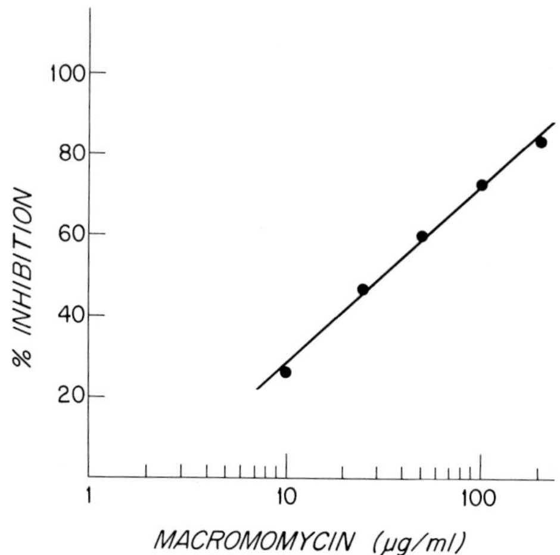

Fig. 15. Inhibition of auromomycin-induced scission of pMB9 DNA by macromomycin. Incubations (100 μl) contained 100 m*M* Tris–HCl, pH 8.0, 0.38 μg of superhelical DNA (1×10^4 cpm), and varying amounts of macromomycin at a constant level of auromomycin (10 μg/ml). Incubation was for 20 minutes at 37°C. The reaction mixture was then analyzed on 5–20% alkaline sucrose gradients. The radioactivity present in the peaks of supercoiled (form I) and the nicked forms of DNA was quantitated. Sixty-eight percent of form I DNA was nicked by auromomycin. From Napier *et al.* (23).

Ovchinnikov) was not inhibitory for either NCS- or auromomycin-induced DNA breakage.

Since the various treatments (i.e., heating, incubation with 2-mercapto-ethanol, treatment with guanidine–HCl, exposure to long-wavelength UV light (or to fluorescent light), methanol extraction, and Amberlite XAD-7 chromatography) used to generate the inhibitory species of NCS all lead to loss of biological activity and chromophore destruction and/or release or removal from the protein (20,23,24), it appeared that the apoprotein of NCS completed with DNA for interaction with the nonprotein chromophore. Furthermore, the ability of macromomycin to block the *in vitro* DNA scission activity of auromomycin seemed to be another instance where the chromophore-free protein bound the active form of the drug (the nonprotein chromophore) so that it was no longer available to complex with the DNA.

L. Is Preneocarzinostatin a Chromophore-free Form of Neocarzinostatin?

It is also of interest that these several different treatments produce a protein with a lower pI as revealed by polyacrylamide gel isoelectric focusing (23). A more acidic form of NCS (pI 3.2, compared to 3.3 for active NCS), which is biologically inactive itself (19,35) but can block NCS action *in vivo,* has been identified as a likely biosynthetic precursor of active drug and has been called pre-NCS (19). Maeda and Kuromizu (18) have proposed that this form of the drug, as well as that generated from native NCS by treatment at an acidic pH, differs from native NCS in having an aspartic acid instead of an asparagine in position 83 of the protein. In order to study the possible role of chromophore removal in generating the species with the lower pI, we rechromatographed a dialyzed preparation of clinical NCS and a previously purified (10) preparation of NCS stored in powder form in a freezer for 2 years (courtesy of T. S. A. Samy) on CM-cellulose (Figs. 16 and 17) (23). The latter material was a single, homogeneous protein at the time of original purification by the criteria listed in [10]. The fraction eluting at a pH of 3.4 [corresponding to pre-NCS (10,18,19)] represents 33 and 55% of the total protein (correcting for extinction coefficients) derived from clinical NCS and purified NCS, respectively. These values are in good agreement with the respective fractions (30 and 60% of the total protein as determined by the relative intensities of Coomassie blue staining) migrating on an isoelectric focusing gel at a pI of 3.2 (Fig. 18). Furthermore, these results agree with *in vitro* DNA scission experiments where the purified NCS had about one-half the activity of the clinical material in converting form I pMB9 DNA to form II (0.12 and 0.06 μg/ml for 50% conversion, respectively). In each case, the protein behaving on CM-cellulose chromatography and isoelectric focusing

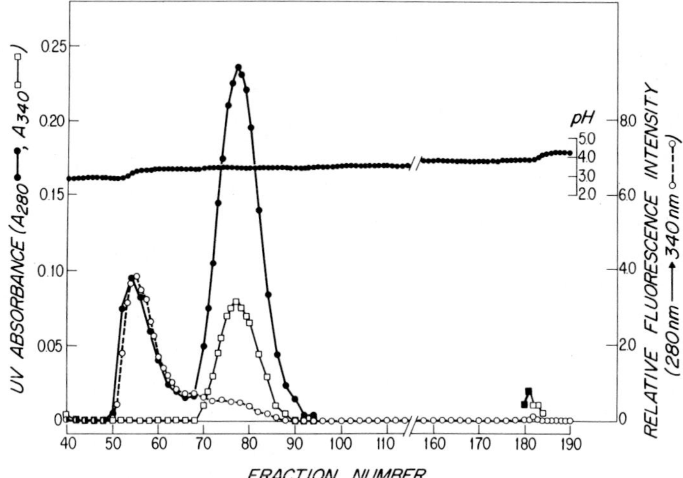

Fig. 16. Chromatography of clinical NCS (3.0 mg) on a CM-cellulose column (1.5 × 75 cm). The sample was first dialyzed against water, lyophilized, and redissolved in 0.1 *N* acetic acid. After sample addition, the column was washed in 0.05 *M* acetic acid and eluted with a pH gradient of 0.1 *M* sodium acetate, pH 3.2–3.7 (500 ml) and pH 3.7–4.7 (500 ml). Fractions (5 ml) were collected at 43 ml/hour. Chromatography was at 4°C in the dark. From Napier *et al.* (23).

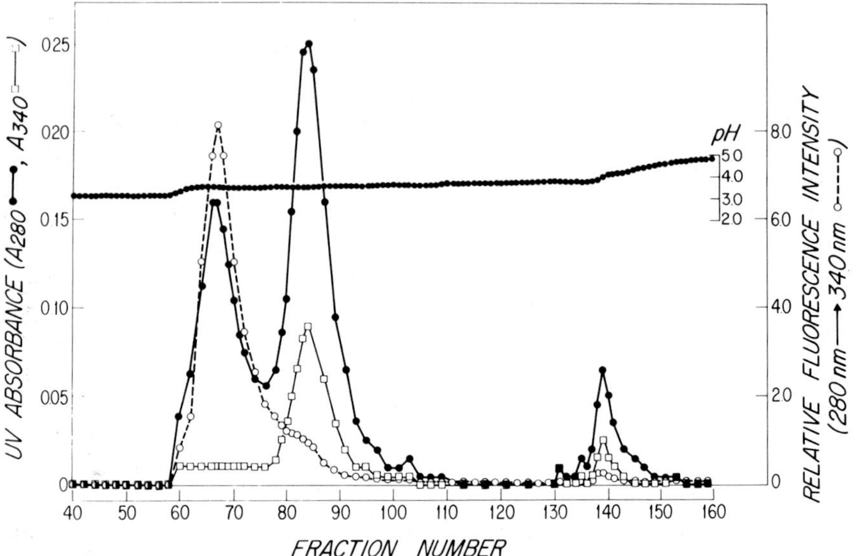

Fig. 17. Chromatography of stored, purified NCS (3.7 mg) on a CM-cellulose column (1.5 × 75 cm). The column was washed with 0.05 *M* acetic acid after sample addition and eluted with a pH gradient of 0.1 *M* sodium acetate, pH 3.2–3.7 (400 ml) and pH 3.7–4.7 (200 ml). Fractions (5 ml) were collected at 43 ml/hour. Chromatography was at 4°C in the dark. From Napier *et al.* (23).

like pre-NCS differs from the active drug by lacking the 340-nm absorption (Figs. 16 and 17) but has an identical amino acid composition. The UV and visible light absorption spectra of the peak tubes of eluted fractions are shown in Figs. 19 and 20. Furthermore, eluting from the CM-cellulose column at pH 3.8–4.0 is a fraction with a uv absorption at 280 and 340 nm and with fluorescent properties similar to those of methanol-extracted chromophore. This material lacks the fluorescence characteristic of tryptophan and is protein-free as determined by amino acid analysis. Since the chromophore is less negatively charged than the chromophore-free protein (pI 3.2) or NCS (pI 3.3), it is conceivable that it is the combination of the chromophore with the apoprotein that determines the characteristic intermediate pI of native NCS. The recovery of less chromophore with the clinical material is probably due to its having been thoroughly dialyzed before application on the column. These several results indicate that chromophore loss is associated with formation of the inactive fraction. We do not know if this is also associated with deamidation of aspargine 83. In order to explain the precursor–product kinetic relationship between pre-NCS and NCS, it has been proposed (18) that amidation of aspartic acid 83 takes place after ribosomal protein synthesis and release of the precursor form. This would be very unusual for protein biosynthesis, since asparagine has its own triplet codon. The above

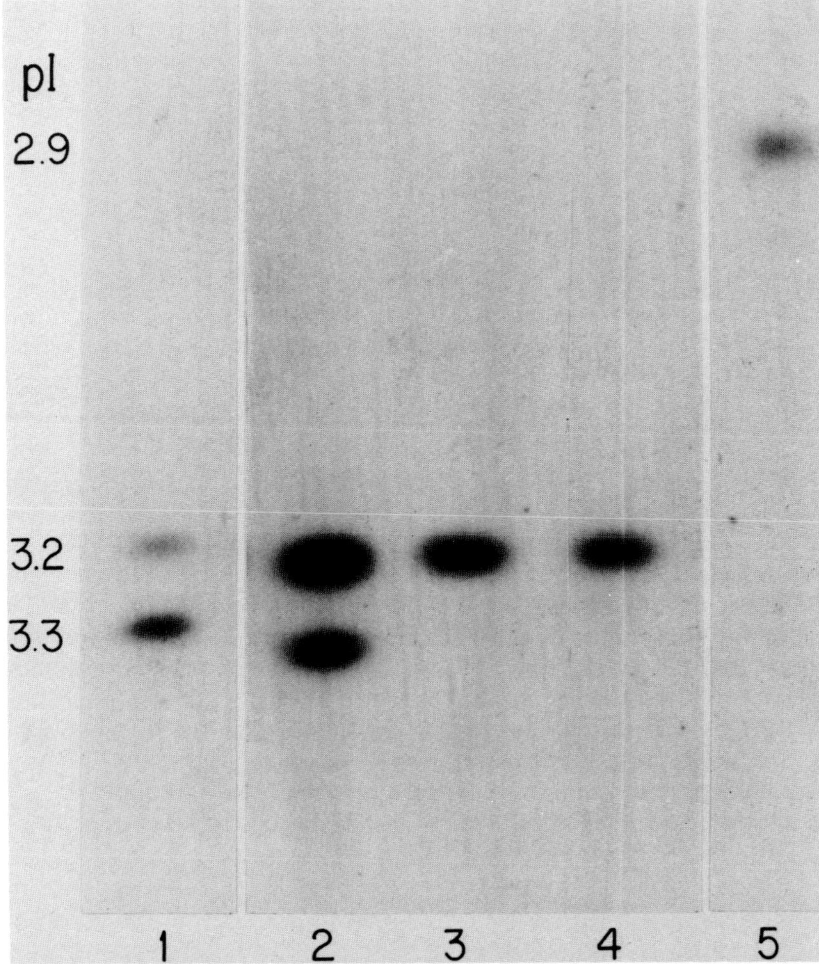

Fig. 18. Isoelectric focusing in polyacrylamide gels of NCS and fractions from Amberlite XAD-7 chromatography of NCS. Acrylamide gel (5%) containing 1% ampholine, pH 2.5–4, was prepared as per specifications given in the LKB manual. The gel was prefocused at 10 W for 45 minutes before application of the sample. Electrofocusing was at 2°C in the dark for 4 hours at 25 W. In order to determine the pH gradient of the gel at the end of the experiment, 0.5-cm-wide slices were made from strips (1 cm) cut out from either end of the gel. The gel slices were homogenized in 1 ml of distilled water, and the pH of the supernatant fraction was measured. The pI values of the Coomassie blue-stained protein bands are indicated on the left. The samples and the approximate amounts of material applied are as follows. (1) Clinical NCS (12 μg); (2) stored, purified NCS (40 μg); (3) water-eluted fraction (12 μg); (4) 30% ethanol-eluted (12 μg); (5) pepsin (48 μg). From Napier *et al.* (23).

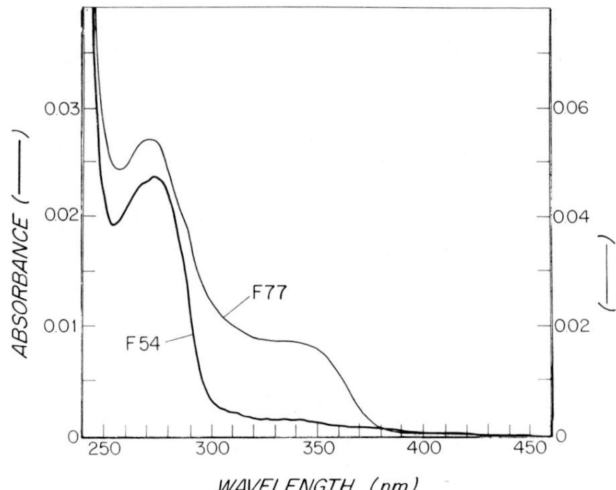

Fig. 19. The uv and visible light absorption spectra of fractions F54 and F77 eluted from the CM-cellulose chromatography of clinical NCS (Fig. 16). From Napier *et al.* (23).

data suggest instead that the active antibiotic is generated by addition of the chromophore to the apoprotein, pre-NCS. Consistent with this proposal are our findings that the chromophore-free protein isolated by chromatography on Amberlite XAD-7 has a CD spectrum (23) and a pI virtually identical with those

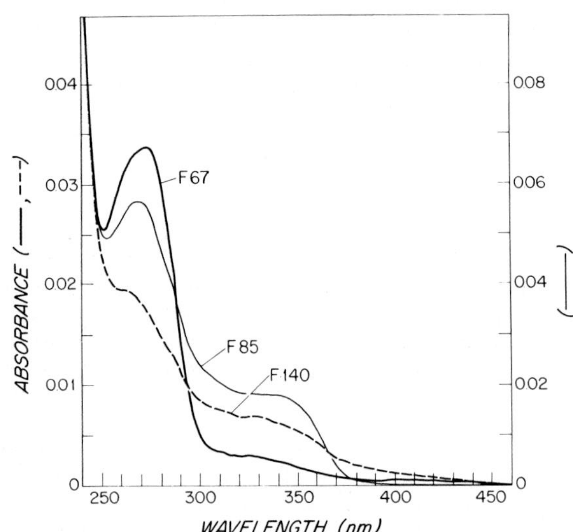

Fig. 20. The UV and visible light absorption spectra of fractions F67, F85, and F140 eluted from the CM-cellulose chromatography of stored, purified NCS (Fig. 17). From Napier *et al.* (23).

reported for pre-NCS (18). Finally, reconstitution of NCS from the isolated chromophore and apoprotein (see Section II,M) provides conclusive evidence for this proposition.

M. Roles of Nonprotein Chromophore and Apoprotein in NCS Action

We have recently succeeded in extracting and purifying the nonprotein chromophore from NCS in a form that possesses the full biological activity of the holo-antibiotic (76). The apoprotein of NCS is inactive by itself but specifically complexes with the chromophore so as to regulate its availability for interaction with DNA. The isolated chromophore is very labile in aqueous solution but is markedly stabilized by binding to its apoprotein (76,77). Reconstitution of NCS from chromophore and apoprotein was shown by both activity studies, isoelectric focusing on polyacrylamide gels, and by CD measurements. As expected, the DNA scission reaction by the isolated chromophore depends markedly on the presence of a reducing compound, and, unlike native NCS, is very active at 0°C. The chromophore has a strong affinity for DNA as shown by (1) quenching by DNA of the 440 nm fluorescence and shifting of the emission peak to 420 nm, (2) protection by DNA against spontaneous loss of activity in aqueous solution, and (3) inhibition by DNA of the spontaneous degradation of active chromophore to a highly fluorescent (490 nm) product (78). The chromophore showed a preference for DNA high in adenine + thymine content in both fluorescence quenching and protection studies. A Scatchard analysis of fluorescence quenching by calf thymus DNA revealed a $K_d = 0.25\ \mu M$ and a binding site on the DNA of about six nucleotides (Fig. 21). Both active and 2-mercaptoethanol-treated chromophore unwind supercoiled DNA, suggesting that intercalation is involved

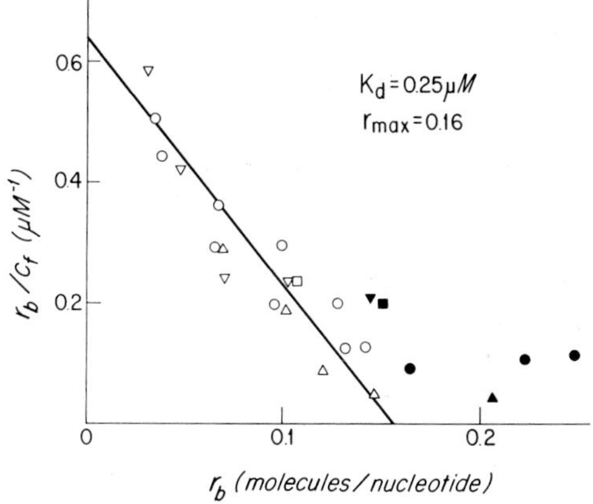

Fig. 21. Scatchard analysis of fluorescence quenching data for NCS chromophore and calf thymus DNA. From Povirk and Goldberg (78).

in the binding reaction. Similar studies with NCS apoprotein showed extremely tight binding (K_d ~0.1 n*M*) of the chromophore. While isopropanol stabilized the chromophore against degradation, it destabilized NCS. These results support the proposal (24,76) that isopropanol accelerates NCS-induced DNA degradation by partially unfolding the protein, thus facilitating chromophore release (see Section II,I).

III. Concluding Remarks

It should be mentioned that many of the consequences of the action of NCS are also seen with ionizing radiation. Thus NCS produces direct DNA sugar damage, induces mutagenesis by nonexcisable, misrepair damage to cellular DNA, causes single-strand breaks in DNA *in vivo* and *in vitro,* and inhibits selectively the initiation of replicons in mammalian DNA.

Finally, it remains to be demonstrated that the mechanism for NCS-induced DNA damage discovered in the *in vitro* system occurs in the intact cell. Mechanisms for cell killing not involving direct effects on DNA have also been proposed for NCS (79,80), as well as for macromomycin (49). Thus studies using NCS covalently bound to Agarose or Sepharose suggested the possibility that the cytotoxic effect may be a membrane-mediated event (79,80). With the finding that the nonprotein chromophore is the active drug, these results can instead be explained by release of the chromophore from the insoluble support at the cell surface and its uptake into the cell for delivery into the cell nucleus. Furthermore, we have obtained similar results with the isolated chromophore of auromomycin (76,81). Also, very high levels of NCS inhibit the vinblastine-induced formation of microtubular paracrystals (82) and cap formation and cell spreading in mammalian cells (83), but these effects are probably not responsible for the killing of cells.

For some time evidence from *in vivo* and *in vitro* studies has strongly implicated DNA as the target in the action of NCS and related antitumor, protein antibiotics. The data, however, were incomplete since it could not be shown that NCS binds to DNA. The demonstration that the nonprotein chromophore complexes with DNA, probably by an intercalative mechanism, with the same base specificity as in the DNA scission reaction provides strong support for this proposal. The precise mechanism whereby these agents damage DNA and the nature of the geometry formed between drug and DNA will await elucidation of the chemical structure of the active chromophoric drug. These efforts are underway and have recently led to a proposed partial structure of the chromophore (molecular weight 661, $C_{35}H_{35}NO_{12}$), consisting, in part, of a 2,6-dideoxy-2-methylamino-galactose moiety and a naphthoic acid derivative (84).

Acknowledgment

This work was supported by U.S. Public Health Service Research Grant GM 12573 from the National Institutes of Health.

References

1. N. Ishida, K. Miyazaki, K. Kumagai, and M. Rikimaru, *J. Antibiot.* **18,** 29 (1965).
2. T. Yamashita, N. Naoi, T. Hedaka, K. Watanabe, Y. Kumada, T. Takeuchi, and H. Umezawa, *J. Antibiot.* **32,** 330 (1979).
3. H. Chimura, M. Ishizuka, M. Hamada, S. Hori, K. Kimura, J. Iwanaga, T. Takeuchi, and H. Umezawa, *J. Antibiot.* **21,** 44 (1968).
4. A. S. Khokhlov, B. Z. Cherches, P. D. Reshetov, G. M. Smirnova, I. B. Sorokina, T. A. Prokoptzeva, T. A. Koloditskaya, V. V. Smirnov, S. M. Navashin, and I. P. Fomina, *J. Antibiot.* **22,** 541 (1969).
5. J. Meienhofer, H. Maeda, C. B. Glaser, J. Czombos, and K. Kuromizu, *Science* **178,** 875 (1972).
6. A. S. Khokhlov, P. D. Reshetov, L. A. Chupova, B. Z. Cherches, L. S. Zhigis, and I. A. Stoyachenko, *J. Antibiot.* **29,** 1026 (1976).
7. T. H. Sawyer, K. Guetzow, M. O. J. Olson, H. Busch, A. W. Prestayko, and S. T. Crooke, *Biochem. Biophys. Res. Commun.* **86,** 1133 (1979).
8. J. Meienhofer, H. Maeda, C. B. Glaser, and J. Czombos, *Prog. Pept. Res.* **2,** 295 (1972).
9. H. Maeda, C. B. Glaser, J. Czombos, and J. Meienhofer, *Arch. Biochem. Biophys.* **164,** 369 (1974).
10. T. S. A. Samy, J.-M. Hu, J. Meienhofer, H. Lazarus, and R. K. Johnson, *J. Natl. Cancer Inst.* **58,** 1765 (1977).
11. H. Maeda, H. Shiraishi, S. Onodera, and N. Ishida, *Int. J. Pept. Protein Res.* **5,** 19 (1973).
12. T. S. A. Samy and J. Meienhofer, *in* "Proceedings of the International Workshop on Hormones and Proteins" (T. A. Bewley, M. Lin, and J. Ramachandran, eds.), p. 143. Chinese University of Hong Kong, Hong Kong, 1974.
13. L. C. Sieker, L. H. Jensen, and T. S. A. Samy, *Biochem. Biophys. Res. Commun.* **68,** 358 (1976).
14. T. S. A. Samy, L. S. Kappen, and I. H. Goldberg, *J. Biol. Chem.* 225, 3420 (1980).
15. T. S. A. Samy, M. Atreyi, H. Maeda, and J. Meienhofer, *Biochemistry* **13,** 1007 (1974).
16. H. Maeda, *J. Antibiot.* **27,** 303 (1974).
17. T. S. A. Samy, *Biochemistry* **16,** 5573 (1977).
18. H. Maeda and K. Kuromizu, *J. Biochem. (Tokyo)* **81,** 25 (1977).
19. M. Kikuchi, M. Shoji, and N. Ishida, *J. Antibiot.* **27,** 766 (1974).
20. M. A. Napier, B. Holmquist, D. J. Strydom, and I. H. Goldberg, *Biochem. Biophys. Res. Commun.* **89,** 635 (1979).
21. M. Kohno, I. Haneda, Y. Koyama, and M. Kikuchi, *Jpn. J. Antibiot.* **27,** 707 (1974).
22. R. M. Burger, J. Peisach, S. B. Horwitz, *J. Biol. Chem.* **253,** 4830 (1978).
23. M. A. Napier, L. S. Kappen, and I. H. Goldberg, *Biochemistry* 19, 1767 (1980).
24. L. S. Kappen and I. H. Goldberg, *Biochemistry* 18, 5647 (1979).
25. J. Shoji, *J. Antibiot.* **14,** 27 (1961).
26. Y. Ono, Y. Watanabe, and N. Ishida, *Biochim. Biophys. Acta* **119,** 46 (1966).
27. M. Homma, T. Koida, T. Saito-Koide, I. Kamo, M. Seto, K. Kumagai, and N. Ishida, *Proc.*

Antimicrob. Anticancer Chemother., Proc. Int. Congr. Chemother., 6th, 1969 Vol. 2, p. 410 (1970).

28. H. Sawada, K. Tatsumi, M. Sasada, S. Shirakawa, T. Nakamura, and G. Wakisaka, *Cancer Res.* **34,** 3341 (1974).
29. T. A. Beerman and I. H. Goldberg, *Biochim. Biophys. Acta* **475,** 281 (1977).
30. T. Hatayama and I. H. Goldberg, *Biochim. Biophys. Acta* **563,** 59 (1979).
31. K. Ohtsuki and N. Ishida, *J. Antibiot.* **28,** 229 (1975).
32. T. A. Beerman and I. H. Goldberg, *Biochem. Biophys. Res. Commun.* **59,** 1254 (1974).
33. K. Tatsumi, T. Nakamura, and G. Wakisaka, *Gann* **65,** 459 (1974).
34. K. Ohtsuki and N. Ishida, *J. Antibiot.* **28,** 143 (1975).
35. T. A. Beerman, R. Poon, and I. H. Goldberg, *Biochim. Biophys. Acta* **475,** 294 (1977).
36. K. Tatsumi, T. Sakane, H. Sawada, S. Shirakawa, T. Nakamura, and G. Wakisaka, *Gann* **66,** 441 (1975).
37. L. S. Kappen and I. H. Goldberg, *Biochim. Biophys. Acta* **520,** 481 (1978).
38. T. Ebina, K. Ohtsuki, M. Seto, and N. Ishida, *Eur. J. Cancer* **11,** 155 (1975).
39. A. P. Rao and P. N. Rao, *J. Natl. Cancer Inst.* **57,** 1139 (1976).
40. K. Kumagai, Y. Ono, T. Nishikawa, and N. Ishida, *J. Antibiot.* **19,** 69 (1966).
41. K. Tatsumi and H. Nishioka, *Mutat. Res.* **48,** 195 (1977).
42. E. Eisenstadt, M. Wolf, and I. H. Goldberg, *Environ. Mutagenesis* **1,** 139 (1979).
43. E. Eisenstadt, M. Wolf, and I. H. Goldberg, *J. Bacteriol.*, in press.
44. M. Sasada, H. Sawada, T. Nakamura, and H. Uchino, *Gann* **67,** 447 (1976).
45. K. Tatsumi, M. Tashima, S. Shirakawa, T. Nakamura, and H. Uchino, *Cancer Res.* **39,** 1623 (1979).
46. T. Yamashita, N. Naoi, K. Watanabe, T. Takeuchi, and H. Umezawa, *J. Antibiot.* **29,** 415 (1976).
47. W. B. Im, C.-K. Chiang, and R. Montgomery, *J. Biol. Chem.* **253,** 3259 (1978).
48. T. H. Sawyer, A. W. Prestayko, and S. T. Crooke, *Cancer Res.* **39,** 1180 (1979).
49. T. Kunimoto, M. Hori, and H. Umezawa, *Cancer Res.* **32,** 1251 (1972).
50. T. Hidaka, Y. Yano, T. Yamashita, and K. Watanabe, *J. Antibiot.* **32,** 340 (1979).
51. M. M. Lippman, W. R. Laster, B. J. Abbott, J. Venditti, and M. Baratta, *Cancer Res.* **35,** 939 (1975).
52. I. H. Goldberg, T. A. Beerman, and R. Poon, *in* "Cancer: A Comprehensive Treatise" (F. F. Becker, ed.), p. 427. Plenum, New York, 1977.
53. H. Suzuki, T. Nishimura, K. Muto, and N. Tanaka, *J. Antibiot.* **31,** 875 (1978).
54. T. A. Beerman, *Biochem. Biophys. Res. Commun.* **83,** 908 (1978).
55. L. S. Kappen, I. H. Goldberg, and T. S. A. Samy, *Biochemistry* 18, 5123 (1979).
56. D. Vandré and R. Montgomery, *Arch. Biochem. Biophys.* **193,** 560 (1979).
57. H. Suzuki, T. Nishimura, and N. Tanaka, *J. Antibiot.* **32,** 706 (1979).
58. H. Suzuki, T. Nishimura, and N. Tanaka, *Cancer Res.* **39,** 2787 (1979).
59. R. Ishida and T. Takahashi, *Biochem. Biophys. Res. Commun.* **68,** 256 (1976).
60. R. Poon, T. A. Beerman, and I. H. Goldberg, *Biochemistry* **16,** 486 (1977).
61. L. S. Kappen and I. H. Goldberg, *Biochemistry* **16,** 479 (1977).
62. L. S. Kappen and I. H. Goldberg, *Nucleic Acids Res.* **5,** 2959 (1978).
63. S.-K. Sim and J. W. Lown, *Biochem. Biophys. Res. Commun.* **81,** 99 (1978).
64. R. Ishida and T. Takahashi, *Cancer Res.* **38,** 2617 (1978).
65. H. Suzuki, K. Miura, and N. Tanaka *Biochem. Biophys. Res. Commun.* **89,** 1281 (1979).
66. T. Tsuruo, H. Satoh, and T. Ukita, *J. Antibiot.* **24,** 423 (1971).
67. L. S. Kappen and I. H. Goldberg, *Biochemistry* **17,** 729 (1978).
68. A. M. Maxam and W. Gilbert, *Proc. Natl. Acad. Sci. U.S.A.* **74,** 560 (1977).

69. T. Hatayama, I. H. Goldberg, M. Takeshita, and A. P. Grollman, *Proc. Natl. Acad. Sci. U.S.A.* **75,** 3603 (1978).
70. A. D. D'Andrea and W. A. Haseltine, *Proc. Natl. Acad. Sci. U.S.A.* **75,** 3608 (1978).
71. D. Freifelder, *J. Mol. Biol.* **35,** 303–309 (1968).
72. H. P. Leenhouts and K. H. Chadwick, *Adv. Radiat. Biol.* **7,** 55 (1978).
73. T. Hatayama and I. H. Goldberg, Biochemistry, in press (1980).
74. H. Maeda, S. Aikawa, and A. Yamashita, *Cancer Res.* **35,** 554 (1975).
75. H. Maeda and M. Matsumoto, *Tohoku J. Exp. Med.* **128,** 313 (1979).
76. L. S. Kappen, M. A. Napier and I. H. Goldberg, *Proc. Natl. Acad. Sci. U.S.A.* 77, 1970 (1980).
77. L. S. Kappen and I. H. Goldberg, *Biochemistry* **19,** 4786 (1980).
78. L. F. Povirk and I. H. Goldberg, *Biochemistry* **19,** 4773 (1980).
79. H. Nakamura and K. Ono, *Proc. Jpn. Cancer Assoc., 33rd Annu. Meet.* p. 112 (1974).
80. H. Lazarus, V. Raso, and T. S. A. Samy, *Cancer Res.* **37,** 3731 (1977).
81. L. S. Kappen, M. A. Napier, I. H. Goldberg and T. S. A. Samy, *Biochemistry* **19,** 4780 (1980).
82. T. Ebina and N. Ishida, *Cancer Res.* **35,** 3705 (1975).
83. T. Ebina, M. Sataki, and N. Ishida, *Cancer Res.* **37,** 4423 (1977).
84. G. Albers-Schönberg, R. S. Dewey, Hensens, O. D., J. M. Liesch, M. A. Napier and I. H. Goldberg, *Biochem. Biophys. Res. Commun.* **95,** 1351 (1980).

9

The Action of Bleomycin on DNA in Solution and in Cells

FRANKLIN HUTCHINSON, LAWRENCE F. POVIRK, AND KAZUO YAMAMOTO

MOLECULAR ACTIONS AND TARGETS FOR CANCER CHEMOTHERAPEUTIC AGENTS

ISBN 0-12-619280-4

I. Introduction

A. Bleomycin and Its Uses

Bleomycin is a glycopeptide antibiotic found in cultures of *Streptomyces verticillus* by Ichikawa *et al.* (1). Its chief use is as a chemotherapeutic agent for the treatment of malignant tumors. Recent reviews of clinical experience with bleomycin are given in reference (2).

In radiation therapy, the selective action of X rays is partly a result of the greater sensitivity of tumor cells and partly a consequence of irradiating only the area containing the tumor. The nature of the highly selective action of bleomycin on some cells such as cancerous ones, and not on others, is not yet understood. It is known that bleomycin concentrates selectively in certain tumors, and it is reasonable to assume that this is responsible for at least part of its differential effect. The concentrating action is great enough so that localization of some tumors is possible with radioactively labeled bleomycin and the imaging techniques used in nuclear medicine. This represents a second clinical use of bleomycin, one that will not be covered in this chapter (3,4).

Bleomycin acts on DNA in solution to produce single- and double-strand breaks and to release bases. This chapter will summarize our knowledge of this effect and of the effect of bleomycin on DNA in cells. A much more extensive coverage of this material is given in a recent monograph (5).

B. Structure of Bleomycin

Bleomycin is a group of compounds having the structure shown in Fig. 1 (5,6), with various side chains attached. The commercial preparations widely used in chemotherapy are a mixture mainly of A_2 and B_2, with smaller quantities of other components. The extent to which different side chains affect biological action is unclear. Generally, the bulk of the evidence suggests that the two major components in the commercial mixture, bleomycin A_2, and B_2, act quite similarly with respect to their effects on cells in culture and on DNA in solution, and in their ability to concentrate in various tissues in animals and humans. The data on other components are too confusing to draw any strong conclusions, but as yet there is little evidence that one particular component is strikingly more effective than the others.

A closely related drug is phleomycin (6,7), which differs from bleomycin in having one of the double bonds in the bithiazole portion saturated. Other derivatives of the basic bleomycin structure are also currently under intensive investigation for possible widespread clinical use, notably tallysomycin (8). It is generally thought that these drugs are similar in action.

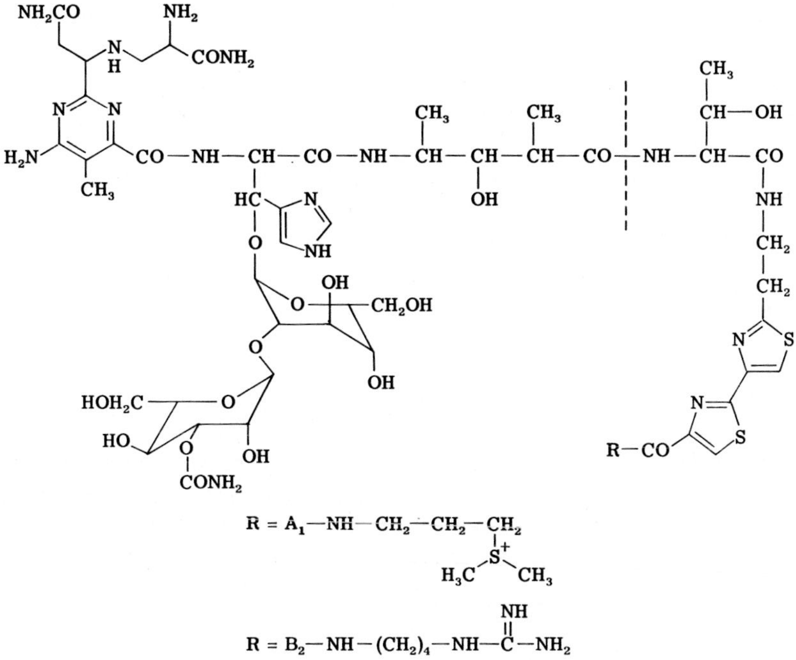

Fig. 1. The structure of bleomycins [6]. Different bleomycins have various groups attached at R; the groups for the most common bleomycins, A2 and B2, are shown. The structure to the right of the vertical dashed line is known as tripeptide S.

C. Biological Effects of Bleomycin

Bleomycin causes a loss of the ability of mammalian and bacterial cells to form colonies (9), induces chromosomal aberrations (10,11), degrades intracellular DNA (12,13), inhibits DNA synthesis in cells (14), releases DNA from complexes with cell membranes (15), induces prophages in bacteria (16,17), and induces synthesis of the *recA* protein in *Escherichia coli* cells (18). All these effects are characteristic of agents which attack the DNA in cells, and it is well-established that bleomycin produces DNA lesions.

A number of experiments suggest that bleomycin does not attack RNA (19–21). Its effects on the action of a variety of enzymes related to nucleic acid metabolism (for a review, see 22) can be interpreted as being the result of lesions in DNA. A few marginal effects of bleomycin on certain specific enzyme systems (e.g., 23) can be interpreted most easily as side effects, such as chelation by bleomycin of metal ions and/or effects on redox potentials. Aside from these, no effect of bleomycin on proteins has been reported.

II. The Role of Iron and Oxygen in the Activity of Bleomycin

There are numerous reports of the effects of sulfhydryl reagents, ascorbic acid, H_2O_2, and so on, in activating bleomycin, and of the activating or inactivating effect of various metal ions and of chelating agents such as EDTA. Two key articles have made it possible to systematize these results. The first was that of Onishi *et al.* (24), showing that oxygen was required for the activity of bleomycin. The second was that of Sausville *et al.* (25), who provided strong evidence that the key reaction was the oxidation of Fe(II) to Fe(III), forming some as yet unidentified reactive species involving oxygen. A series of later papers (26–28) have shown conclusively that the effect of various reducing agents, such as sulfhydryl groups and H_2O_2, is to form Fe(II) from Fe(III). The effect of various metal ions is that of adding or displacing iron at the active site in bleomycin, as is the effect of metal ion chelating agents. The action of bleomycin in solutions to which iron has not been specifically added is caused by low concentrations of adventitious iron, particularly that adsorbed to most DNA preparations. The residual activity of bleomycin found in the absence of added reducing agents is either from traces of such compounds or from the low concentration of Fe(II) in thermodynamic equilibrium with Fe(III) and oxygen. Further discussion of this aspect is given after a description of the products formed by the action of bleomycin on DNA.

III. Products Formed by the Action of Bleomycin on DNA in Solution

A. Base Release

All four bases are released by the action of bleomycin on DNA (29), the pyrimidines being released at a much faster rate than the purines, as shown in Table I. There is a strong preference for the release of bases attached to C-3′ of deoxyguanosine (30,31). The relative rate of release of the four bases is quite independent of the conditions used, apparently being unaffected by the amount of iron added or the amount of reducing agent used (28). The ratios given in Table I are for treatments in which only a very low percentage of the total bases in a DNA sample have been released, but the ratios after extensive digestion are similar (26,29,30).

Ninety percent of the bases released are chemically unchanged, showing that the major effect is hydrolysis of the glycosylic bond between the N-1 position of the base and the C-1′ position of the sugar. About 10% of each of the released bases are modified in some way which has not as yet been established. The modified base is not the nucleoside or the 3′- or 5′-nucleotide (29).

TABLE I

Relative Yields of Various Products from DNA Containing Roughly Equal Quantities of all Four Bases (e.g., *Escherichia coli* DNA) after Exposure to Bleomycin

Product	Relative yield	Reference
Thymine	1.0	29
Thymine minor product	0.10 ± 0.03	29
Cytosine	0.63 ± 0.07	29
Cytosine minor product	0.09 ± 0.03	29
Adenine	0.15 ± 0.02	29
Guanine	0.08 ± 0.01	29
Purine minor product[a]	0.04 ± 0.02	29
Base release (total)	1.0	29
Unaltered bases	0.89	29
Minor products	0.11	29
Single-strand break (in alkali)	1.0	28
True single-strand break	0.17–1.0	32, 33
Alkali-labile bond	0–0.83	32, 33
Double-strand break	0.05–0.2	32, 33

[a] As a fraction of total purine label.

B. Strand Breaks

When a small, supercoiled DNA plasmid (base ratio G-C/A-T = 1) containing radioisotopically labeled thymine was treated with bleomycin and sedimented on alkaline sucrose gradients, 0.49 thymine bases were released per single-strand break produced. For *E. coli* DNA (G-C/A-T = 1), thymine was 47% of the total bases released by bleomycin. Thus, within an accuracy of a few percent, one base is released for each single-strand break for breaks measured under alkaline conditions (28).

After treatment with bleomycin, sedimentation of such supercoiled DNA plasmids on neutral sucrose gradients measures actual strand interruptions, whereas sedimentation on alkaline gradients measures the sum of true breaks plus alkali-labile bonds in the backbone. The ratio of alkali-labile bonds to actual single-strand breaks has been reported by various investigators as ranging from one to five (32–34). The conditions which control this ratio are not yet understood.

Schyns *et al.* (35) have shown that there is a lesion in bleomycin-treated DNA which has the same rate of alkaline hydrolysis as the alkali-labile apurinic (AP) site formed by gentle heating of the DNA. Furthermore, they showed that sites in bleomycin-treated DNA and in alkylated, depurinated DNA were opened at identical rates by a purified rat liver endonuclease believed to be specific for AP sites; exposure to NaOH of bleomycin-treated DNA after it had been incubated with the enzyme yielded the same number of breaks in the DNA as treatment with alkali alone, showing that the same sites were opened by the enzyme and by alkali. Thus the alkali-labile bond is very similar to that left by thermal hydrolysis of the glycosylic bond, a result consistent with the finding that most of the bases released by bleomycin are not chemically modified.

Treatment of DNA with bleomycin causes the appearance of an aldehyde function, as determined either by iodine titration (21) or by reaction with thiobarbituric acid (36,37). The compound with the aldehyde function is released from the DNA during the reaction with bleomycin, and the amount is proportional to the number of Fe(II) atoms oxidized (37). The compound may well be malondialdehyde.

At the breaks, evidence suggests that there is no 3′-phosphate; exonuclease III does not release phosphate (36), and DNA fragments formed by the action of bleomycin do not move on acrylamide gels like those with 3′-phosphates (31). Both 5′-hydroxyl and 5′-phosphate were found in DNA which had been heated to 65°C for 45 minutes (pH 6–8) (36); in this case the breaks may have been only the actual strand interruptions or may have also included some labile bonds which had hydrolyzed.

An interesting characteristic of the action of bleomycin on DNA is that it produces double-strand breaks, the number being linear in the number of single-strand breaks and equal to about 10% of those found after treatment with alkali (32). The linearity of the yield shows that the double-strand breaks are not produced by coincidences between randomly produced single-strand breaks but by some specific process. It so happens that the yield is consistent either with one double-strand break being produced per purine released or per chemically modified base (see Table I).

An even more remarkable fact is that there are "hot spots" for the production of double-strand breaks, such that if certain DNA exposed to bleomycin is subjected to electrophoresis on neutral agarose gels, identifiable bands appear showing the production of double-strand breaks near specific sites (38,39). There are several such sites in PM2 DNA (38), one in SV40 DNA (P. Farnham, unpublished results), and none in pBR322 (L. F. Povirk and P. Farnham, unpublished observations).

IV. The Interaction of Bleomycin with DNA

A. The Structure of the Bleomycin–Metal Chelation Complex

The structure of greatest interest to determine is that of Fe(II) chelated with bleomycin. This is difficult to do because of the rate at which Fe(II) is oxidized in the presence of air. It is known that Cu(II) forms chelation complexes with many

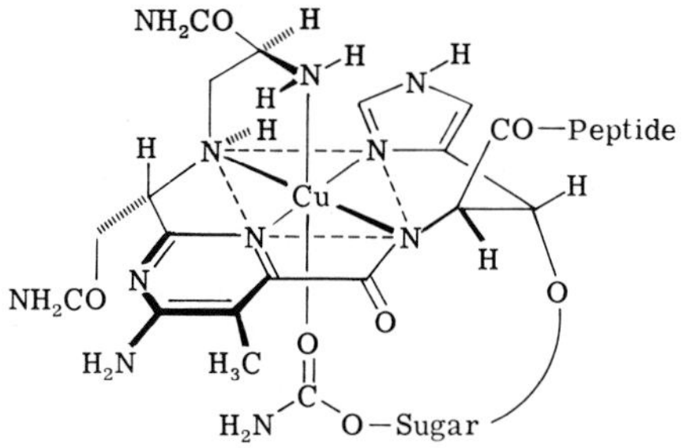

Fig. 2. The structure of bleomycin complexed with Cu(II). Reprinted with permission from (45).

substances which resemble those of Fe(II). Iitaka *et al.* (40) have crystallized the Cu(II) complex of a fragment of the bleomycin molecule and deduced the structure shown in Fig. 2 from X-ray diffraction data. This structure is consistent with esr studies on several metal complexes of bleomycin (41–43), as well as optical spectra of such complexes (37,44,45). Also, nmr spectra of bleomycin–metal complexes confirm that protons near the chelated ion (Fig. 2) have magnetic moments strongly perturbed by the electron magnetic moment on the metal ion; other groups far from the chelation complex, such as the bithiazole rings, do not contain protons with perturbed magnetic moments (46–48). Thus there is good reason to believe that the structure shown in Fig. 2 is close to that which exists in the intact bleomycin molecule.

B. The Bleomycin-Metal-DNA Complex

Bleomycin binds tightly to DNA, with binding constants or the order of 10^5/mole at millimolar salt concentrations, which decrease at higher salt concentrations (46,49). The binding seems to proceed in two steps, with a fast and a slow component (49). Such two-step binding is typical of compounds which intercalate, with the fast reaction involving binding to the outside of the double helix and the slow reaction being the intercalating one. Metal–bleomycin complexes bind even more tightly (50, L. Povirk, unpublished results).

Direct evidence for intercalation of the bithiazole part of the molecule has been obtained by Povirk *et al.* (49). Intercalation was shown both by measuring an increase in the length of the molecule of 3.2 Å per bleomycin molecule bound and by the ability of bleomycin to unwind supercoiled plasmid DNA. Tripeptide S (Fig. 1), which is essentially the part of the molecule which does not participate in metal ion chelation (Fig. 2), intercalates in DNA in the same way as the intact bleomycin molecule, as shown both by lengthening of the DNA molecule and by unwinding of supercoiled plasmid DNA. Studies on the dichroic ratio of the absorption associated with the bithiazole moiety of bound bleomycin show that

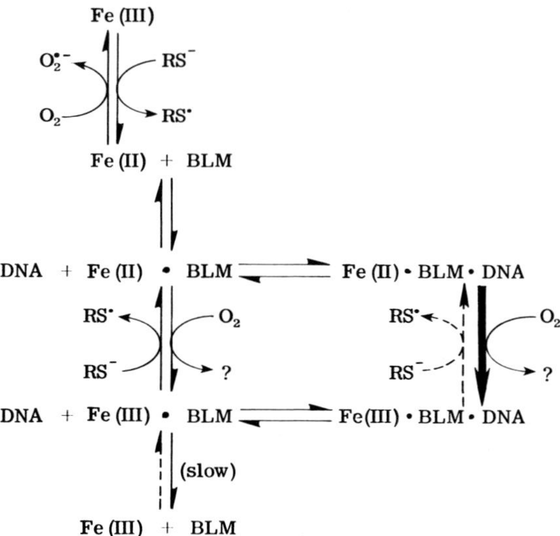

Fig. 3. The reaction sequences involved in the attack of bleomycin (BLM) on DNA. Reactions shown by solid lines have been observed; those shown by dashed lines have not. The reaction indicated by the heavy arrow, the oxidation of Fe(II) in the complex Fe(II)-BLM-DNA, is 60-fold more rapid than the oxidation of Fe(II) or Fe(II)-Blm. Reprinted with permission from (28).

the normal to the plane of the rings makes about the same angle with the DNA axis as the normal to the plane of the stacked bases, as expected for an intercalator (49).

The sterospecificity of the binding of bleomycin to DNA is shown by esr measurements on Cu(II)–bleomycin bound to oriented fibers of DNA. The spectra show unequivocally that the square planar array surrounding the Cu(II) in the chelation complex (Fig. 2) is oriented so that the normal to this plane is parallel to the axis of the DNA (H. M. Shields, unpublished observations).

Many of the details of the formation of various complexes between iron, bleomycin, and DNA have been studied and lead to the scheme shown in Fig. 3 (28). All the reactions shown in solid lines have been demonstrated directly. The most significant point is the very rapid rate of oxidation of Fe(II) when it is complexed with bleomycin and DNA—60 times faster than in the Fe(II)–bleomycin complex. These relative rates greatly favor the oxidation of Fe(II) when it is complexed with bleomycin in DNA, leading to high efficiency for each oxidation event.

C. A Model of the Mechanism of Bleomycin Action on DNA

The oxidation of Fe(II) by oxygen is well known to produce O_2^- and the OH-radical. O_2^- is known to be relatively nonreactive with DNA (51). Freely diffusing OH radicals are unlikely to be the active species for two reasons. First, the products resulting from the action of bleomycin on DNA are more specific and are different from those produced by the action of X rays on dilute DNA solutions; in the latter case it is known that the OH free radical is the major reactive intermediate (51). Second, the results of adding free-radical scavengers to DNA–bleomycin solutions, although somewhat confusing (e.g., 52,53), do not fit the idea that these substances scavenge the OH radicals; it is more likely that the effects they produce are the result of altering the Fe(II) available to the bleomycin. The reactive intermediates are probably some radical complex of iron and oxygen, held in certain sterically defined configurations on the DNA molecule.

The major action must be on the deoxyribose sugar. One effect is probably hydrogen abstraction from C-1′ which Rhaese and Freese (54) have already shown to be the site for the action of H_2O_2 on DNA in releasing free bases and forming strand breaks. This fits with the release of one base per single-strand break measured under alkaline conditions. The variable ratio of alkali-labile bonds to true strand breaks could be the result of alternative modes of decay for a free radical on a particular sugar carbon, as already demonstrated by van Sonntag and Schulte-Fröhlinde (55) for the attack of OH radicals on DNA in solution (55). Alternatively, the ratio of alkali-labile bonds to true breaks could vary because of large increases in bond breakage with small pH changes.

Currently, an important aspect of the action of bleomycin on DNA which needs clarification are the steps by which the chelated Fe(II) forms a reactive intermediate during oxidation and the way in which this intermediate interacts with the sugar. Iron chelated to bleomycin resembles iron in various heme compounds (43) which suggests a way in which the chemistry of bleomycin can be correlated with that of hemoglobin and of various heme enzymes.

The one result which does not fit readily into the picture is the formation of DNA double-strand breaks by a process which is more efficient than that of coincidences between randomly created single-strand breaks.

A free-radical process attacking one strand might give rise to another free radical which could attack the other strand; an analogous situation may exist with uv-induced double-strand breaks in DNA containing bromouracil (56). Alternatively, DNA may bind two bleomycin molecules close together, each one of which would give rise to a single-strand break in the opposite strand. A third possibility, that a bleomycin molecule bound to DNA undergoes successive cycles of oxidation and reduction and thus creates two or more chemical events near the same place, seems unlikely. The number of double-strand breaks per single-strand break is the same whether the bleomycin reaction is activated by adding Fe(II) or by adding sulfhydryl compounds to encourage reduction of Fe(III) (57).

The stoichiometry of the reaction of Fe(II)–bleomycin with DNA is interesting. Addition of Fe(II) to a solution of bleomycin and DNA gives 0.36 bases released per Fe(II) oxidized (28). Addition of excess sulfhydryl moieties and Fe(II) to a DNA–bleomycin solution can release a maximum of 2.82 bases per bleomycin molecule in solution (this value has been corrected for a small release of bases at zero bleomycin concentration [28]). These bases are not released by a chain reaction at a few DNA sites, since exactly one base is released per single-strand break in a small DNA plasmid, even under conditions where there is an average of less than one single-strand break per plasmid. Thus bleomycin must act catalytically. Using the measured yield per Fe(II) oxidation, the bleomycin molecule is capable of going through a minimum of eight (equal to 2.82/0.36) oxidation–reduction cycles.

The oxidation of Fe(II) can inactivate bleomycin, and the addition of DNA greatly reduces this rate of inactivation of bleomycin (43). These results are consistent with the idea that oxidation forms a free radical capable of reacting with a number of chemical groups, including those in the bleomycin molecule itself. The addition of DNA gives this reactive intermediate a substrate to work on, thereby in effect protecting the bleomycin molecule.

V. Effects of Bleomycin on DNA in *Escherichia coli* Cells

A. Single- and Double-Strand Breaks in Intracellular DNA

The effects described in Sections I,C,III, and IV of this chapter strongly suggest that bleomycin acts on cells by damaging their DNA. It was therefore surprising to obtain results such as those shown in Figs. 4 and 5 for DNA from *E. coli* cells treated with bleomycin to 10–20% survival of colony-forming ability. No change could be seen in the DNA sedimentation patterns in alkaline gradients, suggesting less than four single-strand breaks per single-strand genome. In neutral gradients, there was a decrease in a fast-sedimenting component consisting of DNA with an unknown structure (58). The situation is too technical to discuss at length here (see 58), but the data in Fig. 5 show no detectible double-strand breaks, i.e., less than two per genome. The figures also show sedimentation patterns (interpolated from previous results) for DNA from cells which had been treated with X rays to a comparable level of colony-forming ability.

Quite different sedimentation patterns are found in both neutral and alkaline gradients of DNA from cells treated with three- to fourfold more bleomycin, with a colony-forming ability of less than 1%. There is now extensive DNA degradation, with an increase of more than an order of magnitude in the number of single- and double-strand breaks (data not shown).

The data in the literature on the degradation of DNA in *E. coli* cells treated with bleomycin do not contradict the results shown in Figs. 4 and 5. Most experiments on intracellular DNA strand breakage by various agents (such as X

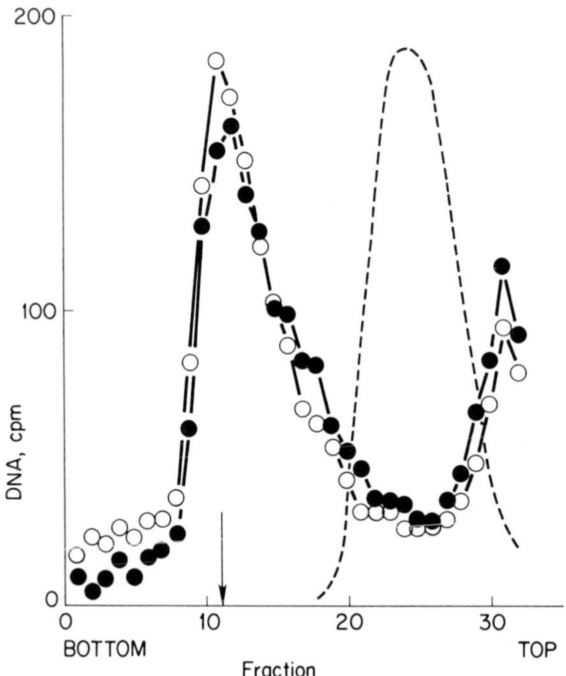

Fig. 4. Alkaline sucrose gradient (5–20% sucrose, 0.2 *M* NaOH) sedimentation of [^{14}C]DNA from *E. coli* AB2497 cells treated with 5 μg/ml bleomycin for 10 minutes at 37°C; colony-forming ability was 20% of controls (●). Sedimentation of DNA from untreated cells is also shown (○). Sedimentation was for 2 hours at 26,000 rpm in an SW50.1 rotor. Lysis conditions were as described in (58). The arrow at fraction 11 shows the sedimentation position of linear single-strand DNA of molecular weight ~4×10^8 and greater. Thus the sharp peak at this position is an artifact (58). The dashed line is an approximate sedimentation pattern for DNA from cells given 22 krads of γ rays (which will give colony-forming ability of about 20% of controls), interpolated from previous data (58).

rays) use exposures at which cell colony-forming ability is low but the number of strand breaks high. Only when special techniques are used to prevent DNA degradation during extraction and to minimize sedimentation artifacts can strand breaks be measured for 10–20% survival after X rays, for example (59). In the absence of specific mention of these precautions, we assume that published data on DNA degradation in bleomycin-treated cells refer to cells with very low levels of colony-forming ability (12,13,15).

B. The Effects of Mutations in Genes Related to DNA Repair

The effects of the *E. coli* mutations *recA*, *lexA*, *polA*, and *uvrA* in bleomycin-treated cells are listed in Table II (60). In exponentially growing cells, these

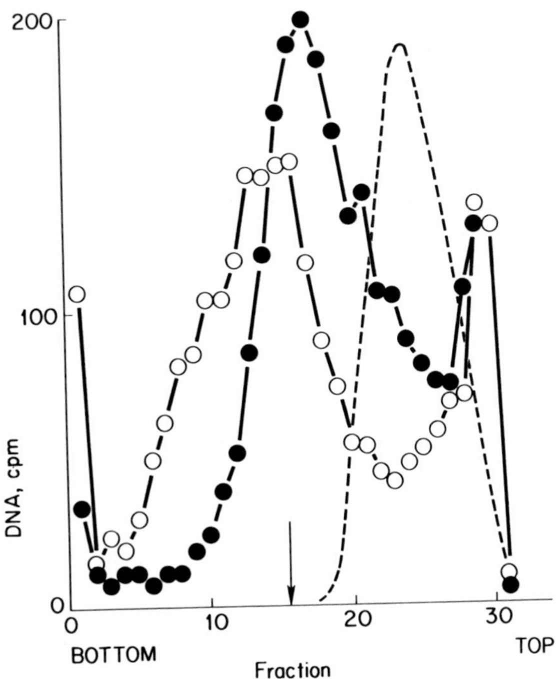

Fig. 5. Neutral sucrose gradient (5–20% sucrose) sedimentation of [^{14}C]DNA from *E. coli* AB2497 cells treated with 5 μg/ml bleomycin for 10 minutes at 37°C; colony-forming ability was 10% of controls (●). Sedimentation of DNA from untreated cells is also shown (○). Sedimentation was for 42 hours at 3700 rpm in an SW50.1 rotor. Lysis conditions were as described in (58). The arrow at fraction 16 shows the position of linear double-strand DNA of molecular weight $\sim 1.5 \times 10^9$ and greater. DNA from untreated cells sedimenting beyond this point cannot be linear but must have a more compact structure. It is known that this structure contains very little if any cellular material aside from DNA. A complete discussion of these points is given in Krasin and Hutchinson (58). The dashed line shows the sedimentation pattern, interpolated from previous data (58), for cells receiving 30 krads of γ rays, which reduces colony-forming ability to 10%.

mutations do not affect the ability of the cells to survive bleomycin treatment. The lack of an effect of the *uvr* gene is reasonable, since there is no known lesion of bleomycin which might be acted upon by this enzymatic repair system. However, *recA, lexA,* and *polA* are all known to be involved in the repair of strand breaks, which seems to be the lesion in the DNA that would predominate in the biological action of bleomycin. For cells starved for amino acids, the *recA* gene makes the cell somewhat more sensitive, but the lack of an effect in introducing *lexA* or *polA* is puzzling.

TABLE II

Response of *Escherichia coli* Repair Mutants to Bleomycin and γ Rays[a]

Strain	Exponential cells and exponential wild-type cells	Starved cells and exponential wild-type cells	Starved cells and starved wild-type cells
AB2497 wild type	1.0 (1)	8.0 ± 2	1.0 (1)
AB2487 *recA13*	1.0 ± 0.3 (0.2)	2.0 ± 0.2 (0.26)	0.2 ± 0.02 (0.35)
Z-7 *lexAl*	1.0 ± 0.3 (0.15)	7.2 ± 3	0.9 ± 0.4 (0.11)
m22 *polAl*	1.1 ± 0.14 (0.35)	8.0 ± 2	1.0 ± 0.2 (0.46)
AB2500 *uvrA6*	0.8 ± 0.2 (1)	6.4 ± 2	0.8 ± 0.2 (1)

[a] The figure given is the amount of bleomycin which reduces the colony-forming ability of the cell to the same level as one unit of bleomycin acting on the wild-type strain, either exponentially growing or starved for amino acids as shown. The figure in parentheses is the experimental value for the γ-ray exposure of the mutant at 37°C which reduces colony-forming ability to the same level as one unit of exposure of the wild type. Note that sensitivity to X rays is the same for cells in exponential growth and starved for amino acids, so the figure in parentheses for any particular mutant, e.g., *recA*, should be about the same for all three columns (59).

C. Physiological Factors Affecting the Sensitivity of *Escherichia coli* Cells

Adding rifampicin or chloramphenicol to cell cultures (61), starving cells for amino acids (see Table II), or holding cells with temperature-dependent *dnaA* or *dnaC* mutations at the nonpermissive temperature (K. Yamamoto, unpublished data) all make *E. coli* cells an order of magnitude more resistant to bleomycin. These treatments cause *E. coli* cells to complete the ongoing round of DNA replication but then fail to initiate a new round. However, stopping the DNA replication fork by starving for thymine, or by holding a *dnaB* temperature-sensitive mutant at the nonpermissive temperature, has no effect on the cells' sensitivity to bleomycin (K. Yamamoto, unpublished data).

Cohen and I (61) reported that a "relaxed" strain of *E. coli* was not made more resistant to bleomycin by blocking protein synthesis. However, these authors (61), as well as we, have relaxed strains which increase their bleomycin resistance when protein synthesis is blocked, very much like "stringent" strains.

D. *Escherichia coli* Mutants with Altered Sensitivity to Bleomycin

A mutant has been described which is more sensitive to bleomycin and in which a *recA* variant is always more sensitive than the corresponding rec^+ allele (62); this mutant may have a cell wall which is more permeable to bleomycin. Another sensitive mutant is also resistant to colicins (63).

Several mutants have been isolated which are an order of magnitude more resistant to bleomycin than usual (K. Yamamoto, unpublished observations). One strain is a double mutant about two orders of magnitude more resistant than wild-type cells. This suggests that bleomycin resistance may involve two or more loci in *E. coli* cells.

E. Does Bleomycin Act on *Escherichia coli* Cells by Damaging DNA?

This is a reasonable question to ask in light of some of the results described above (e.g., Figs. 4 and 5, and Table II). DNA degradation in heavily treated cells (colony-forming ability <1%) could result from the activation of cell nucleases or a breakdown in the cell membrane which allows bleomycin to enter freely. However, the effects of bleomycin on DNA in solution and the lack of reports of effects on other cell components suggest that the answer to the question posed is yes. In addition, there is the following evidence: (1) Bleomycin breaks up the fast-sedimenting intracellular component (Fig. 5) known to be mostly (or entirely) DNA (58); and (2) bleomycin activates two "SOS functions"—prophage induction (16,17) and synthesis of the *recA* protein (18)—both induced by other agents known to act on DNA.

F. A Working Hypothesis for the Action of Bleomycin on *Escherichia coli* Cells

The results just described rule out a picture in which bleomycin affects cells by randomly producing DNA damage such as single- and double-strand breaks, like X rays. A reasonable working hypothesis is that bleomycin adsorbs to the surface of *E. coli* cells and acts on DNA located on this surface. As yet, there is no direct evidence for this mode of action. However, the hypothesis does fit with the following.

1. The lack of detectable intracellular DNA double-strand breaks and single-strand breaks in alkali (true strand breaks plus alkali-labile bonds). Postulating a different kind of lesion for intracellular DNA is unsatisfactory. However, single- and double-strand breaks concentrated in a small part of the genome would not be detected as such in experiments such as those shown in Figs. 4 and 5. Such concentrated damage might well, however, affect the properties of the fast-sedimenting DNA structure, as shown in Fig. 5.
2. The mutagenic action of bleomycin on bacterial cells has not yet been detected (64). This would be expected for an agent which concentrated extensive (and frequently lethal) damage in a small section of the chromosome.
3. Bleomycin is a large molecule for which it is hard to visualize a suitable mechanism to introduce the drug into bacterial cells.

4. The differences in the effects of genetic defects in DNA repair for strand breaks produced by X rays and by bleomycin (Table II) are easier to reconcile if the distribution of the lesions is assumed to differ.

VI. Action of Bleomycin on the DNA of Mammalian Cells

Cultured mammalian cells treated with bleomycin show degraded DNA with both single- and double-strand breaks (14,65,66). However, in most published experiments the cells have been treated so heavily that the level of colony-forming ability is very low. For example, Lehmann and Stevens (67) found that treating cells of human origin with 3 μg/ml bleomycin reduced colony-forming ability to 4% of that of controls; analogous cells from patients with ataxia telangiectasia were reduced to 0.9% colony-forming ability by the same treatment. To measure DNA single-strand breaks (including alkali-labile bonds), they used cells of these two strains treated with 100 μg/ml bleomycin under the same conditions; double-strand breaks were measured after similar treatment with 500 μg/ml. Thus no statement can be made concerning DNA damage in cells treated to reduce colony-forming ability to about 10%.

The most revealing measurements are from Kohn's laboratory, in which mammalian cells showed a rapid drop to 20% colony-forming ability after treatment with 20 μg/ml bleomycin, with a slow further decrease to 10% at 125 μg/ml (68). When single-strand breaks in DNA from these cells were measured by the sensitive alkaline elution technique, the results suggested "the possibility that the DNA of treated cells consists of a mixture of undamaged and severely damaged components" (68). If the severely damaged DNA came from the rapidly inactivated cell component shown by the survival curve, these results would agree with the *E. coli* results.

When both the amount of bleomycin and the pH of the medium were varied, a reasonable correlation was found between the fraction of mammalian cells able to form colonies and the fraction of DNA retained on the filter like undamaged DNA (69). This and the production of chromosomal aberrations in mammalian cells treated with bleomycin (10,11, and many subsequent papers) suggest that bleomycin may act on mammalian cell DNA.

It is interesting to speculate on possible correlations between the high sensitivity to bleomycin of exponentially growing *E. coli* cells and the known sensitivity of some types of rapidly proliferating tumor cells. Other mechanisms which would affect the relative sensitivity of tumor and normal cells are the concentration of bleomycin in tumor cells (Section I,A) and a possible difference in redox potentials which could favor higher levels of Fe(II) in tumor cells.

Acknowledgments

The preparation of the manuscript for this chapter and the original research reported here was supported by grant CA-17938 awarded by the National Cancer Institute, U.S. Public Health Service.

References

1. T. Ichikawa, A. Matsuka, K. Yamamoto, M. Tsubosaki, T. Kaihora, K. Sakamoto, and H. Umezawa, *J. Antibiot.* **20,** 149 (1967).
2. A series of papers by M. A. Friedman, M. Abe *et al.*, T. Miyamoto *et al.*, A. Matsuda *et al.*, N. Yamanaka *et al.*, and S. T. Crooke *et al.*, in *Recent Results Cancer Res.* **63,** 152 (1978).
3. D. A. Goodwin, M. W. Sundberg, C. I. Diamanti, and C. F. Meares, *in* "18th Annual Clinical Conference Monograph, Radiologic and Other Biophysical Methods in Tumor Diagnosis," p. 57. Yearbook Publ. Chicago, Illinois, 1975.
4. J. P. Nouel, *GANN Monogr. Cancer Res.* **19,** 301 (1976).
5. S. M. Hecht, ed., "Bleomycin: Chemical, Biochemical and Biological Aspects." Springer-Verlag, Berlin and New York, 1979.
6. T. Takita, Y. Muraoka, T. Nakatani, A. Fujii, Y. Umezawa, H. Naganawa, and H. Umezawa, *J. Antibiot.* **31,** 801 (1978).
7. T. Takita, K. Maeda, and H. Umezawa, *J. Antibiot.* **12,** 111 (1959).
8. M. Konishi, K. Saito, K. Numata, T. Tsuno, K. Asama, H. Tsukiura, T. Naito, and H. Kawaguchi, *J. Antibiot.* **30,** 789 (1977).
9. H. Umezawa, M. Ishizuka, K. Maeda, and T. Takeuchi, *Cancer* **20,** 891 (1967).
10. K. Ohama and T. Kadotani, *Jpn. J. Hum. Genet.* **14,** 293 (1970).
11. R. S. Bornstein, D. A. Hungerford, G. Haller, P. F. Engstrom, and J. W. Yarbro, *Cancer Res.* **31,** 2004 (1971).
12. H. Suzuki, K. Nagai, H. Yamaki, N. Tanaka, and H. Umezawa, *J. Antibiot.* **22,** 446 (1969).
13. T. Onishi, K. Shimada, and Y. Takagi, *Biochim. Biophys. Acta* **312,** 248 (1973).
14. H. Suzuki, K. Nagai, H. Yamaki, N. Tanaka, and H. Umezawa, *J. Antibiot.* **21,** 379 (1968).
15. M. Miyaki, T. Kitayama, and T. Ono, *J. Antibiot.* **27,** 647 (1974).
16. H. Aoki and H. Sakai, *J. Antibiot.* **22,** 87 (1967).
17. C. W. Haidle, K. K. Weiss, and M. L. Mace, Jr., *Biochem. Biophys. Res. Commun.* **48,** 1179 (1972).
18. L. J. Gudas and A. B. Pardee, *J. Mol. Biol.* **101,** 459 (1976).
19. H. Suzuki, K. Nagai, E. Akutsu, H. Yamaki, N. Tanaka, and H. Umezawa, *J. Antibiot.* **23,** 473 (1970).
20. H. Umezawa, H. Asakura, K. Oda, S. Hori, and M. Hori, *J. Antibiot.* **26,** 521 (1973).
21. W. E. G. Müller, Z. Yamazaki, H.-J. Breter, and R. K. Zahn, *Eur. J. Biochem.* **31,** 518 (1972).
22. W. E. G. Müller, H. J. Rohde, and R. K. Zahn, *J. Mol. Med.* **1,** 173 (1976).
23. M. Griffin, R. N. Barnes, J. Wynne, and C. Williams, *Biochem. Pharmacol.* **27,** 1211 (1978).
24. T. Onishi, H. Iwata, and Y. Takagi, *J. Biochem.* (*Tokyo*) **77,** 745 (1975).
25. E. A. Sausville, J. Peisach, and S. B. Horwitz, *Biochem. Biophys. Res. Commun.* **73,** 814 (1976).
26. E. A. Sausville, R. W. Stein, J. Peisach, and S. B. Horwitz, *Biochemistry* **17,** 2746 (1978).
27. E. A. Sausville, J. Peisach, and S. B. Horwitz, *Biochemistry* **17,** 2740 (1978).
28. L. F. Povirk, *Biochemistry* **18,** 3989 (1979).
29. L. F. Povirk, W. Köhnlein, and F. Hutchinson, *Biochim. Biophys. Acta* **521,** 126 (1978).
30. M. Takeshita, A. P. Grollman, E. Ohtsubo, and H. Ohtsubo, *Proc. Natl. Acad. Sci. U.S.A.* **75,** 5983 (1978).
31. A. D. D'Andrea and W. A. Haseltine, *Proc. Natl. Acad. Sci. U.S.A.* **75,** 3608 (1978).

32. L. F. Povirk, W. Wübker, W. Köhnlein, and F. Hutchinson, *Nucleic Acids Res.* **4,** 3573 (1977).
33. S. L. Ross and R. E. Moses, *Biochemistry* **17,** 581 (1978).
34. R. S. Lloyd, C. W. Haidle, and R. R. Hewitt, *Cancer Res.* **38,** 3191 (1978).
35. R. Schyns, M. Mulquet, and W. G. Verly, *FEBS Lett.* **93,** 47 (1978).
36. M. T. Kuo and C. W. Haidle, *Biochim. Biophys. Acta* **335,** 109 (1974).
37. S. B. Horwitz, E. A. Sausville, and J. Peisach, *in* "Bleomycin: Chemical, Biochemical and Biological Aspects" (S. M. Hecht, ed.), p. 168. Springer-Verlag, Berlin and New York, 1979.
38. R. S. Lloyd, C. W. Haidle, and D. L. Robberson, *Biochemistry* **17,** 1890 (1978).
39. R. S. Lloyd, C. W. Haidle, D. L. Robberson, and M. L. Dodson, Jr., *Curr. Microbiol.* **1,** 45 (1978).
40. Y. Iitaka, H. Nakamura, T. Nakatani, Y. Muraoka, A. Fujii, T. Takita, and H. Umezawa, *J. Antibiot.* **31,** 1070 (1978).
41. Y. Sugiura, *J. Antibiot.* **31,** 1206 (1978).
42. Y. Sugiura, *Biochem. Biophys. Res. Commun.* **87,** 643 (1979).
43. R. M. Burger, J. Peisach, W. E. Blumberg, and S. B. Horwitz, *Biophys. J.* **25,** Abstr., p. 37a (1979).
44. J. C. Dabrowiak, R. T. Greenway, W. E. Longo, M. Van Heusen, and S. T. Crooke, *Biochim. Biophys. Acta* **517,** 517 (1978).
45. T. Takita, Y. Muraoka, T. Nakatani, A. Fujii, Y. Citaka, and H. Umezawa, *J. Antibiot.* **31,** 1073 (1978).
46. M. Chien, A. P. Grollman, and S. B. Horwitz, *Biochemistry* **16,** 3641 (1977).
47. J. C. Dabrowiak, F. T. Greenway, and R. Grulich, *Biochemistry* **17,** 4090 (1978).
48. A. E. G. Cass, A. Goldes, H. A. O. Hill, C. E. McClelland, and C. B. Storm *FEBS Lett.* **94,** 311 (1978).
49. L. F. Povirk, M. Hogan, and N. Dattagupta, *Biochemistry* **18,** 96 (1979).
50. H. Kasai, H. Naganawa, T. Takita, and H. Umezawa, *J. Antibiot.* **31,** 1316 (1978).
51. G. Scholes, *in* "Effects of Ionizing Radiation on DNA" (J. Hütterman, W. Köhnlein, R. Teoule, and A. J. Bertinchamps, eds.), p. 153. Springer-Verlag, Berlin and New York, 1978.
52. M. J. Sleigh, *Nucleic Acids Res.* **3,** 891 (1976).
53. J. W. Lown and S.-K. Sim, *Biochem. Biophys. Res. Commun.* **77,** 1150 (1977).
54. H. J. Rhaese and E. Freese, *Biochim. Biophys. Acta* **155,** 476 (1968).
55. C. von Sonntag and D. Schulte-Fröhlinde, *in* "Effects of Ionizing Radiation on DNA" (J. Hütterman, W. Köhnlein, R. Teoule, and A. J. Bertinchamps, eds.) p. 204. Springer-Verlag, Berlin and New York, 1978.
56. F. Krasin and F. Hutchinson, *Biophys. J.* **24,** 645 (1978).
57. F. Hutchinson and L. F. Povirk, *in* "Bleomycin: Chemical, Biochemical and Biological Aspects" (S. M. Hecht, ed.), p. 253. Springer-Verlag, Berlin and New York, 1979.
58. F. Krasin and F. Hutchinson, *J. Mol. Biol.* **116,** 81 (1977).
59. F. Hutchinson, *in* "DNA Repair Mechanisms" (P. C. Hanawalt, E. C. Friedberg, and C. F. Fox, eds.), p. 457. Academic Press, New York, 1978.
60. K. Yamamoto and F. Hutchinson, *J. Antibiot.* **32,** 1181 (1979).
61. S. S. Cohen and J. I. *Cancer Res.* **36,** 2768 (1976).
62. H. Yamagami, M. Ishizawa, and H. Endo, *GANN* **65,** 61 (1974).
63. N. Otsuji, T. Horiuchi, A. Nakata, and J. Kawamata, *J. Antibiot.* **31,** 794 (1978).
64. W. F. Benedict, M. S. Baker, L. Haroun, E. Choi, and B. N. Ames, *Cancer Res.* **37,** 2209 (1977).
65. Y. Fujiwara and T. Kondo, *Biochem. Pharmacol.* **22,** 323 (1973).
66. M. Miyaki, S. Morohashi, and T. Ono, *J. Antibiot.* **26,** 369 (1973).
67. A. R. Lehmann and S. Stevens, *Nucleic Acids Res.* **6,** 1953 (1979).
68. Z. M. Iqbal, K. W. Kohn, R. A. G. Ewig, and A. J. Fornace, *Cancer Res.* **36,** 3834 (1976).
69. K. W. Kohn and R. A. G. Ewig, *Cancer Res.* **36,** 3839 (1976).

PART III

Antimetabolites—Nucleoside Analogs

10

Transport of Nucleosides and Nucleoside Analogs by Animal Cells

ALAN R. P. PATERSON

I. Introduction

In the search for antineoplastic agents, many analogs of naturally occurring purine and pyrimidine nucleosides have been synthesized; certain of these analogues have impressive biological activity (notably toxicity), and some have current use in the treatment of viral and neoplastic disease. This chapter examines the idea that a basic determinant of biological activity in compounds of this class is transportability, that is, acceptability as a substrate for the transport machinery by which nucleosides enter animal cells. (In this chapter nucleoside "transport" refers to the transporter-mediated passage of nucleoside molecules across the plasma membrane, the initial event in the multistep process of cellular

MOLECULAR ACTIONS AND TARGETS FOR CANCER CHEMOTHERAPEUTIC AGENTS

ISBN 0-12-619280-4

nucleoside uptake. Because various metabolic transformations follow the transport of most nucleosides, measurements of nucleoside "uptake" refer to the total cellular content of a permeant and of the metabolites formed therefrom.) Experimental work is described which suggests that it may be possible to manipulate to some extent nucleoside transporter activity in animal tissues by means of inhibitors of nucleoside transport such as nitrobenzylthioinosine (6-[(-nitrobenzyl)-thio]-9-β-D-ribofuranosylpurine; NBMPR).

II. Nucleoside Transport—An Overview

Upon entry into animal cells, most nucleosides are metabolized, principally to phosphate esters. By phosphorylation, influent nucleoside molecules are removed from permeation equilibria and are, in effect, trapped intracellularly because of the low permeability of the plasma membrane to nucleotides. Nucleoside-specific transporter elements of the plasma membrane mediate nucleoside fluxes in either direction across the membrane, and it has become evident that such fluxes are rapid relative to the metabolic trapping processes (1–6). With the advent of rapid sampling methods (2,6–9), definitive, early time courses of nucleoside permeation in cultured cells and blood cells were obtained, and the measurement of initial rates of nucleoside uptake in such cells became possible. Since transport is the initial step in the multistep process of nucleoside uptake by cells, initial rates of cellular nucleoside uptake are those of transport. Thus, nucleoside transport in cultured cells and blood cells has been explored and characterized through initial rate kinetics of nucleoside uptake in studies which have employed rapid sampling technology.

With the initial rate methods, kinetic characteristics of nucleoside transport in cells that phosphorylate the nucleoside permeants have been found to be similar to those in nonphosphorylating cells of the same type, as shown in the studies of Plagemann *et al.* (10) on uridine transport (Table I).

In a departure from the initial rate approach, Wohlhueter *et al.* (5) have extracted kinetic characteristics of transport from extended time courses of nucleoside uptake in nonphosphorylating cells by fitting the uptake data to an integrated rate equation derived from a transport model. Cell phosphorylation of nucleoside permeants may be reduced by (1) ATP depletion of cells (2,5,10), (2) use of kinase-deficient cells (5,7,10), and (3) use of nucleoside analog permeants which are not kinase substrates (3,11).

The above approach, that is, the assay of nucleoside transport under conditions in which permeant phosphorylation is impaired, has led to the recognition of "high"-K_m facilitated diffusion transport mechanisms in several types of cultured cells; examples are listed in Table I (5,10,12–14). This type of nucleoside transport mechanism mediates exchange phenomena such as countertransport (10,13), appears to be nonconcentrative, and is of low specificity in that a variety

TABLE I

Examples of Nucleoside Transport in Cells Other Than Erythrocytes

Cells	K_m (μM)	Reference
Uridine influx[a]		
3T3, mouse fibroblasts	220	12
3T3-SV40, mouse fibroblasts, transformed	323	12
NIL-8, hamster fibroblasts	550	12
NIL-8SV, hamster fibroblasts, transformed	400	12
N1S1-67, rat hepatoma	137[b]	10
N1S1-67, rat hepatoma, ATP-depleted	125[b]	10
N1S1-67(UK$^-$), rat hepatoma, uridine, kinase-deficient	72[b]	10
Thymidine influx[a]		
N1S1-67, rat hepatoma, ATP-depleted	245	5
N1S1-67(TK$^-$), rat hepatoma, thymidine, kinase-deficient	262	5
HeLa, human carcinoma, ATP-depleted	125	5

[a] Countertransport (10,13) and inhibition of transport by other nucleosides (5,10) and by NBMPR (5,10,14) have also been demonstrated with these permeants in high-K_m systems.
[b] These values may be low because of the curve-fitting method employed (5).

of nucleosides are substrates. These properties were recognized earlier in the uridine–thymidine transport mechanism of human red cells (7,15). The sensitivity of the high-K_m nucleoside transporters to NBMPR and related compounds (7,10,14–16) and to dipyridamole [2,6-bis(diethanolamino)-4,8-dipiperidino-pyrimido-[5,4-*d*]pyrimidine] (10,13) has been demonstrated. Apparent K_m values for transport of naturally occurring nucleosides by this mechanism (Table I) exceed nucleoside concentrations in blood plasma (17–19); however, Jarvis *et al.* (19) have shown that a nucleoside transport system of high capacity (V) may mediate inward nucleoside fluxes of physiological significance under such conditions. Jarvis *et al.* have demonstrated that the nucleoside transport system of pig erythrocytes is of such capacity that, at a physiological concentration of inosine (1.7 μM), the calculated rate of inosine inflow (mediated) would be in apparent excess of the inosine utilized by these cells assuming that their entire energy requirement was derived from inosine metabolism, as is likely. The kinetic characteristics of inosine transport in this system at 25°C were as follows: K_m 180 μM, and V_{max} 16 pmoles/μl cells per second (19); the latter value is comparable to those reported by Lum *et al.* (20) for the transport of adenosine and inosine in P388 mouse leukemia cells.

Saturable processes for the inward transport of adenosine with K_m values somewhat lower than those listed in Table I have been reported for various cell types (Table II). The adenosine transport processes are sensitive to the potent inhibitors of nucleoside transport, NBMPR and dipyridamole. The latter do not interfere with nucleoside permeation through effects on nucleoside phosphorylation (21–23), but do so by binding to specific transporter sites with the result that transport function is blocked with respect to nucleoside permeants in general. Earlier reports of "low"-K_m processes for adenosine uptake (9,24) were from studies in which uptake rates were derived from the cellular content of adenosine acquired during brief intervals of incubation, rather than from time courses of uptake, and it is less certain than in the present study (or in other recent studies [8,20,25]) that initial rates were measured.

Figure 1 illustrates the application of an initial rate method to the assay of adenosine transport by HeLa cells. Two aspects of this procedure are noteworthy: (1) Intervals of adenosine uptake were ended by the addition of NBMPR (7,8) and cells were immediately pelleted under an oil layer, and (2) time courses of adenosine uptake in the presence of 5–10 μM NBMPR were extrapolated to obtain a time-zero value which was then used as the origin for the time course of adenosine uptake in the absence of NBMPR. Saturation of the initial rates of adenosine uptake in this experiment is apparent in Fig. 1B and C. The saturable process is identified as transport by the initial rate criterion and by NBMPR sensitivity. Mean values (±S.D.) of the kinetic constants for this process obtained in 11 experiments were K_m 26 ± 11 μM, and V_{max} 11 ± 5 pmoles/10^6 cells per second.

In the adenosine transport studies cited in Table II, it is noteworthy that (1) Strauss *et al.* (24) showed the presence in mouse lymphocytes of both low- and high-K_m adenosine transport mechanisms, reporting K_m values of 17 and 125 μM for these processes, and (2) Kolassa *et al.* (8) reported K_m values of 1.4 and 260 μM for adenosine transport processes in human erythrocytes. The permeant specificity of the low-K_m adenosine transport processes have yet to be defined, although it is likely that transport of adenosine simply reflects the activity of a nucleoside transport mechanism that is able to accommodate a variety of nucleosides as substrates.

It may be noted that Lum *et al.* (20), in a study of adenosine transport in P388 mouse leukemia cells using a rapid sampling, time course method, reported K_m

TABLE II

Adenosine Transport, 20–25°C

Cells	K_m (μM)	Reference
HeLa (monolayers)	2.5	9
Lymphocytes (mouse)	17	24
Erythrocytes (human)	1.4	8
HeLa (suspension)	26	this study
L5178Y (mouse lymphoma)	16	25

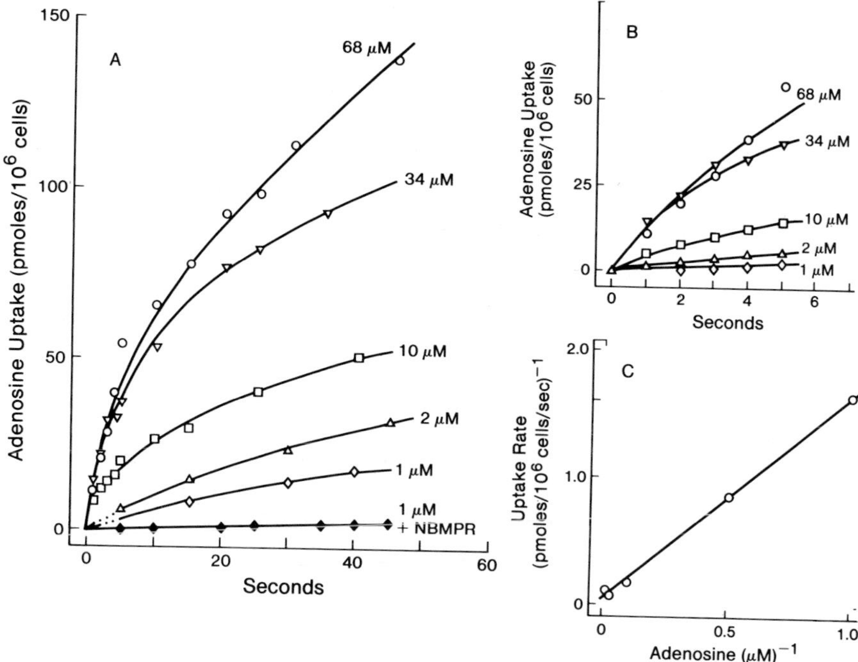

Fig. 1. Transport of adenosine by HeLa cells in suspension. To determine time courses of adenosine uptake, HeLa cells in replicate incubation mixtures were exposed for graded intervals to various concentrations of [2-^{3}H]adenosine. With a procedure described in more detail elsewhere (31), intervals of adenosine uptake were ended by the addition of NBMPR and cells were pelleted at once under an oil layer; cells were solubilized in KOH and assayed for ^{3}H content by liquid scintillation counting. Time courses of adenosine uptake at each concentration were started from the zero-time intercept obtained by back-extrapolation of the time course in the presence of 5 μM NBMPR. Time courses for uptake of adenosine in the presence and absence of NBMPR were obtained for each adenosine concentration, but only the time course of ^{3}H uptake from 1 μM [2-^{3}H]adenosine in the presence of 5 μM NBMPR is shown. Cellular uptake of adenosine in excess of the zero-time values so obtained is plotted in (A) and (B). Uptake data for intervals of 5 seconds and less are shown in (B). Initial rates of adenosine uptake were obtained from the first order terms of least squares parabolas fitted to uptake data. Such rates saturated with increasing adenosine concentration (C). Values of K_m and V_{max} (±S.E.) were 20 ± 5 μM and 11 ± 2.4 pmoles/10^6 cells/second, respectively, at 22°C.

values for adenosine transport (influx) of about 150 μM; a low-K_m adenosine transport mechanism was not detected.

III. Tightly Bound Inhibitors of Nucleoside Transport

Along with various related S^6-substituted 6-thiopurine nucleosides, NBMPR is a potent, tightly bound inhibitor of nucleoside transport. These compounds are proving to be important tools in the exploration of nucleoside transport processes. Erythrocytes and cultured cells of several types possess sites which bind NBMPR and congeners with high affinity; these sites are evidently on the nucleoside transporter, because their occupancy by NBMPR correlates with inhibition of transporter function (16,26). HeLa cells bind about 10^5 NBMPR molecules per cell at these sites; this result has been suggested to be an estimate of the number of transport sites per cell (26). The dissociation constant of NBMPR at these sites on HeLa cells is about 10^{-10} *M* (26).

The inhibitor sites also bind dipyridamole, a potent inhibitor of nucleoside transport (1,8). Dipyridamole inhibited site-specific binding of NBMPR in an apparently competitive manner and, as well, displaced site-bound NBMPR; the dissociation constant of dipyridamole at these sites on HeLa cells was found to be about 3×10^{-8} *M* (27). The implication in these results that NBMPR and dipyridamole interact with the same binding sites on the nucleoside transport mechanism appears to be at odds with the great disparity in the chemical structures of the two inhibitors.

The 5′-monophosphate of NBMPR (NBMPR-P) inhibits nucleoside transport in HeLa cells with a potency comparable to that of NBMPR because of conversion to the latter by cellular ecto 5′-nucleotidase activity (28). The solubility of NBMPR-P and its ready dephosphorylation have facilitated *in vivo* exploration of NBMPR effects.

IV. Nitrobenzylthioinosine Inhibition of Nucleoside Transport in Tissues

As might be expected from the potent effects of NBMPR and congeners on nucleoside transport in erythrocytes and cultured cells, these compounds also have inhibitory effects on nucleoside permeation in animal tissues. Olsson *et al.* (23) showed that nitrobenzylthioguanosine (2-amino-6-[(4-nitrobenzyl)thio]-9-β-D-ribofuranosylpurine) an NBMPR congener with potency in the inhibition of nucleoside transport comparable to that of NBMPR (9,22), inhibited adenosine uptake by dog myocardium, as did dipyridamole. The experiment in Fig. 2 measured the time course of cytidine uptake by mouse liver during *in situ* perfusion of that tissue; it is seen that, when mice received NBMPR-P (50 mg/kg body weight) by intraperitoneal injection about 30 minutes prior to perfusion, cytidine uptake by the liver was greatly reduced. In the perfused livers of NBMPR-P-treated mice, the "cytidine space" was similar to the "inulin space" (a measure of extracellular space), indicating that the permeability of hepatic cells to cytidine had been greatly reduced by the NBMPR-P treatment. These observations suggest that the pharmacokinetics and tissue distribution of nucleoside drugs and of physiological nucleosides might well be influenced by NBMPR and related inhibitors of nucleoside transport.

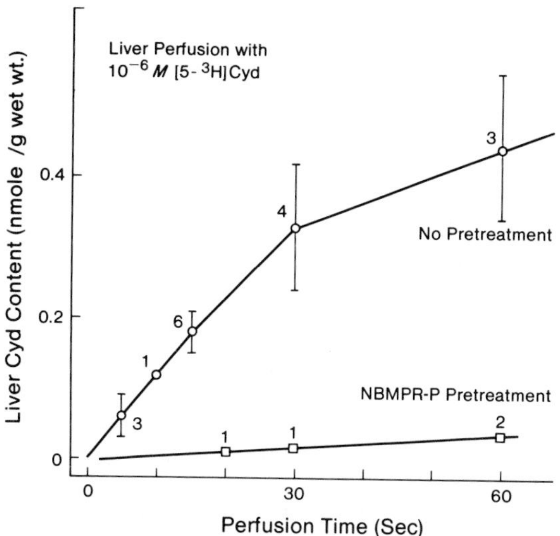

Fig. 2. Perfusion of mouse liver with [5-^{3}H]cytidine. Livers of male BD2F$_1$ mice under pentobarbital anesthesia were perfused with Krebs–Henseleit medium containing heparin (30 units/ml) and saturated with oxygen and 5% CO_2. Livers were perfused for 3 minutes prior to switching (time zero) to medium containing 1 μM [5-^{3}H]cytidine and [*carboxyl*-^{14}C]inulin (20 μg/ml). Perfusion was via the portal vein at 4 ml/minute. At the end of perfusion intervals, livers were weighed, dried, and assayed for ^{14}C and ^{3}H content by a combustion–liquid scintillation procedure employing a Packard Model 306 sample oxidizer. The [5-^{3}H]cytidine (Cyd) content of each sample was corrected for that present in its inulin space. The data presented are means (±S.D.), and the numbers of samples represented by each mean are indicated. Mice were either untreated or treated with disodium NBMPR-P (50 mg/kg) by intraperitoneal injection 30 minutes before perfusion. These data were obtained by N. Kolassa (University of Vienna) during a study leave at the University of Alberta.

V. Nitrobenzylthioinosine Protection against Cytotoxic Nucleosides

A. Protection of Cultured Cells

We reported that, in the presence of NBMPR, cultured cells of several types were protected against the antiproliferative effects of various nucleoside analogues (27,29–31). Our interpretation of these results was that (1) inhibition of cell proliferation signified cellular uptake of the toxic analog, and (2) NBMPR protection against this manifestation of toxicity indicated that cellular uptake of the analogue was mediated by the nucleoside transport mechanism. Consistent with this interpretation was the demonstration that, during culture of RPMI 6410 cells under NBMPR protection from otherwise inhibitory concentrations of nebularine, cellular concentrations of the analogue were much lower in protected cells throughout the 72 hours of culture than in unprotected, growth-inhibited cells (30). Protection was afforded by NBMPR against nucleosides of

TABLE III

Nitrobenzylthioinosine Protection of RPMI 6410 Cells against Cytotoxic Analogs of Adenosine[a]

Analog (μM)	Cell proliferation rate (% of control)[b] Without NBMPR	With NBMPR[c]	Source[d]
2-Azaadenosine (1.0)	−13	98	A
Carbocyclic adenosine (5.0)	−10	84	B
Formycin (6.0)	−18	98	C
6-Methylthioinosine (0.2)	− 1	72	D
Nebularine (1.0)	9	88	D
Tricyclicnucleoside (0.01)	− 1.0	98	E
Xylosyladenine (300)	13	59	F

[a] Data from Paterson (27) and Paterson *et al.* (31).

[b] Population doublings in 72 hours as a percentage of rates in cultures without additives (3.3-3.8 doublings in 72 hours).

[c] This concentration, 5 μM NBMPR, did not significantly affect cell proliferation rates.

[d] Analog sources: (A) J. A. Montgomery; (B) Y. F. Shealy; (C) H. Umezawa; (D) commercial; (E) L. B. Townsend; (F) G. A. LePage.

very different structure (Table III; Fig. 3), indicating that the specificity of the nucleoside transport processes in these cells was low. Although exceptions are known (31), it is also apparent with various other nucleoside analogs (31) that a determinant of toxicity is transportability, that is, acceptance as a substrate by the nucleoside transport mechanism.

B. *In Vivo* Protection

As earlier reports have indicated, mice are protected against potentially lethal dosages of nebularine and other toxic nucleoside analogues by coadministration of NBMPR or NBMPR-P (30,32). For example, the lethality (apparently due to intestinal injury) caused in mice by particular treatment regimens employing 3-deazauridine and arabinosylcytosine was not manifested when NBMPR was administered with either agent (30). In other examples, mice survived otherwise lethal treatment schedules with nebularine, tubercidin, or toyocamycin when these agents were administered with protecting dosages of NBMPR or NBMPR-P (30). The experiments summarized in Fig. 4 illustrate protection of mice by NBMPR-P against potentially lethal nebularine treatments; NBMPR-P protection against single, lethal dosages of nebularine or tubercidin has also been demonstrated.

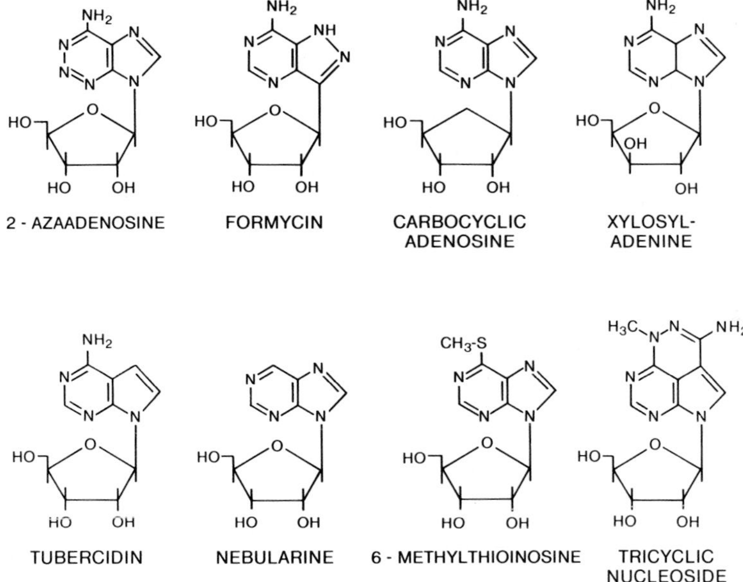

Fig. 3. Structural formulas of adenosine analogs.

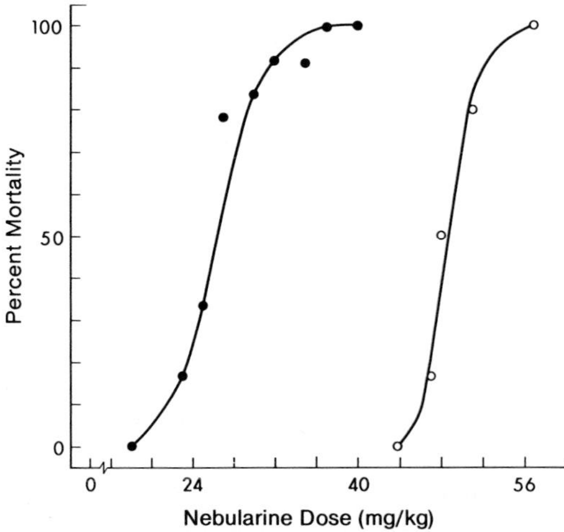

Fig. 4. NBMPR-P protection of $BD2F_1$ mice against nebularine lethality. Data from Lynch *et al.* (33). $BD2F_1$ mice in groups of six were treated with nebularine alone (●) or with nebularine plus monoammonium NBMPR-P [25 mg/kg, (○)]; nebularine was administered at the dosages indicated. Treatments were administered by intraperitoneal injection daily for 5 days, and treatment groups were of one sex or the other. Mortality by day 20 is recorded.

It is seen in Fig. 4 that, when NBMPR-P was administered together with nebularine, the dosage of nebularine which resulted in 50% mortality was about twice that without the protecting agent. When administration of nebularine followed that of NBMPR-P, the protecting effect of the latter was diminished in a manner related to the interval between the administration of each agent. The half-life of the NBMPR-P protection effect was about 4 hours (33). It may be noted that the NBMPR-P dosage (25 mg/kg) employed in these experiments was above the minimum dosage [about 0.5 mg/kg (30)] that would afford protection of mice against nebularine.

In similar experiments, we have demonstrated that the tolerance of male $BD2F_1$ mice toward tubercidin was markedly increased by coadministration of NBMPR-P. When tubercidin was administered by the intraperitoneal route in four doses each 24 hours apart, the dosage which resulted in 50% mortality was about 2.5 mg/kg; this dosage was 3.4 times higher for mice which received NBMPR-P (25 mg/kg) coadministered with tubercidin (34).

Because of (1) the NBMPR inhibition of nucleoside transport, and (2) the protection by NBMPR of cultured cells against toxic nucleosides, it is likely that the *in vivo* protection phenomenon is due to NBMPR-induced changes in the pharmacokinetics and tissue distribution of the toxic nucleosides. This view is supported by current experiments which show that treatment of mice with NBMPR-P (25 mg/kg) 10 minutes prior to the intraperitoneal administration of a lethal dose of [G-^{3}H]tubercidin causes pronounced changes in the blood and urine kinetics of tubercidin and in its tissue distribution (E. S. Jakobs, N. Kolassa, T. P. Lynch, and A. R. P. Paterson). It remains to relate NBMPR-P-induced changes in tubercidin distribution to the protection phenomenon and to histological evidence of tissue damage by tubercidin.

VI. Experimental Chemotherapy with Potentially Lethal Doses of Nebularine

The foregoing *in vivo* protection experiments demonstrated that the tolerance of normal mice for toxic nucleoside analogs was increased in the presence of NBMPR-P. Table IV summarizes an experiment in which potentially lethal dosages of nebularine were administered together with NBMPR-P protection in the treatment of mice bearing leukemia L1210.

The experiment of Table IV demonstrated that survival times of mice implanted with 10^6 leukemia L1210 cells were not increased by treatment with nebularine at 37 mg/kg (a potentially lethal dosage) together with NBMPR-P at a low dosage which protected nonleukemic mice from nebularine lethality. Under these circumstances, mice died leukemic deaths. However, at higher dosages of

TABLE IV

Therapy of Mouse Leukemia L1210 with Potentially Lethal Doses of Nebularine[a,b]

Therapy (mg/kg)				
Nebularine	NBMPR-P[c]	6-Thioinosine	Mean survival time of mice that died (days ± S.D.)	Survivors on day 50
37	50	0	18.7 ± 4.7	3/6
37	25	0	22.4 ± 4.6	1/6
37	13	0	17.5 ± 6.1	0/6
37	1	0	7.7 ± 1.5	0.6[d]
37	0	12	8.7 ± 2.7	0/6[d]
37	1	12	18.0 ± 3.0	2/6
37	1	6	11.8 ± 2.7	1/6
37	1	3	18.4 ± 8.9	1/6
0	1	0	6.5 ± 1.2	0/6
0	0	15	9.3 ± 1.2	0/6
0	0	0	6.5 ± 0.7	0/6

[a] Data from Lynch *et al.* (33).

[b] Female BD2F$_1$ mice were implanted intraperitoneally with 10^6 leukemia L1210 cells, and 24 hours later therapy was begun; therapeutic agents were dissolved in 0.15 *M* NaCl solution and administered by intraperitoneal injection in five doses each 24 hours apart.

[c] Monoammonium salt (35).

[d] Comparison of these mortalities with those in the toxicity control groups (following) shows that NBMPR-P in excess of 1 mg/kg was required for the therapeutic effect (see text). Toxicity controls: When nonleukemic mice were treated (1) with nebularine alone, no mice survived [mean survival time (MST), 7.0 ± 0.9 days]; (2) with nebularine plus NBMPR-P (1 mg/kg), no mice died; and (3) with nebularine plus 6-thioinosine (15 mg/kg), no mice survived (MST, 6.8 ± 1.2 days).

NBMPR-P, substantial kill of leukemic cells was achieved, and some mice, apparently "cured," were alive on day 50. Under these circumstances, mice that did not survive died of leukemia with survival times that were increased about threefold over those of untreated mice. It is seen in Table IV that (1) treatment with dosages of NBMPR-P in excess of that required for protection against nebularine lethality was a necessary condition for the therapeutic effect, and (2) a similar therapeutic effect was achieved when 6-thioinosine replaced the "excess" NBMPR-P (Table IV dosages: nebularine, 37 mg/kg; NBMPR-P, 1 mg/kg; 6-thioinosine, 12 mg/kg). Thus it appears that the therapeutic effect derived from the conjoint presence of nebularine and a 6-thiopurine metabolite formed from NBMPR-P. The NBMPR-P component of the regimen evidently protected a vital, nebularine-sensitive tissue of the mouse and yet allowed nebularine and a 6-thiopurine derivative to interact with the leukemia L1210 cells. In experiments similar to that of Table IV, therapy with nebularine alone at dosages near the maximum tolerated dosage was not effective against leukemia L1210. Nebularine cytotoxicity may well have a basis in perturbations in the area of purine nucleotide metabolism caused by the intracellular presence of mono-, di-, and triphosphates of nebularine (36). The metabolic consequences of the conjoint intracellular presence of nebularine and thiopurine metabolites are unknown.

In the experiments of Tables V and VI, mice bearing transplanted neoplasms, mouse leukemia L1210/TG8, or colon carcinoma 26, were treated with potentially lethal dosages of tubercidin administered together with protecting dosages of NBMPR-P. Treatment with NBMPR-P at 25 mg/kg protected mice from tubercidin lethality yet allowed the killing of neoplastic cells by tubercidin–NBMPR-P combinations to the extent that substantial numbers of long-term survivors resulted. It is not known whether NBMPR-P dosages in excess of the requirement for host protection (less than 1 mg/kg) contributed to the therapeutic effect, as with the nebularine–NBMPR-P combination (Table IV). Mouse leuke-

TABLE V

Treatment of Mice Bearing a Thioguanine-Resistant Variant of Mouse Leukemia L1210 with Potentially Lethal Dosages of Tubercidin[a,b]

Dosages (mg/kg)			
Tubercidin	NBMPR-P[c]	Mean survival time of mice that died (days)[d]	50-day survivors
0	0	6.6 ± 1.3	0/6
0.5	0	7.7 ± 0.9	0/6
1.0	0	11.0 ± 3.6	0/6
1.5	0	9.0 ± 1.3	1/7
5.0[e]	25	13.5 ± 6.5	4/6[f]

[a] Data from Lynch *et al.* (34).

[b] A subline of leukemia L1210 selected for *in vivo* resistance to thioguanine and characterized as deficient in hypoxanthine-guanine phosphoribosyltransferase activity was provided by G. A. LePage. These cells were adapted to culture, a clone (L1210/TG8) was established by the soft agar method, and the line was then returned to *in vivo* passage. Male BD2F$_1$ mice were implanted intraperitoneally with 10^6 L1210/TG8 cells and 24 hours later received the first of four intraperitoneal treatments (specified below) repeated at 24-hour intervals.

[c] Monoammonium salt.

[d] Average deviation from the mean.

[e] Lethal without NBMPR-P.

[f] The parental cell type, L1210/0, did not respond to this therapeutic regimen.

TABLE VI

Treatment of Mice Bearing Colon Carcinoma 26 with Potentially Lethal Dosages of Tubercidin[a,b]

Therapy (mg/kg)			
Tubercidin	NBMPR-P[c]	Mean survival time (days ± S.D.)	Alive on day 98
0	0	24.6 ± 11.2	0/7
1	0	47.8 ± 7.8	1/7
0	50	30.9 ± 3.9	0/7
5[d]	25	38.5 ± 17.2	4/8

[a] Data from Lynch *et al.* (34).

[b] Male BALB/c mice were implanted intraperitoneally, each with 1.9×10^6 cells of colon carcinoma 26 in suspension. Starting 72 hours after implantation, drugs were given by intraperitoneal injection in four doses each 24 hours apart.

[c] Monoammonium salt.

[d] Lethal without NBMPR-P.

mia L1210/0, the parental type from which the L1210/TG8 clone was derived, was much less responsive than the latter to tubercidin–NBMPR-P therapy (data not shown), suggesting that purine salvage via hypoxanthine-guanine phosphoribosyltransferase may ameliorate the consequences of cellular exposure to the tubercidin–NBMPR-P combination; by this reasoning, inhibition of purine nucleotide synthesis *de novo* appears to be a consequence of such exposure. As the data of Table VI indicate, the tubercidin–NBMPR-P protocol (Table V) was effective against colon carcinoma 26 implanted intraperitoneally.

VII. Summary and Conclusions

The entry of nucleosides into animal cells is mediated by nucleoside-specific transporter elements of the plasma membrane. An NBMPR-sensitive facilitated diffusion transport process of low specificity for nucleosides has been recognized in various cell types; that mechanism probably mediates the inward transport of adenosine, a process which in HeLa cells and L5178Y cells had K_m values of 26–16 μm.

Cells proliferating in culture were protected by NBMPR against the growth-inhibitory effects of a variety of cytotoxic nucleoside analogs. Such protection indicated that entry of the analogs was mediated by a nucleoside transport process (or processes) with broad substrate specificity. Protection of mice by NBMPR-P against otherwise lethal treatment regimens with toxic nucleoside analogues (including nebularine and tubercidin) has also been demonstrated and is interpreted to mean that the transport inhibitors protect vital tissues of the mouse by causing changes in the tissue distribution of the toxic analogs.

Mice bearing transplanted neoplasms were treated with combinations of NBMPR-P and potentially lethal dosages of nebularine or tubercidin. In the treatment of mice bearing leukemia L1210, effective therapy required dosages of NBMPR-P in excess of minimal dosages that protected normal mice against nebularine lethality; treatment regimens were found which protected the leukemic hosts against nebularine lethality and yet allowed substantial kill of leukemic cells. Treatment with nebularine alone at tolerated doses was not effective. Tubercidin–NBMPR-P therapeutic regimens were also effective against a thioguanine-resistant subline of leukemia L1210 and against colon carcinoma 26.

"Host protection" with nucleoside transport inhibitors such as NBMPR may allow therapy with otherwise toxic dosages of nucleoside drugs, and it is possible that the transport inhibitors may enable manipulation to some extent of the pharmacokinetics and tissue distribution of nucleoside drugs. It is possible that the *in vivo* availability or salvage of endogenous nucleosides may be also influenced by the inhibitors of nucleoside transport.

Acknowledgments

Support by the National Cancer Institute of Canada and the Medical Research Council of Canada is acknowledged. Drs. Carol E. Cass, Norbert Kolassa, and Thomas P. Lynch provided helpful discussions during the preparation of this chapter, and their contributions to the data presented are acknowledged with gratitude.

References

1. R. D. Berlin and J. M. Oliver, *Int. Rev. Cytol.* **42,** 287 (1975).
2. R. M. Wohlhueter, R. Marz, J. C. Graff, and P. G. W. Plagemann, *Methods Cell Biol.* **20,** 211 (1978).
3. O. Heichal, D. Ish-Shalom, R. Koren, and W. D. Stein, *Biochim. Biophys. Acta* **551,** 169 (1979).
4. E. Rozengurt, W. D. Stein, and N. M. Wigglesworth, *Nature (London)* **267,** 442 (1977).
5. R. M. Wohlhueter, R. Marz, and P. G. W. Plagemann, *Biochim. Biophys. Acta* **553,** 262 (1979).
6. D. Bowen, R. B. Diasio, and I. D. Goldman, *J. Biol. Chem.* **254,** 5333 (1979).
7. Z. I. Cabantchik and H. Ginsburg, *J. Gen. Physiol.* **69,** 75 (1977).
8. N. Kolassa, B. Plank, and K. Turnheim, *Eur. J. Pharmacol.* **52,** 345 (1978).
9. A. R. P. Paterson, L. R. Babb, J. H. Paran, and C. E. Cass, *Mol. Pharmacol.* **13,** 1147 (1977).
10. P. G. W. Plagemann, R. Marz, and R. M. Wohlhueter, *J. Cell. Physiol.* **97,** 49 (1978).

11. D. Kessel, *J. Biol. Chem.* **253,** 400 (1978).
12. R. Koren, E. Shohami, O. Bibi, and W. D. Stein, *FEBS Lett.* **86,** 71 (1978).
13. P. G. W. Plagemann, R. Marz, and J. Erbe, *J. Cell. Physiol.* **89,** 1 (1976).
14. R. M. Wohlhueter, R. Marz, and P. G. W. Plagemann, *J. Membr. Biol.* **42,** 247 (1978).
15. C. E. Cass and A. R. P. Paterson, *J. Biol. Chem.* **247,** 3314 (1972).
16. C. E. Cass, L. A. Gaudette, and A. R. P. Paterson, *Biochim. Biophys. Acta* **345,** 1 (1975).
17. W. L. Hughes, M. Christine, and B. D. Stollar, *Anal. Biochem.* **55,** 468 (1973).
18. S. B. Howell, W. D. Ensminger, A. Krishnan, and E. Frei, III, *Cancer Res.* **38,** 325 (1978).
19. S. M. Jarvis, J. D. Young, M. Ansay, A. L. Archibald, R. A. Harkness, and R. J. Simmonds, *Biochim. Biophys. Acta* **597,** 183 (1980).
20. C. T. Lum, R. Marz, P. G. W. Plagemann, and R. M. Wohlhueter, *J. Cell Physiol.* **101,** 173 (1979).
21. C. E. Cass and A. R. P. Paterson, *Exp. Cell Res.* **105,** 427 (1977).
22. A. R. P. Paterson, S. R. Naik, and C. E. Cass, *Mol. Pharmacol.* **13,** 1014 (1977).
23. R. A. Olsson, J. A. Snow, M. K. Gentry, and G. P. Frick, *Circ. Res.* **31,** 767 (1972).
24. P. R. Strauss, J. M. Sheehan, and E. R. Kashket, *J. Immunol.* **118,** 1328 (1977).
25. E. R. Harley, C. E. Cass, and A. R. P. Paterson, *Cancer Res.* (submitted for publication).
26. G. J. Lauzon and A. R. P. Paterson, *Mol. Pharmacol.* **13,** 883 (1977).
27. A. R. P. Paterson, *in* "Physiological and Regulatory Functions of Adenosine and Adenine Nucleotides" (H. P. Baer and I. Drummond, eds.), p. 305. Raven, New York, 1979.
28. P. O. J. Ogbunude, M. Sc. Thesis, University of Alberta, Edmonton, Alberta, Canada (1979).
29. C. T. Warnick, H. Muzik, and A. R. P. Paterson, *Cancer Res.* **32,** 2017 (1972).
30. A. R. P. Paterson, J. H. Paran, S. Yang, and T. P. Lynch, *Cancer Res.* **39,** 3607 (1979).
31. A. R. P. Paterson, S. Yang, E. Y. Lau, and C. E. Cass, *Mol. Pharmacol.* **16,** 900 (1979).
32. A. R. P. Paterson, E. S. Jakobs, G. J. Lauzon, and W. M. Weinstein, *Cancer Res.* **39,** 2216 (1979).
33. T. P. Lynch, J. H. Paran, and A. R. P. Paterson, *Cancer Res.* in press.
34. T. P. Lynch, E. S. Jakobs, and A. R. P. Paterson, *Cancer Res.* (submitted for publication).
35. T. P. Lynch, G. J. Lauzon, S. R. Naik, C. E. Cass, and A. R. P. Paterson, *Biochem. Pharmacol.* **27,** 1303 (1978).
36. M. P. Gordon and G. B. Brown, *J. Biol. Chem.* **220,** 927 (1956).

11

Purine Nucleoside Phosphorylase and 5′-Methylthioadenosine Phosphorylase: Targets of Chemotherapy

ROBERT E. PARKS, JR., JOHANNA D. STOECKLER, CAROLYN CAMBOR, TODD M. SAVARESE, GERALD W. CRABTREE, AND SHIH-HSI CHU

I. Introduction

Although extensive studies on antimetabolites of purine bases and nucleosides have yielded a rich harvest of clinically useful antineoplastic, immunosuppres-

MOLECULAR ACTIONS AND TARGETS FOR CANCER CHEMOTHERAPEUTIC AGENTS

ISBN 0-12-619280-4

sive, and antiviral drugs, until recently it was widely assumed that agents of this class must be converted to the nucleotide level for activity. Except for xanthine oxidase, whose inhibition by allopurinol increases both the antitumor activity and the toxicity of 6-mercaptopurine (1), other enzymes of purine catabolism, e.g., purine nucleoside phosphorylase (PNP) and adenosine deaminase (ADA), were not considered likely chemotherapeutic targets. During recent years, however, this view was drastically altered by the discovery of congenital immunodeficiency syndromes associated with impairments or deletions of ADA or PNP (2–6). Furthermore, ADA inhibitors have been found that not only potentiate the antineoplastic activity of adenosine analogs, but one of these, deoxycoformycin (Pentostatin), when administered alone, has produced partial or complete remissions in patients with acute leukemias derived from T lymphocytes (7).

The recent discovery that PNP deficiency results in a specific defect in cellular but not humoral immunity and the finding of high PNP activity in T lymphocytes but low activity in B lymphocytes (8) direct attention to PNP as a target in the design of inhibitors that could have specific action against T lymphocytes, both normal and neoplastic. Also, as noted previously (9), nucleosides of chemotherapeutically active purine antimetabolites (e.g., β-deoxythioguanosine) are readily cleaved by PNP, producing the respective free base analogs. It must be appreciated that human erythrocytes have very high PNP activity and also have an active nucleoside transport system that facilitates entry of nucleosides into the cell. Therefore inhibitors of PNP might not only have activity against T lymphocytes but also might potentiate the cytotoxicity of guanine or hypoxanthine deoxynucleoside analogs.

Although PNP and ADA have been studied for many years, only recently has methylthioadenosine phosphorylase (MTA-Pase) been recognized as a potential chemotherapeutic target. This enzyme is essential for salvage of adenine from the 5′-deoxy-5′-methylthioadenosine (MTA) formed from *S*-adenosylmethionine (SAM) during polyamine synthesis (10). The finding of MTA-Pase in most mammalian tissues explains the source of intracellular free adenine and the almost ubiquitous occurrence of adenine phosphoribosyltransferase (APRT).

This chapter deals with recent studies on these two nucleoside phosphorylases. We have undertaken an analysis of the effects of substrate modifications in both the sugar (11,12) and the aglycone moieties, with the intent of finding specific potent PNP inhibitors.

II. Purine Nucleoside Phosphorylase

A. Introduction

This enzyme is the primary mechanism by which animal tissues degrade the ribonucleosides and deoxyribonucleosides of guanine and hypoxanthine to free bases and the respective pentose 1-phosphates. The reaction is readily reversible,

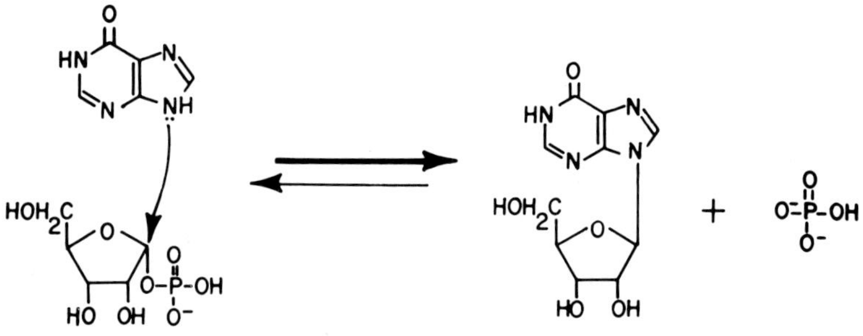

Fig. 1. Reaction mechanism of PNP.

with the equilibrium favoring nucleoside synthesis. The reaction mechanism is S_N2 with a Walden inversion about C-1′ of the pentose (Fig. 1).

The first definitive studies on PNP were performed by Kalckar (13) in the years following World War II. Comprehensive reviews of investigations of PNP reported prior to 1972 have been published (14,15). For more than a dozen years, our laboratory has studied human erythrocytic PNP. Methods have been developed for large-scale isolation of PNP and other enzymes from human erythrocytes, and the enzyme has been obtained in the homogeneous, crystalline state (16–19). In a recent report, we have described the physical properties of PNP, which is among the few enzymes identified to date as a homologous trimer. The molecular weight is about 91,000, i.e., 30,000 per subunit (20,21). Isoelectric focusing of PNP purified from pooled human erythrocytes demonstrates microheterogeneity, presumably due to progressive protein degradation during aging of the erythrocytes (22,23). Several laboratories have reported that PNPs from different tissues and species, e.g., chicken liver, beef brain, and rabbit liver, vary significantly from the human erythrocytic enzyme in physical properties and subunit structures (24–26). Kinetic analyses indicate that human erythrocytic PNP follows an ordered Bi Bi reaction sequence with the nucleoside substrate the first to add to the catalytic site and the purine base the last to leave (27). It is interesting to speculate that, if the tertiary structure of PNP includes a substrate-binding pocket at the active site, as has been identified for several other enzymes, one would expect the purine base to enter the pocket first and to occupy the deepest position with the pentose moiety more exterior. We anticipate that soon X-ray crystallographic and amino acid sequence studies will be initiated with the objective of defining precisely the structure of the active center. This information might enable future investigators to design potent inhibitors based on knowledge of the binding groups in the enzyme.

B. Rationale for the Design of Purine Nucleoside Phosphorylase Inhibitors

Several lines of evidence indicate that PNP inhibitors might have therapeutic activity either alone or in combination with other agents. Since children with heritable PNP deficiencies display normal humoral but defective cellular immunity (3), and the activity of PNP in T lymphocytes is higher than in B lymphocytes (8), one may predict that inhibition of PNP will have specific effects on T lymphocytes and cell-mediated immunity. It has been proposed that high PNP activity is required to degrade 2′-deoxyribonucleosides and thereby prevent phosphorylation by deoxyguanosine kinase of 2′-deoxyguanosine derived from the degradation of DNA during tissue breakdown (28). Once formed, dGMP is converted to dGTP, a potent feedback inhibitor of ribonucleotide reductase, an essential enzyme for the synthesis of deoxynucleotides during DNA synthesis. Accumulation of excessive amounts of dGTP, as occurs in PNP-deficient individuals (29), would be cytotoxic to rapidly dividing cells. Administration of a PNP inhibitor alone or in combination with 2′-deoxyguanosine might provide therapeutic activity in autoimmune diseases and in preventing rejection of foreign tissues during organ transplantation.

It had been expected that β-2′-deoxynucleosides of analogues such as 6-thioguanine would have unique activity through direct conversion to analog-containing 2′-deoxynucleotides by reaction with deoxynucleoside kinases. In clinical trials to date, these compounds have not shown clear-cut advantages over the purine base analogs. One may speculate that the high activity of PNP in human erythrocytes (10–15 units/ml of cells), coupled with the highly active erythrocytic nucleoside transport system, is responsible for very rapid degradation of potentially cytotoxic β-2′-deoxynucleoside analogs during transit to the desired site of action. Thus a potent PNP inhibitor, by preventing this degradation, might permit therapeutic quantities of intact nucleosides to reach the target tissues. Another approach that might decrease the undesired degradation of nucleoside analogs is the use of a PNP inhibitor in combination with a specific nucleoside transport inhibitor such as *p*-nitrobenzylthioinosine (NBMPR) (30). Furthermore, if sufficient understanding of the PNP reaction can be achieved, it may be possible to design nucleoside analogs that are good substrates for enzymes such as deoxyguanosine kinase but have little or no reactivity with PNP. Such analogs might display specific toxicity against T lymphocytes and their derivatives.

Another area where potent inhibitors of PNP may find therapeutic use is in the treatment of hyperuricemic states, i.e., primary and secondary gout. This is suggested by the unusual metabolic disturbances observed in congenital PNP deficiency (31). Children with this condition display hypouricosuria, hypouricemia, increased rates of purine nucleotide biosynthesis *de novo,* and marked elevations in plasma and urinary ribonucleosides and deoxyribonucleosides of guanine and hypoxanthine. Because of the lack of PNP, cells are incapable of degrading nucleosides to free bases, and therefore the enzymes guanase and xanthine oxidase cannot produce xanthine or uric acid. Thus, during rapid cellular breakdown and nucleic acid degradation, inhibition of PNP would

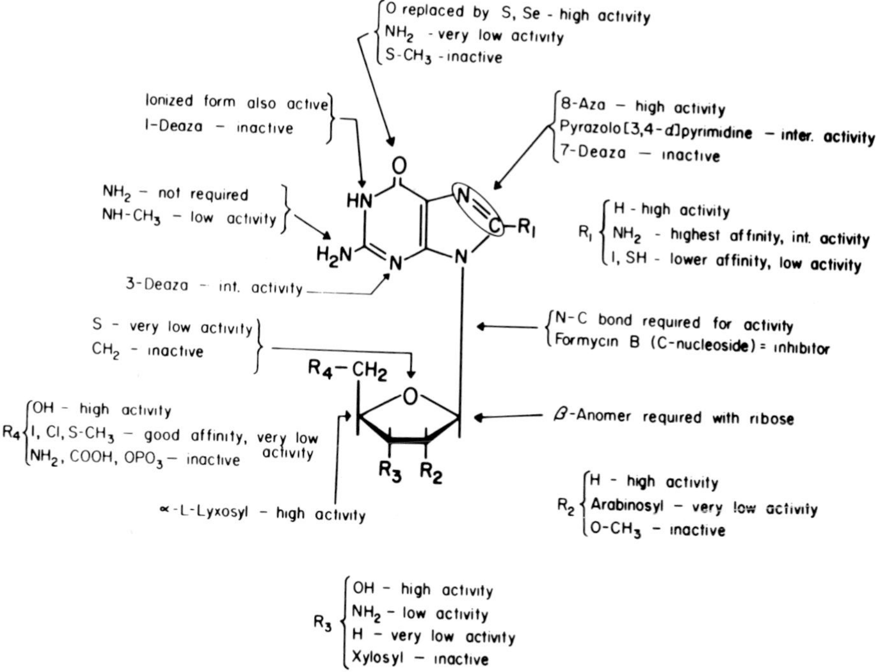

Fig. 2. Structure–activity relationships of substrates for human erythrocytic PNP.

allow purines to be excreted in the form of relatively soluble nucleosides. The recent development of reversed-phase high-pressure liquid chromatography (HPLC) should facilitate the testing of this concept when effective inhibitors are developed. It may also be worthwhile to explore the utility of administering a PNP inhibitor together with the xanthine oxidase inhibitor allopurinol, since under certain conditions additive or synergistic effects might be observed.

In view of the above, we have undertaken a systematic study of the structure–activity relationships of base and nucleoside analogs with PNP. Figure 2 summarizes many of the findings discussed below.

C. Structure–Activity Relationships

1. Sugar Modifications

Recently we have examined various analogs of inosine and guanosine with specific modifications in the ribose moiety (11,12). Representative compounds are shown in Table I. For substrate activity, the ribose must be attached from C-1′ to N-9 of the purine ring in the β-configuration. The only exception to this rule identified to date is the nucleoside α-L-lyxosylhypoxanthine which, as seen in

TABLE I

Effect of Sugar Modification on Substrate or Inhibitory Activity with Purine Nucleoside Phosphorylase[a]

Compound	K_m or K_i (μM)	V_{max}
Inosine	30–35	100
C-1′		
α-L-Lyxosylhypoxanthine	180	38
Formycin B	100(K_i)	
5′-Chloro-5′-deoxyformycin B	10(K_i)	
C-2′		
2′-Deoxyinosine	45	53
Arabinosylhypoxanthine	2000	1
2′-*O*-Methylguanosine		0
C-3′		
3′-Deoxyinosine	1100	2
Xylosylhypoxanthine		0
3′-Amino-3′-deoxyinosine	305	10
C-4′		
Carbocyclic inosine		0
4′-Thioinosine	1900	1
C-5′		
5′-Deoxyinosine	31	45
2′,5′-Dideoxyinosine	120	53
5′-Amino-5′-deoxyinosine		0
5′-Chloro-5′-deoxyinosine	10	0.8
5′-Deoxy-5′-iodoinosine	12	0.1
5′-Deoxy-5′-methylthioinosine	15	0.7
5′-Deoxy-5′-isobutylthioinosine	42	0.2

[a] Some of the data presented in this table have been reported elsewhere (12).

molecular models, resembles inosine but has C-5′ and its substituents cis rather than trans to the hydroxyls on C-2′ and C-3′. Substrate activity is lost in formycin B, where a C—C bond replaces the normal N—C glycosidic bond. This analogue, however, is a moderately good inhibitor of PNP (32).

The C-2′ of ribose is a key determinant of substrate activity. If the hydroxyl of inosine is replaced by a hydrogen atom, (e.g., as in 2′-deoxyinosine), the V_{max} is reduced by only about 50%. On the other hand, marked decreases in velocity and affinity occur if the C-2′ hydroxyl is trans relative to C-3′ as in arabinosylhypoxanthine, and activity is completely lost if it is replaced by a methoxy group as in 2′-*O*-methylguanosine. Especially intriguing are preliminary findings which indicate that 2′-deoxy-2′-fluoroinosine reacts very slowly with PNP. This analog has been available only in limited amounts (prepared by deamination of 2′-deoxy-2′-fluoroadenosine, which was a gift from Murio Ikehara), and detailed kinetic and other studies have not yet been possible. Because the van der Waals radius of fluorine is similar to that of the hydrogen atom, it is likely that analog nucleosides that contain 2′-deoxy-2′-fluororibose will resemble natural 2′-deoxyribonucleosides and will be accepted as substrates for deoxyribonucleoside kinases. We plan to pursue this interesting approach in the future.

The substituents on C-3′ also play a crucial role. If the hydroxyl is absent (e.g., as in 3′-deoxyinosine) substrate activity is markedly decreased; whereas, when the hydroxyl is in the trans configuration (e.g., as in xylosylhypoxanthine), no activity is detectable. Replacement of the C-3′ hydroxyl by an amino group decreases the V_{max} to 10% and increases the K_m about sixfold. If the bridge oxygen is replaced by sulfur as in 4′-thioinosine, substrate activity is greatly decreased, and if it is replaced by a methylene group, as in carbocyclic inosine, activity is abolished.

Modifications at C-5′ are especially interesting. It is well established that phosphorylation (e.g., as in 5′-IMP), or substitution by a carboxyl or amino group, destroys substrate activity. On the other hand, if the hydroxyl is replaced by a hydrogen atom, as in 5′-deoxyinosine, good substrate activity is retained. Also, if the C-5′ hydroxyl of inosine is replaced by a chlorine, bromine, or iodine atom, or by a methylthio group, the V_{max} is greatly decreased but affinity is enhanced. Therefore future attention will be focused on modifications at C-5′ and its substituents in the development of inhibitors. The 5′-chloro-5′-deoxy derivative of formycin B has recently been synthesized, and its K_i (10 μM) is 10-fold lower than that of the parent compound.

2. *Modifications in the Purine Ring and Its Substituents*

To date the study of analogs modified in the purine ring has not identified changes that provide increased affinity for the enzyme. If N-1 is replaced by a carbon atom (e.g., as in 1-deazaguanine), substrate activity is lost; whereas exchange of a carbon atom for N-3, as in 3-deazaguanine, results in greatly diminished substrate activity (33). If C-2 and N-3 are exchanged, as in 2-aza-3-deazahypoxanthine, weak but definite substrate activity is observed (J. D. Stoeckler, R. E. Parks, Jr., and R. P. Panzica, unpublished results).

The results of modifications in the imidazole ring are complex. The inosine analog of tubercidin, 7-deazainosine, and the inosine analog of the formycin series, formycin B, are devoid of substrate activity. On the other hand, formycin B is a competitive inhibitor with a K_i (100 μM) about three times the K_m of inosine (30 μM) (12,32). Good substrate activities with PNP are seen in 8-azaguanine (34) and the guanine analog of allopurinol (4-hydroxy-6-amino-pyrazolo[3,4-*d*]pyrimidine) (J. D. Stoeckler, R. E. Parks, Jr., and L. B. Townsend, unpublished results). From these and other observations, it appears unlikely that modifications of the carbon or nitrogen atoms of the purine ring will yield potent PNP inhibitors. On the other hand, analogs that are poor substrates for PNP may have chemotherapeutic activity in the form of the 2′-deoxyribonucleosides, by serving as substrates for deoxynucleoside kinases.

When considering substituents on the purine ring, N-1 and C-6 are best viewed as a single entity, since they function as a keto-enol tautomer. Recent evidence indicates that ionization of this tautomer does not markedly affect the ability of either the base or the nucleoside to bind to PNP (E. Chu, J. D. Stoeckler, and R. E. Parks, Jr., unpublished observations). This finding is in striking contrast to results with human erythrocytic hypoxanthine-guanine phosphoribosyltransferase (HGPRT), where ionization of this group abolishes the ability of the purine base to bind to the enzyme (35). With regard to binding to PNP, methylation of N-1 greatly reduces the affinity of hypoxanthine (36). An oxygen atom, which is required at C-6 for activity with natural substrates, may be replaced by a sulfur or selenium atom (e.g., as in 6-mercaptopurine and 6-selenoguanine). Substitution at C-6 by an amino group as in adenosine (37) or a methylthio group as in 6-methylthioinosine greatly decreases substrate activity.

The amino group on C-2 of guanine may be replaced by a hydrogen atom (e.g., as in hypoxanthine) but, if the amino group is methylated or hydroxylated, substrate activity is markedly decreased (J. D. Stoeckler, R. E. Parks, Jr., and L. B. Townsend, unpublished results). If this amino group is replaced by a hydroxyl (e.g., as in xanthosine) substrate activity is also greatly reduced.

The most promising inhibitors we have identified to date have a substituent on C-8. In the experiments in Table II, the spectrophotometric assays of PNP were performed with 30 μM guanosine (approximately the K_m concentration), with the prospective inhibitors also added at 30 μM. The analogues 8-aminoguanine (8-AG) and 8-aminoguanosine have been examined further (see Section II,D) and hopefully will serve as model compounds for the development of useful inhibitors in this series.

We have had the opportunity to examine the inhibitory activity of a series of

TABLE II

Inhibition of Guanosine Phosphorolysis by 8-Substituted Purine Analogs

Compound	Inhibition (%)	K_i (μM)
Guanine		5
8-Aminoguanine	95	1-2
8-Thioguanine	25	53
8-Iodoguanine	22	51
Hypoxanthine		17
8-Aminohypoxanthine	57	10
8-Amino-6-thiopurine	26	79

N-9-substituted analogues: 9-phenyl-, 9-benzyl-, 9-(*p*-chlorobenzyl)-, 9-(2-naphthyl)-, 9-cyclohexyl-, 9-methyl-, 9-ethyl-, and 9-propyl-substituted guanines. With most of these compounds no inhibition was detected when tested against equimolar concentrations of guanosine (30 μM). Several compounds [9-phenylguanine, 9-benzylguanine, and 9-(2-naphthyl)guanine] were mildly inhibitory, i.e., on the order of 10–25%. In view of this weak inhibition, these compounds were not studied further. In the above test system, 9-butyl-6-thioguanine does not inhibit PNP.

D. Studies with the PNP Inhibitor 8-Aminoguanine

During the past year, 8-AG and 8-aminoguanosine have been subjected to detailed kinetic analyses with PNP and have been tested as substrates for enzymes such as HGPRT, guanase, and xanthine oxidase. No activity was seen for 8-AG with the latter three enzymes. On the other hand, as seen in Table III, 8-AG displays reasonably good inhibitory activity against PNP and also serves as a substrate. It should be noted that the K_i (1–2 μM) of 8-AG is about 50-fold lower than that of formycin B (100 μM), to our knowledge the most potent PNP inhibitor described previously (32), and 5-fold lower than that of 5′-chloro-5′-deoxyformycin B. Reasonably good inhibitory activity has also been observed with 8-aminoguanosine (Table III), and future efforts will be directed toward the synthesis of 5′-substituted derivatives of this analogue with the purpose of generating a potent inhibitor that has negligible substrate activity. However, 8-aminoguanosine itself could be an agent of some interest because it may have favorable solubility properties and may also be transported selectively into cells via nucleoside transport systems. Furthermore, if cleaved intracellularly by PNP, it would generate 8-AG, a good PNP inhibitor that should be incapable of further metabolism by enzymes such as HGPRT and guanase. The details of these studies will be documented elsewhere.

We have not yet had the opportunity to perform extensive chemotherapeutic studies with 8-AG and plan to devote considerable attention to this area in the immediate future. Results to date, however, have been very promising. For

TABLE III

Kinetic Parameters of 8-Aminoguanine and 8-Aminoguanosine

Compound	K_i (μM)	K_m (μM)	V_{max} (%)
8-Aminoguanine	1-2	11	16 (relative to guanine)
8-Aminoguanosine	17	7	12 (relative to guanosine)

example, when Sarcoma 180 cells were incubated with 100 μM guanosine and then examined by HPLC for both guanosine disappearance and guanine nucleotide production, within 15 minutes all added guanosine had disappeared and had been converted stoichiometrically to intracellular guanine nucleotides. When the same experiment was performed in the presence of 100 μM 8-AG, both the disappearance of guanosine and the formation of guanine nucleotides were markedly inhibited. Experiments planned with 8-AG in the immediate future will include attempts to inhibit the blastogenesis of lymphocytes and to potentiate the cytotoxicity of analogs such as β-2′-deoxythioguanosine.

III. Methylthioadenosine Phosphorylase

A. Introduction

A question that has long puzzled purine biochemists is the source of free adenine in animal tissues. The salvage enzyme APRT is found at relatively high activity in most cells, and its kinetic characteristics [i.e., a K_m for adenine of less than 1μM (38)] seem designed to prevent accumulation of free adenine, which upon reaction with xanthine oxidase forms 2,8-dihydroxyadenine, a highly insoluble analog of uric acid (39). This compound, if produced in substantial quantities, can crystallize in the renal tubules and result in fatal anuria (40). Thus the presence of APRT at relatively high activity in erythrocytes may serve to scavenge adenine that escapes from the tissues into the blood. Both APRT and PNP have been regarded as possible sources of free adenine. No evidence has been uncovered, however, for reversal of the APRT reaction under physiological conditions. Also, although PNP can react with adenosine, the kinetics are so unfavorable that it is unlikely that this reaction plays a significant role in mammalian tissues (37).

The first evidence of a mechanism for liberating free adenine in mammals was reported in 1969 when Pegg and Williams-Ashman (41) discovered an enzyme in rat ventral prostate that catalyzed the phosphate-dependent cleavage of free adenine from MTA, a by-product of the biosynthesis of spermine and spermidine from putrescine and SAM. The presence of this enzyme, now referred to as methylthioadenosine phosphorylase (MTA-Pase), in other mammalian tissues including tumors, has been established only within the past 1 or 2 years (42–46). The PNP and MTA-Pase reactions are analogous. Both are reversible and, when reacting with nucleosides, generate a purine base and a pentose 1-phosphate (Fig. 3).

B. Explanation of the Metabolic Effects of 5′-Deoxyadenosine

Recently, puzzling findings were reported by Hunting and Henderson (47) indicating that 5′-deoxyadenosine (5′-dAdo; Fig. 4) produces major metabolic

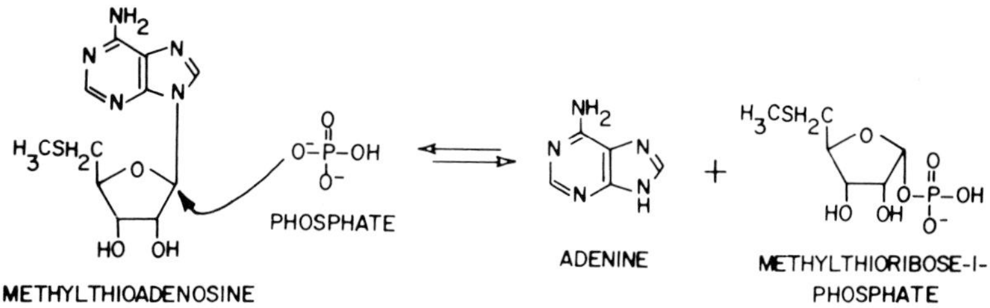

Fig. 3. Proposed reaction mechanism of MTA-Pase.

disturbances when incubated with Ehrlich ascites cells. They described profound decreases in intracellular levels of 5-phosphoribosyl 1-pyrophosphate (PRPP), inhibition of purine nucleotide biosynthesis *de novo,* and inhibition of glycolysis with a "crossover" at the phosphofructokinase reaction. Since 5′-dAdo cannot be converted directly to adenine 5′-nucleotides, it was proposed that this compound exerted its metabolic actions at the nucleoside level without prior conversion to nucleotides. It was not possible, however, to demonstrate direct effects of 5′-dAdo on PRPP synthetase or phosphofructokinase (47).

Our investigations of this problem originated with attempts to confirm the reports of Hunting and Henderson (47). When Sarcoma 180 ascites cells were incubated with 5′-dAdo, marked inhibition of PRPP synthesis was observed. In this system, 5′-dAdo is the most potent of many adenosine analogs examined to date. The nucleotide profiles of Fig. 5 (48) were obtained with Sarcoma 180 cells that had been incubated for 3 hours with 500 μM 5′-dAdo. In comparison with profiles from control cells, the levels of ATP and ADP were increased 2 to 3-fold in cells incubated with 5′-dAdo, with little effect on other nucleotides. This suggested that free adenine was cleaved from 5′-dAdo, with subsequent conversion to adenine nucleotides via reaction with APRT and the respective nucleotide kinases. Therefore several methods were employed to demonstrate the liberation of free adenine from 5′-dAdo in extracts of Sarcoma 180 cells. As shown in Fig. 6, when 5′-dAdo was incubated with high-speed supernatant fractions of Sarcoma 180 cells, the progressive formation of free adenine was readily demonstrated by reversed-phase HPLC. The identity of the new peak as

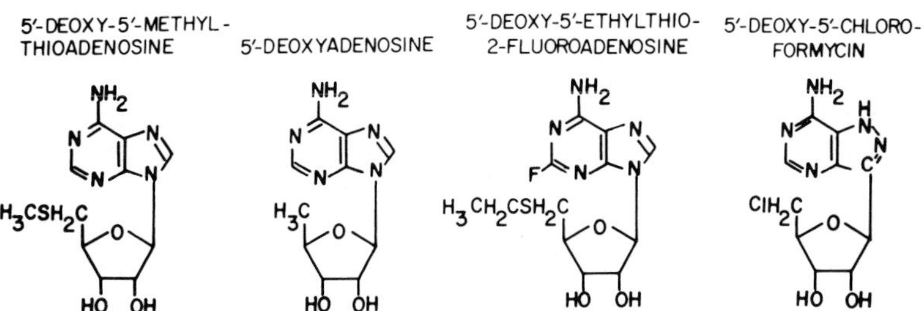

Fig. 4. Structures of some substrates and an inhibitor of MTA-Pase.

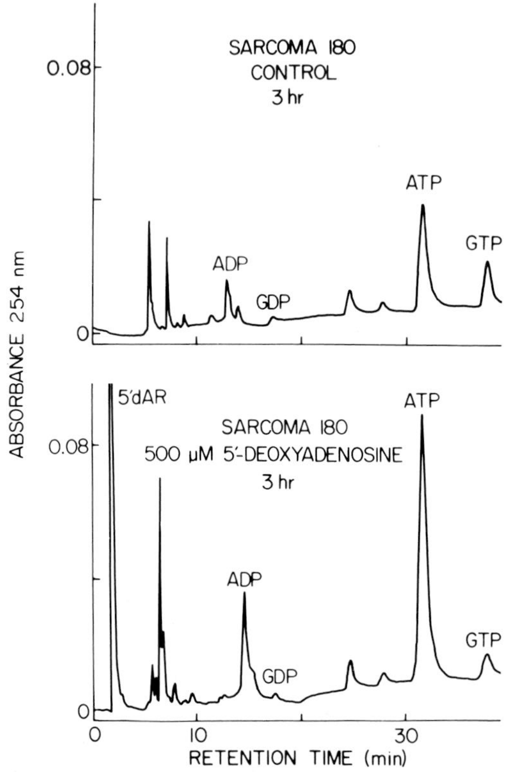

Fig. 5. Nucleotide profiles of Sarcoma 180 cells in the absence (upper) and presence (lower) of 500 μM 5′-dAdo after 3 hours of incubation. Cells were isolated from CD-1 mice bearing the ascites cell form of the tumor, washed, and suspended (3% final cell concentration) in a minimal salt medium consisting of 50 m*M* potassium phosphate, pH 7.4, 75 m*M* NaCl, 2 m*M* $MgSO_4$, and 10 m*M* dextrose to which was added 5′-dAdo. The suspensions were incubated in a shaking water bath (37°C), and aliquots were extracted with perchloric acid (final concentration 4%) at 4°C. After centrifugation, supernatant solutions were neutralized with 5 *N* KOH and frozen (−20°C) for HPLC analysis. Anion-exchange HPLC was carried out as previously described (48). Peaks were identified and quantitated by comparison with the chromatographic behavior of authentic nucleotides.

adenine was established by comparing its retention time with that of authentic adenine, by its UV spectral characteristics (λ_{max} at 260 nm), by its reaction with xanthine oxidase resulting in the formation of 2,8-dihydroxyadenine (λ_{max} at 305 nm), and by its reaction with endogenous APRT in the presence of excess PRPP to yield 5′-AMP as detected by anion-exchange HPLC. No adenine was formed in the absence of the tissue extract.

These observations explain the metabolic effects of 5′-dAdo reported previously (47). Specifically, the increased consumption of PRPP through its reac-

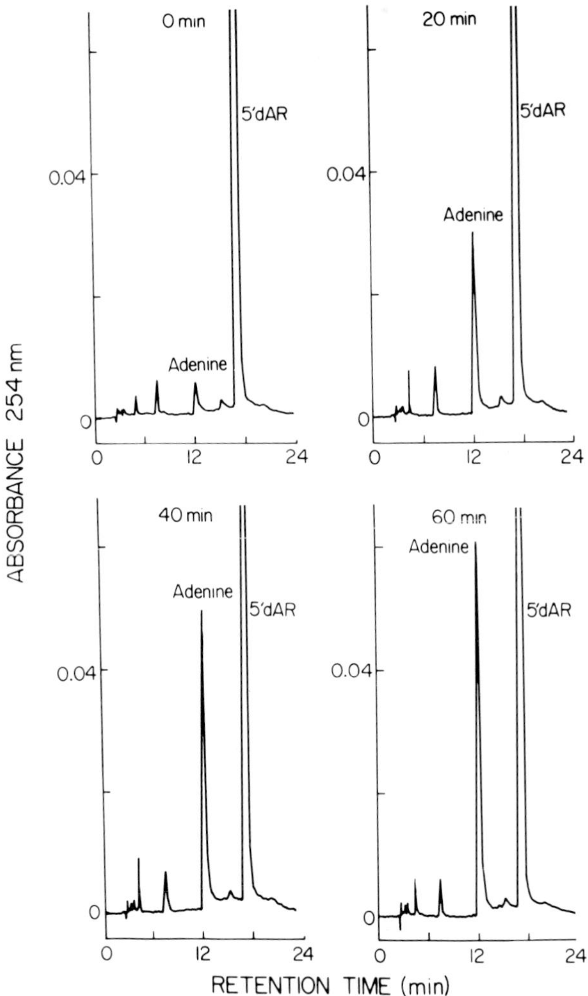

Fig. 6. Time-dependent formation of adenine from 5′-dAdo in the presence of Sarcoma 180 extracts. A reaction mixture (1.3 ml) containing 800 μM 5′-dAdo, 20 mM potassium phosphate, pH 7.4, and 105,000 g supernatant fractions of Sarcoma 180 homogenates (1.2 mg protein) was incubated in a shaking water bath (37°C). At appropriate times, aliquots were deproteinized with perchloric acid (4% final concentration) at 4°C. Following centrifugation, the supernatant fluids were neutralized to pH 6.5–7.5 with 5 N KOH and frozen (−20°C). The samples were chromatographed on a Varian 4200 high-pressure liquid chromatograph under the following conditions. Column: Waters μBondapak C_{18} (4.5 mm × 30 cm); low-concentrate eluent (eluent A): 0.01 M potassium phosphate, pH 5.5; high-concentrate eluent (eluent B): 20% methanol in eluent A (v/v); gradient: linear increase of eluent B from 0 to 100% at a rate of 9%/minute; flow rate: 1.0 ml/minute. The adenine peak was identified using criteria outlined in the text.

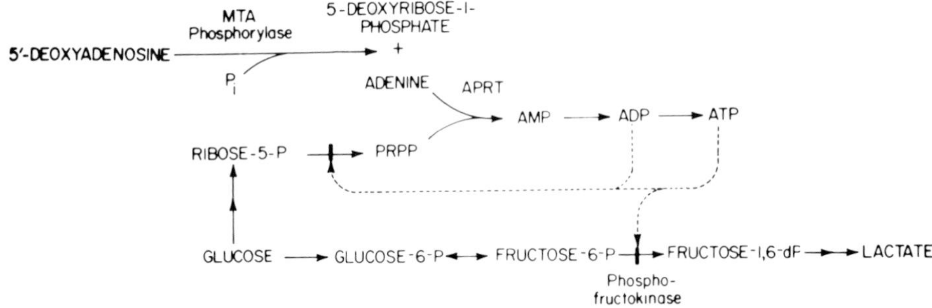

Fig. 7. Proposed mechanism of the metabolic alterations produced by 5′-dAdo. Inhibitory effects are represented by dotted lines.

tion with adenine in the APRT reaction would deplete the steady-state levels of this compound, while increased levels of ADP (49) and ATP (50) would block PRPP synthesis through inhibition of PRPP synthetase. This combined effect of increased consumption and decreased synthesis would result in marked decreases in PRPP availability, which in turn would lead to inhibition of purine nucleotide biosynthesis *de novo*. Also, the inhibition of glycolysis is readily explained by the well-established block of the phosphofructokinase reaction by ATP (51,52). These interrelationships are illustrated in Fig. 7.

C. The Identity of 5′-Deoxyadenosine Cleaving Activity with Methythioadenosine Phosphorylase

To establish the identity of the enzyme responsible for 5′-dAdo cleavage, various possibilities were examined. First, 5′-dAdo has very weak but definite activity with adenosine deaminase, forming 5′-deoxyinosine, an excellent substrate for purine nucleoside phosphorylase (see above). However, no substrate activity with PNP was detected with 5′-dAdo. While mycoplasma-infected cells are known to have adenosine phosphorylase activity (53), the Sarcoma 180 cells were known to be free of this infection. In view of the earlier observations of Pegg and Williams-Ashman (41), we wondered whether MTA-Pase was present in Sarcoma 180 cells and, if so, whether it could react with 5′-dAdo. Therefore experiments were performed with MTA to evaluate this question.

The liberation of free adenine from MTA by extracts from Sarcoma 180 cells was demonstrated by reversed-phase HPLC and the enzymatic procedures noted above for studies with 5′-dAdo. A spectrophotometric assay for MTA-Pase was developed that is a modification of the procedure of Pegg and Williams- Ashman (41). The adenine liberated from MTA is measured dynamically by coupling MTA-Pase to the xanthine oxidase reaction which converts adenine to 2,8-dihydroxyadenine (λ_{max} 305 nm, $\Delta \epsilon$ 15.5 × 10^3). This assay has been employed routinely in continuing studies of MTA-Pase and will be described in detail elsewhere.

The identity of the MTA-cleaving activity of Sarcoma 180 cells as a phosphorylase was established by phosphate dependency studies as shown in Fig. 8. No reaction was detected in the absence of phosphate, but phosphate could be partially replaced by arsenate. The K_m of phosphate determined from Lineweaver–Burk plots is about 3.5 m*M*. In order to demonstrate reversibility of the reaction, an aliquot of 5′-dAdo was converted to 5′-deoxyinosine by reaction with calf intestinal ADA. Upon reaction with highly purified PNP, 5-deoxyribose 1-phosphate was produced and purified (12). When this sugar phosphate was incubated with partially purified Sarcoma 180 MTA-Pase with an excess of adenine in 10 m*M* HEPES buffer, pH 7.4, the time-dependent formation of 5′-dAdo was readily demonstrated by reversed-phase HPLC (Fig. 9).

Following this demonstration that MTA-Pase occurred in Sarcoma 180 cells, several additional pieces of evidence were uncovered that established that this enzyme was responsible for the cleavage of adenine from 5′-dAdo. When

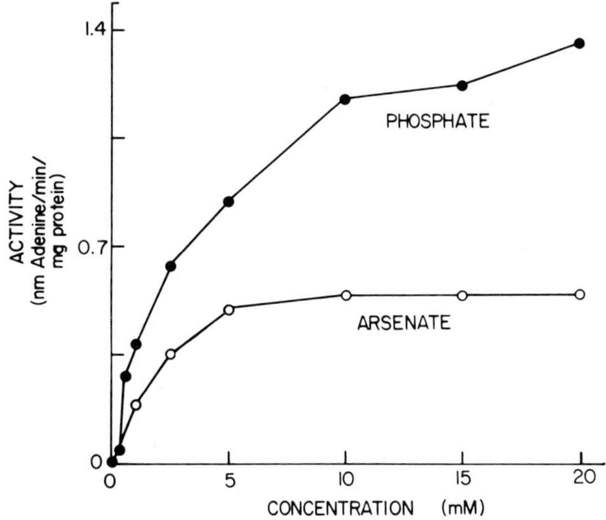

Fig. 8. The dependency of MTA-Pase from Sarcoma 180 cells on the phosphate and arsenate concentration. The activity of MTA-Pase was determined using a coupled xanthine oxidase assay (41) on a Gilford recording spectrophotometer at 305 nm and 37°C. Each reaction mixture (1 ml) contained 20 m*M* HEPES, pH 7.4, 200 μ*M* MTA, 0.8 unit xanthine oxidase (Grade III, Sigma Chemical Company), partially purified enzyme preparation (340 μg protein), and appropriate concentrations of either potassium phosphate or sodium arsenate. The MTA-Pase from Sarcoma 180 cells was partially purified as described previously (46) and dialyzed against several changes of a solution consisting of 10 m*M* HEPES, pH 7.2, 1 m*M* dithiothreitol, 50 m*M* KCl, and 1 m*M* EDTA (3 hours) prior to assay.

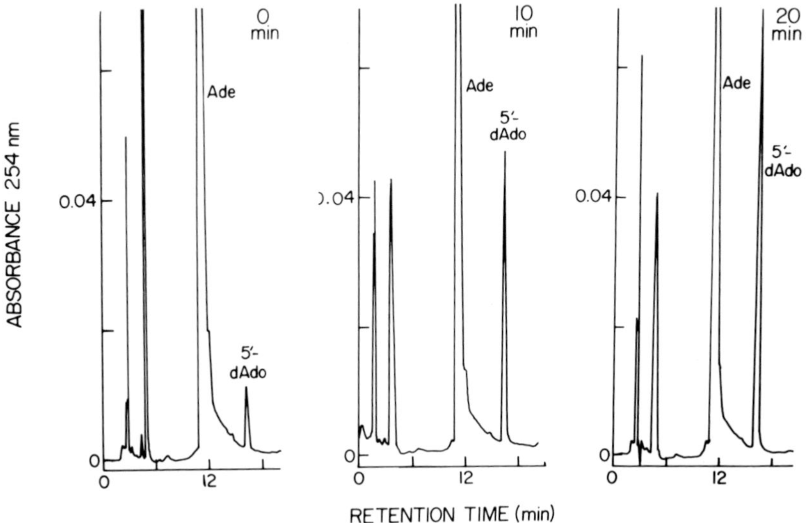

Fig. 9. Reversed-phase HPLC profiles demonstrating the time-dependent formation of 5′-dAdo from adenine and 5-deoxyribose 1-phosphate in the presence of MTA-Pase partially purified from Sarcoma 180 cells. A reaction mixture (2 ml) containing 475 μM adenine, 250 μM 5-deoxyribose 1-phosphate, 12.5 mM HEPES, pH 7.3, and partially purified MTA-Pase prepared from Sarcoma 180 cells (2.15 mg protein) was incubated at 37°C in a shaking water bath. Samples were prepared for reversed-phase HPLC and chromatographed as described in Fig. 6. The 5′-dAdo peak was identified using authentic 5′-dAdo as a standard.

saturating concentrations of MTA and 5′-dAdo were incubated with MTA-Pase, reaction velocities were determined that were intermediate between the V_{max} values with either substrate. If a different enzyme for each substrate had been present, one would have observed additive velocities. With the use of alternative substrate kinetic methodology (54), Lineweaver–Burk plots were obtained that were characteristic of competing alternative substrates with different V_{max} values. When partially purified extracts from Sarcoma 180 cells were subjected to molecular sieving on Sephadex G-100 columns, complete separation of MTA-Pase and PNP activities was accomplished. Furthermore, the ratios of reactivity with MTA and 5′-dAdo were constant throughout the peak of MTA activity. Other points supporting this conclusion are the identical K_m values for phosphate determined with both substrates and the fact that the same K_i value was found for the inhibitor 5′-chloroformycin (see Section III,D) when determined with both substrates.

D. Substrate Specificity of Methylthioadenosine Phosphorylase

Because we have studied MTA-Pase for less than 1 year and have had limited access to all appropriate analogues, it is not yet possible to present a complete evaluation of structure–activity relationships. However, a number of important points, especially in relation to the sugar moiety, have emerged. Table IV presents the kinetic constants of a number of analogues examined to date. The only aglycone-modified structures studied have been 5′-deoxy-5′-ethylthio-2-fluoroadenosine and 5′-chloroformycin, which are a good substrate and a potent inhibitor, respectively. Each of these compounds may have chemotherapeutic potential.

Adenosine itself can react with good velocity (V_{max} 115%) but binds poorly (K_m 1400 μM), i.e., 350-fold more weakly than MTA. The low but definite affinity of adenosine for MTA-Pase explains the earlier report of an adenosine phosphorylase in Sarcoma 180 cells (55). The fact that 5′-deoxy-5′-methylthioarabinosyladenine, 2′-deoxyadenosine, arabinosyladenine, 3′-deoxyadenosine, and xylosyladenine are not substrates for MTA-Pase indicates the importance of cis hydroxyls on C-2′ and C-3′. On the other hand, substantial modifications are possible at C-5′. Good substrate activity is found if the methylthio group is replaced by adducts ranging from a hydrogen atom to a 2° isobutyl-

TABLE IV

Kinetic Constants of Methyladenosine Phosphorylase Partially Purified from Sarcoma 180 Cells for 5′-Methyladenosine, 5′-Deoxyadenosine, Adenosine, and a Number of Their Derivatives[a]

Compound	K_m (μM)	Relative V_{max}
5′-Deoxy-5′-methylthio-adenosine	4	100
5′-Deoxyadenosine	23	180
5′-Deoxy-5′-s-isobutyl-adenosine	8	89
5′-Deoxy-5′-ethylthio-2-fluoradenosine[b]	20	73
5′-Chloro-5′-deoxyadenosine	21	46
5′-Bromo-5′-deoxyadenosine	8	38
5′-Deoxy-5′-iodoadenosine	10	25
adenosine[c]	1417	115
2′-Deoxyadenosine	N.A.	N.A.
3′-Deoxyadenosine	N.A.	N.A.
Arabinosyladenine	N.A.	N.A.
5′-Deoxy-5′-methylthioarabino-syladenine	N.A.	
Xylosyladenine	N.A.	N.A.

[a] Enzyme purification and kinetic studies performed as previously described (46). N.A., No activity at a substrate concentration of 1000 μM or greater.

[b] Values determined by following the formation of 2-fluoroadenine by reversed-phase HPLC (unpublished methods).

[c] Determined using a MTA-Pase preparation in which PNP activity had been removed by gel filtration chromatography (Sephadex G-100, unpublished method).

thio group. Interestingly, halogenation of C-5′ is acceptable, since replacement with a bulky iodine atom permits reasonably good substrate activity. The reaction of these compounds should result in formation of the respective halogenated sugar phosphates (e.g., 5-iodoribose 1-phosphate). The possible metabolic consequences of intracellular accumulation of such analogue sugar phosphates will be considered below.

E. Speculations on Methylthioadenosine Phosphorylase as a Chemotherapeutic Target Enzyme

Although MTA-Pase has attracted investigative attention only recently, it is apparent that it must play a crucial role in the salvage of adenine from MTA formed during the synthesis of polyamines. As illustrated in Fig. 10, the synthesis of 1 mole of spermidine requires 1 mole of SAM and results in the formation of 1 mole of MTA, and the synthesis of spermine requires 2 moles of SAM and results in the formation of 2 moles of MTA. Since SAM is synthesized from ATP, the absence of a mechanism for salvaging adenine from MTA would

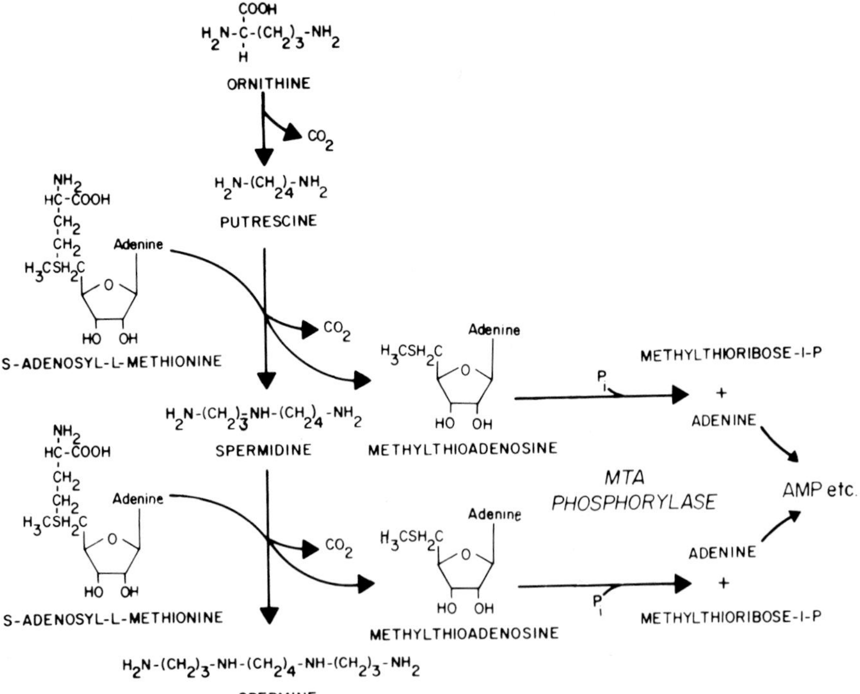

Fig. 10. The role of MTA-Pase in the salvage of adenine moieties from SAM during polyamine biosynthesis.

result in the depletion of adenine nucleotide pools during polyamine biosynthesis. Polyamine production is greatly accelerated by a variety of biological stimuli associated with cellular replication (e.g., hepatectomy, lymphocytic blastogenesis, and stimulation of breast tissue by prolactin) and increases greatly during late G_1 and early S phase of the cell cycle (56). Enzymes of polyamine synthesis, such as ornithine decarboxylase and SAM decarboxylase, are induced rapidly by such events, and furthermore have unusually short half-lives (for recent reviews, see 10, 57, 58). Although the precise biological functions of polyamines are not yet understood, it is clear that there is a relationship between polyamines and cell division (59).

A number of intriguing questions related to MTA-Pase may be asked, all of which have important implications for chemotherapy. One wonders, for example, whether the activity of MTA-Pase modulates in conjunction with that of ornithine decarboxylase and whether it is highest in cells undergoing rapid division or responding to growth stimulation. An indication that this occurs is the 2- to 20-fold higher MTA-Pase activity found in various tumor tissues of human and murine origin in comparison with normal tissues (unpublished data, this laboratory). Also, it has been reported that the activity of MTA-Pase doubles during blastogenesis of lymphocytes (60). If this enzyme increases in activity in specific phases of the cell cycle, it might provide a specific chemotherapeutic target in tissues with high-growth fractions. Several approaches could be considered. First, it may be possible to design analogs of MTA in which the adenine portion of the nucleoside is replaced by an adenine analogue, such as 2-fluoroadenine, 8-azaadenine, 4-aminopyrazolo[3,4-*d*]pyrimidine, and 2,6-diaminopurine, that may have substrate activity for MTA-Pase. Such analogues, upon reaction with intracellular MTA-Pase, would liberate adenine analogues which in turn would be converted to cytotoxic nucleotides by reaction with APRT and other enzymes of adenine nucleotide formation. The synthesis of cytotoxic analog adenine nucleotides might occur in cells that are in the cell cycle, including the proliferating portion of a tumor cell population. Cells not in cycle, like those present in most tissues with low-growth fractions, might have lower MTA-Pase activity and therefore synthesize little or no analog nucleotides from MTA analogs.

In order to test one of these concepts we have performed preliminary studies with 5′-deoxy-5′-ethylthio-2-fluoroadenosine (5′-ETFAR; provided by John Montgomery), an MTA analog that is highly cytotoxic to H.Ep.2 cells (61). As shown in Fig. 11, when 3% suspensions of Sarcoma 180 cells were incubated with 5′-ETFAR (500 μM), a sizable peak corresponding to 2-fluoroadenosine 5′-triphosphate (FATP) appeared in nucleotide profiles. In contrast, when the same concentration of 5′-ETFAR was incubated with 3% suspensions of human erythrocytes (a cell with little or no MTA-Pase activity), only trace amounts of FATP were detected. These studies indicate that this class of MTA analogs has

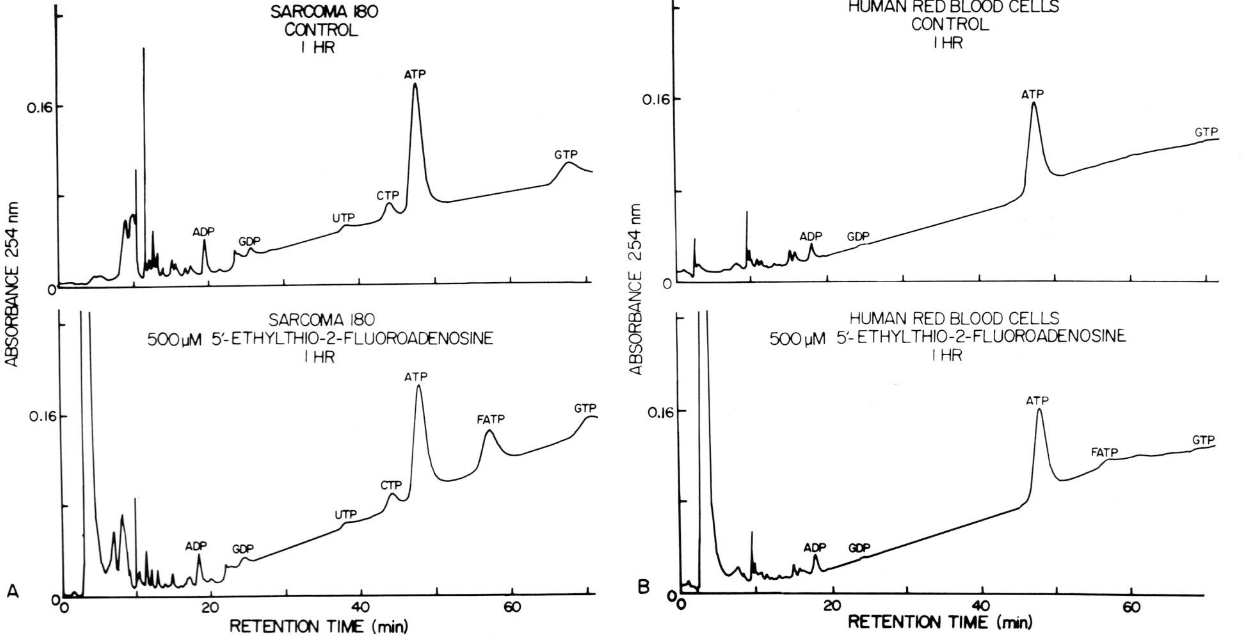

Fig. 11. Anion-exchange HPLC nucleotide profiles demonstrating the incorporation of 5′-ETFAR into 2-fluoroadenine nucleotides in Sarcoma 180 cells (A) and human erythrocytes (B). Sarcoma 180 cell preparation and incubation were performed in the same manner as described in Fig. 5. Human erythrocytes were obtained in a heparinized syringe from a normal, healthy donor, the white cell layer removed by centrifugation, and cells suspended (3% final cell concentration) in the minimal salt medium described in Fig. 5 to which 5′-ETFAR (500 μM final concentration) had been added. Incubation of these erythrocyte suspensions was identical to that described for the Sarcoma 180 cells. Nucleotide analysis by anion-exchange HPLC was performed using the method of Crabtree *et al.* (48), except that low- and high-concentrate eluting buffers of pH 3.5 instead of pH 4.5 were employed. The identity of the peak corresponding to FATP was based on the chromatographic behavior of previously prepared FATP (unpublished method).

the potential for interacting specifically with MTA-Pase-containing cells and, in addition, that these compounds would not be degraded in the bloodstream in transit to the target tissue.

In addition to base-modified analogs of MTA, substrates containing modifications in the sugar moiety (e.g., 5′-deoxy-5′-iodoadenosine) would, upon reaction with MTA-Pase, generate substantial quantities of C-5-substituted ribose 1-phosphates (e.g., 5-iodoribose 1-phosphate) which could have adverse effects on various metabolic reactions. Preliminary evidence indicates that rabbit muscle phosphoglucomutase is inhibited by 5-deoxyribose 1-phosphate (K_i 75 μM; E. Chu and R. E. Parks, Jr., unpublished data). Although information is now emerging on the metabolic disposition of MTA, little is known about the metabolism of 5-methylthioribose 1-phosphate. In a report of an enzyme that splits the methylthio group from 5-methylthioribose 1-phosphate, it has been postulated that the methylthio group is required for cell growth (45). Because MTA and 5-methylthioribose 1-phosphate are derived from the essential amino acid methionine (one of the limiting amino acids in most diets), one must assume that animal tissues have evolved an efficient mechanism for salvaging the methylthio group. This is an obvious area for future study. One wonders, for example, whether intracellular production of analogues of 5-methylthioribose 1-phosphate, (e.g., 5-iodoribose 1-phosphate) would interfere with this postulated mechanism.

Another area of study is the blockade of MTA-Pase by an inhibitor such as 5′-chloroformycin. This could produce various adverse metabolic events including accumulation of MTA, which could inhibit SAM metabolism, and depletion of intracellular adenine nucleotide pools by preventing the salvage of adenine from MTA. It may be that such effects could cause profound metabolic disturbances and cellular death.

These speculations are under investigation in our laboratory. Information on the distribution and modulation of MTA-Pase in normal and malignant human tissues is of crucial importance. Since MTA-Pase activity is high in human prostate (43), the approaches discussed above may find application in prostatic diseases such as hypertrophy and neoplasia.

Certain of these concepts may apply to other areas of chemotherapy. For example, 5′-*S*-isobutyladenosine is active against *Plasmodium falciparum* in culture (62). In this experimental system, the malarial parasite grows in human erythrocytes, cells that have negligible MTA-Pase activity. It would be of interest to see whether *Plasmodium*-infected cells have MTA-Pase and thus are responsive to the type of agent discussed above. Another intriguing observation is a report of elevated levels of ornithine decarboxylase in animal cells infected with vaccinia virus (63). Perhaps these cells also have elevated levels of MTA-Pase and thus will suffer damage if exposed to MTA analogues.

Acknowledgments

The authors are grateful to Drs. L. B. Townsend of the University of Michigan, R. P. Panzica of the University of Rhode Island, J. A. Montgomery and L. L. Bennett, Jr., of the Southern Research Institute, M. Ikehara of Osaka University, Dr. Cory of the University of South Florida, and F. White and other members of the Drug Synthesis and Chemistry Branch, Division of Cancer Treatment, National Cancer Institute, for providing many of the compounds used in these studies. We are also indebted to Ms. A. Shiragian and Ms. V. Kuhns for their excellent technical assistance.

This work was supported by the following grants: ACS CH-7S and CH-7T from the American Cancer Society; CA-07340, CA-20892, and CA-13943 from the U.S. Public Health Service; and a 1979 Predoctoral Fellowship from the Pharmaceutical Manufacturers Association.

References

1. G. B. Elion, S. W. Callahan, R. W. Rundles, and G. H. Hitchings, *Cancer Res.* **23,** 1207 (1963).
2. E. R. Giblett, J. E. Anderson, F. Cohen, B. Pollara, and H. J. Meuwissen, *Lancet* **2,** 1067 (1972).
3. E. R. Giblett, A. J. Ammann, R. Sandman, D. W. Wara, and L. K. Diamond, *Lancet* **1,** 1010 (1975).
4. L. H. Siegenbeek van Heukelom, G. E. J. Staal, J. W. Stoop, and B. J. M. Zegers, *Clin. Chim. Acta* **72,** 117 (1976).
5. W. R. A. Osborne, S.-H. Chen, E. R. Giblett, W. D. Biggar, A. J. Ammann, and C. R. Scott, *J. Clin. Invest.* **60,** 741 (1977).
6. J.-L. Virelizier, M. Hamet, J.-J. Ballet, P. Reinert, and C. Griscelli, *J. Pediatr.* **92,** 358 (1978).
7. J. F. Smyth, M. M. Chassin, K. R. Harrap, R. H. Adamson, and D. G. Johns, *Proc. Am. Assoc. Cancer Res.* **20,** 47 (1979).
8. M. Borgers, H. Verhaegen, M. DeBrabander, F. Thone, J. Van Reempts, and G. Geuens, *J. Immunol. Methods* **16,** 101 (1977).
9. R. E. Parks, Jr., G. W. Crabtree, C. M. Kong, R. P. Agarwal, K. C. Agarwal, and E. M. Scholar, *Ann. N.Y. Acad. Sci.* **255,** 412 (1975).
10. H. G. Williams-Ashman, *in* "Biochemical Regulatory Mechanisms in Eukaroytic Cells" (E. Kun and S. Grisolia, eds.), p. 245. Wiley, New York, 1972.
11. R. E. Parks, Jr., K. C. Agarwal, R. P. Agarwal, G. W. Crabtree, T. Rogler-Brown, T. M. Savarese, and J. D. Stoeckler, *in* "Nucleosides, Nucleotides and Their Biological Applications" (J.-L. Barascut and J.-L. Imbach, eds.), Vol. 81, p. 209. INSERM, Paris, France, 1978.
12. J. D. Stoeckler, C. Cambor, and R. E. Parks, Jr., *Biochemistry* 19, 102 (1980).
13. H. M. Kalckar, *J. Biol. Chem.* **158,** 723 (1945).
14. M. Friedkin and H. M. Kalckar, *in* "The Enyzmes" (P. D. Boyer, H. Lardy, and K. Myrbäck, eds.), 2nd rev. ed., Vol. 5, p. 237. Academic Press, New York, 1961.
15. R. E. Parks, Jr. and R. P. Agarwal, *in* "The Enzymes" (P. D. Boyer, ed.), 3rd ed., Vol. 7, p. 483. Academic Press, New York, 1972.
16. B. K. Kim, S. Cha, and R. E. Parks, Jr., *J. Biol. Chem.* **243,** 1763 (1968).
17. R. P. Agarwal and R. E. Parks, Jr., *J. Biol. Chem.* **244,** 644 (1969).
18. R. P. Agarwal, K. C. Agarwal, and R. E. Parks, Jr., *in* "Methods in Enzymology" (P. A. Hoffee and M. E. Jones, eds.), Vol. 51, p. 581. Academic Press, New York, 1978.
19. J. D. Stoeckler, R. P. Agarwal, and R. E. Parks, Jr., *in* "Methods in Enzymology" (P. A. Hoffee and M. E. Jones, eds.), Vol. 51, p. 530. Academic Press, New York, 1978.

20. J. D. Stoeckler, R. P. Agarwal, K. C. Agarwal, K. Schmid, and R. E. Parks, Jr., *Biochemistry* **17,** 278 (1978).
21. V. Zannis, D. Doyle, and D. W. Martin, Jr., *J. Biol. Chem.* **253,** 504 (1978).
22. B. M. Turner, R. A. Fisher, and H. Harris, *Eur. J. Biochem.* **24,** 288 (1971).
23. K. C. Agarwal, R. P. Agarwal, J. D. Stoeckler, and R. E. Parks, Jr., *Biochemistry* **14,** 79 (1975).
24. K. Murakami and K. Tsushima, *Biochim. Biophys. Acta* **453,** 205 (1976).
25. A. S. Lewis and M. D. Glantz, *Biochemistry* **15,** 4451 (1976).
26. A. S. Lewis and M. D. Glantz, *J. Biol. Chem.* **251,** 407 (1976).
27. B. K. Kim, S. Cha, and R. E. Parks, Jr., *J. Biol. Chem.* **243,** 1771 (1968).
28. L. J. Gudas, B. Ullman, A. Cohen, and D. W. Martin, Jr., *Cell* **14,** 531 (1978).
29. A. Cohen, L. J. Gudas, A. J. Amman, G. E. J. Staal, and D. W. Martin, Jr., *J. Clin. Invest.* **61,** 1405 (1978).
30. A. R. P. Paterson and J. M. Oliver, *Can. J. Biochem.* **49,** 271 (1971).
31. A. Cohen, D. Doyle, D. W. Martin, Jr., and A. J. Ammann, *N. Engl. J. Med.* **295,** 1449 (1976).
32. M. R. Sheen, B. K. Kim, and R. E. Parks, Jr., *Mol. Pharmacol.* **4,** 293 (1968).
33. L. B. Townsend, B. L. Cline, R. P. Panzica, P. E. Fagerness, L. W. Roti Roti, J. D. Stoeckler, G. W. Crabtree, and R. E. Parks, Jr., *Heterocycl. Chem. Ser.* **3,** S-79 (1978).
34. M. Friedkin, *J. Biol. Chem.* **209,** 295 (1954).
35. C. M. Kong and R. E. Parks, Jr., *Mol. Pharmacol.* **10,** 648 (1974).
36. T. A. Krenitsky, G. B. Elion, A. M. Henderson, and G. H. Hitchings, *J. Biol. Chem.* **243,** 2876 (1968).
37. T. P. Zimmerman, N. Gersten, A. F. Ross, and R. P. Miech, *Can. J. Biochem.* **49,** 1050 (1971).
38. M. Hori and J. F. Henderson, *J. Biol. Chem.* **241,** 3404 (1966).
39. H. Klenow, *Biochem. J.* **50,** 404 (1952).
40. A. Bendich, G. B. Brown, F. S. Philips, and J. B. Thiersch, *J. Biol. Chem.* **183,** 367 (1950).
41. A. E. Pegg and H. G. Williams-Ashman, *Biochem. J.* **115,** 241 (1969).
42. V. Zappia, A. Oliva, G. Cacciapuoti, P. Galletti, G. Mignucci, and M. Carteni-Farina, *Biochem. J.* **15,** 1043 (1978).
43. G. Cacciapuoti, A. Oliva, and V. Zappia, *Int. J. Biochem.* **9,** 35 (1978).
44. D. L. Garbers, *Biochim. Biophys. Acta* **523,** 82 (1978).
45. J. I. Toohey, *Biochem. Biophys. Res. Commun.* **83,** 27 (1978).
46. T. M. Savarese, G. W. Crabtree, and R. E. Parks, Jr., *Biochem. Pharmacol.* **28,** 2227 (1979).
47. D. Hunting and J. F. Henderson, *Biochem. Pharmacol.* **27,** 2163 (1978).
48. G. W. Crabtree, R. P. Agarwal, R. E. Parks, Jr., A. F. Lewis, L. L. Wotring, and L. B. Townsend, *Biochem. Pharmacol.* **28,** 1491 (1979).
49. L. C. Yip, S. Roome, and M. E. Balis, *Biochemistry* **17,** 3286 (1978).
50. A. S. Bagnara, A. A. Letter, and J. F. Henderson, *Biochim. Biophys. Acta* **438,** 259 (1974).
51. H. A. Lardy and R. E. Parks, Jr., *in* "Enzymes: Units of Biological Structure and Function" (O. H. Gaebler, ed.), p. 584. Academic Press, New York, 1956.
52. A. Ramaiah, *Curr. Top. Cell. Regul.* **8,** 297 (1974).
53. M. Hatanaka, R. Del Giudice, and C. W. Long, *Proc. Natl. Acad. Sci. U.S.A.* **72,** 1401 (1975).
54. S. Cha, *Mol. Pharmacol.* **4,** 621 (1968).
55. A. Y. Divekar, *Biochim. Biophys. Acta* **422,** 15 (1976).
56. C. W. Tabor and H. Tabor, *Annu. Rev. Biochem.* **45,** 285 (1976).
57. H. G. Williams-Ashman and Z. N. Canellakis, *Perspect. Biol. Med.* **22,** 421 (1979).
58. D. H. Russell, ed., "Polyamines in Normal and Neoplastic Growth." Raven, New York, 1973.

59. D. H. Russell, *in* "Polyamines in Normal and Neoplastic Growth" (D. H. Russell, ed.), p. 1. Raven, New York, 1973.
60. A. J. Ferro, *in* "Transmethylation" (E. Usdin, R. Borchardt, and C. Creveling, eds.), p. 117. Am. Elsevier, New York, 1979.
61. J. A. Montgomery, A. T. Shortnacy, and H. J. Thomas, *J. Med. Chem.* **17,** 1197 (1974).
62. W. Trager, M. Robert-Gero, and E. Lederer, *FEBS Lett.* **85,** 246 (1978).
63. J. Hodgson and J. D. Williamson, *Biochem. Biophys. Res. Commun.* **63,** 308 (1975).

12

In Vitro and *in Vivo* Effects of 5′-Thioadenosine Nucleosides

JAMES K. COWARD

I. Biosynthesis and Utilization of *S*-Adenosylmethionine

In nearly all biochemical reactions involving the transfer of intact alkyl groups, the nucleoside amino acids *S*-adenosylmethionine (SAM) (4) and its decarboxylated derivative (DSAM) (7) are the requisite alkyl donors. Only in the methylation of homocysteine (6) to form methionine (3) is another alkyl donor, 5-methyltetrahydrofolate or betaine, utilized. The methionine thus synthesized is converted to SAM as a result of nucleophilic attack by the sulfur atom of methionine on the 5′-methylene carbon of ATP. Then SAM either is employed directly as the methyl donor in a wide variety of enzyme-catalyzed methylation reactions or is first decarboxylated to DSAM which serves as a source of aminopropyl groups in the biosynthesis of the polyamines spermidine and spermine (1). The nucleoside products of enzyme-catalyzed methyl transfer and aminopropyl transfer are *S*-adenosylhomocysteine (SAH) (5) and 5′-deoxy-5′-methylthioadenosine (MTA) (9), respectively. As discussed later, both SAH and MTA are potent product inhibitors of the respective group transfer reactions. Cellular levels of these nucleosides are controlled by further metabolism; SAH is

MOLECULAR ACTIONS AND TARGETS FOR CANCER CHEMOTHERAPEUTIC AGENTS

ISBN 0-12-619280-4

hydrolyzed at the 5′-thioether bond to adenosine (1) and homocysteine (6), whereas MTA is cleaved at the purine–ribose bond to adenine (11) and 5-deoxy-5-methylthioribose (MTR) (12). These biochemical reactions are summarized in Fig. 1. In this brief chapter, the effects of specifically designed, metabolically stable, synthetic analogs of SAH and MTA on enzymes isolated from mammalian cells, and on selected mammalian cells in culture, will be described. Since most of the data considered have been fully discussed in published articles, only a summary of the experimental results will be presented; for further details, the reader is referred to the original publications cited in the reference list.

II. Design and Synthesis of Metabolically Stable Analogs

Kinetic studies in our laboratory and in others (2) have shown that SAH is a potent, reversible inhibitor of almost all SAM-dependent methylases. These observations stimulated the synthesis of many SAH analogs for use in probing the topography of the SAH-binding site on these enzymes (3). However, consideration of transport and metabolism of the analogs, critical for their eventual use as methylation inhibitors in cell culture and whole animals, was largely ignored. The transport of SAH has not been well studied, and in only one article has the subject been addressed experimentally; this report describes the formation of *S*-adenosyl-4-thio-2-ketobutyrate in the urine, and the lack of intracellular SAH, after intravenous administration of SAH to rats and dogs and concludes that SAH does not penetrate mammalian cells (4,5). Our approach has been to design and synthesize metabolically stable analogs of SAH, based on knowledge of the chemistry and biochemistry of purine nucleoside analogs and SAH. At the time we started this work, SAH-metabolizing enzymes had been isolated from both prokaryotes [SAH nucleosidase (6)] and eukaryotes [SAH hydrolase (7)]. However, metabolic studies on SAH in mammalian cells had not been carried out. Therefore we synthesized only SAH analogs which we predicted, based on chemical and/or biochemical data, would not be substrates for one or more of the following enzymes: SAH nucleosidase, SAH hydrolase, and adenosine deaminase (8–11). The most effective of these synthetic analogs is 7-deaza-SAH or *S*-tubercidinylhomocysteine (STH) (10), chosen for synthesis because the parent nucleoside, tubercidin, is known to be resistent to both acid- and enzyme-catalyzed hydrolysis of the purine–ribose bond and is not a substrate for adenosine deaminase (12). Another SAH analogue in which the sulfur atom of SAH is replaced by a —NH— group [N^{γ}-adenosyl-α, γ-diaminobutyric acid (NADABA)] (11), although not a very effective methylase inhibitor, proved to be the most effective nonsubstrate inhibitor of SAH hydrolase (13).

In contrast, earlier kinetic studies on partially purified spermidine synthase

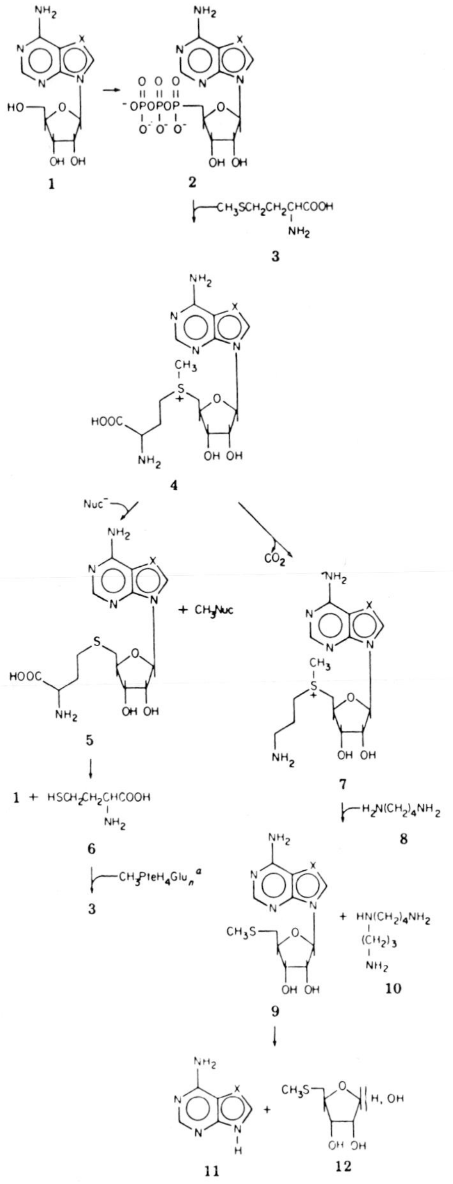

a, X = N; b, X = CH

Fig. 1. Biosynthesis and utilization of SAM (*4*). [a] CH_3 Pte H_4 Glu*n* = 5-methyl-5,6,7,8 = tetrahydropteroyl poly-λ-L-glutamate. Reprinted from (14).

from rat ventral prostate showed no product inhibition by MTA (14). Based on the results mentioned above with 7-deaza-SAH, and considering the metabolic fate of MTA, we synthesized 7-deaza-MTA or 5′-deoxy-5′-methylthiotubercidin (MTT) and showed that it was not a substrate but an inhibitor of MTA phosphorylase (14). The associated observation that MTA did not inhibit spermidine synthase decreased our interest in MTT. However, recent studies have shown that purified spermidine and spermine synthase, free of MTA phosphorylase, are both strongly inhibited by MTA (15,16).

III. Enzymology and Metabolism

Our studies with synthetic SAH analogs revealed that structural modifications in the sugar and amino acid portion of SAH resulted in a drastic reduction in inhibitory activity (8,9,11). However, certain modifications in the heterocyclic base were tolerated (9) and, in particular, replacement of the N-7 with a —CH— group gave a very potent inhibitor (10). This compound, 7-deaza-SAH or STH, is a potent inhibitor of every SAM-dependent methylase tested to date, with K_i values close to that of the natural product inhibitor, SAH, in almost all enzymes studied (17). Furthermore, synthesis of ^{14}C-labeled SAH and STH has allowed study of their metabolism in cultured murine neuroblastoma cells (18). These studies show that, although SAH is rapidly and extensively metabolized by cell cultures, STH is completely inert under the same conditions (18). Thus our initial design criteria, namely, the development of a potent, nonmetabolizable analog of SAH, have been fulfilled.

Similarly, the demonstration that 7-deaza-MTA or MTT was an effective inhibitor and not a substrate of MTA phosphorylase (14) meant that we had a compound which would not be susceptible to metabolic degradation via the route known for MTA. The recent demonstration of potent product inhibition by MTA of purified spermidine and spermine synthase (15,16) led us to study MTT as an inhibitor of these two enzymes. Although complete kinetic data are not yet available, it is already clear that MTT is nearly equipotent with MTA as an inhibitor; ID_{50} for MTT = 45 μM versus ID_{50} for MTA = 30 μM for spermidine synthase, and ID_{50} for MTT = 15 μM versus ID_{50} for MTA = 10 μM for spermine synthase (16). A detailed study of MTT metabolism has not yet been carried out and, although another 5′-deoxy adenosine derivative, *S*-isobutyladenosine (SIBA; see Section IV) has been shown to be metabolized by both deamination (adenosine deaminase?) and hydrolysis (MTA phosphorylase?) (19), MTT has been shown to be resistant to the latter pathway and is also probably not a substrate for adenosine deaminase. However, these tentative conclusions must await verification by studies on MTT metabolism in cell culture.

IV. Effects of 5′-Thioadenosine Derivatives in Cultured Cells

Our initial results with STH in isolated cell-free systems were obtained with the enzymes catechol-O-methyltransferase (COMT) and mixed tRNA methylases (tRNAMT), both from rat liver (10). Therefore our initial studies with STH in cultured cells involved tRNA methylation (20) and dopamine methylation (21) in phytohemagglutinin (PHA)-stimulated rat lymphocytes and murine neuroblastoma cells, respectively. In both these studies, SAH and STH at concentrations of 50' μM were each able to inhibit methylation in intact, viable cells. An interesting finding was that STH was consistently about twice as effective as SAH and that the SAH effects could be mimicked by equal concentrations of adenosine or homocysteine. These two facts are in accord with the hypothesis that SAH is metabolized via cleavage of the 5′-thioether bond to give adenosine and homocysteine. This is an equilibrium reaction in which synthesis of SAH is favored thermodynamically (7); in the cell, deamination of adenosine normally drives the equilibrium in the hydrolytic direction. Recent experiments by others have used a similar approach, in combination with adenosine deaminase inhibitors, to generate elevated levels of SAH (22) and 3-deaza-SAH (23) in cultured cells. In both cases, inhibition of intracellular methylation reactions was observed. The fact that STH is more effective than SAH is in accord with the hypothesis that STH is more resistant to metabolic degradation than SAH. This has subsequently been shown to be the case, as described in Section III.

More recently, in collaboration with M. Kaehler and F. Rottman of Michigan State University, we have studied the effects of STH on RNA methylation in Novikoff hepatoma cells (24–27). In these studies, we have shown that STH can inhibit the methylation of cytoplasmic mRNA (24), resulting in about 70–80% inhibition of N^6-methyladenosine (m^6A) and cap-two structures, about 50% inhibition of cap-one structures, and accumulation of a small amount of cap-zero structures. Cap-two, -one, and -zero structures contain two, one, and zero 2′-*O*-methyl groups, respectively, in the two terminal residues of the mRNA (28,29). Cap-zero structures could also be detected on polysomes (26), thereby suggesting that these methyl-deficient mRNAs may be competent to direct protein synthesis. Thus STH is able to block the methylation of both adenosine N-6 and 2′-hydroxyl groups during the maturation of hnRNA to mRNA. Surprisingly, no inhibition of 7-methylguanosine (m^7G) formation was observed in this work. Furthermore, STH is a potent inhibitor of the enzyme which catalyzes m^7G synthesis in the cap of Newcastle disease virus (NDV) RNA (30). It is possible that the NDV N-7 methylase is very different from the Novikoff enzyme, or it may be that methylation at N-7 of guanine is required for mRNA transport from the nucleus to the cytoplasm. rRNA isolated from the same cells was not affected by STH; sugar methylated dinucleotides were identical in both STH-treated and control cells (25). This result suggests that processing of larger precursors (45 S) to mature 28 and 18 S rRNA may require methylation; analysis of large nuclear precursors would be informative in this regard. Finally, analysis of total 4 S RNA from STH-treated and untreated Novikoff tumor cells showed a large difference in the pattern of methylated nucleosides isolated following enzyme-catalyzed hydrolysis of the RNA. The action of STH ranges from about 90% inhibition of N^2-dimethylguanosine (m^2_2G) and m^7G formation to little or no effect on 5-methyluridine (m^5U, ribothymine) formation (27). The ability to block RNA methylation effectively in whole cells should allow us to produce RNA which is undermethylated at specific sites and then to ask questions concerning the function of a methylated residue in a particular step in nucleic acid replication and/or protein synthesis.

These types of questions are perhaps better addressed in a system which yields a reasonable number of defined mRNAs. Tumor viruses such as Rous sarcoma virus (RSV) contain genetic information for only a small number of virus-coded proteins. Thus the RSV system can be used to probe the role of methylation in RNA structure and function. While on sabbatical leave (1977–1978) at the Salk Institute, I collaborated with Karen Beemon on such a study. In previous work, she had located the m^6A as being close to the 3′-end of the 10-kb 38 S RSV RNA (31). In addition, approximately 50% of the m^6A were located in the region of the genome (*src*) required for transformation of chick embryo fibroblasts (CEF). Thus a possible relationship between RNA methylation and RSV transformation of CEFs was suggested. If STH could inhibit RSV RNA methylation as effectively as it inhibited Novikoff tumor cytoplasmic RNA methylation (see above), it might be possible to study the effects of this methylation on production of the *src* gene product and its effect on transformation of CEF by RSV. As shown in Table I, STH slightly inhibits (20–35%) the formation of cap-one (m^7GpppG^m) and m^6A, and a small amount of cap-zero (m^7GpppG) was seen in a similar but not nearly as convincing manner as with Novikoff tumor cytoplasmic mRNA. The results with STH were not encouraging, but two articles published at that time suggested the use of other agents as possible inhibitors of RNA methylation. Sinefungin and A9145C, two natural products isolated by scientists at Eli Lilly and shown to be structurally similar to SAH (the sulfur of SAH being replaced by —$CHNH_2$— in sinefungin) are poor inhibitors of COMT (32), in agreement with our earlier work on modifications at the sulfur atom, e.g., NADABA (11). However, these two compounds are very potent inhibitors of two capping enzymes isolated from vaccinia virus (33). In addition, cycloleucine, a weak inhibitor of SAM synthetase (34,35), has been shown to inhibit RNA methylation in Chinese hamster ovary cells (36,37). As can be seen in Table I, although sinefungin and A9145C (32,33) had some slight effects on RSV RNA methylation, they were not significantly different from STH, except at the higher concentration of A9145C which significantly inhibited 70 S RNA synthesis. Similarly, cycloleucine at the very high concentrations required to produce inhibition of

TABLE I

Methylation of Rous Sarcoma Virus 38 S RNA[a]

		RSV 38 S [^{32}P] RNA					
		P_1 (One-dimensional electrophoresis)		A, T_1, T_2 (Two-dimensional electrophoresis)			
Addition	μM	m^7GpppG^m	m^7GpppG	$GpppG^m$	m^7GpppG^mpCp[b]	m^6Ap	70 S RNA synthesis (%)
Control	—	0.048	0.005	0.003	0.05	0.11	100
STH	200/182	0.040	0.011	0.011	0.032	0.071	70/100
Sinefungin	200/209	0.044	0.007	0.005	0.032	0.132	75/75
A9145C	200/233	0.064	0.010	0.026	0.032	0.154	43/40
A9145C	50/—	0.041	0.001	0.009	N.D.	N.D.	64/—
Cycloleucine	45,000/—	0.043	0.008	0.009	N.D.	N.D.	38/—

[a] Virus added to CEFs about 5-7 days prior to drug and ^{32}P. Data are presented as percentages of ^{32}P in 10-kb 38 S RNA.

[b] Cap structures $m^7GpppGp$ and $GpppGp^{(m)}$ are included in this number.

methylation in earlier work (36,37) markedly inhibited 70 S RNA synthesis. Whether the observed inhibition of 70 S RSV RNA synthesis really reflects inhibition of virus assembly or inhibition of the RNA polymerase is not yet known. Translation of RSV 70 S RNA (denatured) in the messenger-dependent lysate (MDL) system clearly shows the 60K *src* gene product in addition to the related 25K and 17K proteins (38). Denatured 70 S RSV RNA isolated from cells treated with STH, Sinefungin, A9145C, and cycloleucine were translated in the MDL system. No significant differences were seen in the amount of 60K, 25K, or 17K proteins synthesized in this system, which could not be attributed to a drug-related decrease in 70 S RNA synthesis (Table I). However, studies on the ability of STH, Sinefungin, and A9145C to inhibit RSV transformation of CEF, as measured by a focus assay (39), showed that these drugs inhibited focus formation by about 50, 80, and >90%, respectively. Thus, although these compounds affect RSV transformation of CEF, we have been unable to obtain evidence that this parallels inhibition of methylation.

Recent work in collaboration with A. Pegg of Pennsylvania State University has shown that MTT, the synthetic phosphorylase-resistant MTA analogue, decreases polyamine concentrations in mouse 3T3 cells. Thus 300 μM MTT decreases spermidine and spermine levels by approximately 70 and 20%, respectively, over a 3-day growth period. These decreases in intracellular polyamine concentration parallel a retardation of cell growth, and it is not yet clear whether the decreased polyamine levels are a cause or an effect of diminished cell growth. Much more work remains to be done with MTT, but it is already clear that this phosphorylase-resistant analogue of MTA is capable of affecting polyamine levels in whole cells, much as it does with isolated purified enzymes (Section III). It should be noted that MTT also has been shown to inhibit PHA-stimulated lymphocyte transformation irreversibly, a process thought to be dependent on MTA metabolism mediated by MTA phosphorylase (40).

Another 5′-deoxy-5′-thioadenosine derivative which has been studied extensively over the past several years is *S*-isobutyladenosine (SIBA) (41). Although this compound has been described as a methylase inhibitor and was originally synthesized as a SAH analog , *in vitro* assays of the effects of SIBA on isolated tRNA methylases and protein methylase I (42) show that it is a poor inhibitor of these enzymes (K_i = ca. 3.6 and 0.6 mM, respectively). An alternative explanation of the observed biological effects of SIBA is that it is an alternate substrate for MTA phosphorylase (17), competing with endogenous MTA for this enzyme. Recent support for this proposal has come from two different laboratories; SIBA is a substrate for MTA phosphorylase from human placenta (43) and sarcoma 180 cells (44). Thus SIBA might affect the levels of the polyamines by interfering with the normal metabolic degradation of MTA. Since polyamines are involved in a myriad of biological processes, it is not surprising that SIBA evokes such a wide variety of biological responses.

A working hypothesis for the action of 5′-thioadenosine analogues *in vivo* is summarized in Fig. 2. In this scheme, 5-′-thioadenosine derivatives such as SAH, Sinefungin, and MTA can undergo several metabolic conversions. In a reversible reaction, SAH is hydrolyzed to adenosine and homocysteine, hydrolysis being favored *in vivo* by the removal of adenosine via enzyme-catalyzed deamination to inosine or phosphorylation to AMP (18). Neither direct deamination of SAH nor cleavage of the purine–ribose bond of SAH is observed. Adenosine kinase-negative (AK^-) mutants of mouse lymphoma cells, which are given adenosine deaminase (ADA) inhibitors together with adenosine and homocysteine thiolactone, synthesize SAH in sufficient quantities to inhibit DNA methylation significantly (22). This inhibition of DNA methylation is proposed as one way in which adenosine toxicity might be mediated *in vivo*. A similar approach, using 3-deazaadenosine, results in synthesis of 3-deaza-SAH and SAH, since 3-deazaadenosine is a potent ADA inhibitor and is not converted to the nucleotide (23). Thus it is now possible to increase intracellular synthesis of SAH, 3-deaza-SAH, and other SAH analogs (45) by these techniques. In

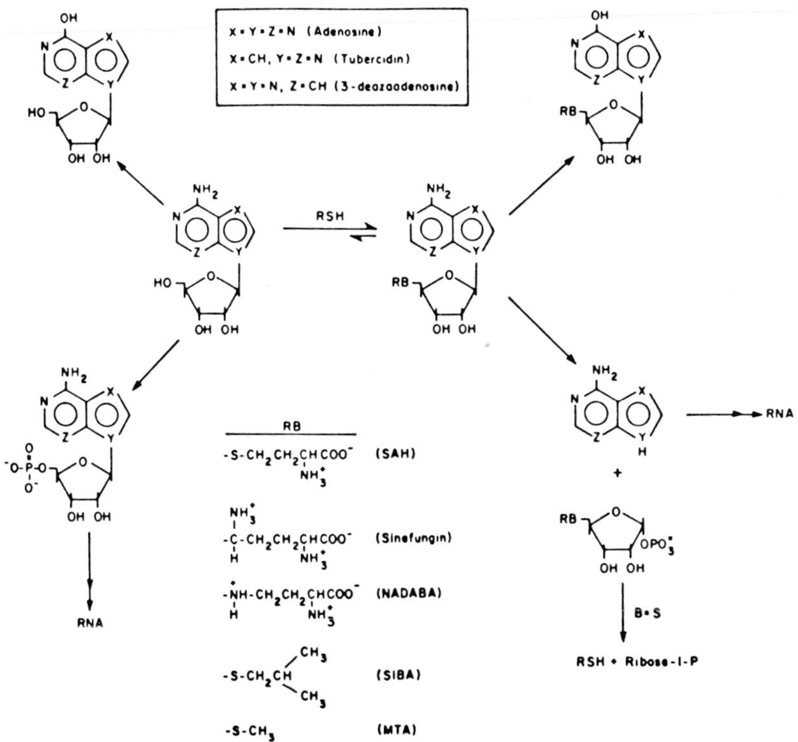

Fig. 2. Possible metabolic fates of 5′-substituted purine nucleosides.

contrast, STH which was designed to resist metabolic degradation, is completely stable under cell culture conditions and affects intracellular methylation reactions as described above. Therefore STH apparently is transported into the cell intact and inhibits SAH-dependent methylation of a wide variety of cellular nucleophiles. The metabolic fates of Sinefungin and NADABA are not yet known, although the latter is not a substrate for SAH hydrolase (13).

In contrast, MTA and SIBA are metabolized by either cleavage of the purine–ribose bond and/or deamination to the inosine derivative (19,40). Thus adding an inhibitor (MTT) or an alternate substrate (SIBA) of MTA phosphorylase may lead to an accumulation of intracellular MTA. The consequences of increasing MTA concentrations in the cell have only recently been studied and it would be premature to propose any biochemical mechanisms. However, it should be noted that the observed potent inhibition of spermidine and spermine synthase by MTA suggests that alteration in MTA levels in the cell may be an effective way of controlling polyamine biosynthesis *in vivo*.

Acknowledgment

The research described here was supported by grants MH-34195 and CA-28097 from the National Institutes of Health.

References

1. E. Usdin, R. T. Borchardt, and C. R. Creveling, eds., "Transmethylation." Am Elsevier, New York, 1979.
2. J. K. Coward, E. P. Slisz, and F. Y.-H. Wu, *Biochemistry* **12,** 2291 (1973).
3. R. T. Borchardt, *in* "The Biochemistry of S-Adenosylmethionine" (F. Salvatore *et al.*, eds.), p. 151. Columbia Univ. Press, New York, 1977.
4. J. A. Duerre, C. H. Miller, and G. G. Reams, *J. Biol. Chem.* **244,** 107 (1969).
5. R. D. Walker and J. A. Duerre, *Can. J. Biochem.* **53,** 312 (1975).
6. J. A. Duerre, *J. Biol. Chem.* **237,** 3737 (1962).
7. G. Dela Haba and G. L. Cantoni, *J. Biol. Chem.* **234,** 603 (1959).
8. J. K. Coward and W. D. Sweet, *J. Med. Chem.* **15,** 381 (1972).
9. J. K. Coward and E. P. Slisz, *J. Med. Chem.* **16,** 460 (1973).
10. J. K. Coward, D. L. Bussolotti, and C.-D. Chang, *J. Med. Chem.* **17,** 1286 (1974).
11. C.-D. Chang and J. K. Coward, *J. Med. Chem.* **19,** 684 (1976).
12. R. J. Suhadolnik, "Nucleoside Antibiotics," Chapter 9. Wiley (Interscience), New York, 1970.
13. P. K. Chiang, H. H. Richards, and G. L. Cantoni, *Mol. Pharmacol.* **11,** 701 (1977).
14. J. K. Coward, N. C. Motola, and J. D. Moyer, *J. Med. Chem.* **20,** 500 (1977).
15. R. L. Pajula and A. Raina, *FEBS Lett.* **99,** 343 (1979).
16. H. Hibasami, R. T. Borchardt, S. Y. Chen, J. K. Coward, and A. E. Pegg, *Biochem. J.*, *187* 419 (1980).
17. J. K. Coward and P. A. Crooks, *in* "Transmethylation" (E. Usdin, R. T. Borchardt, and C. R. Creveling, eds.), p. 215. Am. Elsevier, New York, 1979.

18. P. A. Crooks, R. N. Dreyer, and J. K. Coward, *Biochemistry* **18,** 2601 (1979).
19. F. Lawrence, M. Richou, M. Vedel, G. Farrugia, P. Blanchard, and M. Robert-Gero, *Eur. J. Biochem.* **87,** 257 (1978).
20. C.-D. Chang and J. K. Coward, *Mol. Pharmacol.* **11,** 701 (1975).
21. R. J. Michelot, N. Lesko, R. W. Stout, and J. K. Coward, *Mol. Pharmacol.* **13,** 368 (1977).
22. N. M. Kredich and D. W. Martin, Jr., *Cell* **12,** 931 (1977).
23. P. K. Chiang and G. L. Cantoni, *Biochem. Pharmacol.* **28,** 1897 (1979).
24. M. Kaehler, J. Coward, and F. Rottman, *Biochemistry* **16,** 5770 (1977).
25. F. Rottman, M. Kaehler, and J. Coward, *in* "Transmethylation" (E. Usdin, R. T. Borchardt, and C. R. Creveling, eds.), p. 361. Am. Elsevier, New York, 1979.
26. M. Kaehler, J. Coward, and F. Rottman, *Nucleic Acids Res.* **6,** 1161 (1979).
27. P. A. Crooks, M. Kaehler, F. M. Rottman, and J. K. Coward, (submitted for publication).
28. A. J. Shatkin, *Cell* **9,** 645 (1976).
29. F. Rottman, *Trends Biochem. Sci.* **1,** 217 (1976).
30. C. S. G. Pugh, R. T. Borchardt, and H. O. Stone, *Biochemistry* **16,** 3928 (1977).
31. K. Beemon and J. Keith, *J. Mol. Biol.* **113,** 165 (1977).
32. R. W. Fuller and R. Nagarajan, *Biochem. Pharmacol.* **27,** 1981 (1978).
33. C. S. G. Pugh, R. T. Borchardt, and H. O. Stone, *J. Biol. Chem.* **253,** 4075 (1978).
34. J. B. Lombardini, A. W. Coulter, and P. Talalay, *Mol. Pharmacol.* **6,** 481 (1970).
35. J. B. Lombardini, T.-C. Chou, and P. Talalay, *Biochem. J.* **135,** 43 (1973).
36. M. Caboche and J.-P. Bachellerie, *Eur. J. Biochem.* **74,** 19 (1977).
37. K. Dimmock and C. M. Stoltzfus, *Biochemistry* **17,** 3627 (1978).
38. K. Beemon and T. Hunter, *J. Virol.* **28,** 551 (1978).
39. J. Tooze, "The Molecular Biology of Tumor Viruses," p. 99. Cold Spring Harbor Lab., Cold Spring Harbor, New York, 1973.
40. A. J. Ferro, *in* "Transmethylation" (E. Usdin, R. T. Borchardt, and C. R. Creveling, eds.), p. 117. Am. Elsevier, New York, 1979.
41. M. Robert-Gero, P. Blanchard, F. Lawrence, A. Pierre, M. Vedel, M. Vuilhorgne, and E. Lederer, *in* "Transmethylation" (E. Usdin, R. T. Borchardt, and C. R. Creveling, eds.), p. 207. Am. Elsevier, New York, 1979.
42. M. Legraverend, S. Ibañez, P. Blanchard, J. Enouf, F. Lawrence, M. Robert-Gero, and E. Lederer, *Eur. J. Med. Chem.* **12,** 105 (1977).
43. M. Carteni-Farina, F. Della Ragione, G. Ragosta, A. Oliva, and V. Zappia, *FEBS Lett.* **104,** 266 (1979).
44. T. M. Savarese, G. W. Crabtree, and R. E. Parks, Jr., *Biochem. Pharmacol.* **28,** 2227 (1979).
45. J. L. Hoffman, *J. Biol. Chem.* **253,** 2905 (1978).

13

Studies on Identifying the Locus of Action of Fluorouracil*

FRANK MALEY AND GLADYS F. MALEY

*The following abbreviations are used: FU, 5-fluorouracil; FUR, 5-fluorouridine; FUMP, FUDP, FUTP, the corresponding 5-mono-, 5-di-, and 5-triphosphate derivatives of FUR: FUdR, 5-fluoro-2′-deoxyuridine; FdUMP, FdUDP, FdUTP, the corresponding 5′-mono-, 5′-di-, triphosphate derivatives of FUdR; dUMP, 2′-deoxyuridine 5′-monophosphate; PRPP, 5′-phosphoribosyl pyrophosphate; 5,10-CH_2H_4PteGlu, 5,10-methylene tetrahydropteroylmonoglutamate; H_2PteGlu, dihydrofolate; MTX, methotrexate; CPase, carboxypeptidase; NEM, *N*-ethylmaleimide; DTNB, 5,5′-dithiobis(2-nitrobenzoic acid); SCM, *S*-carboxymethyl; CNBr, cyanogen bromide; PGA, phenylglyoxal; BNPS, 2-(2-nitrophenylsulfenyl)-3-methyl-3-bromoindolenine.

MOLECULAR ACTIONS AND TARGETS FOR CANCER CHEMOTHERAPEUTIC AGENTS

ISBN 0-12-619280-4

I. Introduction

A. Metabolic Interconversion of Fluorouracil

Since the introduction of FU (1) as an antitumor agent, numerous attempts have been made to define clearly the mechanism by which this drug elicits its chemotherapeutic response. An explanation appeared to be provided by the discovery of the enzyme thymidylate synthetase (EC 2.1.1.45) (2), which turned out to be extremely sensitive to a metabolic product of FU, FdUMP (3,4), and in effect explained why FU impaired the synthesis of the methyl group of thymine *in vivo* (5). Thus, with a K_i that exceeds by at least three orders of magnitude the K_m for the enzyme substrate dUMP, FdUMP can very effectively impair DNA synthesis in rapidly dividing normal and tumor tissue. It is this lack of selectivity which has been used to rationalize the toxic side effects often observed on treating patients with FU.

It has since become evident, however, that FU can be metabolized to other products (6), as shown below, which might contribute to many of the apparent conflicting responses obtained with this drug.

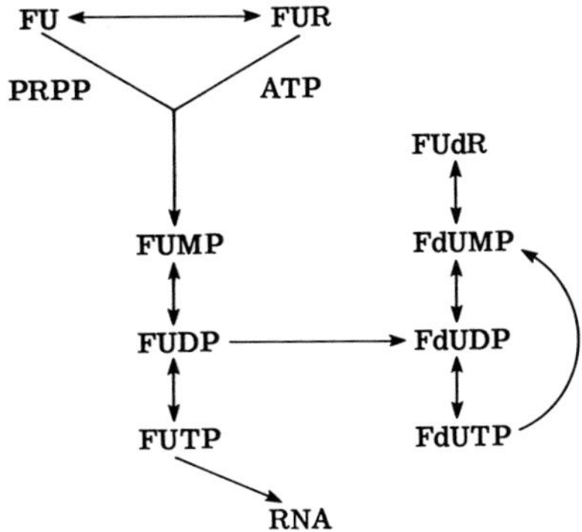

Thus, by the appropriate addition and scheduling of MTX prior to the addition of FU, an antagonistic (7) or synergistic (8) effect can be evoked in L1210 mouse leukemia cells. In the former instance the depletion of intracellular folate was rationalized as impairing the inhibition of thymidylate synthetase, while in the latter case MTX was shown to effect an increase in the intracellular levels of PRPP and as a consequence the FUR nucleotide pool. Since FUTP is incorporated into RNA as FUMP (9), in contrast to FdUTP which is broken down to FdUMP too rapidly to be incorporated into DNA (5), some of the toxic effects obtained with FU can be attributed to its impairment of RNA maturation (10). While it is important to recognize these additional reactions as possibly contributing to the biological effects obtained with FU, it still appears that the major response of this drug is elicited through its inhibition of thymidylate synthetase.

B. The Mechanism of Thymidylate Synthetase Inhibition by FdUMP

Kinetic studies were required initially to understand better the mechanism of this inhibition, because of the lack of sufficient amounts of highly purified enzyme to undertake more refined studies. These studies revealed that the inhibition could be either competitive (11,12) or noncompetitive (12,13), depending on the order of addition of the substrate and inhibitor to the enzyme-containing reaction mixture. Thus, when FdUMP was preincubated with the synthetase, the compound appeared to act as an irreversible noncompetitive inhibitor but, when added to the reaction mixture in the presence of dUMP, the inhibition observed was strictly competitive (12). Even when the enzyme is irreversibly inhibited, this effect is more apparent than real, since dUMP can slowly reverse the inhibition (14). The implications of this finding become apparent when it is realized that, as the intracellular levels of dUMP rise as a consequence of the FU treatment, the inhibition can be eventually overridden. A similar elevation of dUMP by MTX might also be used as an explanation for the antagonism observed when FU is scheduled after MTX.

In general, the basic tenet of the kinetic studies was that the two substrates added to the enzyme in an ordered manner, with dUMP adding first followed by 5,10-CH_2H_4PteGlu (12). The stabilizing influence of dUMP on the synthetase, in contrast to that of 5,10-CH_2H_4PteGlu and folate analogs, supports this proposal (12,15).

II. *Lactobacillus casei* Thymidylate Synthetase: A Model Enzyme for Studying the Dynamics of a Reaction

A. The Nature of dUMP and FdUMP Binding

Much of what we know today regarding the mechanism of the thymidylate synthetase reaction was made possible by the isolation of large quantities of crystalline enzyme from MTX-resistant strains of *L. casei* (16,17). Although it might be anticipated that the kinetics of the reaction of the synthetase from diverse phylogenetic sources might differ, most of the studies to date have revealed that enzymes from animal (12,13,18–20) and bacterial sources (11,21,22) do not differ greatly in their physical or catalytic properties. With respect to the inhibition effected by FdUMP, enzymes from all sources form an almost irreversible ternary complex consisting of enzyme, FdUMP, and 5,10-CH_2H_4PteGlu (23,24), with as many as three forms of the enzyme observed on gel electrophoresis (25). These result from the fact that each of the two enzyme subunits can react individually to form a ternary complex so that in any reaction mixture, depending on the ratio of FdUMP and 5,10-CH_2H_4PteGlu to enzyme, there exist uncomplexed enzyme, a 1:1:1 complex of enzyme–FdUMP–5,10-CH_2H_4PteGlu, and a 1:2:2 complex of the same components. The initiation of formation of this complex is believed to result from the reaction of a nucleophilic residue in the enzyme with the 6-position of the pyrimidine ring (Fig. 1), which can be detected in the case of dUMP as a change in ellipticity at 267 nm (26). On addition of 5,10-CH_2H_4PteGlu, which is believed to add to the 5-position of the pyrimidine ring, the complex is so stabilized that it can be detected by means of UV difference spectra (23,24), fluorescence (27,28), circular dichroism (CD) (27,29), gel electrophoresis (25,27), and ^{19}F NMR spectra (30) and is sufficiently stable to be used as a quantitative measure of thymidylate synthetase in animal cells (7,31). Although stable in 6 *M* guanidine (21,24), the complex does, however, exchange bound and unbound FdUMP (24,32) and is partially dissociated in 3 *M* urea (21). The degree to which ternary complex formation affects the enzyme protein conformation is shown in Fig. 2 where the crystal structure of the T_2 phage synthetase in the presence (Fig. 2A) and absence (Fig. 2B) of FdUMP plus 5,10-CH_2H_4PteGlu is shown. The differences in the crystal structures are self-evident.

The validity of earlier kinetic studies, which attempted to establish the order of binding, were verified in equilibrium dialysis studies (33) where it was shown that folate derivatives did not bind to the enzyme until the nucleotide derivatives were added (Table I) (12,33,34). The significance of this interplay is made evident by the fact that the dissociation constant of FdUMP decreases from 2.20×10^{-6} *M* (33) (Table II) to 5×10^{-11} *M* (24) in the ternary complex.

Since the enzyme is composed of two identical subunits, it is not surprising to find that 2 moles of FdUMP are bound to completely inhibited enzyme (24,27,33). However, this finding is not consistent with the observation (33) that only 1 mole of the substrate, dUMP, binds to the enzyme. This anomaly is

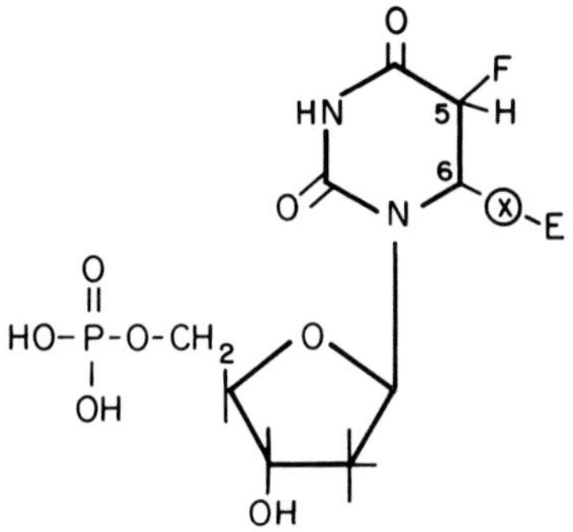

Fig. 1. Proposed binary complex of thymidylate synthetase and FdUMP. The enzyme nucleophile (×) initiates the dissociable complex by adding to C-6 of the pyrimidine ring to saturate the double bond between C-5 and C-6.

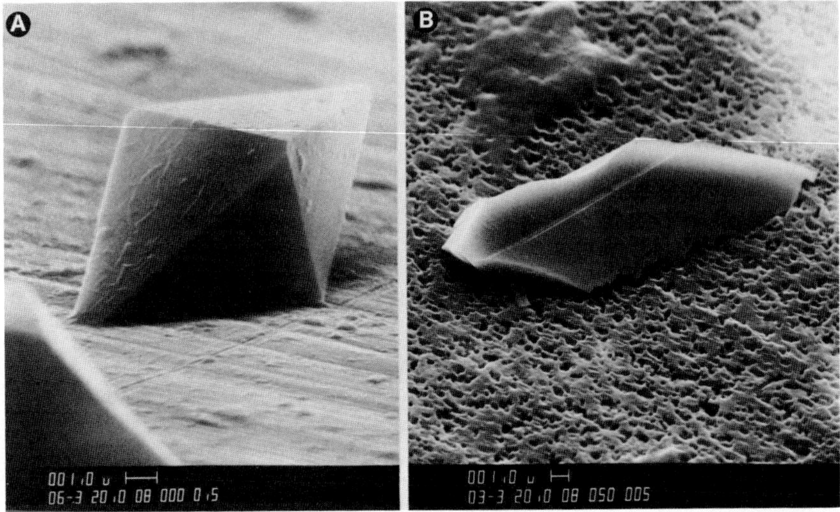

Fig. 2. Scanning electron micrographs of T_2 phage-induced thymidylate synthetase. Crystal formation in the absence (A) and presence (B) of FdUMP and 5,10-Ch_2H_4PteGlu.

further compounded by the fact that FdUMP appears to be bound to each site with a different dissociation constant (2,3). It is possible a second site is available for dUMP but it is so weak that it is not detectable except by extraordinary procedures (35). Alternatively, the enzyme may belong to a class where only half of the sites are reactive (36).

Although the (−) isomer of 5,10-CH_2H_4PteGlu inhibits the synthetase reaction

TABLE I

Factors Affecting Binding of Folate to *Lactobacillus casei* Thymidylate Synthetase

Folate	Binding sites	K_D ($\times 10^6$)
(+)-5,10-CH_2H_4PteGlu	0.0	0.0
Plus 4N-HO-dCMP[a]	1.10	1.9
Plus FdUMP	1.82	<0.01
(+)-5,10-CH_2H_4PteGlu$_4$	0.99	18
Plus CPase-E[b]	0.0	0.0
Plus NEM-E[b]	0.83	5.1
Plus 4N-HO-dCMP	1.0	<0.01
Plus FdUMP	1.6	<0.01

[a] The 4N-hydroxy derivative of deoxycytidine 5′-monophosphate is a nonreactive competitive inhibitor of thymidylate synthetase (12). On preincubation, however, it becomes noncompetitive.

[b] CPase-E and NEM-E represent carboxypeptidase A and NEM-treated thymidylate synthetase, respectively. For additional details see Galivan *et al.* (34).

TABLE II

Factors Affecting the Binding of dUMP and FdUMP to *Lactobacillus casei* Thymidylate Synthetase[a]

Nucleotide	Binding sites	K_D ($\times 10^6$)
dUMP	1.16 ± 0.16	1.80 ± 0.25
Plus CPase-E[b]	1.10 ± 0.09	0.51 ± 0.05
Plus NEM-E[b]	0	0
Plus H_2PteGlu	1.10 ± 0.09	0.52 ± 0.03
Plus (−)-CH_2H_4PteGlu	0.90 ± 0.14	3.20 ± 0.54
FdUMP	2.20 ± 0.21	37.2 ± 3.6
Plus (+)-CH_2H_4PteGlu	1.75 ± 0.15	< 0.01
Plus (−)-CH_2H_4PteGlu	1.52 ± 0.16	2.26 ± 0.17

[a] For additional details see Galivan *et al.* (33,34).
[b] See Table I, footnote *b*, for abbreviations.

(37), it too can bind to the FdUMP–enzyme complex to form a ternary complex (Table II) (33). However, as seen in the CD difference spectra in Fig. 3, there are distinct differences in the spectral properties of the two ternary complexes at 285 and 332 nm, suggesting the presence of conformational isomers.

B. The Nature of Folate Binding

As indicated above, 5,10-CH_2H_4PteGlu does not bind to the synthetase unless a binary complex of the nucleotide substrate or inhibitor is available. However, even the binding of folate derivatives which cannot add to the 5-position of the

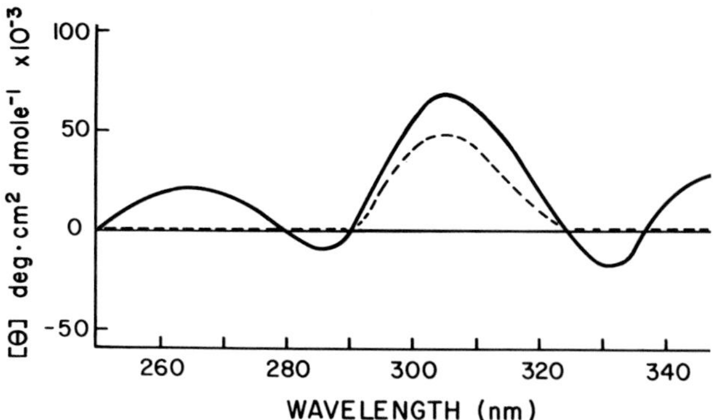

Fig. 3. The CD difference spectra for free *L. casei* thymidylate synthetase and enzyme in the presence of FdUMP and (+)-5,10-CH_2H_4PteGlu (solid line). The corresponding spectrum resulting from the presence of FdUMP and (−)-5,10-CH_2H_4PteGlu is indicated by a dashed line. For additional details see Galivan *et al.* (29).

pyrimidine ring, such as MTX, H_2PteGlu, and 2-amino-4-hydroxyquinazoline, is enhanced. In contrast, the folylpolyglutamates can bind to the enzyme in the absence of FdUMP, but the binding is greatly increased on addition of a nucleotide analog of dUMP (Table II). As indicated, the binding of folylpolyglutamates is accompanied by protection against proteolytic inactivation by CPase A, trypsin, and chymotrypsin (38). In the absence of the protective compound, CPase, by removing a single COOH-terminal valine, completely inactivates the synthetase (39) and eliminates its capacity to bind folate but not dUMP (Table II) (34). The binding of the latter, however, can be prevented by thiol reagents such as NEM and iodoacetate, an effect which does not apparently impair the binding of folylpolyglutamates (Table I). It is clear from these studies that each substrate possesses a separate, distinct binding site of its own and that, if either is impaired, binding at the other site is not greatly affected. Still, the structural change effected by CPase treatment must be a subtle one, for although dUMP can promote the binding of 5,10-CH_2H_4PteGlu$_4$ to the modified enzyme, these compounds are not apparently in a conformation that can overcome the activation energy barrier required for catalysis.

It should perhaps be emphasized that, while most of the kinetic studies with thymidylate synthetase have been derived with 5,10-CH_2H_4PteGlu and its corresponding analogues, naturally occurring folates exist predominantly as polyglutamates. As such, these compounds may yield entirely different kinetic responses *in situ* than are obtained with the corresponding monoglutamates. Some evidence in support of this view has been found recently in studies with highly purified human leukemic cell thymidylate synthetase (19,40). Also as indicated in Table I, folylpolyglutamates bind much more effectively to the synthetase than monoglutamates and can be, under the appropriate conditions, quite inhibitory to the synthetase (37). As a consequence, any conclusions regarding the nature and the extent of inhibition of thymidylate synthetase effected by dUMP analogues *in vitro* should if possible be extrapolated to *in vivo* conditions, where folylpolyglutamates prevail.

Inhibition studies with folylpolyglutamates of varying chain length revealed a degree of selectivity with synthetases from various sources that has not been encountered with nucleotide inhibitors (41). Thus the *L. casei* synthetase was inhibited to a greater extent by PteGlu$_{3-7}$ than that from *Escherichia coli,* which in turn was more inhibited than the T_2 bacteriophage-induced synthetase. Recent studies showed that, when Mg^{2+} was excluded from the reactions, the synthetase from T_2 phage was almost completely inhibited by PteGlu$_6$ but only marginally impaired in the case of the *E. coli* enzyme (42). This effect, however, could be reversed in part by the addition of Mg^{2+}. The nature of the inhibition effected by PteGlu$_6$ is clearly noncompetitive (Fig. 4), having a K_i of 8×10^{-7} M. Although this degree of selectivity may not be encountered with synthetases from normal and tumor tissue, these results suggest that the folate site might be a more

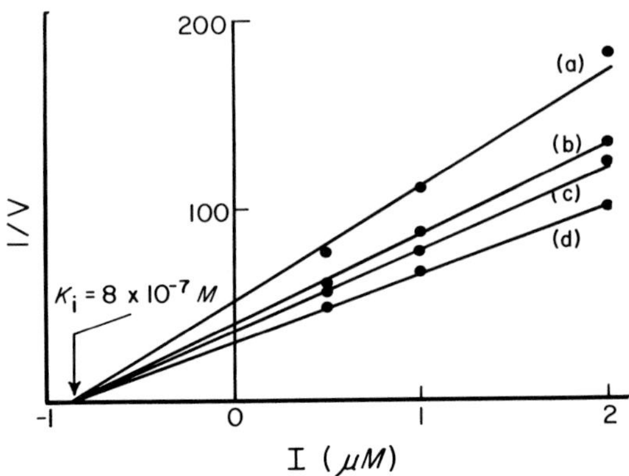

Fig. 4. Kinetics of inhibition of T_2 phage-induced thymidylate synthetase by $PteGlu_6$. The variable substrate, (±)-5,10-CH_2H_4PteGlu, is represented by (a–d) and the inhibitor by I.

desirable target for selective chemotherapy than the nucleotide site, particularly in cases where comparable host and parasite enzymes are involved.

C. Structural Comparisons of Synthetase from Various Sources

The fact that the synthetases from *L. casei*, *E. coli*, and T_2 phage respond so differently to folylpolyglutamates suggests that significant structural differences exist among these enzymes and appear to have surfaced so far in their amino acid compositions and molecular weights. Thus it is seen in Table III (43) that, although the enzymes from these sources contain two identical subunits, there are obvious differences in their size; the *L. casei* enzyme is the largest with molecular weight of about 73,000, as compared to the *E. coli* and T_2 phage synthetases with respective molecular weights of 59,000 and 64,000.

Except for significant differences in Gly, Val, Tyr, Lys, His, and Arg the amino acid compositions of the *E. coli* and T_2 synthetases appear to be quite similar. An analogous case can be made for the *L. casei* and T_2 phage enzymes, where striking similarities exist except for Cys, Pro, His, and Arg.

A comparison of the fingerprint patterns of the three enzymes, however, reveals a surprising number of similarities but also distinctive differences among them. As indicated by the arrow in Fig. 5, the active site peptide in each case is located in almost identical regions.

D. Studies on Clarifying the Nucleophile at the Nucleotide-Binding Site

Because of the analogy between model studies (44), which demonstrated that nucleophiles by attacking the C-6 position of the pyrimidine ring promoted exchange reactions at the C-5 position, it was proposed that a comparable reaction was promoted by thymidylate synthetase. The most likely candidate for this nucleophile appeared to be a cysteinyl residue, since sulfhydryl compounds can promote comparable exchange reactions (45) and because of the sensitivity of the synthetase to sulfhydryl reagents (16,23,26,46). In addition, as indicated in Table II, the binding of dUMP can be prevented by NEM. That the sulfhydryl inhibitor and substrate-binding site may be synonomous is indicated by the data in Fig. 6 which reveal that the titration of but one of the enzyme's four sulfhydryl groups results in complete inactivation. These results are consistent with the fact that only 1 mole of dUMP binds per mole of enzyme and protects against the inhibition effected by the sulfhydryl reagent. Although others (23,26) have obtained similar results, these findings were questioned recently when two NEM-binding sites could be demonstrated in the *L. casei* synthetase (47). More re-

TABLE III

Amino Acid Composition of Thymidylate Synthetase from Different Sources

	Average residues per mole		
Amino acid	*L. casei*, MW = 73,176[c]	*E. coli* B, MW = 59,000	T_2-phage-induced MW = 64,000
Cysteic acid[a]	4	9	8
Aspartic acid	76	62	60
Threonine	32	28	22
Serine	25 (26)	23	26
Glutamic acid	56	59	56
Proline	36	28	24
Glycine	36	37	44
Alanine	40	28	32
Valine	32	31	38
Methionine	12	13	10
Isoleucine	29 (30)	31	34
Leucine	70	56	56
Tyrosine	28	13	28
Phenylalanine	38	24	22
Lysine	40	23	40
Histidine	36 (38)	20	14
Arginine	24	24	34
Tryptophan[b]	12 (14)	8	10

[a] Determined after hydrolysis in dimethyl sulfoxide plus 6 *N* HCl at 107°C for 21 hours.

[b] Determined after hydrolysis in 4 *N* methanesulfonic acid at 107° for 24 hours. All other amino acids were obtained from the average of 24-, 48-, and 72-hour hydrolyzates in 6 *N* HCl at 107°C.

[c] Figures in parentheses were obtained from the sequence of the enzyme protein (43), Fig. 8.

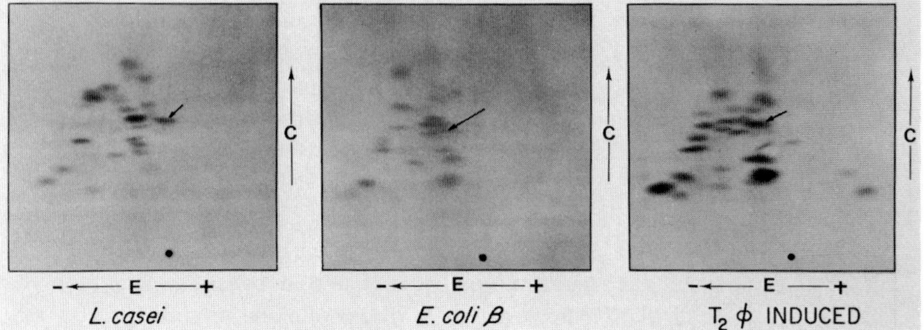

Fig. 5. Tryptic peptide maps of *L. casei, E. coli,* and T_2 phage synthetases (left to right). The arrow in each case reveals the location of the [2-^{14}C]FdUMP-containing peptide following trypsin digestion of the respective ternary complexes and their subjection to two-dimensional chromatography. E, Electrophoresis; C, chromatography.

cently, however, confirmation of the single-site thesis was obtained by measuring the binding of DTNB in the presence and absence of FdUMP (48). It was shown that, while only 1 mole of DTNB could be bound per mole of enzyme, a second DTNB reactive site could be uncovered following the formation of 1:1:1 enzyme–FdUMP–5,10-CH_2H_4PteGlu ternary complex. It was therefore proposed that the second sulfhydryl site became accessible as the result of a conformational change on formation of the ternary complex.

More convincing data implicating a cysteinyl residue as the substrate reactive nucleophile came from an amino acid analysis of a 1:2:2 enzyme–FdUMP–5,10-CH_2H_4PteGlu ternary complex which had been reacted with iodoacetate

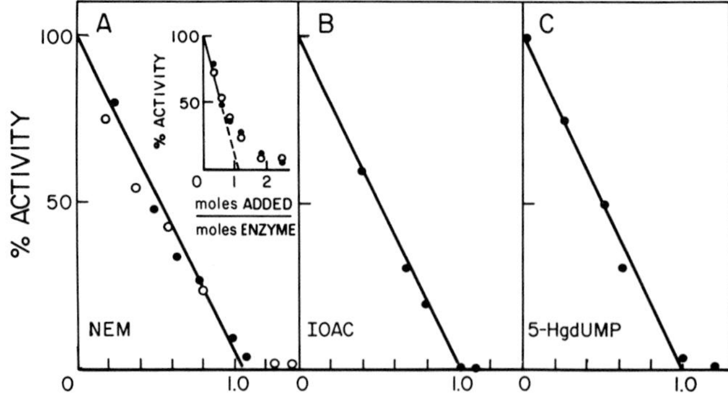

Fig. 6. Stoichiometry of binding of sulfhydryl reagents to *L. casei* thymidylate synthetase. The inset in (A) represents the relationship between the extent of binding and enzyme activity. For additional details see Galivan *et al.* (46).

TABLE IV

Number of Sulfhydryl Reactive Groups in Intact Enzyme and CNBr 4 before and after Treatment with FdUMP

	SCM cysteine residues per mole	
Treatment	Holoenzyme	CNBr 4
Iodoacetate[a]	3.71	1.80
Iodoacetate plus FdUMP[b]	2.05	1.03

[a] Thymidylate synthetase was *S*-carboxymethylated following denaturation with 6 *M* guanidine-HCl (49).

[b] The enzyme was first converted to a ternary complex with FdUMP and 5,10-CH_2H_4-PteGlu and then *S*-carboxymethylated; CNBr 4 was isolated as described (49, 50).

under denaturing conditions. As indicated in Table IV (49,50), only two of the enzyme's four cysteines could be recovered as SCM cysteine, confirming the association of the substrate analog with a cysteinyl residue.

E. Isolation of the Active Site or Ternary Complex Peptide

To establish cysteine firmly as the nucleophilic amino acid residue responsible for the binding of dUMP, and for the formation of the ternary inhibitor complex, the enzyme was labeled with [2-^{14}C]FdUMP in the presence of 5,10-CH_2H_4PteGlu. The residual sulfhydryl groups were blocked by *S*-carboxymethylation, and the resulting protein was cleaved with CNBr to yield five peptides. The largest peptide, with a molecular weight of about 12,000, was found to contain the radioactive nucleotide and was further digested with chymotrypsin. A labeled nonapeptide was isolated from the resulting peptide mixture by a combination of BioGel-P2 and two-dimensional paper chromatography. The sequence (49) Ala-Leu-Pro-Pro-Cys-His-Thr-Leu-Tyr was established by a modified dansyl Edman procedure and was in agreement with that also reported by Pogolotti *et al.* (51).

To confirm the association of FdUMP with the same residue that is sensitive to sulfhydryl reagents, the enzyme was first inactivated with 1 mole of iodo[1−^{14}C]acetate (Fig. 6) and dialyzed to remove excess label; the residual sulfhydryl groups were *S*-carboxymethylated with cold iodoacetate following denaturation of the labeled enzyme. The same procedures that provided the FdUMP-containing nonapeptide were employed and yielded an identical peptide, except that the cysteinyl residue was labeled with a radioactive SCM group. The fact that the specific activity of the isolated SCM cysteine was one-half that of the iodoacetate employed supports the dUMP-binding data indicating that, although the enzyme is composed of two identical subunits, only one is reactive under nondenaturing conditions.

III. Location of the Active Site Peptide within the Primary Sequence of *Lactobacillus casei* Thymidylate Synthetase

A. Isolation of Cyanogen Bromide Peptides

In an effort to establish the placement of the active site peptide within the primary sequence of the enzyme, its location within a series of CNBr peptides was examined prior to our undertaking their structural analysis. The cleavage reaction was directed at either the completely *S*-carboxymethylated protein or one that contained both FdUMP and SCM groups. Although a maximum of seven should have been obtained, since the enzyme contains six methionines, only five were isolated. This apparent anomaly has been resolved by the finding that one residue of methionine is on the NH_2-terminal end and another is resistant to cleavage. The peptides were separated by a novel extraction and BioGel elution scheme (50) which is shown in Fig. 7. The largest peptide, CNBr 4, remained insoluble following ammonium acetate and pyridine acetate extractions of the lyophilized CNBr peptides but could be solubilized in 30% acetic acid and purified on BioGel P-100 as shown. The molecular weights and number of amino acid residues in each of the CNBr peptides are presented in Table V. Each of the enzyme's identical subunits contains two cysteines, both of which were found in CNBr 4 (Table IV).

B. Placement of the Active Site Region in the Primary Sequence

On sequencing CNBr 4 (52), it was quickly established that the active site nonapeptide was located on the NH_2-terminal end immediately following the COOH-terminal methionine of CNBr 3. Through the use of BNPS-skatole and *N*-bromosuccinimide, it was possible to establish the methionine overlap peptides essential for ordering the CNBr peptides and for completing the primary sequence (43) of this protein (Fig. 8). The outlined region of this structure reveals the location of the active site nonapeptide (residues 194–202), with the nucleophilic cysteinyl residue at position 198 and its less reactive mate at residue 244.

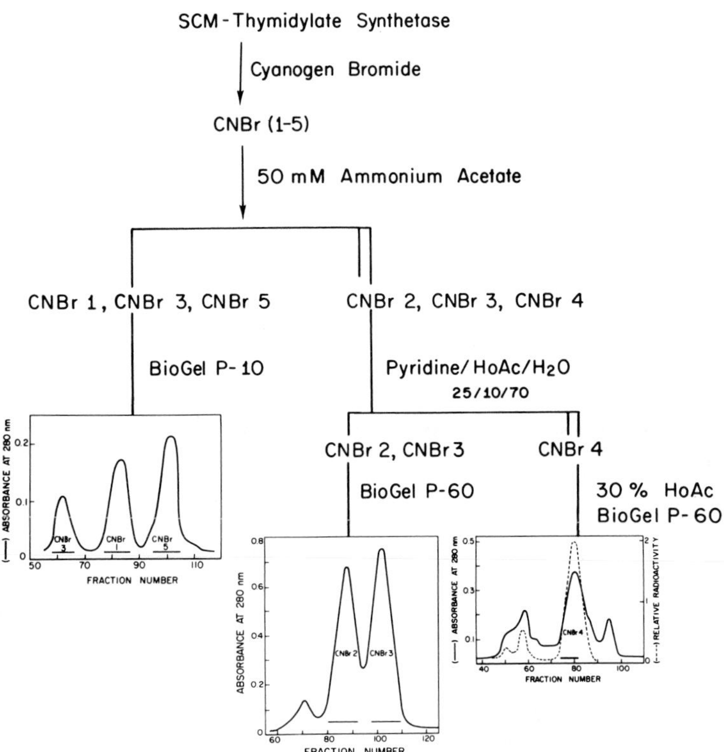

Fig. 7. Scheme employed for separation of the five CnBr peptides obtained on cleavage of *S*-carboxymethylated *L. casei* thymidylate synthetase. For additional details see Maley *et al.* (50).

TABLE V

Amino Acid Content and Molecular Weight of the Cyanogen Bromide Peptides from *Lactobacillus casei* Thymidylate Synthetase[a]

CNBr peptide	Number of residues	Molecular weight
1 (NH_2-end)	36	4,100
2	86	10,300
3	71	8,100
4	103	11,800
5 (COOH-end)	20	2,200
Total	316	36,500

[a] Isolated as described in Fig. 7 (50).

10 20
H-Met-Leu-Glu-Gln-Pro-Tyr-Leu-Asp-Leu-Ala-Lys-Lys-Val-Leu-Asp-Glu-Gly-His-Phe-Lys-
30 40
Pro-Asp-Arg-Thr-His-Thr-Gly-Thr-Tyr-Ser-Ile-Phe-Gly-His-Gln-Met-Arg-Phe-Asp-Leu-
50 60
Ser-Lys-Gly-Phe-Pro-Leu-Leu-Thr-Thr-Lys-Lys-Val-Pro-Phe-Gly-Leu-Ile-Lys-Ser-Glu-
70 80
Leu-Leu-Trp-Phe-Leu-His-Gly-Asp-Thr-Asn-Ile-Arg-Phe-Leu-Leu-Gln-His-Arg-Asn-His-
90 100
Ile-Trp-Asp-Glu-Trp-Ala-Phe-Glu-Lys-Trp-Val-Lys-Ser-Asp-Glu-Tyr-His-Gly-Pro-Asp-
110 120
Met-Thr-Asp-Phe-Gly-His-Arg-Ser-Gln-Lys-Asp-Pro-Glu-Phe-Ala-Ala-Val-Tyr-His-Glu-
130 140
Glu-Met-Ala-Lys-Phe-Asp-Asp-Arg-Val-Leu-His-Asp-Asp-Ala-Phe-Ala-Ala-Lys-Tyr-Gly-
150 160
Asp-Leu-Gly-Leu-Val-Tyr-Gly-Ser-Gln-Trp-Arg-Ala-Trp-His-Thr-Ser-Lys-Gly-Asp-Thr-
170 180
Ile-Asp-Gln-Leu-Gly-Asp-Val-Ile-Glu-Gln-Ile-Lys-Thr-His-Pro-Tyr-Ser-Arg-Arg-Leu-
190 200
Ile-Val-Ser-Ala-Trp-Asn-Pro-Glu-Asp-Val-Pro-Thr-Met-Ala-Leu-Pro-Pro-Cys-His-Thr-
210 220
Leu-Tyr-Gln-Phe-Tyr-Val-Asn-Asp-Gly-Lys-Leu-Ser-Leu-Gln-Leu-Tyr-Gln-Arg-Ser-Ala-
230 240
Asp-Ile-Phe-Leu-Gly-Val-Pro-Phe-Asn-Ile-Ala-Ser-Tyr-Ala-Leu-Leu-Thr-His-Leu-Val-
250 260
Ala-His-Glu-Cys-Gly-Leu-Glu-Val-Gly-Glu-Phe-Ile-His-Thr-Phe-Gly-Asp-Ala-His-Leu-
270 280
Tyr-Val-Asn-His-Leu-Asp-Gln-Ile-Lys-Glu-Gln-Leu-Ser-Arg-Thr-Pro-Arg-Pro-Ala-Pro-
290 300
Thr-Leu-Gln-Leu-Asn-Pro-Asp-Lys-His-Asp-Ile-Phe-Asp-Phe-Asp-Met-Lys-Asp-Ile-Lys-
310
Leu-Leu-Asn-Tyr-Asp-Pro-Tyr-Pro-Ala-Ile-Lys-Ala-Pro-Val-Ala-Val-OH

Fig. 8. Primary amino acid sequence of *L. casei* thymidylate synthetase. The outlined region represents the active site nonapeptide originally isolated as described in Bellisario *et al.* (49).

IV. Identifying Amino Acids Essential for Catalytic Activity

With the primary sequence of the *L. casei* thymidylate synthetase now available, it should be possible with the appropriate functional group reagents to establish not only which amino acids are essential for catalytic activity but their location within the enzyme. Thus agents such as phenylglyoxal and diethylpyrocarbonate, which are relatively specific in their ability to modify arginine (53) and histidine residues (54), respectively, should reveal the degree to which these amino acids contribute to the catalytic process. The merit of this approach is apparent from studies with sulfhydryl reagents which clearly revealed the role of cysteine in promoting the binding of nucleotide substrates and analogues to the enzyme.

A. Effect of Arginine Modification on Enzyme Activity

As indicated earlier by Cipollo and Dunlap (55), treatment of the *L. casei* synthetase with 2,3-butanedione, a compound that modifies arginine, inactivates the enzyme by a pseudo-first-order process. Although the inactivation could be prevented by dUMP, 5,10-CH_2H_4PteGlu and other folate analogues were clearly ineffective. Similar studies were undertaken in our laboratory with phenylglyoxal, since this reagent appeared to be much more effective in its ability to inactivate thymidylate synthetase.

As indicated in Table VI, when the two reagents were compared with respect to their capacity to inactivate the synthetase, phenylglyoxal inactivated 50% of the enzyme in 30 seconds relative to 120 minutes for butanedione, providing both were present at a 500:1 molar ratio of compound to enzyme. That an active site-associated amino acid may be involved is suggested by the finding that 85% of the enzyme could be protected from phenylglyoxal inactivation by dUMP, as compared to only 24% for butanedione. Even more striking is the demonstration that the incorporation of 2 moles of phenylglyoxal is required for complete inactivation of 1 mole of the synthetase and that the course of this reaction follows a linear relationship (Fig. 9). The apparent requirement for 2 moles of phenylglyoxal per mole of enzyme is consistent with the finding that two molecules of phenylglyoxal are needed to irreversibly modify one molecule of arginine (53).

It should be emphasized that, if the incorporation of phenylglyoxal is measured with time, many more than 2 moles of phenylglyoxal can be incorporated per mole of protein but that dUMP, as shown by amino acid analysis (Table VII), protects only one mole of arginine from being modified.

It is probably not a coincidence that a single sulfhydryl group and a single

TABLE VI

Characteristics of Phenylglyoxal and Butanedione Inactivation of Thymidylate Synthetase

Characteristic	Butanedione in 50 m*M* borate, pH 8.2	Phenylglyoxal in 200 m*M* NEM, pH 8.2
Time required to reach 50% activity in the presence of a 500-fold molar excess of reagent over enzyme	120 minutes	0.5 minute
Molar excess of reagent required to achieve 99% inactivation in 60 minutes	>8000-fold	175-fold
Kinetics of inactivation	First-order	> First-order
Number of arginine residues modified to achieve complete inactivation	4	1.2
Protection from inactivation by 100-fold excess of dUMP when unprotected enzyme retained 2% activity	24% activity retained	85% activity retained
Number of arginine residues protected from modification by dUMP as determined by amino acid analysis	1.1	0.9

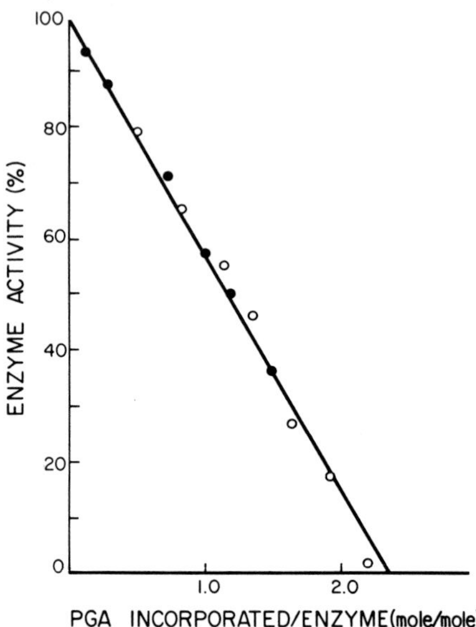

Fig. 9. Relationship between thymidylate synthetase activity and the moles of [^{14}C]phenylglyoxal fixed per mole of enzyme.

arginine residue per two subunits of enzyme are essential for activity when it is considered that the binding of the anionic substrate, dUMP, to cysteine 198 should be greatly stabilized by the proximity of a cationic arginine residue. Recent ^{31}P nmr studies by Beckage *et al.* (56) reveal that the pK_a of the phosphate in the dUMP–thymidylate complex is less that 5.0, relative to that of dUMP alone, which is 6.25. Thus, at the optimal pH of the reaction, the

TABLE VII

Phenylglyoxal Modification of Thymidylate Synthetase

Conditions	Incubation time (minutes)	Arginine residues modified[a]	[^{14}C]PGA incorporated[b]
Without dUMP	30	3.2	6.0
	60	4.2	8.8
With dUMP	30	2.2 (1.0)	4.2
	60	3.2 (1.0)	7.0

[a] From residues of arginine per mole of enzyme; figures in parentheses represent the number of arginine residues (determined by amino acid analysis) protected by dUMP per mole of enzyme.

[b] Moles of phenylglyoxal incorporated per mole of enzyme.

dianionic form of dUMP should predominate and greatly enhance its interaction with the phenylglyoxal-sensitive arginine. The location of the latter residue is currently under investigation.

B. Studies on Clarifying the Folate-Binding Site

Since the enzyme was not protected from the deleterious effects of the arginine-modifying reagents by 5,10-CH_2H_4PteGlu (55) or PteGlu (57), the influence of these compounds on protecting the enzyme from diethylpyrocarbonate was examined. In the presence of this compound, a progressive loss of activity was encountered until, at the point where 8 moles of histidine per mole of enzyme were destroyed, no enzyme activity remained. Neither dUMP nor PteGlu could prevent the loss in enzyme activity, which was somewhat surprising in view of the presence of a histidine residue adjacent to cysteine 198.

To pursue the question of which sites might be involved in folate binding, Pte[^{14}C]Glu_7 was activated by a water-soluble carbodiimide (58) in the hope that the folate would couple specifically to its binding site. As shown in Fig. 10, the folate was fixed at a ratio of 2 moles/mole of enzyme providing dUMP was present in the reaction mixture. Since in the absence of dUMP even greater amounts of folate are fixed, it appears that the nucleotide enhances the specificity of the reaction. The extent to which the Pte[^{14}C]Glu_7 was incorporated into protein is shown in the inset in Fig. 10, where it is seen that about half of the radioactivity was associated with the protein in the void volume of the gel filtration column. On treatment of this protein with proteolytic enzymes a labeled peptide was obtained, which should on sequencing reveal its location within the structure of the enzyme. However, it should be cautioned that the unreduced

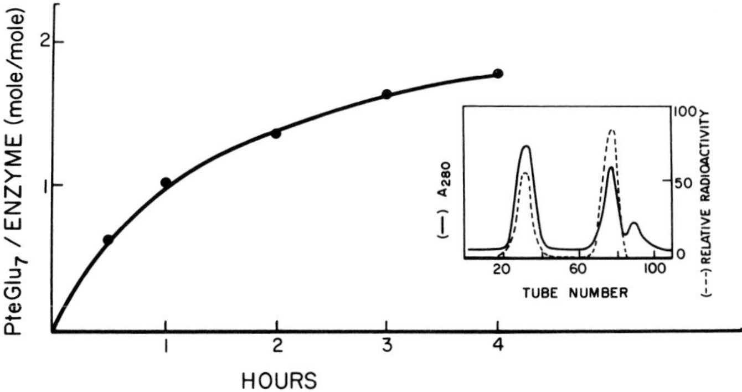

Fig. 10. Fixation of Pte[^{14}C]Glu$[Glu]_6$ to *L. casei* thymidylate synthetase in the presence of dUMP and a water-soluble carbodiimide. The inset indicates the extent to which the labeled folate is associated with the protein in the void volume of the Sexphadex G-100 column and that which is retarded by the column elution procedure.

folylpolyglutamates may not bind to the same site as the corresponding reduced folate substrate. Some evidence on this point has been presented already, which indicates that the synthetase from human leukemia cells may have two distinct folate-binding sites (40) and, as shown in Fig. 4, $PteGlu_6$ behaves as a noncompetitive inhibitor with respect to 5,10-CH_2H_4PteGlu. Further clarification of this question is necessary and is currently under investigation.

Acknowledgments

Our appreciation is expressed to Drs. Ronald Bellisario, Marlene Belfort, and Charles Baugh, and to Judith Reidl and Don Guarino for their invaluable contributions. This work was supported in part by United States Public Health Service grants GM-20371 and GM-26387, in addition to PCM 77-24662 from the National Science Foundation.

References

1. R. Duschinsky, E. Plevan, and C. Heidelberger, *J. Am. Chem. Soc.* **79,** 4559 (1957).
2. M. Friedken and A. Kornberg, in "Chemical Basis of Heredity" (W. D. McElroy and B. Glass, eds.), p. 609. Johns Hopkins Press, Baltimore, Maryland, 1957.
3. S. S. Cohen, J. G. Flaks, H. D. Barner, M. R. Loeb, and J. Lichtenstein, *Proc. Natl. Acad. Sci. U.S.A.* **44,** 1004 (1958).
4. P. B. Dannenberg, B. J. Montag, and C. Heidelberger, *Cancer Res.* **18,** 329 (1958).
5. L. Bosch, E. Habers, and C. Heidelberger, *Cancer Res.* **18,** 355 (1958).
6. C. Heidelberger. *in* "Cancer Medicine" (J. F. Holland and E. Frei, III, eds.), p. 768. Lea & Febiger, Philadelphia, Pennsylvania, 1973.
7. 8. Ullman, M. Lea, D. Martin, Jr., and D. V. Santi, *Proc. Natl. Acad. Sci. U.S.A.* **75,** 980 (1978).
8. E. Cadman, R. Heimer, and L. Davis, *Science* **205,** 1135 (1979).
9. H. G. Mandel, *Prog. Mol. Subcell. Biol.* **1,** 82 (1969).
10. D. S. Wilkinson, R. D. Tlsty, and R. J. Hanas, *Cancer Res.* **35,** 3014 (1975).
11. C. K. Mathews and S. S. Cohen, *J. Biol. Chem.* **238,** 367 (1963).
12. M. Y. Lorenson, G. F. Maley, and F. Maley, *J. Biol. Chem.* **242,** 3332 (1967).
13. P. Reyes and C. Heidelberger, *Mol. Pharmacol.* **1,** 14 (1965).
14. C. E. Myers, R. C. Young, D. G. Johns, and B. A. Chabner, *Cancer Res.* **34,** 2686 (1974).
15. R. J. Bonney and F. Maley, *Cancer Res.* **35,** 1950 (1975).
16. R. B. Dunlap, N. G. L. Harding, and F. M. Huennekens, *Biochemistry* **10,** 88 (1971).
17. R. P. Leary and R. L. Kisliuk, *Prep. Biochem.* **1,** 47 (1971).
18. A. Fridland, R. J. Langenbach, and C. Heidelberger, *J. Biol. Chem.* **246,** 7100 (1971).
19. B. J. Dolnick and Y. C. Cheng, *J. Biol. Chem.* **252,** 7697, (1977).
20. H. Horinishi and D. Greenberg, *Biochim. Biophys. Acta* **258,** 741 (1972).
21. J. Galivan, G. F. Maley, and F. Maley, *Biochemistry* **13,** 2282 (1974).
22. H. H. Daron and J. L. Aull, *J. Biol. Chem.* **253,** 940 (1978).
23. P. V. Danenberg, R. J. Langenbach, and C. Heidelberger, *Biochemistry* **13,** 927 (1974).
24. D. V. Santi, C. S. McHenry, and H. Sommer, *Biochemistry* **13,** 471 (1974).
25. J. L. Aull, J. A. Lyon, and R. B. Dunlap, *Michrochem. J.* **19,** 210 (1974).
26. R. P. Leary, N. Beaudette, and R. L. Kisliuk, *J. Biol. Chem.* **250,** 4864 (1975).

27. H. Donato Jr., J. L. Aull, J. A. Lyon, J. W. Reinsch, and R. B. Dunlap, *J. Biol. Chem.* **251,** 1303 (1976).
28. R. K. Sharma and R. L. Kisliuk, *Biochem. Biophys. Res. Commun.* **64,** 648 (1975).
29. J. H. Galivan, G. F. Maley, and F. Maley, *Biochemistry* **14,** 338 (1975).
30. T. L. James, A. L. Pogolotti, K. M. Ivanetich, Y. Wataya, S. S. M. Lam, and D. V. Santi, *Biochem. Biophys. Res. Commun.* **72,** 404 (1976).
31. R. Langenbach, *Biochim. Biophys. Acta* **422,** 295 (1976).
32. P. V. Danenberg and K. D. Danenberg, *Biochemistry* **17,** 4018 (1978).
33. J. H. Galivan, G. F. Maley, and F. Maley, *Biochemistry* **15,** 356 (1976).
34. J. H. Galivan, F. Maley, and C. M. Baugh, *Biochem. Biophys. Res. Commun.* **71,** 527 (1976).
35. N. V. Beaudette, N. Langerman, R. L. Kisliuk, and Y. Gaumont, *Arch. Biochem. Biophys.* **179,** 272 (1977).
36. A. Levitzski, W. B. Stallcup, and D. E. Koshland, Jr., *Biochemistry* **10,** 3371 (1971).
37. R. L. Kisliuk, Y. Gaumont, and C. M. Baugh, *J. Biol. Chem.* **249,** 4100 (1974).
38. J. Galivan, F. Maley, and C. M. Baugh, *Arch. Biochem. Biophys.* **184,** 346 (1977).
39. J. L. Aull, R. B. Loeble, and R. B. Dunlap, *J. Biol. Chem.* **249,** 1167 (1974).
40. B. J. Dolnick and Y. C. Cheng, *J. Biol. Chem.* **253,** 3563 (1978).
41. R. L. Kisliuk, Y. Gaumont, C. M. Baugh, J. H. Galivan, G. F. Maley, and F. Maley, in *Developments in Biochemistry* (R. L. Kisluik and G. M. Brown eds.) Vol. 4, p. 431. Elsevier/North Holland, Amsterdam, (1979).
42. G. F. Maley, F. Maley, and C. M. Baugh, *J. Biol. Chem.* **254,** 7485 (1979).
43. G. F. Maley, R. L. Bellisario, D. U. Guarino, and F. Maley, *J. Biol. Chem.* **254,** 1301 (1979).
44. A. L. Pogolotti and D. V. Santi, *Bioorg. Chem.* **1,** 277 (1977).
45. T. I. Kalman, *Biochemistry* **10,** 2567 (1971).
46. J. H. Galivan, J. Noonan, and F. Maley, *Arch. Biochem. Biophys.* **184,** 336 (1977).
47. P. C. Plese and R. B. Dunlap, *J. Biol. Chem.* **252,** 6139 (1977).
48. K. D. Danenberg and P. V. Danenberg, *J. Biol. Chem.* **254,** 4345 (1979).
49. R. L. Bellisario, G. F. Maley, J. H. Galivan, and F. Maley, *Proc. Natl. Acad. Sci. U.S.A.* **73,** 1848 (1976).
50. G. F. Maley, R. L. Bellisario, D. U. Guarino, and F. Maley, *J. Biol. Chem.* **254,** 1288 (1979).
51. A. L. Pogolotti, K. M. Ivanetich, H. Sommer, and D. V. Santi, *Biochem. Biophys. Res. Commun.* **70,** 972 (1976).
52. R. L. Bellisario, G. F. Maley, D. U. Guarino, and F. Maley, *J. Biol. Chem.* **254,** 1296 (1979).
53. K. Takahashi, *J. Biol. Chem.* **243,** 6171 (1968).
54. E. W. Miles, *in* "Methods in Enzymology" (C. H. W. Hirs, ed.), Vol. 47, p. 6171. Academic Press, New York, 1977.
55. K. L. Cipollo and R. B. Dunlap, *Biochem. Biophys. Res. Commun.* **81,** 1139 (1978).
56. M. J. Beckage, M. Blumenstein, and R. L. Kisluik, *Biochem. Biophys. Acta* **571,** 157 (1979).
57. M. Belfort, G. F. Maley, and F. Maley, *Arch. Biochem. Biophys.,* **204,** 340 (1980).
58. B. C. F. Chu and J. M. Whiteley, *Mol. Pharmacol.* **13,** 80 (1977).

14

Inhibition of Thymidylate Synthetase: Mechanism, Methods, and Metabolic Consequences

DANIEL V. SANTI

I. Introduction

Thymidylate (dTMP) synthetase (EC 2.1.1.45) catalyzes the reductive methylation of 2′-deoxyuridylate (dUMP) to dTMP, with concomitant conversion of 5,10-methylenetetrahydrofolate (CH_2H_4folate) to 7,8-dihydrofolate (H_2folate). This enzyme is unique among those which utilize H_4 folate cofactors in that CH_2-H_4folate serves the dual function of both one-carbon donor and reductant. As a result, the synthesis of dTMP (Eq. 1)

$$\text{dUMP} + CH_2\text{-}H_4\text{folate} \rightarrow H_2\ \text{folate} + \text{dTMP} \qquad (1)$$

consumes an equivalent amount of H_4folate, and the dihydrofolate reductase-

MOLECULAR ACTIONS AND TARGETS FOR CANCER CHEMOTHERAPEUTIC AGENTS

ISBN 0-12-619280-4

catalyzed conversion of H_2folate to H_4folate is required for continued dTMP synthesis as well as for purine nucleotide biosynthesis. Various aspects of this enzyme have been extensively reviewed (1–3). Since dTMP synthetase represents the sole *de novo* pathway for dTMP synthesis, it is not surprising that it has been of major interest as a target of anticancer agents. In this chapter, a review is presented of the most pertinent inhibitors of this enzyme, as well as their mechanism of action. Consideration is also given to possible methods of manipulating the metabolic consequences of the *in vivo* action of important precursors of such inhibitors.

II. Analogs of dUMP as Inhibitors of Thymidylate Synthetase

A. Reversible Inhibitors

Although a systematic study of the structural features involved in the binding of dUMP analogs to dTMP synthetase has not been performed, certain generalizations may be gleaned from known, effective inhibitors. The ensuing is specifically directed toward factors involved in the formation of *reversible* enzyme inhibitor complexes which do not involve covalent bond formation; some of the inhibitors undergo subsequent covalent bond formation with the enzyme and are considered in detail later in this chapter. It is relevant to the discussion here that the affinity of many dUMP analogues for dTMP synthetase appears to be enhanced by the presence of CH_2-H_4folate or folate analogues (4,5). That is, the affinity of binary enzyme inhibitor complexes (E–I) may be equal to or lower than that of corresponding ternary complexes (E–I–CH_2-H_4folate). The structural features of dUMP analogs which govern this synergism are currently unknown. The K_d values of binary enzyme–dUMP analogue complexes are most accurately determined by equilibrium binding methods [e.g., equilibrium dialysis (4)] but may be approximated kinetically as K_i values using the enzyme-catalyzed dehalogenation of bromodeoxyuridylate in the absence of CH_2-H_4folate (5). The K_d of the ternary complex is most easily approximated as the K_i of the dUMP analog in the normal enzymatic reaction using high concentrations of the cofactor CH_2-H_4folate (5). Unless otherwise specified, K_i values reported here have been determined by initial velocity experiments of dTMP formation.

From what is currently known, the 5′-phospho-2′-deoxyribosyl-, the 2-keto, and the 3-NH moieties of dUMP analogs appear to be important for the binding of dUMP analogs to dTMP synthetase. Virtually all modifications of these moieties lead to a decrease in affinity for the enzyme. 6-Substituted dUMP analogues have not been examined as inhibitors or substrates of this enzyme but represent prime candidates for potential new inhibitors. Almost all chemical modifications at the 4-position of dUMP result in tautomerization of the heterocycle to the "enol" form and loss of the 3-NH group essential for reversible binding. Thus, in general, 4-substituted dUMP analogues have not provided potent inhibitors of dTMP synthetase. The one exception to this is N^4-hydrox-2′-deoxycytidylate (N^4-HO-dCMP). When assayed rapidly, this compound is a potent competitive inhibitor with $K_i = 1 \mu M$ (6). Interestingly, upon incubation, the inhibition becomes noncompetitive with respect to dUMP, suggesting a time-dependent inactivation of the enzyme. The mechanism of inhibition of N^4-HO-dCMP has not been investigated in detail, but it is possible that it ultimately forms a covalent bond with the enzyme as described later.

The most extensively studied inhibitors of dTMP synthetase are 5-substituted derivatives of dUMP. Once reversibly bound to the enyzme, many of these compounds undergo subsequent reactions which make them much more potent inhibitors. Nevertheless, a number of observations have emerged which point out factors important for reversible binding to this enzyme.

It has been recognized for some time that electron-withdrawing groups at the 5-position of dUMP enhance the affinity of such analogs for the enzyme (5,7,8). This is illustrated in Table I, which shows reversible K_i values of a number of 5-substituted derivatives of dUMP as inhibitors of *Lactobacillus casei* dTMP synthetase. Multiple regression analysis of these values has provided the following equation:

$$\log 1/K_i = 1.58(\pm 1.17)\sigma^- + 3.49(\pm 2.33)\mathscr{F} - 1.43(\pm 1.11)MR + 5.88(\pm 0.84) \quad (2)$$

which relates the experimentally determined K_i values to physical properties of the 5-substituent (5). It is noted that the K_i values used to derive Eq. (2) were

TABLE I

Inhibition of Thymidylate Synthetase by 5-Substituted Derivations of dUMP and QSAR-Calculated Values[a]

Compound	5-Substituent	K_i (μM)	Log $1/K_i$, obsd	Log $1/K_i$, calcd
dTMP	CH_3	15.5	4.80	4.67
$HOCH_2$-dUMP	CH_2OH	8.3	5.08	4.84
dUMP	H	5.2	5.29	5.73
IdUMP	I	1.6	5.79	5.56
BrdUMP	Br	1.4	5.85	6.50
CldUMP	Cl	0.19	6.72	6.81
CF_3-dUMP	CF_3	0.039	7.41	7.51
FdUMP	F	0.014	7.85	7.33
CHO-dUMP	CHO	0.017	7.77	7.75

[a] Data taken from Wataya *et al.* (5); all inhibitors were competitive with respect to dUMP.

obtained in the standard assay containing CH_2-H_4folate; all K_i values obtained in the absence of CH_2H_4 folate were in the range of about 1–10 μM and could not be correlated.

The first and second most important variables in Eq. (2) are σ and $\mathcal{F}$, respectively. The positive coefficients associated with these terms indicate that electron withdrawal from the uracil heterocycle is the *most* important factor in enhancing the affinity of these analogues for the enzyme. The manifestations of electron withdrawal directly responsible for the different affinities of the inhibitors are unknown but likely are a result of increasing the acidity of the 3-NH group and affecting the electronic properties of the heterocycle. The other important factor in inhibition of dTMP formation by 5-substituted nucleotides is the size of the 5-substituent; from the quantitative structure–activity relationship (QSAR) in Eq. (2), it appears that larger 5-substitutents are more detrimental to binding. The hydrophobicity of the substituents examined does not appear to play an important role in affinity of the analog for the enzyme–H_4 folate complex. It is of interest to note that the factors involved in the binding of 5-substituted 2′-deoxyuridylates to thymidylate synthetase, which we are able to ascertain with QSAR, are analogous to some which were proposed by empirical observations of a few similar inhibitors (7–9).

The aforementioned QSAR provides insight into the binding of 5-substituted derivatives of dUMP to dTMP synthetase but should not be considered final. As more data become available, the equation will almost certainly be expanded or modified. However, it does provide a useful starting point for future design of inhibitors. For example, Eq. (2) was used to calculate that NO_2-dUMP should have a K_i value of 0.54×10^{-8} M, and when this compound was examined the apparent K_i value was about 2×10^{-8} M (10,11). While at first glance this appears to support the validity of the QSAR relationship, the K_i of NO_2-dUMP was not affected by the presence of CH_2-H_4folate. As previously noted, the QSAR described in Eq. (2) was developed using the standard assay and does not apply to interaction of these analogs in the absence of CH_2H_4 folate.

One of the more interesting reversible inhibitors of dTMP synthetase is 5-mercapto-dUMP, which has a reversible $K_i = 4 \times 10^{-8}$ M (7). This affinity is similar to those of 5-CF_3-, 5-F-, 5-CHO-, and 5-NO_2-dUMP; however, in contrast to these inhibitors, preincubation of 5-mercapto-dUMP does not alter the kinetic pattern of inhibition or decrease the K_i value. Thus 5-mercapto-dUMP is currently the most potent of all the strictly competitive inhibitors of this enzyme. It has been proposed that the high affinity of this compound for dTMP synthetase results from a favorable interaction of the ionized sulfhydryl group with a positively charged group of the enzyme.

B. Mechanism-Based Inhibitors

In recent years, there has been much interest in the development of mechanism-based inhibitors of enzymatic reactions. These inhibitors reversibly bind to the active site of an enzyme and then undergo events in a manner analogous to one or more steps of the normal catalytic reaction, ultimately leading to formation of a covalent E–I complex. Although the combined requirements of reversible binding and enzyme-induced covalent bond changes place restrictions on the design of such inhibitors, once these are fulfilled, the resultant inhibitors are extremely specific for their target enzymes. For optimal efficacy, mechanism-based inhibitors of dTMP synthetase should be derived from dUMP analogs which form tight, reversible complexes with the enzyme (Section II,A). Understanding of the subsequent changes which lead to the formation of covalent complexes requires consideration of the catalytic mechanism of the enzyme. The currently accepted minimal mechanism of dTMP synthetase is depicted in Fig. 1 (2,12). It is most relevant that an early event in catalysis involves attack of a nucleophile of the enzyme at the 6-position of dUMP; as a consequence, a variety of 5,6-dihydropyrimidine intermediates are formed which

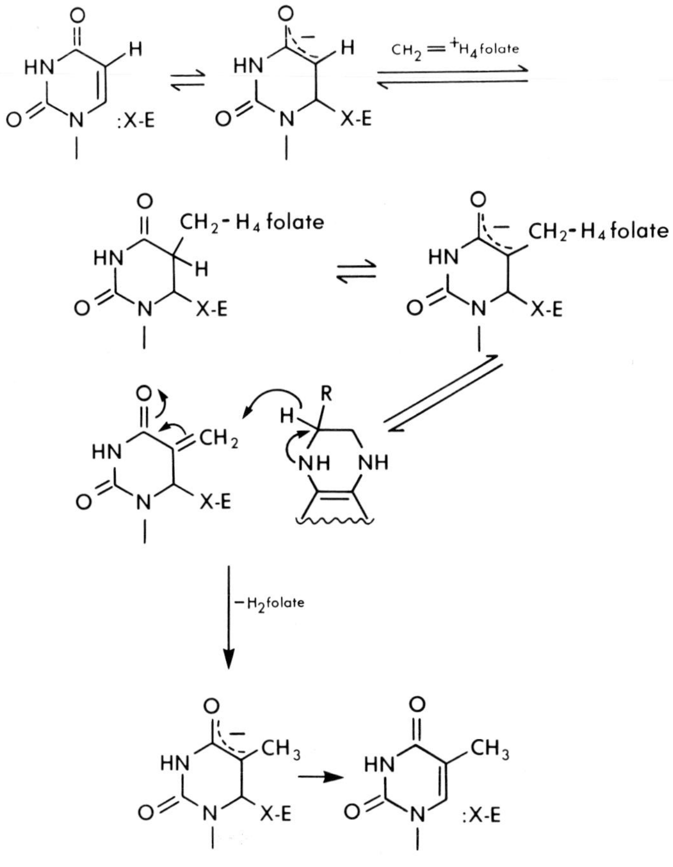

Fig. 1. Catalytic mechanism of dTMP synthetase.

remain covalently bound to the enzyme throughout the catalytic sequence and serve to activate moieties of dUMP which normally are inert. This early step of the reaction provides the basis for the design and action of mechanism-based inhibitors of this enzyme. After formation of a noncovalent reversible complex, a nucleophile of the enzyme attacks the 6-position of the heterocycle of the inhibitor in a manner directly analogous to the normal enzymatic reaction. The inhibitors remain covalently attached to the nucleophile of the enzyme; covalent bond formation may activate a latent chemically reactive group at the 5-position of the heterocycle which subsequently inactivates the enzyme.

1. *5-Fluoro-2′-deoxyuridylate (FdUMP)*

The prototype mechanism-based inhibitor of dTMP synthetase is FdUMP (2,3). In the presence of the cofactor, CH_2-H_4folate, this compound rapidly reacts with the enzyme in a manner analogous to the first two steps depicted in Fig. 1. At this stage, the C-5 proton of the covalently bound dUMP is removed in the normal enzymatic reaction; however, as shown in Fig. 2, the C—F bond of the analogous intermediate formed with FdUMP cannot be broken, and what may be considered an analog of a steady-state intermediate accumulates. In this tight ternary complex ($K_d \simeq 10^{-13}$ M), the 6-position of FdUMP and a nucleophile of the enzyme are covalently bound, and the cofactor, CH_2-H_4folate, is linked to the 5-position of FdUMP. In the absence of the cofactor, binding of FdUMP is noncovalent and weak ($K_i \simeq 10^{-5}$ M). In the presence of CH_2-H_4folate, 2 equivalents of FdUMP are bound to dTMP synthetase, one per subunit of the dimeric enzyme of molecular weight 70,000. Reversal of covalent bond formation is slow ($t_{1/2} \simeq 10$ hours at 25°C) and requires integrity of the 3° structure of the enzyme. When the complex is treated with protein denaturants, covalent bonds appear to be indefinitely stable. However, the complex irreversibly dissociates upon heat treatment (e.g., 65°C, 15 minutes) (13). This results from rapid dissociation of the ligands at higher temperature and subsequent denaturation of the free enzyme.

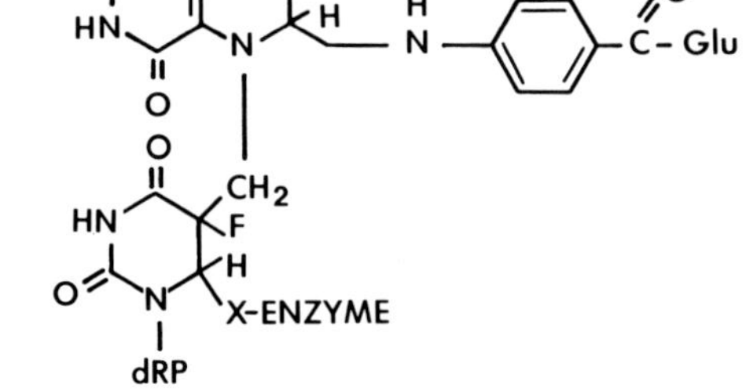

Fig. 2. Structure of the FdUMP-CH_2-H_4folate-dTMP synthetase complex.

2. *5-Trifluoromethyl-2′-deoxyuridylate (CF_3-dUMP) and trans-5-(3,3,3,-Trifluoro-1-propenyl)-2′-deoxyuridylate ($CF_3CH{=}CH$-dUMP)*

CF_3-dUMP, a potent inhibitor of dTMP synthetase, has been reported to modify irreversibly the enzyme from Ehrlich ascites cells (14). Although C—F bonds are generally quite strong, a number of compounds have been reported to have labile C—F linkages. These were summarized in a report in 1973 (15) in which a common feature of most of the C—F bond cleavages was recognized; when a transient or stable negative charge exists on the carbon adjacent to a C—F bond, β-elimination of fluoride ion may occur.

The activation of CF_3 moieties of 1-substituted 5-CF_3- and 5-$CF_3CH{=}CH$-uracils has been shown to proceed by the mechanism depicted in Scheme I, which shows the pathway leading to hydrolysis of the CF_3 moiety of

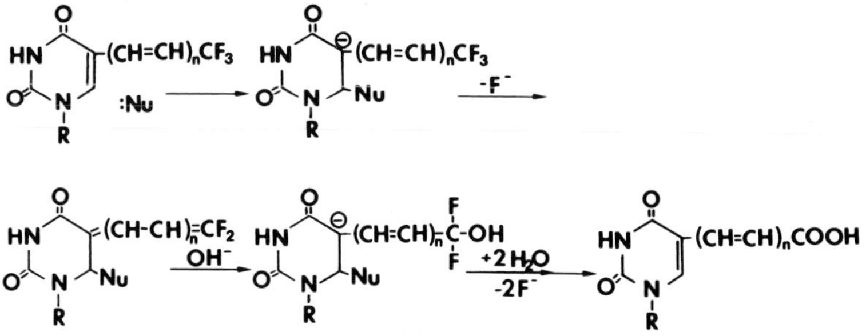

Scheme I

such compounds (16,17). The first step involves addition of a nucleophile to the 6-position to generate an incipient negative charge at C-5. This modification activates the latently reactive CF_3 group which undergoes a series of elimination–addition reactions to provide the corresponding carboxylic acid or acylated nucleophile. Regarding the interaction of CF_3dUMP with dTMP synthetase, it is clear that the normally inert CF_3 group would behave as an acylating agent or be hydrolyzed *only* when a nucleophile is first added to the 6-position of the heterocycle to produce a transient carbanion at C-5. Currently, the exact mechanism of interaction of CF_3-dUMP and dTMP synthetase is poorly understood, but it is clear that nucleophilic attack at the 6-position of CF_3-dUMP, fluoride ion release, and activation of the CF_3 moiety are catalyzed by dTMP synthetase (18). As with CF_3-dUMP, $CF_3CH{=}CH$-dUMP also irreversibly inactivates dTMP synthetase (17). When variable excess amounts of $CF_3CH{=}CH$-dUMP are incubated with dTMP synthetase at 25°C, there is a first-order decrease in enzyme activity which can be protected by dUMP. Kinetic analyses of such data have demonstrated that, in the absence of cofactor, the dissociation constant of the reversible E–I complex is 2.5×10^{-5} *M* and that the unimolecular rate constant for inactivation is 0.133 min^{-1}. As with CF_3-dUMP, difference spectra indicate that the CF_3 moiety has been transformed by the enzyme to an acyl derivative. While these results are too preliminary to allow definitive mechanistic conclusions, they clearly demonstrate an irreversible or pseudo-irreversible inhibition of dTMP synthetase initiated by nucleophilic attack at the 6-position of $CF_3CH{=}CH$-dUMP. It is likely that the mechanism of inhibition by this analogue is similar to that of CF_3-dUMP.

3. *5-Nitro-2′-deoxyuridylate (NO_2dUMP)*

We have recently reported (10), that NO_2-dUMP forms a reversible complex with dTMP synthetase, with an apparent $K_i \simeq 2 \times 10^{-8}\ M$. Since the electron-withdrawing NO_2 moiety also polarizes the 6-position of the heterocycle, it was anticipated that nucleophilic attack at that site would be facilitated. Indeed, 1,3-dimethyl-5-NO_2-uracil and NO_2-dUMP react with a variety of nucleophiles at the 6-position to form the corresponding 5,6-dihydropyrimidines with favorable equilibrium constants. Two groups have independently reported that NO_2-dUMP rapidly inactivates dTMP synthetase (10,11). At 25°C, at least 80% of enzyme activity is lost within 1 minute (Fig. 3), and at 0°C the half-life of the first-order inactivation at saturating NO_2-dUMP is about 13 minutes. It was not experimentally feasible to obtain complete inactivation kinetics even at 0°C, and dUMP was included in the reaction mixture to slow the reaction. The results of such experiments are shown in Fig. 3. Two relevant points emerged from these experiments. First, it is clear that dUMP protects the enzyme against inactivation by NO_2-dUMP, which suggests that the inhibitor binds at the same site as the substrate. Second, the inactivation of dTMP synthetase by NO_2-dUMP clearly follows first-order kinetics, indicative of reversible binding of the inhibitor, followed by irreversible (or pseudoirreversible) inhibition. The fact that the nucleoside 5-NO_2-dUrd does *not* inactivate the enzyme (10) supports the notion that NO_2-dUMP acts upon the active site of the enzyme, since it has been well-established that the 5′-phosphate moiety of nucleotides is required for binding to the active site of this enzyme.

Further evidence that structural changes occur in the heterocycle of NO_2-dUMP was obtained by uv difference spectra (10). The difference spectrum of enzyme and NO_2-dUMP versus enzyme shows that the λ_{max} of bound NO_2-dUMP is 11 nm higher than that of NO_2-dUMP in a reaction buffer containing 6 m*M* dithiothreitol (λ_{max} 326 versus 337 nm). When the samples are subsequently treated with sodium dodecyl sulfate, there is a rapid, albeit observable, reversion of the difference spectra to one identical to that of NO_2-dUMP, and NO_2-dUMP can be recovered unchanged. The covalently bound NO_2-dUMP is not irreversibly modified, and the covalent bond can readily be disrupted when the enzyme is denatured. While this is expected based on model studies, it is in contrast to the FdUMP–CH_2H_4 folate–enzyme complex in which denaturation stabilizes the covalent bonds. We have also observed that dissociation of the NO_2-[2-^{14}C,6-

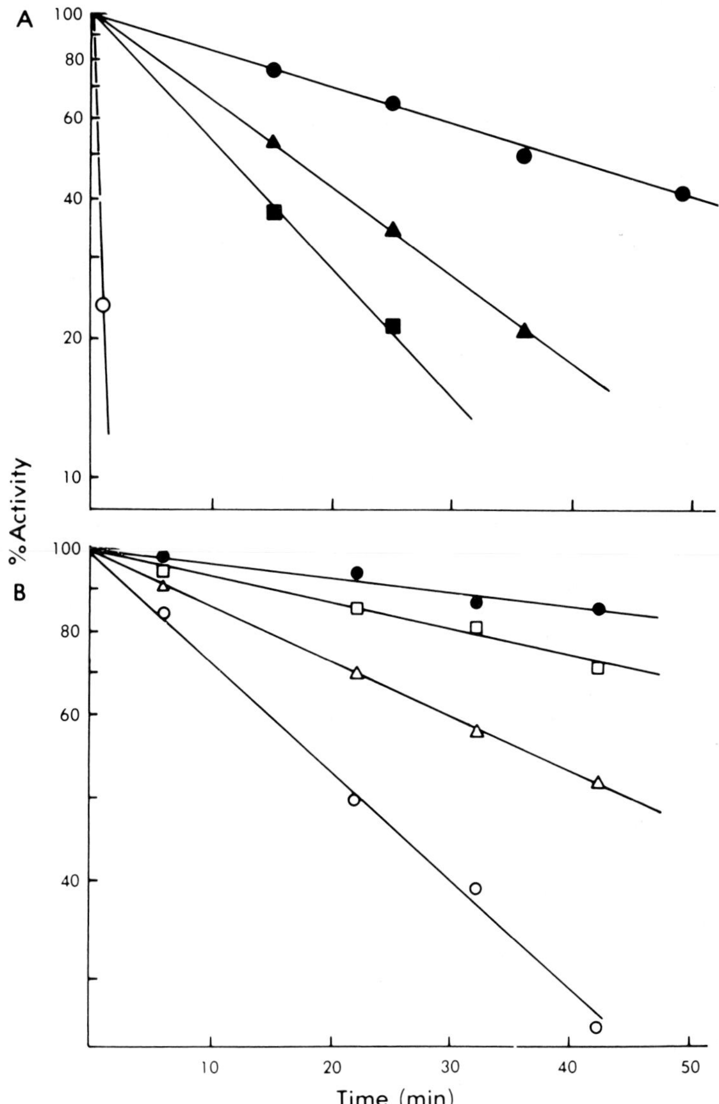

Fig. 3. (A) Inactivation of dTMP plus NO_2dUMP at concentrations of 0.6 μM (●), 1.1 μM (▲), and 1.7 μM (■). (B) 0.3 μM NO_2-dUMP plus dUMP at concentrations of 0.19 mM (○), 0.37 mM (△), 0.55 mM (□), and 0.92 mM (●).

^{3}H]dUMP–dTMP synthetase complex proceeds with a secondary isotope effect of $k_H/k_T = 1.18$ (unpublished results); this demonstrates that within the covalent complex the 6-carbon of NO_2-dUMP is sp^3-hybridized as it would be if a nucleophile of the enzyme were covalently attached at this position. An important difference between FdUMP and NO_2-dUMP inhibition is that the interaction of NO_2dUMP with dTMP synthetase neither requires nor is facilitated by the presence of the cofactor, CH_2H_4 folate.

Taken together, these data support the mechanism of inhibition shown in Fig. 4. Simply stated, once a reversible complex has been formed, the active site nucleophile adds to the 6-position of NO_2-dUMP to form a tight but reversible covalent bond. A large portion of the driving force for the overall reaction is probably provided by reversible interactions ($\triangle G^{\circ} \simeq 10$ kcal), and denaturation of the protein results in a less stable covalent bond.

4. *4-Hydroxy-2′-deoxycytidylate (*N^4*-HO-dCMP)*

This compound was reported to be a competitive inhibitor of dTMP synthetase from chick embryo, but on incubation it showed noncompetitive kinetics (6). This pattern of competitive changing to noncompetitive inhibition has been observed for *all* mechanism-based inhibitors of dTMP synthetase thus far reported. While not proven, it is possible, perhaps likely, that N^4-HO-dCMP is also a mechanism-based inhibitor of dTMP synthetase.

5. *5-Formyl-2′-deoxyuridylate (CHO-dUMP)*

This compound is a potent reversible inhibitor of dTMP synthetase ($K_i \simeq 10^{-8}$ M) and causes a time-dependent inactivation of the enzyme (19). Two possible mechanisms may be envisioned for this inactivation (Fig. 5). As originally proposed (19), the 5-formyl group may simply form a Schiff base with an amino group of the enzyme. Alternatively, and perhaps more likely, as with other mechanism-based inhibitors of dTMP synthetase, a nucleophile of the enzyme may form a covalent bond at the 6-position of the heterocycle; if this is the case, the 5-CHO group may or may not be involved in additional interactions. The mechanism of this inhibitor is currently being further investigated.

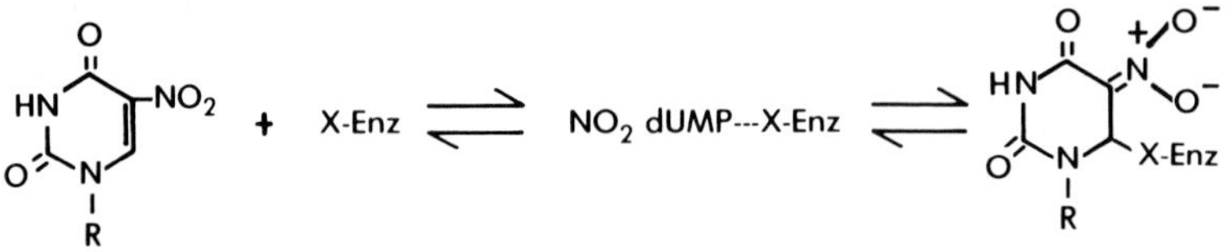

Fig. 4. Mechanism of interaction of NO_2-dUMP with dTMP synthetase.

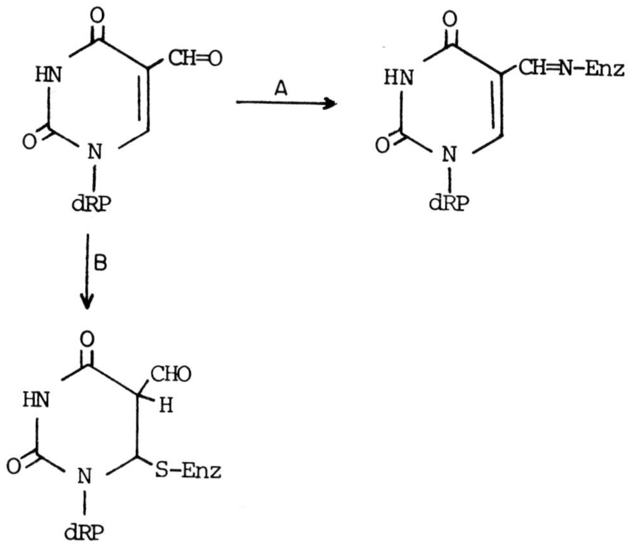

Fig. 5. Possible mechanisms for inhibition of dTMP synthetase by CHO-dUMP: (A) formation of Shiff base; (B) covalent bond formation at C-6 with sulfhydryl group of enzyme.

III. Metabolic Manipulation of the Action of 5-Fluorouracil

In this section consideration is given to approaches which might be used to alter the metabolism and/or action of the anticancer agent 5-fluorouracil (FUra). It is becoming increasingly clear that the cytotoxicity of FUra may result from its incorporation into RNA, or through FdUMP inhibition of dTMP synthetase (13,19,20). Furthermore, the mechanism of FUra action may vary in different cells or under different metabolic conditions. Thus it may be possible to amplify or alter FUra action in specific cells by exploiting quantitative differences in enzymes involved in its metabolism and differing susceptibilities of cells toward the effects of FdUMP inhibition of dTMP synthetase and FUra incorporation into RNA.

The metabolism of FUra is shown in Scheme II. Three enzymes can readily be identified as primary targets for amplifying or altering the metabolism of FUra:

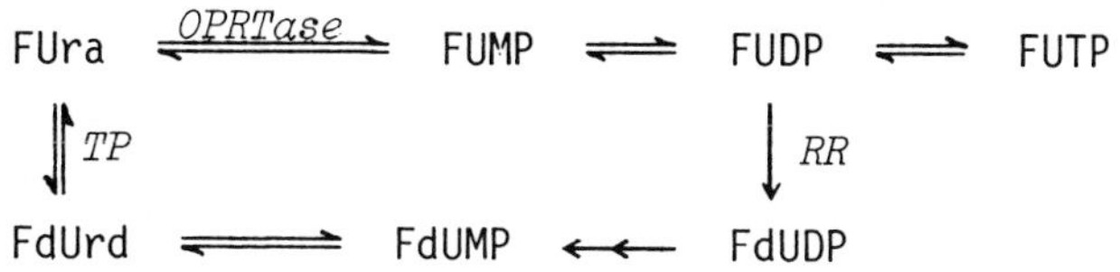

FUra $\underset{}{\overset{OPRTase}{\rightleftharpoons}}$ FUMP $\rightleftharpoons$ FUDP $\rightleftharpoons$ FUTP

FUra $\updownarrow$ *TP* FdUrd; FUDP $\downarrow$ *RR* FdUDP

FdUrd $\rightleftharpoons$ FdUMP $\leftarrow$ FdUDP

thymidine phosphoprylase (TP), orotidine phosphoribosyltransferase (OPRTase), and ribonucleotide reductase (RR). In addition, alterations in H_4

folate pools can effect the action of FUra. The rationale for choosing and manipulating these targets is outlined below.

A. Thymidine Phosphorylase

This enzyme catalyzes the reversible conversion of thymine (Thy) and 2-deoxyribose 1-phosphate (dR-1-P) to thymidine and P_i [Eg. (3)]; it also utilizes FUra and FdUrd as substrates. It has primary importance in the catabolism of FdUrd, but if suitable donors of dR-1-P could be supplied, the

$$\begin{array}{l} \text{Thy} + \text{dR-1-P} \rightleftharpoons \text{dThd} + P_i \\ \text{(FUra)} \qquad\qquad\qquad \text{(FdUrd)} \end{array} \tag{3}$$

metabolism of FUra might be "pushed" toward FdUrd and subsequently to FdUMP rather than FUMP. This would result in an increase in the FdUMP/FUTP ratio and would favor inhibition of dTMP synthetase rather than FUra RNA incorporation. Purine-2′-deoxyribonucleosides which are substrates for purine nucleoside phosphorylase might provide sufficiently high levels of dR-1-P to effect this shunt in the metabolism of FUra. Alternatively, substrates of dThd phosphorylase (e.g., dUrd or 5-substituted derivatives of dUrd) could serve as direct donors of the 2′-deoxyribosyl moiety to FUra (21,22). It should be noted that levels of dThd phosphorylase vary in different tissues of animals and humans (23). Thus, if this enzyme could be exploited in directing the metabolism of FUra, it may be possible to achieve tissue selectivity in the action of this drug.

B. Orotidine Phosphoribosyltransferase

This enzyme represents the major pathway for conversion of FUra into FUMP, and in most cells the major route for metabolism of FUra to its corresponding nucleotides. This pathway is not a branch point in the metabolism of FUra and should *not* alter the FdUMP/FUTP ratio or the relative effects on RNA and dTMP synthetase of this drug. However, since different cells may vary in the rate in which FUra is converted to FUMP, changes in the *in vivo* activity of this enzyme may amplify the effect of FUra and, in effect, provide some degree of selectivity. Theoretically, the conversion of FUra to FUMP may be increased or decreased by manipulating the supply of the natural substrates of OPRTase. It may be increased by inducing *increases* in the levels of 5-phosphoribosyl 1-pyrophosphate (PRPP), the second substrate of the reaction, and/or *decreasing* the levels of orotic acid, thereby decreasing competition of FUra for the natural pyrimidine acceptor of PRPP.

Increases in PRPP may be induced by administration of suitable precursors or by manipulating the metabolism of PRPP. For example, it has recently been reported that exposure of cells to a combination of FUra and Methotrexate (MTX) results in a significant synergistic effect on the number of L1210 cells killed in culture (24). It has also been found that MTX causes an increase in the intracellular concentrations of FUra nucleotides and in the incorporation of FUra into RNA. These changes were correlated with increased concentrations of PRPP. It was reasoned that MTX induced a state of H_4folate depletion sufficient to inhibit purine nucleotide biosynthesis; the resultant increase in PRPP levels stimulated conversion of FUra to FUMP via OPRTase. As H_4folate depletion also diminishes the FdUMP inhibition of dTMP synthetase (20), the MTX–FUra regimen would expectedly result in manifestation of the effect of FUra incorporation into RNA. It may be possible to increase intracellular PRPP levels without using MTX. This would avoid depleting cells of H_4folate and antagonizing the FdUMP inhibition of dTMP synthetase. For example, direct inhibition of purine nucleotide biosynthesis, at an early site which does not result in feedback inhibition of PRPP synthetase, should produce a similar accumulation of intracellular PRPP. It would be interesting to examine the effects of glutamine analogues [e.g., azaserine and diazonorleucine (25)], which inhibit two enzymes of purine nucleotide biosynthesis, and inhibitors of IMP dehydrogenase [e.g., myocophenolic acid (26)], on the metabolism and cytotoxicity of FUra. An alternate approach to increasing the net conversion of FUra to FUMP would be to deplete cells of the natural pyrimidine substrate orotic acid, which competes with FUra for OPRTase. This can be accomplished with the drug *N*-(phosphonoacetyl)-L-aspartate (PALA), a potent inhibitor of aspartate transcarbamoylase (27,28), the first enzyme of pyrimidine biosynthesis. Indeed, treatment of susceptible cells with PALA blocks the formation of orotic acid as well as uracil nucleotides, which would compete in the subsequent steps of FUra nucleotide metabolism. Interestingly, PALA is most cytotoxic toward cells which have low proliferative activity and has little effect on gastrointestinal epithelium and hematopoetic cells. As the latter cells represent major sites of FUra toxicity and, since FUra appears to be most effective against solid tumors, the PALA-FUra combination may provide an additional degree of selective toxicity. From the above, it may be anticipated that proper scheduling of a combination of PALA, MTX, and FUra would decrease orotic acid and increase PRPP levels; as a result, conversion of FUra to FUra nucleotides and incorporation of FUra into RNA would increase, and the effect of FdUMP inhibition of dTMP synthetase would be depressed as a result of H_4folate depletion. This combination might prove effective for treatment of solid tumors in which the FUra RNA is primarily responsible for the cytotoxic effect of FUra and spare cells in which FdUMP inhibition of dTMP synthetase is the initiating cytotoxic event.

Situations may also be envisioned where it would be desirable to reduce the conversion of FUra to FUMP. For example, if qualitative differences in pyrimidine phosphoribosyltransferase activities exist in normal and tumor cells, depression of FUMP formation in normal cells might reduce untoward toxic effects. Furthermore, if as previously described FUra may be converted to FdUMP via dThd phosphorylase, the effects of FUra incorporation into RNA might be reduced. A logical approach to reducing the metabolism of FUra to FUMP would simply involve inducing intracellular effects essentially opposite those described above which increase this conversion; that is, reducing intracellular PRPP pools and increasing the orotic acid levels should depress the conversion of FUra to FUMP. Reduction of PRPP levels could be achieved by administering a purine base which is a substrate for hypoxanthine-guanine phosphoribosyltransferase (HGPRTase). For example, guanine and hypoxanthine rapidly utilize PRPP in the HGPRTase-catalyzed conversion to their corresponding 5′-mononucleotides, and these further depress synthesis of PRPP by feedback inhibition of PRPP synthetase. In addition, as PRPP levels are depressed, orotic acid should accumulate and further inhibit the conversion of FUra to FUMP. An alternative approach to achieving high intracellular orotic acid levels would be to inhibit OMP decarboxylase, the last enzyme of *de novo* pyrimidine nucleotide biosynthesis, and thereby induce the accumulation of precursors of OMP. Chen and Jones (29) have demonstrated that treatment of Ehrlich ascites cells with 6-azauridine (6-aza-UMP), a potent inhibitor of OMP decarboxylase, results in the accumulation of large amounts of orotic acid. It would be interesting to ascertain the effect of this inhibitor on the metabolism of FUra.

C. Ribonucleotide Reductase

The major pathway by which FUra nucleotides diverge toward FUTP (and RNA incorporation) or FdUMP, with subsequent inhibition of dTMP synthetase, involves the enzyme ribonucleotide reductase. This single enzyme is responsible for the production of all 2′-deoxyribonucleotides; it catalyzes reduction of ribonucleoside 5′-diphosphates to corresponding 2′-deoxyribonucleotides, which are ultimately converted to the 5′-triphosphate precursors of DNA synthesis (30). What is most interesting about this enzyme is its intricate feedback control by deoxyribonucleoside 5′-phosphates. Through proper manipulation, it should be possible to increase or decrease the conversion of FUDP to FdUDP. In this manner, FUra could selectively be directed toward FdUMP or toward RNA incorporation. The reduction of UDP, and likely FUDP, is inhibited by dTTP, GTP, and dATP. Thus increased levels of these modifiers should depress reduction of FUDP, whereas decreased levels should enhance it. It should likewise be possible to increase the rate of FUDP reduction by depleting cells of dTTP and/or GTP, providing this can be accomplished without depleting cells of ATP which is a general positive effector of this enzyme. Approaches toward this objective are currently being investigated in our laboratory.

D. Tetrahydrofolate Cofactors

A quite different approach might be taken to amplify the action of FUra in cells or tissues in which FdUMP inhibition of dTMP synthetase is the primary cytotoxic action. As previously discussed, dTMP inhibition by FdUMP requires CH_2-H_4folate. This aspect of FUra action is antagonized by MTX, and it is reasonable to suggest that in such situations a folate cofactor (e.g., folinic acid) might be adiministered with FUra instead of the folate antagonist MTX. It may also be relevant that, as shown for L1210 cells, intracellular H_4folates can be sufficient for optimal growth but not for optimal inhibition of thymidylate synthetase by FdUMP (20). This relationship may vary in different cells for a number of reasons; for example, cells with higher levels of thymidylate synthetase would require higher concentrations of CH_2-H_4folate to achieve optimal inhibition of this enzyme by FdUMP. Thus the possibility exists that intracellular folate cofactors in tumors that are marginally responsive toward FUra may be sufficient for their optimal growth but not for effective inhibition of thymidylate synthetase by FdUMP. Should this be the case, administration of a reduced folate, such as folinic acid, might increase the effectiveness of thymidylate synthetase inhibition by FdUMP while H_4folate-independent effects of FUra would remain unchanged; it is possible that such tumors could be made more responsive toward FUra or FdUrd with a resultant increase in therapeutic index.

Acknowledgments

This work was supported by USPHS Grant CA-14394 from the National Cancer Institute. D.V.S. is the recipient of an NIH Career Development Award.

References

1. M. Friedkin, *Adv. Enzymol.* **38,** (1973).
2. A. L. Pogolotti, Jr. and D. V. Santi, *Bioorg. Chem.* **1,** 277 (1977).
3. P. V. Danenberg, *Biochim. Biophys. Acta* **473,** 73 (1977).
4. J. H. Galivan, G. F. Maley, and F. Maley, *Biochemistry* **13,** 471 (1974).
5. Y. Wataya, D. V. Santi, and C. Hansch, *J. Med. Chem.* **20,** 1469 (1977).
6. M. Y. Lorenson, G. F. Maley, and F. Maley, *J. Biol. Chem.* **242,** 3332 (1967).
7. T. I. Kalman and T. J. Bardos, *Mol. Pharmacol.* **6,** 621 (1970).
8. P. D. Ellis, A. L. Dunlap, K. Pollard, K. Seidman, and A. D. Cardin, *J. Am. Chem. Soc.* **95,** 4398 (1973).
9. B. R. Baker, "Design of Active-Site-Directed Irreversible Enzyme Inhibitors." Wiley, New York, 1967.
10. A. Matsuda, Y. Wataya, and D. V. Santi, *Biochem. Biophys. Res. Commun.* **84,** 654 (1978).
11. M. P. Mertes, C. T.-C. Chang, E. De Clercq, G.-F. Huang, P. F. Torrence, *Biochem. Biophys. Res. Commun.* **84,** 1054 (1978).

12. A. L. Pogolotti, Jr. and D. V. Santi, *Biochemistry* **13,** 456 (1974).
13. W. L. Washtien and D. V. Santi, *Cancer Res.* **39,** 3397 (1979).
14. P. Reyes and C. Heidelberger, *Mol. Pharmacol.* **1,** 14 (1965).
15. T. T. Sakai and D. V. Santi, *J. Med. Chem.* **16,** 1079 (1973).
16. D. V. Santi and T. T. Sakai, *Biochemistry* **10,** 3598 (1971).
17. Y. Wataya, A. Matsuda, D. V. Santi, D. E. Bergstrom, and J. L. Ruth, *J. Med. Chem.* **22,** 339 (1979).
18. D. V. Santi, A. L. Pogolotti, Jr., T. L. James, Y. Wataya, K. M. Ivanetich, and S. S. M. Lam, *ACS Symp. Ser.* **28,** 57 (1978).
19. C. Heidelberger, *in* "Handbuch der Experimentellen Pharmakologie" (A. C. Sartorelli and D. G. Johns, eds.), Vol. 38, Part I, p. 193. Springer-Verlag, Berlin and New York, 1974.
20. B. Ullman, M. Lee, D. W. Martin, and D. V. Santi, *Proc. Natl. Acad. Sci. U.S.A.* **75,** 980 (1978).
21. R. Bose and E. W. Yamada, *Biochemistry* **13,** 2051 (1974).
22. R. C. Gallo and T. R. Breitman, *J. Biol. Chem.* **243,** 4936 (1968).
23. M. Zimmerman and J. Seidenberg, *J. Biol. Chem.* **239,** 2618 (1964).
24. E. Cadman, R. Heimer, and L. Davis, *Science* **205,** 1135 (1979).
25. L. L. Bennett, Jr., *in* "Handbuch der Experimentellen Pharmakologie" (A. C. Sartorelli and D. G. Johns, eds.), Vol. 38, Part II, p. 484. Springer-Verlag, Berlin and New York, 1975.
26. C. A. Nichol, *in* "Handbuch der Experimentellen Pharmakologie" (A. C. Sartorelli and D. G. Johns, eds.), Vol. 38, Part II, p. 434. Springer-Verlag, Berlin and New York, 1975.
27. E. A. Swyryd, S. S. Seaver, and G. R. Stark, *J. Biol. Chem.* **249,** 6945 (1974).
28. R. K. Johnson, E. A. Swyryd, and G. R. Stark, *Cancer Res.* **38,** 371 (1978).
29. J.-J. Chen and M. E. Jones, *J. Biol. Chem.* **254,** 4908 (1979).
30. L. Thelander and P. Reichard, *Annu. Rev. Biochem.* **48,** 133 (1979).

PART IV

Antimetabolites—Folate Analogs

15

The Binding of Ligands to Dihydrofolate Reductase

RAYMOND L. BLAKLEY

Over the last decade considerable research effort has been devoted to study of the structure of dihydrofolate reductase (DHFR), particularly with the hope of disclosing details of the binding of antifolates like methotrexate (MTX) to the active site. The reasons for this concentration of effort on DHFR are twofold.

MOLECULAR ACTIONS AND TARGETS FOR CANCER CHEMOTHERAPEUTIC AGENTS

ISBN 0-12-619280-4

First, there is abundant evidence that this enzyme is the target of the anticancer drug MTX and the antibacterial drug trimethoprim and, second, the modest size of this enzyme (molecular weight about 20,000) permits optimal use of many techniques that are more difficult to employ in elucidation of the structure of larger proteins. Structures of folate, MTX, and related compounds are shown in Fig. 1.

Many laboratories have contributed to this effort, and a formidable array of chemical and physical techniques has been brought to bear. All these efforts have contributed to the structural picture that is emerging, and no one approach could have provided more than a segment of the total information. Nevertheless, the X-ray diffraction results obtained from crystals of bacterial DHFR by Matthews, Kraut, and their colleagues at the University of California at San Diego have been of outstanding significance. Not only have these studies provided a wealth of information about the conformation of the backbone and spatial arrangement of the side chains in the crystals, but they have also been exceedingly informative about the interaction of both MTX and NADPH with the enzyme. Furthermore, the information obtained from the X-ray diffraction studies has allowed the data gathered by several other methods to be interpreted in more specific molecular terms than otherwise would have been possible. Accordingly, it is appropriate in this chapter to start by summarizing the information obtained by the X-ray diffraction approach and to then consider the additional insights obtained by other methods, including such spectroscopic methods as circular dichroism (CD), nmr, fluorescence, and differential electronic spectroscopy, examining whether they confirm the X-ray crystallographic information and what they add

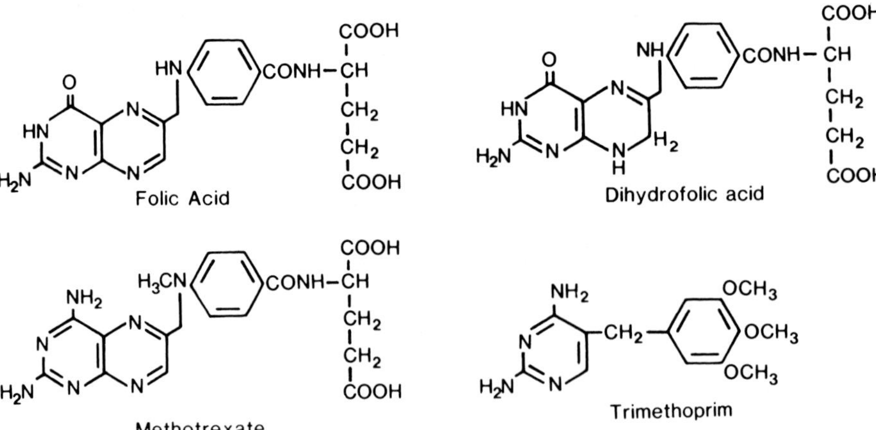

Fig. 1. Structures of some ligands of major interest. Dihydrofolate is the substrate for DHFR from all sources, and folate is an alternative substrate for the enzyme from some sources. Trimethoprim and MTX are well-known examples of many inhibitors having a 2,4-diaminopyrimidine ring.

to our overall understanding of the enzyme and the way it binds ligands. Since more information has been obtained about DHFR from *Lactobacillus casei* than about the enzyme from any other source, structural information about the *L. casei* enzyme will be reviewed first.

I. X-Ray Diffraction Studies on *Lactobacillus casei* Dihydrofolate Reductase

A. General Structure of the Enzyme

The structure of the ternary complex of *L. casei* DHFR with MTX and NADPH has been determined at 2.5-Å resolution (1). Like the backbone of *Escherichia coli* DHFR, described earlier (2), the overall folding of the polypeptide backbone of *L. casei* DHFR is dominated by an eight-stranded β sheet, beginning at the NH_2-terminus and ending with a single antiparallel strand at the COOH-terminus. The residues involved in the successive strands of the sheet are: 74–76 (βD), 57–62 (βC), 38–42 (βB), 95–98 (βE), 1–7 (βA), 111–118 (βF), 151–158 (βH), and 139–146 (βG). There are four helical regions involving approximately residues 25–35 (αB), 43–49 (αC), 78–86 (αE), and 100–108 (αF), although it is difficult to define the limits of the helices exactly. This corresponds to approximately 26% of the backbone chain.

The molecule is very roughly pear-shaped, with the COOH-terminus at the apex and a loop formed by residues 84–93 forming an extension from the surface. The ligand-binding site consists, in part, of a deep cavity that cuts halfway across the base and most of the way up its side. The remainder of the binding site, where the 2′-phosphoadenosine 5′-diphosphate (PADP) moiety of NADPH binds, is a groove part way around the side of the cone. When bound at the catalytic site, MTX has C-2, N-3, and C-4 of the pteridine ring at the bottom of the pocket and the plane of the pteridine ring approximately parallel to the axis of the cone. The 1′-4′ axis of the benzoyl moiety is nearly at right angles to the plane of the pteridine ring, and the glutamate moiety is draped over helix αB. The reduced NMN moiety of NADPH is inserted in the bottom of the cavity so that C-4 of the nicotinamide ring is nearest the pteridine ring (4–6 Å from C-6 of the pteridine), and the rest of the NADPH molecule winds around the surface in the shallow groove already mentioned.

B. Interaction of Methotrexate with the Enzyme

The amino acid side chains that line the active site cavity are, with few exceptions, hydrophobic in nature. Consequently, most of the interactions of the pteridine ring, the N-10 methyl group, and the benzoyl group of MTX with the amino acid residues lining the cavity are also of a hydrophobic nature, as summarized in Table I. It might be expected that the glutamate moiety of MTX would bind by charge interactions between its carboxyl groups and basic residues, and this is the case (Table I), but the other charge interaction is apparently between Asp-26 and N-1 of the pteridine ring. The latter interaction may be related to the much greater affinity shown by MTX for DHFR than shown by folate. As first suggested by Baker (3), the greater affinity of MTX may be at least in part a result of the greater basicity of N-1 due to the 4-amino substituent. It is now seen that this would increase the interaction of N-1 with Asp-26. Additionally, in the ternary complex the nicotinamide ring prevents access of solvent to the hydrophobic cavity in which Asp-26 resides, so that the pK of Asp-26 must be considerably higher than that of solvent-exposed aspartic acid.

It seems likely in view of this interaction between Asp-26 and N-1 of MTX that Asp-26 is also the required proton donor to the pteridine ring of the substrate

TABLE I

Residues of *Lactobacillus casei* Dihydrofolate Reductase Interacting with Methotrexate in th Ternary Complex (1)

Methotrexate component	Residue	Interaction	Residue in DHFR from other sources[a]
Pteridine	Leu–4	Hydrophobic	Ile, Met
	Leu–4, CO	H bond, 4-NH_2 group	Ile, Met
	Peptide 5-6	Hydrophobic or pi–pi	
	Ala–6	Hydrophobic	Ala
	Leu–19	Hydrophobic	Leu, Met
	Asp–26	Charge, H bond	Asp, Glu
	Leu–27	Hydrophobic	Leu, Met, Tyr, Phe
	Phe–30	Hydrophobic	Phe
	Ala–97, CO	Hydrophobic	Val, Gly, Ser
	Thr–116	H bond, 2-NH_2 group	Thr
N^{10}-Methyl	Ser–48	Hydrophobic	Ser, Gly
p-Aminobenzoyl	Leu–27	Hydrophobic	Leu, Met, Tyr, Phe
	Phe–49	Hydrophobic	Ile, Met
	Leu–54	Hydrophobic	Leu
Glutamate	His–28	Charge	Arg, Lys, Ala, Gln
	Arg–57	Charge	Arg

[a] The other sources examined were *E. coli* (4,5), *S. faecium* isoenzyme II (6,7), L1210 muri lymphoma (8,9), bovine liver (10), and chicken liver (11). The *L. casei* sequence has been report by Bitar *et al.* (12) and Freisheim *et al.* (13). Sequences have been aligned so as to align conserv residues, and to cause deletions and insertions to occur in the loops connecting elements of second structure. The bovine liver DHFR sequence has been corrected according to unpublished resu (P. -H Lai and R. L. Blakley), and the *S. faecium* isoenzyme I data are from unpublished work of Pongsamart and R. L. Blakley.

in the enzyme-catalyzed reaction. A difficulty for this view is that, in the enzymatic reduction of DHF, the proton is ultimately added to N-5. However, if the pteridine ring of the substrate were to be turned over, the carboxylate group of Asp-26 would be close to N-5. The pteridine ring could be turned over in this fashion by rotations of 180° and 30° about the C-6—C-9 and C-9—N-10 bonds, respectively. Such a rearrangement does not much alter the close approach between C-4 of the nicotinamide ring of NADPH and C-6 of the pteridine ring. However, as pointed out by Matthews *et al.*, [1], it is not essential to suppose such a rotated position of the pteridine ring of bound dihydrofolate (DHF), since other possibilities are a proton jump from N-1 to N-5 within the pteridine ring and a proton rearrangement mediated by water, either during the enzyme reaction or after the release of products.

C. Interaction of NADPH with the Protein

The ribose-phosphate portions of the coenzyme are involved in numerous specific hydrogen-bonded interactions, the adenine ring binds in a hydrophobic cleft, and the nicotinamide ring binds in the outer end of the hydrophobic cavity in which MTX also binds (14). It may be seen from Table II that, as in the case of the interactions with MTX, many of the residues involved are conserved in DHFR from the other species for which the sequence is known. Where there are replacements, they are almost always conservative in cases where the side chain of a residue (rather than the carboxyl or imide group) is involved in interaction with the ligands.

When the conformation of bound NADPH is examined, one of the major features is that the ribose-phosphate links making up the dinucleotide backbone are in an extended conformation, and as a result the two bases are even farther apart than observed for NAD^+ bound to the four dehydrogenases previously investigated by X-ray diffraction. Second, several of the individual dihedral angles, especially within the adenine nucleotide portion of the coenzyme, differ significantly from their minimum energy conformations.

D. Effect of NADPH Binding on Enzyme Conformation

1. *Effects on Backbone Conformation*

Since the binary complex of MTX with *E. coli* DHFR as well as the ternary complex of MTX and NADPH with *L. casei* DHFR have both been examined by X-ray diffraction, it is possible to attempt to discern changes in DHFR conformation due to NADPH binding by comparing these two structures (14). Obviously care must be taken to distinguish differences in conformation due to differences in the primary sequence from conformational changes that arise as a result of coenzyme binding.

TABLE II

Interactions between *Lactobacillus casei* Dihydrofolate Reductase and NADPH in the Ternary Complex (14)

NADPH component	Residue	Interaction	Residue in DHFR from other sources[a]
Adenine	Leu-62	Hydrophobic	Leu
	His-64	Hydrophobic	Arg, Ser, Thr
	Thr-63	Hydrophobic	Thr, Ser
	Ile-102	Hydrophobic	Ile, Val
	His-77	Hydrophobic	His, Lys
	Asp-78	Hydrophobic	Ser
AMP ribose	Arg-43	Charge, P-2′	Arg
	Thr-63	H bond, O-2 of P-2′	Thr, Ser
	His-64	H bond, O-3 of P-2′	Thr, Ser, Arg
	Gln-101	H bond, O-3′	Arg, Ala, Ser
	Ile-102	Hydrophobic	Ile, Val
	Gly-42	Hydrophobic	Gly
Pyrophosphate	Arg-44	Charge	Lys, His
	Thr-45, NH	H bond, O-1*a*	Thr
	Ala-100, NH	H bond, O	Gly, Thr, Ser
	Thr-45	H bond, O-2*a*	Thr
	Thr-126	H bond, O-2*n*	Thr, Ala
	Gly-99	Hydrophobic	Gly
NMN ribose	Gly-17, CO	H bond, O-2′	Gly, Asn
	Ser-48	H bond, O-2′	Gly, Asn
	His-18, CO	H bond, O-3′	Leu, Asp, Asn, Ala, Gln
	Ile-13	Hydrophobic	Ile
	Gly-14	Hydrophobic	Gly
Nicotinamide	Trp-5	Hydrophobic	Trp, Ala, Val
	Ala-6	Hydrophobic	Ala
	Ala-6, NH	H bond, O-7	Ala
	Ala-6, CO	H bond, N-7	Ala
	Ile-13	Hydrophobic	Ile
	Ile-13, CO	H bond, N-7	Ile
	Leu-19	Hydrophobic	Leu, Met
	Trp-21	Hydrophobic	Trp
	Ala-97, CO	Hydrophobic	Ser, Gly, Val

[a] See Table I, footnote *a*.

When 142 out of the 159 α-carbon coordinates in the binary complex of *E. coli* DHFR (2) are matched by least squares to structurally equivalent α-carbon coordinates for the ternary complex of *L. casei* DHFR (1), the root mean square deviation is 1.7 Å (14). Thus, despite the rather low sequence homology for these bacterial enzymes, the geometry of the peptide backbone is almost identical in the two structures. In three loop regions connecting βA to αB, βF to βG, and

βG to βH, respectively, corresponding parts of the structures differ by 2 Å or more. The last of these loops is on the exterior of the molecule and is not involved in the structure of the active site cavity. In addition, none of its residues interact with ligands bound in the cavity. It was therefore reasonably assumed by Matthews *et al.* (14) that structural variation in this region (residues 143–149 of *L. casei* and residues 140–147 of *E. coli*) were due to differences in the primary structure and to crystal packing effects.

The other two loops form one side of the active site cavity. They are represented by relatively weak electron density on the map of the *E. coli* structure, so that they are probably rather flexible in this molecule. On the other hand, the main-chain and side-chain electron density for these two loops is strong and well-defined in the *L. casei* ternary complex. Moreover, both of these loops are moved slightly in the *L. casei* complex when compared with the corresponding structures in the *E. coli* complex. The largest movements (up to 3 Å) involve residues 12–21 and 125–128 in *L. casei* DHFR. As seen from Table II, residues 13, 14, 17–19, 21, and 126 interact directly with NADPH, and three of them are conserved in all six enzymes and three others in five of the six enzymes. This confirms their functional importance and supports the view that the relative movement of these two loops in the ternary complex is due to NADPH binding.

2. *Effects on Side-Chain Conformations*

Since only 43 side chains are identical in the *L. casei* and *E. coli* structures, only tentative conclusions can be drawn from comparison of the X-ray diffraction results, especially since conserved side chains are located in nonconserved environments created by the nonhomologous side chains. Nevertheless, 21 of the 43 conserved residues have the same side-chain conformation angles. Furthermore, of 10 conserved residues interacting with bound NADPH in the *L. casei* complex, three have unchanged side-chain conformations, three others are invariant glycines, and one is an invariant alanine. The general indication is therefore that side chains retain their conformations to a greater degree than might have been anticipated when NADPH binds, even when the side chains directly interact with the bound NADPH.

II. Correlation of Other Results for *Lactobacillus casei* Dihydrofolate Reductase with the X-Ray Diffraction Model

A. Circular Dichroism

Several reports have appeared on the use of CD to study the binding of ligands to DHFR, since for many ligands large extrinsic Cotton effects are observed. However, it has been impossible to determine whether these effects should be ascribed to changes in particular parts of the protein structure, changes in conformation of the ligand, or immobilization of the ligand. Further, even when it seems probable that changes in protein structure are responsible, it remains open to speculation as to whether major movements of the protein backbone, simple changes in side-chain conformation, or both have occurred.

Hood *et al.* (15) found that changes in CD for *L. casei* DHFR were consistent with the perturbation of one or more aromatic residues, including a tryptophan residue. Differences between the CD for the NADPH–MTX ternary complex and the CD of the two binary complexes were considered to be consistent with direct interaction between the pteridine and dihydronicotinamide chromophores. The X-ray diffraction model of the *L. casei* ternary complex shows hydrophobic interaction between the nicotinamide ring and the pyrazine portion of the pteridine ring. Reddy *et al.* (16) also noted the striking change in the CD and magnetic circular dichroism (MCD) bands centered at 360 nm when either of the binary complexes was converted to the ternary complex and concluded that a conformational change occurred in the environment of the bound ligands. This is also consistent with the NADPH-induced movement of the two loops containing residues 10–22 and 120–139 deduced from the X-ray diffraction data.

B. Difference Spectroscopy

Hood and Roberts (17) concluded that a major component of the UV difference spectrum generated when MTX binds to *L. casei* DHFR closely resembles that observed on protonation of MTX, reflecting an increased degree of protonation on binding, as predicted from the X-ray diffraction results for the interaction of Asp-26 with N-1 of MTX. Quantitative analysis of the pH dependence of this component of the difference spectrum appeared to arise from perturbation of contrast, folate was not protonated when bound to DHFR at neutral pH. Another component of the difference spectrum appeared to arise from perturbation of one or more tryptophan residues of the enzyme. Although the X-ray diffraction model does not appear to involve any tryptophans in direct interaction with MTX, Trp-21 has its indole ring in the side of the hydrophobic cavity and may change its side-chain conformation when MTX binds.

C. Chemical Modification Studies

Treatment of *L. casei* DHFR with *N*-bromosuccinimide under appropriate conditions resulted in modification of one tryptophan residue and loss of enzymatic activity (18,19). This tryptophan was shown to be the conserved Trp-21 (19) and, since it is located on the side of the hydrophobic cavity, it is not surprising that its modification caused loss of activity. Whether this was due to decreased binding of ligands or to loss of catalytic function was not determined. NADPH protects from loss of enzymatic activity against *N*-bromosuccimide (18), but the possibility that this was due to preferential oxidation of NADPH by the reagent was not unambiguously eliminated.

Modification of five arginines of *L. casei* DHFR with phenylglyoxal resulted in loss of catalytic activity but, when NADPH protected two of these arginines, activity was completely retained (20). The identity of the two residues protected by NADPH was not determined but, since Arg-43 and Arg-44 interact with NADPH (Table II), it may be supposed that these were the residues involved. However, it should be noted that coenzyme does not block access to these residues from the solvent and that, if protection is afforded by the coenzyme, it must be due solely to interaction of the coenzyme with these arginine residues.

D. Nuclear Magnetic Resonance Studies

1. *Proton Nuclear Magnetic Resonance of Histidine Residues*

Birdsall *et al.* (21) have reported the effects of binding of substrates (folate, DHF) and inhibitors [5-formyltetrahydrofolate, trimethoprim, MTX, aminopterin, 2,4-diaminopyrimidine, and *p*-aminobenzoyl-L-glutamate (pABG)] to *L. casei* DHFR on the histidine C-2 proton resonances of the enzyme, and Matthews (22) has interpreted these results in terms of the crystal structure. The behavior observed for resonance H_F (Table III) is explained by formation of a hydrogen bond between His-28 and the γ carboxyl of ligands (Table I). The effect of pABG binding to the low-affinity second site on the H_c resonance is that normally occupied by the AMP moiety of NADPH, with which His-64 interacts (Table II). H_D and H_B are assigned to resonances remote from the binding cavity, and the microenvironment of His-77 is consistent with the high p*K* of the residue associated with H_D. His-12 and His-18 are located in one of the flexible loops that form one side of the active site cavity and change conformation when

TABLE III

^{1}H Nuclear Magnetic Resonance Study of Histidines in *Lactobacillus casei* Dihydrofolate Reductase (21)

Resonance	Residue assigned	NMR behavior
H_F	His-28	pK 6.5 increased to 7.5 by pAGB binding
H_C	His-64	Shifted upfield by weak pAGB binding to a second site; unaffected by MTX binding
H_D	His-77	Unaffected by ligand binding; p*K* 7.7
H_B	His-89	Unaffected by ligand binding; p*K* 7.2
H_A	His-12 or His-18	All substrates and inhibitors cause downfield shifts
H_E	His-12 or His-18	Inhibitors cause upfield shifts
Unobserved	His-135	

NADPH binds in the cavity, and it is reasonable to assume ligand-produced changes in chemical shift as observed for H_A and H_E.

2. ^{1}H Nuclear Magnetic Resonance of Tyrosine and ^{19}F Nuclear Magnetic Resonance of 3-Fluorotyrosine Residues

Feeney *et al.* (23) prepared a selectively deuterated DHFR in which all the aromatic protons except the 2,6 protons of the tyrosine residues were replaced by deuterium. Rapid rotation about the $C_\beta—C_\gamma$ bond produced a single resonance for each residue. Unfortunately, the range of the chemical shifts of these resonances was only 0.32 ppm, and ligands induced only small shifts ($\leq$0.15 ppm). This finding is consistent with information obtained from the crystallographic model, which indicates that only one tyrosine side chain is near bound ligands, so that the majority of ligand-induced shifts must be due to conformation changes. Since, in addition to this, the tyrosine residues exist in complex protein environments, interpretation of the ^{1}H nmr data in terms of structure is not possible (22).

In another study Kimber *et al.* (24) grew *L. casei* on medium containing 3-fluorotyrosine and DHFR isotaled from the organism was studied by ^{19}F-nmr. One of the 5-fluorotyrosine resonances, Y_N^F, shows marked downfield shifts (1.06–2.68 ppm) when the enzyme forms binary complexes with folate or substrate analogs (cf. 0.37 ppm for the other three resonances influenced by ligand binding). The largest shift is produced by MTX, and the 2,4-diaminopyrimidine moiety is responsible for most of this effect. Matthews (22) argues convincingly that this effect can be explained by hydrogen bonding of the 2-amino group of the inhibitor to the 3-fluoro group of Tyr^{29} and simultaneous exclusion of solvent from the latter by the inhibitor.

3. ^{19}F Nuclear Magnetic Resonance of 6-Fluorotryptophan Residues

Lactobacillus casei DHFR containing 6-fluorotryptophan residues has been prepared and studied by ^{19}F nmr by Kimber *et al.* (24), and the results analyzed in terms of the crystal structure by Matthews (22). Table IV shows the main characteristics of each resonance and the assignments made by Matthews. Trp-21 is assigned to W_M^F because it is the only tryptophan residue that interacts with ligands, residing on the inner surface of the cavity in which MTX and the nicotinamide portion of NADPH are bound. In the ternary complex, the indole ring is in Van der Waals contact with the carboxamide group of the coenzyme. Downfield movement of the resonance on ligand binding can be understood in terms of solvent exclusion from fluorine by bound ligand. W_K^F is identified with Trp-5, because the latter is the most completely buried residue in the uncomplexed protein, which accounts for the downfield position of the resonance in the spectrum. W_K^F and W_L^F have a double structure in the presence of MTX, the splitting being due to through space $^{19}F–^{19}F$ spin coupling (24,25). Examination

TABLE IV

^{19}F Nuclear Magnetic Resonance Study of Fluorotryptophans in *Lactobacillus casei* Dihydrofolate Reductase (25)

Resonance	Residue assigned	NMR behavior
W_M^F	Trp-21	Large downfield changes in shift on binding MTX and NADPH
W_K^F	Trp-5	Most downfield position in uncomplexed enzyme; doublet structure
W_L^F	Trp-133	Slightly downfield in uncomplexed enzyme; doublet structure
W_N^F	Trp-158	Slightly upfield in uncomplexed enzyme

of the position of tryptophan residues in the crystal model indicates that only Trp-5 and Trp-133 are close enough for 6-fluorine atoms to interact, and even 6-fluorotryptophan residues in these positions would be close enough for F–F coupling only if Trp-5 rotates 30° and 60° about the C_α—C_β and C_β—C_γ bonds, respectively. This rotation would be caused by steric constraints imposed by C_β of Leu-113 and C_γ of Met-128 when the 6-fluorine is present on Trp-5. Assignments for W_L^F and W_N^F appropriately correlate the chemical shifts of these resonances in the uncomplexed enzyme with the accessibility to solvent of the assigned residues.

4. *Nuclear Magnetic Resonance Studies on Bound Ligands*

Roberts *et al.* (26) have observed that the aromatic proton resonances of pABG are shifted upfield when this ligand binds to DHFR. The X-ray structural results show that Phe-49 lines one side of the binding cavity, with its aromatic ring nearly parallel to the phenyl group of MTX in the enzyme–MTX–NADPH ternary complex and positioned so that its center lies above protons ortho and meta to the glutamate group of the inhibitor. Magnetic shielding by ring currents in the Phe-49 side chain explain the shifts of 0.41 and 0.48 ppm for protons ortho and meta to the glutamate moiety, respectively (22). The ^{13}C resonance from folate labeled in the benzoyl carbonyl has been found by Pastore *et al.* (27) to shift upfield by over 2 ppm when folate binds to DHFR. However, this result is not readily ascribed to the ring current of the Phe-49 side chain, since in the ternary MTX–NADPH–DHFR complex the carbonyl is about 3 Å beyond the edge of the Phe-49 ring and the ring current would in this case cause deshielding of the ^{13}C nucleus.

When NADPH bound to *L. casei* DHFR is examined by ^{31}P nmr (28), the 2′-phosphate signal is shown to be shifted downfield by 2.19 ppm. Moreover, this chemical shift is independent of pH within the range 4.7–7.5. Feeney *et al.* (28) have concluded that the 2′-phosphate group binds in the dianionic form and that its pK must be decreased by at least 3 units from its value in the free coenzyme. Similar behavior was found for 2′-AMP (29). These results are consistent with the information provided by X-ray diffraction (Table II), which indicates that (1) a side-chain NH group of His-64 hydrogen-bonds with one oxygen of this phosphate group, and the imidazole pK is increased as a consequence; (2) the side-chain hydroxyl of Thr-63 hydrogen-bonds with another oxygen of the group; (3) the guanidino group of Arg-43 approaches and may interact with two of the phosphate oxygens; and (4) the phosphate group is about 5 Å from the NH_2-terminus of the αC helix, the electric field from which would stabilize the group. The mutual effect of these interactions explains the 100-fold greater association constant for NADPH as compared to that for NADH (21).

Measurement of ^{31}P–O–C–^{1}H coupling constants showed that these differed for the two ^{31}P atoms in the pyrophosphate group (28), and from this it was concluded that in one case the conformation about the C-5′—O-5′ changed by at least 50° upon binding to DHFR. As mentioned earlier, X-ray diffraction data for the ternary complex has indicated that, whereas in free nucleotides the dihedral angle about the C-5′—O-5′ bond is 180° ± 20°, the adenine nucleotide portion of bound NADPH has a dihedral angle of 120°.

When 1 equivalent of [*carboxamido*-^{13}C]NADP$^+$ is added to a solution of *L. casei* DHFR, the single resonance is observed at 1.6 ppm upfield from the position for the free ligand (29). Further addition of MTX or folate to form ternary complexes shifts the resonance further upfield to positions 2.62 and 4.33 ppm, respectively, from free NADP$^+$. Rationalization of these results in terms of structure is less straightforward. Ring current effects are an unlikely cause, since Trp-21 is the only aromatic residue in the vicinity of the carboxamide group of bound NADPH and is unfavorably positioned for a large upfield shift. Matthews (22) has argued that Asp-26, the only group in the binding cavity which might be charged, is unlikely to be the major cause of the upfield shifts, especially in the case of the folate–NADPH ternary complex. The explanation favored by Matthews is that the major factor for the upfield shifts is exclusion from the binding cavity of solvent molecules which hydrogen-bond to the carbonyl and decrease shielding of the ^{13}C nucleus. Since the exclusion of solvent is more complete in the ternary complex, the observed greater upfield shift for this complex is to be expected. This may also be the cause of the upfield shift of the carbonyl resonance of bound folate referred to above.

E. Ligand-Binding Studies

Birdsall *et al.* (30,31) have studied the mutual effects that binding of one ligand to the active site of *L. casei* DHFR has on binding of other ligands. Thus pABG binds 54-fold more tightly to the 2,4-diaminopyrimidine–DHFR complex than to DHFR alone, and this effect is reciprocal. NADPH increases the association constants for diaminopyrimidine and for pABG without substantially altering the cooperativity between them.

Although it is not known how bound 2,4-diaminopyrimidine is located in the active site cavity, it seems reasonable to assume that it adopts a position close to that occupied by the pyrimidine ring of MTX. This would place it within 5 Å of the position occupied by the nicotinamide ring of NADPH in the ternary MTX–NADPH–DHFR complex, and therefore close enough for hydrophobic interactions with this ring. Similarly, it seems likely from the X-ray structure that hydrophobic interactions occur between bound 2,4-diaminopyrimidine and the benzoyl group of bound pABG. These interactions would account for some of the cooperativity in binding. In addition, as discussed above, binding of ligands probably causes changes in the conformation of the two flexible loops (10–22 and 120–139) which form one side of the active site cavity. This would also favor subsequent binding of other ligands.

Dietrich *et al.* (32) have made an extensive comparison of the inhibitory effects of 2,4-diaminotriazines on *L. casei*. DHFR and conclude that the active site contains a substantial hydrophobic cavity with polar groups beyond it. This is in general agreement with the X-ray structure.

F. Transient-State Kinetics

Dunn *et al.* (33) have concluded from stopped-flow measurements of fluorescence changes occurring when NADPH or its analogues bind to *L. casei* DHFR that the enzyme exists in at least two interconvertible forms whose relative proportions are pH-dependent. NADPH binds to only one of these forms. However, there is not presently adequate information to relate this to the X-ray structure.

III. Results with Dihydrofolate Reductase from Other Sources

A. General Considerations

Correlation of structural data obtained with DHFR from sources other than *L. casei* with the X-ray structure obtained for *L. casei* DHFR must be approached with great caution, because differences in primary structure (which may be substantial) may result in differences in the backbone conformation, side-chain conformations, or both. However, in the case of *E. coli* DHFR, for which the structure is also known from X-ray crystallography, it has been pointed out earlier that the backbone conformation is virtually identical with that of the *L. casei* enzyme, despite rather low sequence homology for these two bacterial enzymes. Furthermore, when structurally equivalent backbone atoms in these two enzymes are appropriately aligned, the β-carbon atoms for each amino acid residue involved in secondary structure (α helices and β sheets) must also be aligned, so that the directions of side-chains of such residues in one structure can be predicted from their direction in the other. The same kind of inferences about the position of side-chains of residues involved in secondary structure can be made for DHFR from four other sources for which the complete sequence is available, provided these sequences can be correctly aligned with the sequences of the *L. casei* and *E. coli* enzymes. Through at least the first 130 residues (numbering in the *L. casei* sequence) this is relatively straightforward, because a number of residues that are identical in all six DHFR sequences occur throughout this portion of the sequence and provide markers that can be used for alignment purposes (Table V). The few insertions and deletions that do occur in this region can be located appropriately by requiring that (1) there be strict coincidence of functionally important residues (both homologous and analogous), and (2) insertions (or deletions) occur in loops connecting elements of secondary structure or, alternatively, at the extremities of the structures themselves (for example an extra half-turn of the helix). Comparison of the *E. coli* and *L. casei* DHFR structures showed this to occur in all cases.

Beyond residue 130, alignment becomes more difficult because there are fewer homologous and analogous residues. Although the sequences differ in length, it is unlikely that this results in a "tail" at the carboxyl terminus of the longer sequences. This is confirmed by two observations. In the *E. coli* and *L. casei* structures, the last strand (βH) of the β sheet in each case occurs very close to the COOH-terminus, hence these portions of the sequence are aligned. Since residues analogous or homologous to residues in the βH strands of the *E. coli* and *L. casei* enzymes are present at the COOH-termini of all the other sequences, these regions are also probably aligned with the *L. casei* and *E. coli* carboxyl termini. Furthermore, it is unlikely that either the βG or βH strands would be found in regions of the other sequences containing proline residues, since proline is almost never found in β-sheet structure. Insertions (or deletions) must therefore occur in the loops connecting βF to βG and βG to βH. While alignments in this region are admittedly speculative, reasonable suggestions can be made as shown in Table V.

A point of special interest from the sequence alignments is that in all six sequences the residue corresponding to Asp-26 in the *L. casei* sequence is either aspartic acid or glutamic acid. This provides strong confirmatory evidence of the importance of the side-chain carboxyl of this residue in the catalytic function of the enzyme.

B. *Escherichia coli* Dihydrofolate Reductase

Results obtained by other methods are consistent with the X-ray structure. Small CD changes in the far UV when NADPH, trimethoprim, pyrimethamine, or

TABLE V

Dihydrofolate Reductase Sequences[a]

* * * 10 * * 20 * * *

Val-Arg- Pro-Leu-Asn-Cys- Ile-Val-Ala- Val-Ser-Gln-Asn-Met-Gly- Ile-Gly-Lys-Asn-Gly-Asp-Leu-Pro-Trp-Pro-
Val-Arg- Pro-Leu-Asn-Cys- Ile-Val-Ala- Val-Ser-Gln-Asn-Met-Gly- Ile-Gly-Lys-Asn-Gly-Asp-Leu-Pro-Trp-Pro-
Val-Arg-Asp-Leu-Asn- Ser- Ile-Val-Ala- Val-Cys-Gln-Asn-Met-Gly- Ile-Gly-Lys-Asp- Gly-Asn-Leu-Pro-Trp-Pro-
Met- *Ile-Ser-Leu- Ile-Ala-Ala-Leu-*Ala-Val-Asp-Arg-Val- Ile-Gly-Met-Glu- Asn-Ala-Met-Pro-Trp-Asn-
*Thr- Ala-Phe-Leu-Trp-Ala-Gln-*Asn-Arg-Asp-Gly-Leu- Ile-Gly-Lys-Asp- Gly-His-Leu-Pro-Trp-His-
Met-Phe- Ile- Ser-Met-Trp-Ala- Gln-Asp-Lys-Asn-Gly-Leu-Ile-Gly-Lys-Asp- Gly-Leu-Leu-Pro-Trp-Arg-
Met-Leu- Ala- Ala- Ile-Trp-Ala- Gln-Asp-Gln-Asn-Gly-Leu-Ile-Gly-Lys-Gln- Asn-Gln-Leu- Trp-Asp-

30 * * * * 40 50

Pro-Leu-Arg-Asn-Glu-Phe-Lys-Tyr- Phe-Gln-Arg-Met-Thr-Thr-Thr-Ser-Ser-Val-Glu-Gly-Lys-Gln-Asn-Leu-Val-
Pro-Leu-Arg-Asn-Glu-Phe-Gln-Tyr- Phe-Gln-Arg-Met-Thr-Thr-Val-Ser-Ser-Val-Glu-Gly-Lys-Gln-Asn-Leu-Val-
Pro-Leu-Arg-Asn-Glu-Tyr- Lys-Tyr- Phe-Gln-Arg-Met-Thr-Ser-Thr-Ser-His-Val-Glu-Gly-Lys-Gln-Asn-Ala- Val-
Leu-Pro-Ala-Asp-Leu-Ala-Trp- Phe-Lys-Arg-Asn-Thr-Leu- Asp- Lys- *Pro-Val-*
Leu-Pro-Asp-Asp-Leu-His-Tyr- Phe-Arg-Ala-Gln- Thr-Val- Gly-Lys- *Ile-Met-*
Leu-Pro-Asn-Asp-Met-Arg-Phe-Phe-Arg-Glu-His- Thr-Met- Asp- Lys- Ile-Leu-
Leu- Asn- Leu-Lys- Lys-Glu-Leu

60 70 * * * * * * * * *

Ile-Met-Gly- Arg-Lys-Thr-Trp-Phe-Ser-Ile- Pro-Glu-Lys-Asn-Arg-Pro-Leu-Lys-Asp-Arg- Ile- Asn- Ile-Val-Leu-
Ile-Met-Gly- Arg-Lys-Thr-Trp-Phe-Ser-Ile- Pro-Glu-Lys-Asn-Arg-Pro-Leu-Lys-Asp-Arg- Ile- Asn- Ile-Val-Leu-
Ile-Met-Gly- Lys-Lys-Thr-Trp-Phe-Ser-Ile- Pro-Glu-Lys-Asn-Arg-Pro-Leu-Lys-Asp-Arg- Ile- Asn- Ile-Val-Leu-
Ile-Met-Gly- Arg-His-Thr-Trp- Glu-Ser-Ile- Gly- Arg-Pro-Leu-Pro-Gly-*Arg-Lys-Asn- Ile- Ile-Leu-*
Val- Val-Gly- Arg-Arg-Thr-Tyr- Glu-Ser-Phe-Pro- Lys- Arg-Pro-Leu-Pro-Glu-*Arg-Thr-Asn-Val-Val-Leu-*
Val-Met-Gly- Arg-Lys-Thr-Tyr- Glu-Gly-Met- Gly- Lys- Leu-Ser-Leu-Pro-Tyr-Arg-His- Ile- Ile-Val-Leu-

(continued)

TABLE V—*Continued*
Dihydrofolate Reductase Sequences[a]

* * 80 90 * * 100

Ser-Arg-Glu-Leu-Lys-Glu-Pro-Pro-Arg-Gly-Ala-His-Phe-Leu-Ala-Lys-Ser-Leu-Asp-Asp-Ala-Leu-Arg-Leu-Ile-
Ser-Arg-Glu-Leu-Lys-Glu-Pro-Pro-Lys-Gly-Ala-His-Phe-Leu-Ala-Lys-Ser-Leu-Asn-Asp-Ala-Leu-Glu-Leu-Ile-
Ser-Arg-Glu-Leu-Lys-Glu-Ala-Pro-Lys-Gly-Ala-His-Tyr-Leu-Ser-Lys-Ser-Leu-Asp-Asp-Ala-Leu-Ala-Leu-Leu-
Ser-Ser-Gln-Pro-Gly-Thr-Asp- Asp-Arg-Val- *Thr-Trp-Val-* Lys-Ser-Val-Asp-Glu-Ala- Ile-Ala-Ala-Cys-
Thr-His-Gln-Glu-Asp-Tyr-Gln- Ala-Gln- Gly-Ala- *Val-Val-Val-* His-Asp-Val-Ala-Ala-Val-Phe-Ala-Tyr-Ala-
Thr-Thr-Gln-Lys-Asp-Phe-Lys-Val-Glu-Lys-Asn-Ala-Glu-Val-Leu-His-Ser-Ile-Asp-Glu-Leu-Leu-Ala-Tyr-Ala-

110 * 120 * * *

Glu-Gln-Pro-Glu-Leu-Ala-Ser-Lys-Val-Asp-Met-Val-Trp-Ile-Val-Gly-Gly-Ser-Ser-Val-Tyr-Glu-Gln-Ala-Met-
Gln-Asp-Pro-Glu-Leu-Thr-Asn-Lys-Val-Asx-Met-Val- Ile-Val-Gly-Gly-Ser-Ser-Val-Tyr-Lys-Glx-Ala-Met-
Asp-Ser-Pro-Glu-Leu-Lys-Ser-Lys-Val-Asp-Met-Val-Trp-Ile-Val-Gly-Gly-Thr-Ala-Val-Tyr-Lys-Ala-Ala-Met-
Gly-Asn-Val-Pro-Glu- Ile-*Met-Val-Ile-Gly-* Gly-Gly-Arg-Val-Tyr-Glu-Gln-Phe-Leu-
Lys-Gln-His-Leu-Asp-Gln- Glu- Leu-*Val-Ile-Ala-* *Gly*-Gly-Ala-Gln-Ile-Phe-Thr-Ala-Phe-Lys-
Lys-Asp-Ile-Pro-Glu-Asp- Ile-Tyr-Val-Ser-Gly-Gly-Ser-Arg-Ile-Phe-Gln-Ala-Leu-Leu-

130 * 140 150

Asn-Glu-Pro-Gly-His-Leu-Arg-Leu-Phe-Val-Thr-Arg-Ile-Met-Gln-Glu-Phe-Glu-Ser-Asp-Thr-Phe-Phe- Pro-
Asp-Lys-Pro-Gly-His-Val-Arg-Leu-Phe-Val-Thr-Arg-Ile-Met-Gln-Glu-Phe-Glu-Ser-Asp-Ala-Phe-Phe- Pro-
Glu-Lys-Pro-Ile-Asn-His-Arg-Leu-Phe-Val-Thr-Arg-Ile-Leu-His-Glu-Phe-Glu-Ser-Asp-Thr-Phe-Phe- Pro-
Pro-Lys- Ala-*Gln-Lys-Leu-Tyr-Leu-Thr-His-Ile*-Asp-Ala-Gln-Val-Glu-Gly-Asp-Thr-His-Phe- Pro-
Asp-Asp- Val- *Asp-Thr-Leu-Leu-Val-Thr-Arg-Leu*-Ala-Gly-Ser-Phe-Glu-Gly-Asp-Thr-Lys-Met-Ile-Pro-
Pro-Glu-Thr-Lys-Ile-Ile-Trp-Arg-Thr-Leu-Ile-Asp-Ala-Glu-Phe-Glu-Gly-Asp-Thr- Phe-Ile-Gly-

160 170

Glu- Ile- Asp-Leu -Gly - Lys- Tyr-Lys-Leu -Leu-Pro -Glu -Tyr-Pro-Gly-Val- Leu- Ser- Glu-Val-
Glu- Ile- Asp-Phe -Glu - Lys- Tyr-Lys-Leu -Leu-Pro -Glu -Tyr-Pro-Gly-Val- Pro- Leu-Asp-Val-
Glu- Ile- Asp-Tyr -Asp- Lys- Phe-Lys-Leu -Leu-Thr -Glu -Tyr-Pro-Gly-Val- Pro- Ala-Asp- Ile-
Asp-Tyr- Glu -Pro -Asp- Asp-Trp -Glu- Ser- *Val-Phe-Ser-Gln-Phe-His -Asp- Ala* -
Leu-Asn -Trp -Asn- Asp-Phe-Thr- Lys-*Val- Ser -Ser-Arg-Thr - Val-Glu - Asp*-
Glu- Ile- Asp-Phe-Thr - Ser -Phe-Glu- Leu-Val-Glu -Glu-His -Glu - Gly- Ile- Val-Asn-Gln-Glu-

180 190

Gln-Glu-Glu-Asp-Gly-Ile- Lys- Tyr-Lys- Phe-Glu-Val- Tyr- Glu-Lys-Lys-Asp
Glu-Glu-Asp-Gln-Gly-Ile- Lys- Tyr-Lys- Phe-Glu-Val- Tyr- Glu-Lys-Asn
Gln-Glu-Glu-Asp-Gly-Ile- Gln- Tyr-Lys- Phe-Glu-Val- Tyr- Glu-Lys-Lys-Asn
Asp-Ala-Gln-Asn-Ser-*His-Ser- Tyr-Cys- Phe-Glu****-Ile- Leu*- Glu-Arg-Arg
Thr-Asn-Pro-Ala-*Leu-Thr- His-Thr- Tyr- Glu-Val- Trp*- Gln-Lys-Lys-Ala
Asn-Gln-Tyr-Pro-His-Arg- Phe-Gln-Lys- Trp- Gln-Lys-Met- Ser-Lys- Val-Val
(His,Thr, Phe, Glu,Ala)(Tyr,Ser)-Arg-Lys

---

[a] In order, top to bottom, L1210, bovine liver, chicken liver, *E. coli* (RT500), *L. casei, S. faecium* isoenzyme II, *S. faecium* isoenzyme I. Residues marked with an asterisk are involved in binding NADPH or MTX in the *L. casei* reductase complex. The residue marked with a double asterisk in the *E. coli* sequence is lysine in *E. coli* MB1428. Italicized regions of the *L. casei* and *E. coli* sequences indicate strands of β sheet. Regions underlined indicate portions of the α helix. For references see Table I.

MTX binds to the enzyme are consistent with alterations in backbone conformation (34). NADPH addition to the enzyme produces changes in the near-UV CD that seem to be due to sharpening of tryptophan transitions and are consistent with hydrophobic interaction of Trp-22 (*E. coli* sequence) with bound NADPH (35). Since NADPH and $NADP^+$ induce very similar CD bands when bound to the enzyme–MTX complex, the geometry of the ternary complexes seems very similar (36). The UV difference spectroscopy indicates that, on binding to DHFR, the pyrimidine ring of MTX is protonated by interaction with a side chain on the enzyme (37), presumably Asp-27 (*E. coli* DHFR). Folate does not exhibit evidence of such protonation. This result closely parallels the earlier report of Erickson and Mathews (38) of similarities between changes in the UV spectra of aminopterin, MTX, and 10-formylaminopterin on binding to DHFR of T4 bacteriophage, and changes on acidification of solutions of the free compounds. There was no evidence that DHF binds in the protonated form. Striking similarities have been observed in the Raman spectrum of MTX at pH 2 and that of the complex of MTX with *E. coli* DHFR at pH 7 (39), but these features are not observed in the spectrum of MTX at pH 7 or 13. This finding further suggests binding of MTX in a protonated form.

The binding of two molecules of NADPH per molecule of *E. coli* DHFR has been reported (33,36) based on CD titration, fluorescence titration, and ultrafiltration. $NADP^+$ and NADH also appear to form such complexes (36), and the two molecules of nucleotide can bind either to the enzyme alone (40) or to the enzyme–MTX complex (36,40). This is difficult to reconcile with the X-ray structure. The only likely site for binding a second molecule of NADPH is the portion of the hydrophobic cavity where MTX normally binds, but this would not account for the binding of two molecules of NADPH to the DHFR–MTX complex.

Poe *et al.* (41) have reported the effects of pH upon the ^1H nmr resonances due to the C-2 protons of the five histidine residues of *E. coli* DHFR. Binary complexes of the enzyme with MTX, folate, aminopterin, and trimethoprim were studied, and pK' values were obtained for each histidine in the uncomplexed enzyme and in each of the binary complexes by determining the effect of pH on chemical shift. Titrations of the complexes of DHFR modified by treatment with 5′-dithiobis(2-nitrobenzoate) (DTNB) or with *N*-bromosuccinimide were also carried out. The chemical shift data could all be interpreted in terms of the microenvironment of the five histidines seen in the X-ray structure and permitted assignment of the five resonances in the nmr spectra to specific residues in the sequence. The consistency of these assignments strongly suggests that, as in the case of the *L. casei* enzyme, the solution conformation of the enzyme must closely resemble that in the crystal.

Greenfield (42) reported partial inactivation of DHFR from *E. coli* by treatment with ethoxyformic anhydride. Examination of the modified enzyme by proton nmr confirmed that two histidines reacted extensively, two more slowly, and one slowly if at all (41). NADPH substantially protected against loss of activity, and the K_m for NADPH was increased for the modified enzyme. This is in agreement with the assignment (41) of one of the rapidly modified residues as His-45, which corresponds to Arg-44 in the *L. casei* sequence. This residue has a charge interaction with the pyrophosphate group of bound NADPH (Table II). It is less obvious why MTX affords protection against ethoxyformic anhydride modification, since no histidine residues are involved in the binding of MTX to the *E. coli* enzyme. Treatment of the enzyme with DTNB results in rapid modification of Cys-152 and much slower modification of Cys-85 (43). These modifications do not change enzymatic activity or the binding of MTX or NADPH, and this is not surprising, since neither residue is in or near the active site and both are in regions of secondary structure, Cys-85 being in αE and Cys-152 in βH. Both MTX and NADPH protect Cys-85 from modification. The mechanism involved is unclear but is presumably due to ligand-induced conformational changes.

C. Structural Results for Vertebrate Dihydrofolate Reductase

Comparison of the sequence results for three vertebrate DHFR enzymes with those for three bacterial DHFRs (Table V) indicates that the vertebrate sequences have very high homology with each other and also show sufficient homology within the bacterial sequences that very probable alignments can be made with the *E. coli* and *L. casei* sequences, particularly in regions containing residues that interact with ligands. This strongly suggests that much of the backbone of the vertebrate enzymes will have the same conformation as that of the bacterial DHFRs and that the regions where differences occur are the loops connecting elements of secondary structure. It is particularly noticeable that all side chains in vertebrate DHFR corresponding to residues of *L. casei* DHFR that interact with ligands are either homologous or analogous. This is a strong indication that these residues in the vertebrate structure make similar interactions with bound ligands.

Gupta *et al.* (44) have shown that the binding of folate, DHF, MTX, $NADP^+$, and NADPH to DHFR purified from L1210 murine leukemia produces changes in the UV absorption spectra similar to those observed for the *E. coli* enzyme, suggesting that the environment of the bound ligands is the same for the two enzymes. This is also suggested by the observation that the CD of the binary complexes of the L1210 enzyme with inhibitors or substrates exhibits some homologies with the CD spectra of the *E. coli* enzyme. Perturbation of a tryptophan residue by ligand binding is also indicated. Neef and Huennekens (45) have reported quenching of fluorescence when MTX is added to the binary complex of the 1,N^6-ethenoadenine analog of $NADP^+$ and when the $NADP^+$ analog is added to the binary complex of DHF. If structural analogy between the L1210 and the bacterial enzymes is assumed, this is most readily interpreted by assuming that the binding of the second ligand modifies interaction between the enzyme and the first ligand. Direct interaction between the bound ligands seems unlikely to be the cause, because the adenine ring is more than 14 Å from the pteridine ring in the *L. casei* ternary complex and is presumably also too far for direct interaction when bound to the L1210 enzyme.

From calorimetric and fluorescence measurements, Subramanian and Kaufman (46) determined ΔG, ΔH, and ΔS for the binding of ligands to chicken liver DHFR. Binding of NADPH and $NADP^+$ is characterized by small negative enthalpies and large positive entropies. The latter could be due to dehydration of the ligand or of the binding site, hydrophobic interaction of the ligand with the binding site, a conformational change in the enzyme, or any combination of these. In fact, as discussed above, all these appear to be involved in binding of NADPH to DHFR of *L. casei,* so that interactions responsible for binding of the nucleotides to the two enzymes are probably very similar. In addition, the difference in ΔH^o for binding of NADPH to chicken liver DHFR in phosphate buffer and in Tris buffer indicates that NADPH binds in the dianionic form, as in the case of binding to the *L. casei* enzyme.

The enthalpies of binding of MTX in Tris and in phosphate buffer differ by 10.4 kcal/mole. This is consistent with a proton transfer to MTX during binding (45). In contrast, enthalpies of binding of folate and DHF were identical in the two buffers, so that these ligands are not protonated on binding. These conclusions were confirmed by a study of the changes in the UV spectra of MTX, folate, and DHF upon binding to the chicken liver enzyme.

Modification of Cys-11 in chicken liver DHFR with organic mercurials (47), iodine (48), DTNB, *N*-ethylmaleimide, or tetrathionate (49) causes large increases in activity. This effect probably involves changes in the conformation of side-chains at the active site, since the K_m for NADPH increases 2.5-fold and that for DHF 50-fold after modification with CH_3HgOH (11). If Cys-11 of chicken liver DHFR occupies a position in the structure similar to that of Asn-8 in the *L. casei* DHFR structure (Table V), substitution with a bulky group will cause adjustments in the conformation of the two flexible loops (10–22 and 120–139 in the *L. casei* sequence) which form one side of the active site cavity. Similar but less drastic changes in activity occur under certain conditions when Cys-6 of L1210 DHFR or of bovine liver DHFR is modified (11,50), and the explanation is presumably similar.

D. *Streptococcus faecium* Dihydrofolate Reductase

Streptococcus faecium var. *durans* contains two isoenzymes of DHFR (51), and these differ considerably in the portion of their sequences presently known (Table V). The sequence of isoenzyme II shows about the same degree of homology with the *L. casei* sequence as the *E. coli* sequence (Table V), so that it is not unreasonable to assume a similar backbone conformation for isoenzyme II of *S. faecium* DHFR. As discussed above, this also implies similar conformations for side chains of residues involved in β-sheet structure.

Isoenzyme I has not been studied extensively, but Freisheim and his collaborators (51–53) have reported CD spectra for the enzyme and its complexes. Titration of the enzyme with NADPH, and to a lesser extent with $NADP^+$, decreases the Cotton effect of the protein aromatic side chains and would be consistent with interaction of bound NADPH with such side chains, especially with Trp-22, which is conserved in all sequences and which in the *L. casei* structure interacts hydrophobically with the carboxamide group of bound NADPH. However, as in all such experiments, it is difficult to distinguish such effects from the results of induced asymmetry of the nucleotide on binding. CD effects due to the binding of folate and DHF were also observed, but extrinsic and intrinsic effects were again difficult to distinguish. Warwick and Freisheim (54) have reported inactivation of this isoenzyme on modification of the single cysteine residue, but the position of this residue in the sequence is not yet known.

Isoenzyme II has been more extensively studied by chemical modification and by nmr. The following is an outline of the major results obtained in our laboratory. One strategy has been to enrich ^{13}C in one specific type of residue of the enzyme and then to study the motion and microenvironment of these residues in the free enzyme and in its complexes by the use of ^{13}C nmr. When *S. faecium* strain A, a MTX-resistant strain, is grown on a defined medium containing [*indole*-3-^{13}C, 90%]tryptophan the labeled amino acid is incorporated into DHFR with high efficiency and negligible dilution. The ^{13}C nmr spectrum of the purified DHFR shows four peaks corresponding to the four tryptophan residues in the sequence (55). With the alignments shown in Table V, these *S. faecium* tryptophan residues correspond to residues in the *L. casei* sequence that are all in hydrophobic regions of the structure, where these indole rings are likely to have little internal motion. The spin-lattice relaxation time for the four tryptophan resonances are a little shorter than expected on this assumption, but in general agreement. The two upfield resonances are much broader than predicted, and one of them (W^3) has a double structure which is due to slow exchange of the side chain of this residue between different conformations in which it has different chemical shifts (55). The populations in the two conformations are in the ratio 2:3, and lifetimes are ≥ 0.5 and 0.75 second, respectively.

The upfield resonance (W^4) is unique, being ~3 ppm further upfield than the most upfield tryptophan resonance previously observed in proteins. With a decrease in temperature from 25 to 5°C, this resonance sharpens and moves downfield, a result consistent with a slow exchange process that assumes an intermediate rate at 25°C. This residue therefore also exchanges slowly between two conformational states of the side chain, but in this case the populations are disparate. The major population is in the conformational state corresponding to the observed upfield resonance, whereas the minor population is in a conformational state with a downfield shift, perhaps near that of peaks 1 and 2. The minor resonance component is invisible because of its low concentration and broad peak width. The lifetime of the major species at 15°C is about 0.03 second.

The slow exchange of W^4 between alternative conformations is dramatically affected by the binding of many ligands including MTX, 3′,5′-dichloromethotrexate, and $NADP^+$. This is shown by a marked sharpening of the upfield resonance and a small change in chemical shift and is most plausibly interpreted as due to locking of W^4 in one of the side chain conformations. It seems very likely that W^4 is in the vicinity of the active site and is most probably identified with the conserved residue, Trp-22. This corresponds to Trp-21 in the *L. casei* sequence and therefore is partly exposed on one side of the cavity in which MTX and the nicotinamide moiety of NADPH are bound. If this assignment is correct, the upfield shift of the resonance may be explained by the proximity of Asp-9 to Trp-22. If the side-chain conformation of this residue is the same as for the corresponding residue in *L. casei* (Asn-8), the negative charge would be close enough (7.7 Å) to cause the observed upfield shift if the orientation is favorable.

The resonance of W^3 is also shifted by many ligands, the shift usually being downfield, and it seems likely that W^3 is identified with Trp-6, which corresponds to Trp-5 in the *L. casei* sequence. In the *L. casei* structure this residue is buried in a hydrophobic region just below the active site cavity. In this case, the changes in chemical shift which occur on ligand binding probably reflect ligand-induced conformational changes in this region of the enzyme, with consequent changes in ring currents of adjacent residues (Table VI).

The residues giving the two downfield resonances, W^1 and W^2, must be assigned to Trp-115 and Trp-160, which correspond (Table V) to Leu-114 and Tyr-155 in the *L. casei* sequence, respectively. Both of these *L. casei* DHFR residues are buried in a hydrophobic region forming the end of the active site cavity. Trp-160 may well be stacked with Phe-30, since in the *E. coli* structure the corresponding residues, Phe-153 and Trp-30, are shown by X-ray diffraction results to be stacked. Trp-115 must be located on the other side of Phe-30, and there is a possibility of stacking in this case also. Without X-ray diffraction results for *S. faecium* DHFR, it is impossible to predict which tryptophan residue is more likely to experience edge ring current effects, or linear field effects, which would account for the downfield shift of W^1. On the whole, Trp-160 seems to be in a position where it will be more influenced by inhibitor binding, since (if the alignment in Table V is correct and side-chain conformations are as in the *L. casei* enzyme) the indole ring is at the end of the cavity directly opposite the 2-amino group of bound MTX. This suggests that W^1, which shows small changes in its chemical shift with ligand binding, may correspond to Trp-160.

Table VI

Approximate Distances from *Streptococcus faecium* Dihydrofolate Reductase Tryptophan *Indole*-C^3 to Ligand Rings

Tryptophan residue	Microenvironment	Anticipated effect of ligand binding	Perturbing residues and distance[a]
6	Buried in hydrophobic region below substrate pocket	Some, via conformation	Phe-104 (5.5 Å),[b] Phe-128 (2–6 Å), Phe-134 (9 Å)
22	Partly buried in hydrophobic lining of pocket	Direct effects	Asp-9 (7.7 Å), Asp-27 (7.7 Å), Phe-123 (5.5 Å)[c]
115	Partly buried in hydrophobic pocket	Little	Phe-30 (6 Å), His-34 (6 Å), Lys-162 (4–8 Å)
160	Largely screened from solvent by hydrophobic residues; at end of active site cavity	Some effect anticipated by substrates or inhibitors	Phe-30 (4 Å)[c] His-143 (4 Å)

[a] Approximate distance to center of aromatic ring or center of charged group from indole-C^3.
[b] Probably has edge adjacent, giving deshielding.
[c] Probably has face adjacent, giving shielding.

Trp-115, which is probably further from bound ligands, seems less likely to be influenced by inhibitor binding and is more exposed to solvent, hence corresponds more closely to W^2.

These assignments are supported by studies with a spin-labeled analogue of $NADP^+$ (56). The decreases in relaxation times of the four tryptophan resonances that occur when the enzyme forms a binary complex with the spin-labeled analog instead of with its diamagnetic reduced form, indicate that W^1 and W^2 represent distant residues (Trp-115, Trp-160), whereas W^3 and W^4 represent nearer residues (Trp-6, Trp-22) (57). Neither the nmr data nor the distances estimated by comparison with the *L. casei* structure are accurate enough to assign resonances within each of the two groups.

Streptococcus faecium DHFR labeled with [*guanidine*-^{13}C, 90%]arginine exhibits a ^{13}C nmr spectrum in which three resonances (R^1, R^2, R^4) are resolved, but the remaining five resonances coalesce in a central envelope (58). The average T_1 for resonances in the central envelope is significantly longer than the values for R^1, R^2, and R^4, and the chemical shift of the central envelope is close to that for denatured enzyme, whereas those for R^1 and R^2 are downfield and that for R^4 upfield. The temperature dependence of T_1 for the central envelope is complex, whereas T_1 values for R^1, R^2, and R^4 steadily decrease with temperature. All resonances have very small nuclear Overhauser enhancement values (1.13–1.26). From these data, it is probable that R^1, R^2, and R^4 are immobilized residues, whereas those contributing to the central envelope have significant internal motion. In support of this view, calculations of the correlation time for R^1, R^2, and R^4 based on T_1 values in H_2O and D_2O gave a value of 20 nsec, in good agreement with the rotational correlation time of other proteins of this molecular size.

R^1 is sensitive to ligand binding, the resonance moving 0.14 ppm downfield with nucleotide binding and 0.16 ppm upfield with inhibitor binding. It also shows changes in chemical shift with temperature in the free enzyme, in binary complexes with folate and MTX, and in the ternary NADPH–MTX complex. In all cases, the resonance shifts downfield as the temperature is decreased. The simplest explanation of these results is that this resonance monitors the effects of conformational changes in its microenvironment. The downfield shift, compared with the shift of arginine in the denatured enzyme, is presumably due to edge-on ring current effects from adjacent aromatic residues. When the arginine residues in the *S. faecium* enzyme are compared with corresponding residues in *L. casei* DHFR, only one of them appears to be buried in a hydrophobic region. This is Arg-116, which corresponds to Val-115 in the *L. casei* sequence. The guanidino carbon of this residue must be located reasonably close to Trp-6 and Phe-134 and very possibly experiences edge-on ring currents from these residues.

Although none of the other arginine residues appear to be buried in hydrophobic regions, two others may be largely immobilized by nearby carboxylate groups; these are Arg-44 and Arg-156. The former corresponds to Arg-43 in the *L. casei* sequence, and the guanidino carbon of this residue is only 3.2 Å from C-4 of Glu-47. The latter is conserved in the *S. faecium* sequence and is presumably located at about the same distance from Arg-44. Arg-156 is relatively close to Asp-120 and probably interacts with it, but the intercharge distance cannot be calculated because neither residue is conserved in the *L. casei* sequence. It seems likely, however, that Arg-44 and Arg-156 are the other two immobilized residues corresponding, respectively, to R^4 and R^2. Arg-44 seems more likely to correspond to R^4, because it is located close to the 2′-phosphate group of bound NADPH and is therefore likely to show the change in chemical shift due to NADPH binding exhibited by R^4. Arg-156 is remote from the NADPH-binding site. What is currently unclear is why R^4 is not perturbed by the binding of $NADP^+$ or by bound NADPH in the ternary complex with MTX. Clearly, however, these markedly different effects on the chemical shift of R^4 indicate significant differences in the conformations associated with bound NADPH in the binary and ternary complexes and with $NADP^+$ in the binary complex.

The remaining arginine residues (23, 29, 32, 58, and 102) appear to be rather well-exposed to solvent and, although the distances of potentially perturbing residues can only be roughly approximated from comparison with the *L. casei* structure, it is likely that charged or aromatic residues are not close enough to move the chemical shifts far from the value of arginine in denatured protein. These residues are therefore responsible for the five resonances coalescing in the central peak.

Binding of the spin-labeled nucleotide analogue of $NADP^+$ causes broadening of one of the resonances in the central envelope. By comparison with the *L. casei* structure, the arginine residue of this group nearest the unpaired electron in the nitroxide group is likely to be Arg-102 (~11 Å distant).

Streptococcus faecium DHFR labeled with [*methyl*-^{13}C, 90%]methionine gives a ^{13}C nmr spectrum in which the seven resonances are incompletely separated, although the resolution is improved in the MTX binary complex and improved still further in the ternary complex (59). Relaxation times and nuclear Overhauser enhancements for these resonances indicate that in all the residues there is not only rapid rotation of the methyl groups about the C—S bond but also rapid rotation about the CH_2—S bond through a restricted angle. Different residues differ in the angle through which the latter type of motion occurs, the angles varying from ~100° for the broadest peaks to 180°–360° for the narrower peaks (59,60).

The most marked chemical shift change in the nmr spectrum of the [*methyl*-^{13}C]methionine-labeled enzyme is that due to the binding of $NADP^+$, which causes a single resonance to move downfield by at least 1.7 ppm. The binding of NADPH causes no similar movement of this resonance, and it is not observed in the ternary $NADP^+$–MTX ternary complex. However, MTX and related inhibitors cause significant upfield movement of at least two resonances, and this is even more marked in ternary complexes like the NADPH–MTX complex.

Carboxymethylation studies have assisted in assignment of these resonances. Treatment of *S. faecium* DHFR with iodoacetate at pH 6.3 at 0°C results in modification of only methionine residues (61). Met-28 was most rapidly carboxymethylated, and Met-36 and Met-50 to a considerably lesser degree (62). There was a very small amount of modification at Met-163 and negligible attack on the remaining methionines. The carboxymethylated enzyme has a 25-fold lower association constant for aminopterin and a 10-fold lower association constant for DHF, which suggests that one or more of the modified methionines is in the binding cavity. When the aminopterin–DHFR binary complex was treated with iodoacetate, Met-28 and Met-50 were modified to a negligible extent, an observation suggesting that these two residues are in the binding cavity. Comparison of the *L. casei* and *S. faecium* sequences (Table V) indicates that Met-28 and Met-50 in the latter sequence correspond to Leu-27 and Phe-49, respectively. These residues interact hydrophobically with the pteridine and benzene rings of bound MTX in the NADPH–MTX complex with the *L. casei* enzyme.

When the ^{13}C nmr spectrum of the carboxymethylated [*methyl*-^{13}C]methionine-labeled *S. faecium* DHFR is examined, it may be seen that upfield resonances have been depleted, the resonances for the carboxymethylated methionine residues appearing more than 10 ppm downfield. It therefore appears that Met-28 and Met-50 have upfield resonances in the spectrum, and these small upfield shifts may be attributable to linear field effects. Although the side-chain conformations are unknown, the methyl carbon of Met-28 is only about 4 Å from the Asp-27 carboxyl, and the Met-50 methyl must be about 11 Å from this carboxyl and only slightly further from Arg-23, Arg-29, and Lys-52. The nmr spectrum of the MTX complex of the carboxymethylated [*methyl*-^{13}C]methionine-labeled enzyme shows that the resonances which are shifted further upfield by MTX binding correspond to Met-28 and Met-50. This is to be expected, since they are likely to experience shielding ring current effects from MTX, particularly from the benzene ring.

Carboxymethylation does not affect the residue which is shifted downfield in the NADP$^+$ binary complex. Comparison with the *L. casei* sequence and the X-ray diffraction structure of the latter suggests that this residue must be Met-5, the only other methionine corresponding to a residue of the *L. casei* enzyme present in the active site cavity (Leu-4). Leu-4 is at the bottom of the cavity with its methyl carbons 4.2 and 3.6 Å from N-3 of bound MTX. Since this methionine resonance is not perturbed by NADPH binding, it appears to be the positively charged nicotinamide ring which perturbs this methionine methyl. However, the center of the nicotinamide ring of bound NADPH is 9.7 and 9.0 Å from the methyl carbons of Leu-4 in the *L. casei* structure. If the charged nicotinamide ring were to perturb the methionine methyl directly by linear charge effect, it would have to be a good deal closer than this, and for this to be the case it would have to be assumed that $NADP^+$ binds significantly differently in the binary complex than NADPH does in the ternary complex.

Evidence for possible differences in binding of $NADP^+$ and NADPH to DHFR is fragmentary. The association constant for $NADP^+$ binding is one to three orders of magnitude less than for NADPH, depending on the source of the enzyme. In the calorimetric study by Subramanian and Kaufman (46), the less negative $\Delta G^{o\prime}$ for $NADP^+$ binding was shown to be due to a 2.8 kcal/mole smaller enthalpy decrease on binding, the entropy increase being even larger than for NADPH binding. This might be due *inter alia* to a less favorable interaction of the phosphate groups with positively charged side chains in the $NADP^+$ binary complex. Feeney *et al.* (28,63). have concluded, from a study on the ^{31}P nmr spectra of $NADP^+$ and NADPH bound to *L. casei* DHFR, that the 2′-phosphate and pyrophosphate groups are bound in similar positions on the enzyme. Furthermore, the chemical shift of the adenine 2-proton is the same for both bound nucleotides, so they conclude that differences in binding must be strongly localized at the binding site for the nicotinamide ring. Because of the extended conformation of the bound nucleotide, however, changes in binding of the nicotinamide ring must involve some changes, even if small, in the binding of the rest of the molecule. The most likely cause for a different location for the oxidized nicotinamide ring is attraction by the carboxylate ion of Asp-26, which is the only charged residue in the cavity. This might draw the charged nicotinamide ring further into the cavity, so that instead of its center being 9.0 and 9.7 Å from the methyl carbons of Leu-4 it might be only 6 or 7 Å away. This would in turn cause a linear field effect at Leu-4 (or Met-5 in the *S. faecium* structure). The further intrusion of the nicotinamide ring into the cavity would explain why the internal motion of Trp-22 in the *S. faecium* enzyme is more restricted in the $NADP^+$ complex than in the NADPH complex, and consequent adjustments in the binding of the phosphate groups would account for the difference in the chemical shift of R^4 (Arg-44) in the two nucleotide complexes.

IV. Conclusion

It is clear that a large body of evidence now indicates considerable similarity in the structure of DHFR from various sources, particularly at the active site. It is also clear that the structure of the enzyme in the crystalline state as revealed by X-ray diffraction must closely resemble that in solution. A major puzzle that remains to be solved concerns the mode of binding of folate and DHF at the active site and why there is no protonation of these substrates in the binary complex by the carboxyl group, which clearly plays a major role in the catalytic process and which protonates inhibitors like MTX in their binary complexes.

Clarification of this and other aspects of this important enzyme should not be long in coming.

Acknowledgments

I am indebted to Dr. David A. Matthews for making available the atomic coordinates for the *L. casei* ternary complex and for helpful comments on several aspects of this review. This work was supported by United States Public Health Service research grant CA-13840 from the National Cancer Institute.

References

1. D. A. Matthews, R. A. Alden, J. T. Bolin, D. J. Filman, S. T. Freer, R. Hamlin, W. G. J. Hol, R. L. Kisliuk, E. J. Pastore, L. T. Plante, N.-H. Xuong, and J. Kraut, *J. Biol. Chem.* **253,** 6946 (1978).
2. D. A. Matthews, R. A. Alden, J. T. Bolin, S. T. Freer, R. Hamlin, N. Xuong, J. Kraut, M. Poe, M. Williams, and K. Hoogsteen, *Science* **197,** 452 (1977).
3. B. R. Baker, *Cancer Chemother. Rep.* **4,** 1 (1959).
4. D. Stone, A. W. Phillips, and J. J. Burchall, *Eur. J. Biochem.* **72,** 613 (1977).
5. C. D. Bennett, J. A. Rodkey, J. M. Sondey, and R. Hirschmann, *Biochemistry* **17,** 1328 (1978).
6. J. M. Gleisner, D. L. Peterson, and R. L. Blakley, *Proc. Natl. Acad. Sci. U.S.A.* **71,** 3001 (1974).
7. D. L. Peterson, J. M. Gleisner, and R. L. Blakley, *J. Biol. Chem.* **250,** 4945 (1975).
8. D. Stone and A. W. Phillips, *FEBS Lett.* **74,** 85 (1977).
9. D. Stone, S. J. Paterson, J. H. Raper, and A. W. Phillips, *J. Biol. Chem.* **254,** 480 (1979).
10. P.-H. Lai, Y.-C. Pan, J. M. Gleisner, D. L. Peterson, and R. L. Blakley, *in* "Chemistry and Biology of Pteridines" (R. L. Kisliuk and G. M. Brown, eds.), p. 437. Am. Elsevier, New York, 1979.
11. J. H. Freisheim, A. A. Kumar, and D. T. Blankenship, *in* "Chemistry and Biology of Pteridines" (R. L. Kisliuk and G. M. Brown, eds.), p. 419. Am. Elsevier, New York, 1979.
12. K. G. Bitar, D. T. Blankenship, K. A. Walsh, R. B. Dunlap, A. V. Reddy, and J. H. Freisheim, *FEBS Lett.* **80,** 119 (1977).
13. J. H. Freisheim, K. G. Bitar, A. V. Reddy, and D. T. Blankenship, *J. Biol. Chem.* **253,** 6437 (1978).
14. D. A. Matthews, R. A. Alden, S. T. Freer, N.-H. Xuong, and J. Kraut, *J. Biol. Chem.* **254,** 4144 (1979).
15. K. Hood, P. M. Bayley, and G. C. K. Roberts, *Biochem. J.* **177,** 425 (1979).
16. A. V. Reddy, W. D. Behnke, and J. H. Freisheim, *Biochim. Biophys. Acta* **533,** 415 (1978).
17. K. Hood and G. C. K. Roberts, *Biochem. J.* **171,** 357 (1978).
18. J.-K. Liu, and R. B. Dunlap, *Biochemistry* **13,** 1807 (1974).
19. J. H. Freisheim, L. H. Ericcson, K. G. Bitar, R. B. Dunlap, and A. V. Reddy, *Arch. Biochem. Biophys.* **180,** 310 (1977).
20. G. A. Vehar, and J. H. Freisheim, *Biochem. Biophys. Res. Commun.* **68,** 937 (1976).
21. B. Birdsall, D. V. Griffiths, G. C. K. Roberts, J. Feeney, and A. Burgen, *Proc. R. Soc. London, Ser. B* **196,** 251 (1977).
22. D. A. Matthews, *Biochemistry* **18,** 1602 (1979).

23. J. Feeney, G. C. K. Roberts, B. Birdsall, D. V. Griffiths, R. W. King, P. Scudder, and A. Burgen, *Proc. R. Soc. London, Ser. B* **196,** 267 (1977).
24. B. J. Kimber, D. V. Griffiths, B. Birdsall, R. W. King, P. Scudder, J. Feeney, G. C. K. Roberts, and A. S. V. Burgen, *Biochemistry* **16,** 3492 (1977).
25. B. J. Kimber, J. Feeney, G. C. K. Roberts, D. V. Griffiths, and A. S. V. Burgen, *Nature (London)* **271,** 184 (1978).
26. G. C. K. Roberts, J. Feeney, A. S. V. Burgen, V. Yuferov, J. G. Dann, and R. Bjur, *Biochemistry* **13,** 5351 (1974).
27. E. J. Pastore, L. T. Plante, J. M. Wright, R. L. Kisliuk, and N. O. Kaplan, *Biochem. Biophys. Res. Commun.* **68,** 471 (1976).
28. J. Feeney, B. Birdsall, G. C. K. Roberts, and A. S. V. Burgen, *Nature (London)* **257,** 564 (1975).
29. B. Birdsall, G. C. K. Roberts, J. Feeney, and A. S. V. Burgen, *FEBS Lett.* **80,** 313 (1977).
30. B. Birdsall, A. S. V. Burgen, J. R. Miranda, and G. C. K. Roberts, *Biochemistry* **17,** 2102 (1978).
31. B. Birdsall, *in* "Nuclear Magnetic Resonance Spectroscopy in Molecular Biology" (B. Pullman, ed.), p. 339. Reidel Publ., Dordrecht, Netherlands, 1978.
32. S. W. Dietrich, R. N. Smith, S. Brendler, and C. Hansch, *Arch. Biochem. Biophys.* **194,** 612 (1979).
33. S. M. J. Dunn, J. G. Batchelor, and R. W. King *Biochemistry* **17,** 2357 (1978).
34. B. B. Kitchell, and R. W. Henkens, *Biochim. Biophys. Acta* **534,** 89 (1978).
35. N. J. Greenfield, M. N. Williams, M. Poe, and K. Hoogsteen, *Biochemistry* **11,** 4706 (1972).
36. N. J. Greenfield, *Biochim Biophys. Acta* **403,** 32 (1975).
37. M. Poe, N. J. Greenfield, J. M. Hirshfield, and K. Hoogsteen, *Cancer Biochem. Biophys.* **1,** 7 (1974).
38. J. S. Erickson and C. K. Mathews, *J. Biol. Chem.* **247,** 5661 (1972).
39. D. D. Saperstein, A. J. Rein, M. Poe, and M. F. Leahy, *J. Am. Chem. Soc.* **100,** 4296 (1978).
40. M. N. Williams, N. J. Greenfield, and K. Hoogsteen *J. Biol. Chem.* **248,** 6380 (1973).
41. M. Poe, K. Hoogsteen, and D. A. Matthews, *J. Biol. Chem.* **254,** 8143 (1979).
42. N. J. Greenfield, *Biochemistry* **13,** 4494 (1974).
43. M. N. Williams, and C. D. Bennett, *J. Biol. Chem.* **252,** 6871 (1977).
44. S. V. Gupta, N. J. Greenfield, M. Poe, D. R. Makulu, M. N. Williams, B. A. Moronson, and J. R. Bertino, *Biochemistry* **16,** 3073 (1977).
45. V. G. Neef, and F. M. Huennekens, *Biochemistry* **15,** 4042 (1976).
46. S. Subramanian and B. T. Kaufman, *Proc. Natl. Acad. Sci. U.S.A.* **75,** 3201 (1978).
47. B. T. Kaufman, *J. Biol. Chem.* **239,** PC669 (1964).
48. B. T. Kaufman, *Proc. Natl. Acad. Sci. U.S.A.* **56,** 695 (1966).
49. E. K. Barbehenn and B. T. Kaufman, *Biochem. Biophys. Res. Commun.* **85,** 402 (1978).
50. R. L. Blakley "The Biochemistry of Folic Acid and Related Pteridines," p. 147. North-Holland Publ., Amsterdam, 1969.
51. L. D'Souza, P. E. Warwick, and J. H. Freisheim, *Biochemistry* **11,** 1528 (1972).
52. J. H. Freisheim and L. D'Souza, *Biochem. Biophys. Res. Commun.* **45,** 803 (1971).
53. L. D'Souza and J. H. Freisheim, *Biochemistry* **11,** 3770 (1972).
54. P. E. Warwick and J. H. Freisheim, *Biochemistry* **14,** 664 (1975).
55. R. E. London, J. P. Groff, and R. L. Blakley, *Biochem. Biophys. Res. Commun.* **86,** 779 (1979).
56. L. Cocco and R. L. Blakley, *Biochemistry* **18,** 2414 (1979).
57. J. P. Groff, R. E. London, and R. L. Blakley, unpublished results.
58. L. Cocco, L., R. L. Blakley, T. E. Walker, R. E. London, and N. A. Matwiyoff, *Biochemistry* **17,** 4285 (1978).

59. R. L. Blakley, L. Cocco, R. E. London, T. E. Walker, and N. A. Matwiyoff, *Biochemistry* **17,** 2284 (1978).
60. R. E. London and J. Avitabile, *J. Am. Chem. Soc.* **100,** 7159 (1978).
61. J. M. Gleisner and R. L. Blakley, *J. Biol. Chem.* **250,** 1580 (1975).
62. J. M. Gleisner and R. L. Blakley, *Eur. J. Biochem.* **55,** 141 (1975).
63. J. Feeney, B. Birdsall, G. K. C. Roberts, and A. S. V. Burgen, *in* "NMR in Biology" (R. A. Dwek, I. D. Campbell, R. E. Richards, and R. J. P. Williams, eds.), p. 111. Academic Press, New York, 1977.

16

Transport of Folate Compounds in L1210 Cells: Components and Mechanisms

F. M. HUENNEKENS, K. S. VITOLS, M. R. SURESH, AND
G. B. HENDERSON

I. Introduction

Folic acid is essential for cell replication, and cells unable to synthesize the vitamin have an absolute requirement for an external source. Mammalian cells fall into this category, along with certain bacteria (e.g., *Lactobacillus casei, Streptococcus faecalis,* and *Pediococcus cerevisiae*) that lack the vitamin-synthesizing system. Inside the cell, conversion of folic acid to the metabolically active coenzyme, tetrahydrofolate, is catalyzed by the NADPH-dependent enzyme, dihydrofolate reductase (1,2). Alternative routes to tetrahydrofolate (Fig. 1) also exist (3), e.g., from 5-methyltetrahydrofolate via B_{12}-dependent methionine synthetase and from 5-formyltetrahydrofolate (folinate) via a path-

MOLECULAR ACTIONS AND TARGETS FOR CANCER CHEMOTHERAPEUTIC AGENTS

ISBN 0-12-619280-4

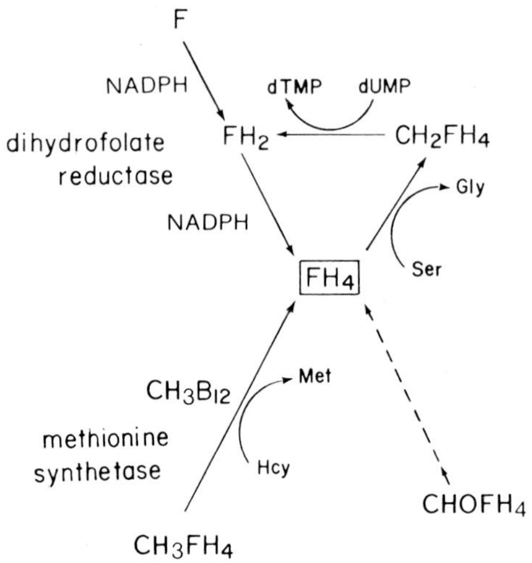

Fig. 1. Metabolic interconversions of folate compounds. F, Folate; FH_2, dihydrofolate; FH_4, tetrahydrofolate; CH_2FH_4, 5,10-methylenetetrahydrofolate; CH_3FH_4, 5-methyltetrahydrofolate; $CHOFH_4$, 5-formyltetrahydrofolate; CH_3B_{12}, methylcobalamin; other abbreviations are standard.

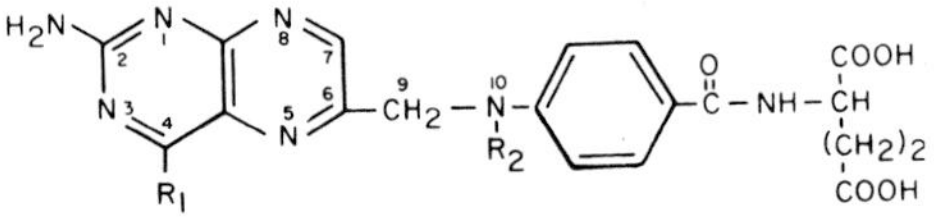

Oxidized Folates

R_1 = OH, R_2 = H ; Folate
R_1 = NH_2, R_2 = H ; Aminopterin
R = NH_2, R_2 = CH_3; Methotrexate

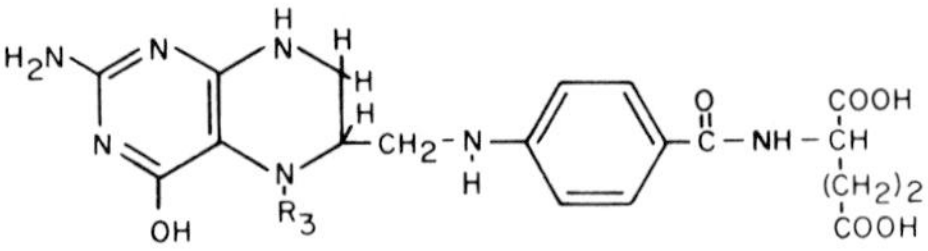

Reduced Folates

R_3 = H ; Tetrahydrofolate
R_3 = CH_3; 5-Methyltetrahydrofolate
R_3 = CHO; 5-Formyltetrahydrofolate

Fig. 2. Structures of oxidized and reduced folate compounds.

way that is still not well understood. Structures of the relevant folate compounds are shown in Fig. 2.

Dihydrofolate reductase is the intracellular target for methotrexate (MTX). The effectiveness of this drug as a cancer chemotherapeutic agent depends upon its ability to prevent replenishment of the tetrahydrofolate pool via the thymidylate synthesis cycle (Fig. 1). This is particularly critical when folate is the vitamin source. Conversion of 5-methyl- or 5-formyltetrahydrofolate to the coenzyme is not directly affected by MTX, but the drug can still block replication of cells supplied with *limiting* amounts of either of these reduced folate compounds.

5-Methyltetrahydrofolate, rather than folate, is the primary circulating form of the vitamin in mammals (4,5). It is not surprising therefore that in most mammalian cells folate is transported poorly and reduced sluggishly. 5-Methyltetrahydrofolate is transported with a high degree of efficiency (6), but its conversion to the coenzyme is controlled by the rate-limiting activity of methionine synthetase (7). 5-Formyltetrahydrofolate is also taken up readily by cells (8), and its effectiveness as a "rescue agent" in high-dose MTX regimens is dependent upon this property and its facile conversion to tetrahydrofolate. As would be expected, 5-methyltetrahydrofolate can also rescue cells from MTX toxicity (9). Despite these considerations, folate at concentrations of approximately 1 μM can serve, and is usually used, as the vitamin source for mammalian cells propagated in culture. Growth on 5-methyltetrahydrofolate occurs at lower levels (about 0.1 μM) which more nearly approximate the physiological situation (10,11).

From the above discussion, it is evident that mammalian cells require both a source of folic acid and some means for its internalization. Transport of folate compounds has been studied in a variety of eukaryotic and prokaryotic cells, and considerable information has accumulated regarding the general characteristics of these systems (reviewed in 6,12,13). However, much less is known about the specific components or the detailed mechanism(s) for translocation of folates across membranes. This chapter will focus upon these parameters, particularly with reference to the transport of MTX in cultured L1210 mouse leukemia cells.

II. Transport of Reduced Folate Compounds and Methotrexate in L1210 Cells

A. General Characteristics

Uptake of reduced folate compounds and MTX by L1210 cells (reviewed in 6,12,13) occurs via an active transport system whose primary substrate is 5-methyltetrahydrofolate. The process is saturable, inhibited competitively by various folate compounds, and highly dependent upon temperature. Energy-dependent uptake can produce concentration gradients of free, unmetabolized substrate. *P*-Chloromercuriphenylsulfonate (pCMS) and other mercurials (14) inhibit uptake, while azide (15) and iodoacetate (14) are stimulatory. This property of pCMS makes it a useful probe for distinguishing carrier-mediated transport from passive diffusion at substrate concentrations relevant to high-dose MTX chemotherapy (16). Regulation of transport appears to occur via the intracellular level of cyclic AMP (17).

B. Binding Component

1. *Lactobacillus casei Model*

Membrane-associated binding proteins have been identified as constituents of many transport systems. A component of this type, having a broad specificity for folate compounds, is present in *L. casei* cells (18–20). This entity was first detected by low-temperature (4°C) binding measurements using [^{3}H]folate, which provided values of 15 n*M* for the dissociation constant (K_D) and 2 × 10^4 for the number of binders per cell (21). It was then solubilized by treatment of cells or membranes with Triton X-100 (in the presence of [^{3}H]folate) and purified by adsorption and elution from microgranular silica followed by filtration through Sephadex G-25 (20,22). Homogeneity of the protein was demonstrated by sodium dodecyl sulfate polyacrylamide gel electrophoresis (Fig. 3), and its molecular weight was estimated to be 25,000 by comparison with the mobility of standard proteins. Noncovalently bound, labeled folate (0.9 mole/mole of protein) was associated with the purified binder (22). The amino acid composition (Table I), which shows a preponderance of hydrophobic residues (22), is consistent with localization in the membrane. Amino acid sequencing of the protein is being performed by J. H. Freisheim, University of Cincinnati. Functionality of the *L. casei*-binding protein, after incorporation into liposomes, has not yet been demonstrated; reconstitution of the system may require the presence of a second component that appears to be responsible for the coupling of energy to the translocation step (23). However, involvement of the binding protein in folate transport seems reasonably certain from other lines of evidence: (1) Cells grown on increasing levels of folate show a parallel loss of transport activity, binding activity, and amount of detergent-extractable binding protein (19); (2) a linear relationship exists between the binding constants (K_D values) and the kinetic constants (K_t values) for various folate compounds (20); and (3) *L. casei* mutants defective in folate transport are equally defective in binding this substrate (20).

2. *Binding Measurements*

Studies with the *L. casei* transport system, summarized above, have provided guidance for a parallel program aimed at isolation of the corresponding binding

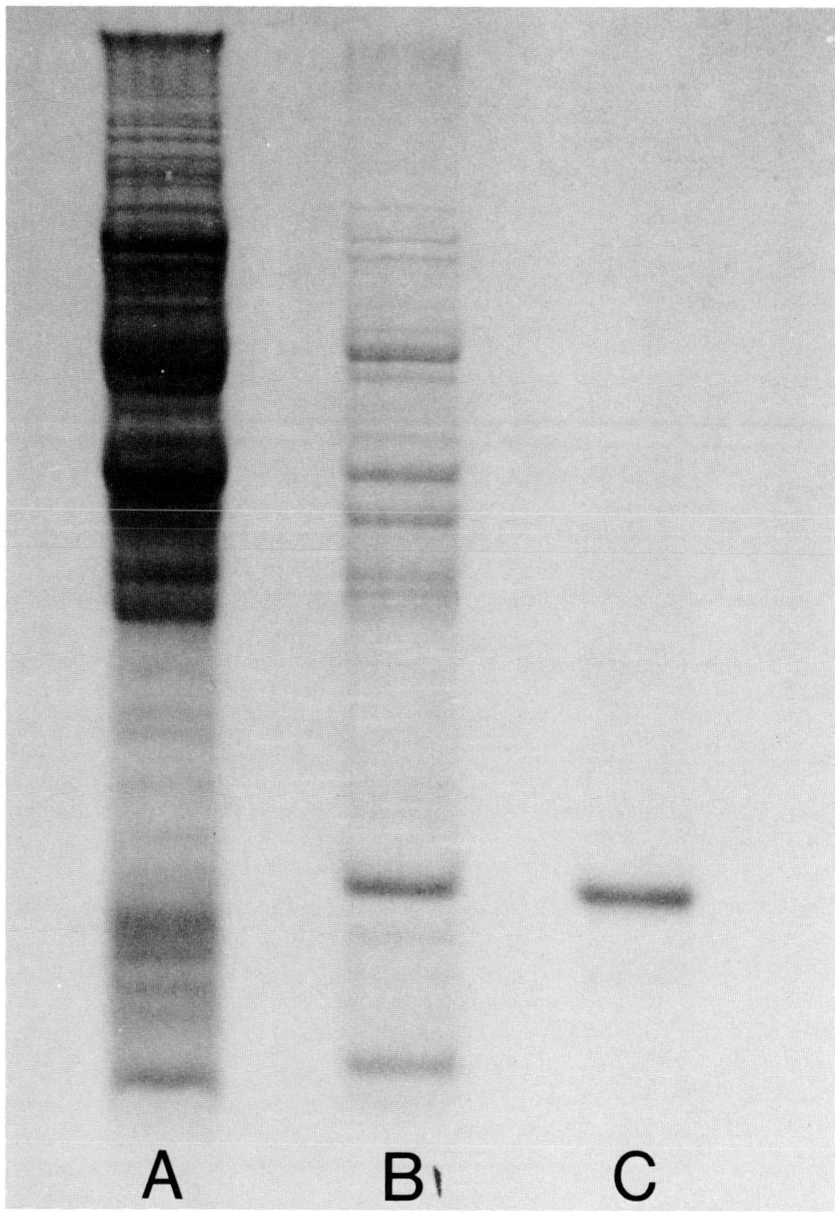

Fig. 3. SDS-gel electrophoresis of the folate-binding protein from *L. casei.* Procedures for purification of the binding protein and SDS gel electrophoresis are described in Henderson *et al.* (22). (A) After extraction from membrane; (B) after silica fractionation; (C) after Sephadex G-150 chromatography.

TABLE I

Amino Acid Composition of the Folate-Binding Protein from *Lactobacillus casei*

Amino acid	Residues per 25,000-*g* protein
Cysteine	0.2
Aspartic acid	14.2
Methionine	17.9
Threonine	15.0
Serine	14.3
Glutamic acid	9.3
Proline	12.1
Glycine	15.5
Alanine	22.2
Valine	12.7
Isoleucine	18.2
Leucine	26.1
Tyrosine	4.9
Phenylalanine	13.1
Histidine	2.7
Lysine	8.3
Arginine	8.0
Tryptophan	10.5

protein from the 5-methyltetrahydrofolate–MTX transport system in L1210 cells. Low-temperature measurements using [*Me*-^{14}C]5-methyltetrahydrofolate in 4-(2-hydroxyethyl)-1-piperazine ethanesulfonic acid (HEPES) buffer (unless otherwise indicated, HEPES buffer will refer to 160 m*M* HEPES adjusted to pH 7.4 with KOH) verified the presence of a binding component with a K_D value of 0.1 μM for this substrate (Fig. 4) (24). The number of binders per cell was 8×10^4, a value similar to that found for *L. casei*. The smaller bacterial cells, however, have a higher density of binding proteins on the membrane. Similar measurements with [^{3}H]MTX yielded a K_D of 0.4 μM for this substrate. Binding could be rapidly and almost completely reversed by the addition of an excess amount of unlabeled substrate, indicating that transport did not occur under the experimental conditions employed. Involvement of the binding component in transport was shown by the fact that aminopterin, 5-formyltetrahydrofolate, MTX, and folate exhibited the same order of effectiveness as inhibitors of both binding and transport of 5-methyltetrahydrofolate (Table II).

3. *Covalent Labeling*

The kinetic constants in Table II were obtained in HEPES buffer, which maximizes interaction between folate substrates and the membrane-associated binding protein (24,25). These constants, however, are considerably larger than

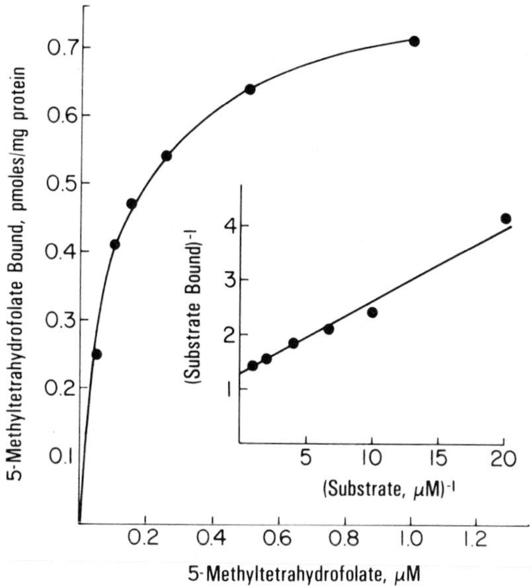

Fig. 4. Binding of [*Me*-^{14}C]5-methyltetrahydrofolate by L1210 cells. After exposure of cells for 5 minutes (at 4°C) to the indicated concentrations of labeled 5-methyltetrahydrofolate in HEPES buffer, samples were centrifuged at 1000 *g* (5 minutes 4°C), supernatant fractions were withdrawn by suction, and residual fluid around the pellets was removed. Pellets were then dissolved in 1.0 ml of water and analyzed for radioactivity in a Triton- and toluene-based scintillation fluid. Results were corrected by a control in which excess unlabeled MTX (100 *μM*) was added prior to the labeled substrate. Inset, double reciprocal plot of substrate bound versus concentration.

TABLE II

Inhibition of [*Me*-^{14}C]5-Methyltetrahydrofolate Binding and Transport in L1210 Cells by Various Folate Compounds[a]

Compound	K_i for binding (*μM*)	K_i for transport (*μM*)
Aminopterin	0.11	0.19
5-Formyltetrahydrofolate	0.36	0.72
MTX	0.44	1.1
Folate	10.	30.

[a] Binding (at 4°C) of 0.2 *μM* [*Me*-^{14}C]5-methyltetrahydrofolate or transport (at 37°C) of 0.5 *μM* [*Me*-^{14}C]5-methyltetrahydrofolate was determined (as in Figs. 4 and 5) in the presence of the indicated unlabeled compounds. K_i values were obtained from Dixon plots of the data.

those of the *L. casei* binder, and it is unlikely that a noncovalently bound, labeled substrate would be retained by the L1210 protein during extraction from the membrane and subsequent purification. Accordingly, an effort has been made to develop procedures for covalent attachment of a marker ligand to the protein prior to its release from the membrane.

One procedure makes use of photoaffinity labeling, a technique that has been utilized extensively for delineating the active site of proteins (reviewed in 26,27). Since adenine nucleotides are inhibitors of both binding (24) and transport (12,25) in the 5-methyltetrahydrofolate–MTX system, it was anticipated that the commercially available 8-azido derivative of AMP would also interact with the membrane protein. Indeed, in the absence of light, 8-azidoadenosine 5′-monophosphate (azido-AMP) inhibited MTX transport competitively with a K_i (140 μM) only slightly higher than the corresponding value (74 μM) for the parent compound, AMP (28). When azido-AMP was irradiated in the presence of cells, a time-dependent, irreversible inhibition of MTX transport was observed (Fig. 5). In order to achieve complete inhibition, cells had to be subjected to several cycles of the azido-AMP treatment. The nitrene (R—$\ddot{N}$) generated by irradiation of azido-AMP (Fig. 6) reacts readily with C—H bonds in proteins: $\left(\text{—C—H} + \text{R—}\ddot{\text{N}} \rightarrow \text{—C—}\underset{\text{H}}{\text{N}}\text{—R}\right)$.

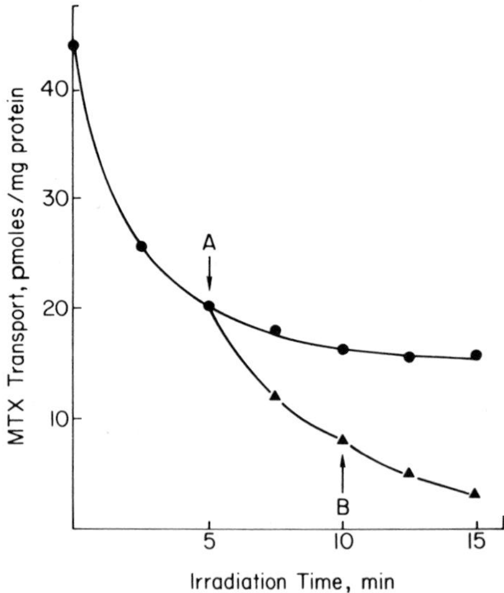

Fig. 5. Time-dependent photoinactivation of MTX transport by 8-azido-AMP. Cell suspensions containing 200 μM azido-AMP were exposed to a mercury lamp (254 nm) for the indicated time intervals, centrifuged at 600 *g* (5 minutes, 4°C), washed with 4 ml of HEPES buffer, and examined for MTX transport activity (●). At arrows A and B, duplicate samples were centrifuged, resuspended in a fresh aliquot of buffer (1.0 ml) containing 200 μM azido-AMP, and irradiated further (▲). From Henderson *et al.* (28).

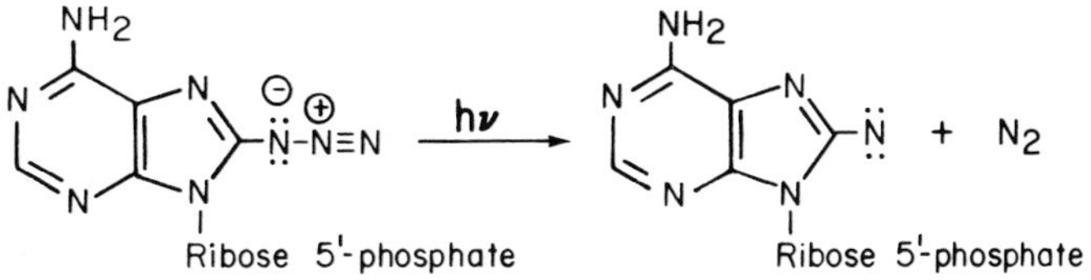

Fig. 6. Photoactivation of azido-AMP.

Treatment of the cells with a carbodiimide-activated derivative of MTX has proved to be an alternative, and even more effective, procedure for irreversibly inhibiting the MTX transport system (29). As observed previously with azido-AMP, specificity of this new reagent has been demonstrated by (1) the ability of a substrate (MTX) or a competitive inhibitor (phosphate) to protect the transport system from inactivation, and (2) failure of the reagent to inhibit other transport systems (e.g., those responsible for uptake of leucine or phosphate).

By employing radiolabeled azido-AMP or activated MTX, it should be possible to identify the 5-methyltetrahydrofolate–MTX transport protein during isolation and purification. When a satisfactory purification procedure has been established, omission of the covalent labeling step would allow the protein to be obtained in a functional state.

C. Energetics and Anion-Exchange Mechanism

Transport of MTX into eukaryotic cells has generally been performed in physiological buffers containing bicarbonate, chloride, and/or phosphate. Under these conditions, rates of uptake are not particularly rapid, and the concentration ratios (C_{in}/C_{out}) barely exceed a value of 1. However, when cells were buffered with HEPES (a large zwitterion that does not appear to interact appreciably with the transport system), uptake rates and steady-state levels of MTX were considerably greater than the corresponding values in phosphate-buffered saline (PBS—138 mM NaCl, 2.7 mM KCl, 8.1 mM Na_2HPO_4, 1.5 mM KH_2PO_4, 1.0 mM $CaCl_2$, and 0.5 mM $MgCl_2$) (Fig. 7). The inhibitory effect of chloride upon these parameters was evident from the intermediate curve. When uptake rates were examined as a function of MTX concentration in L1210 cells buffered with HEPES, HEPES containing KCl, or PBS, double reciprocal plots of these data (Fig. 8) indicated that K_t (rather than V_{max}) was affected. Subsequent observations showed that a wide variety of anions were able to compete with the substrate for the binding site on the membrane protein (Table III). Adenine nucleotides and thiamine pyrophosphate were good inhibitors; the K_i for the latter compound (2.3 μM) approached the K_t value (0.9 μM) for MTX. Each compound listed in Table III was shown to be a competitive inhibitor of MTX transport. Data for inhibition of MTX transport by inorganic phosphate are illustrated in Fig. 9.

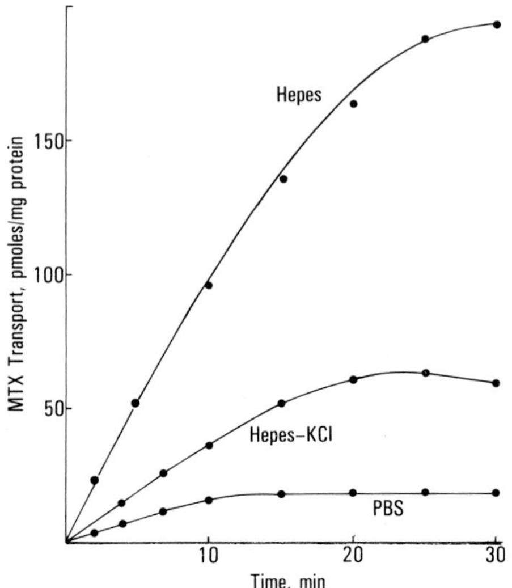

Fig. 7. Time-dependent uptake of MTX by L1210 cells in various buffer systems. For a description of HEPES and PBS buffers see the text; HEPES-KCl is 20 m*M* HEPES and 140 m*M* KCl adjusted with KOH to pH 7.4. From Henderson and Zevely (25).

The improved uptake of MTX and other folate compounds that can be achieved in HEPES buffer has considerable practical value, since it allows concentration ratios as high as 60 to be attained (25). Results of the above experiments have also provided a possible explanation for the energization of transport in this system, namely, that influx of MTX is coupled with efflux of intracellular

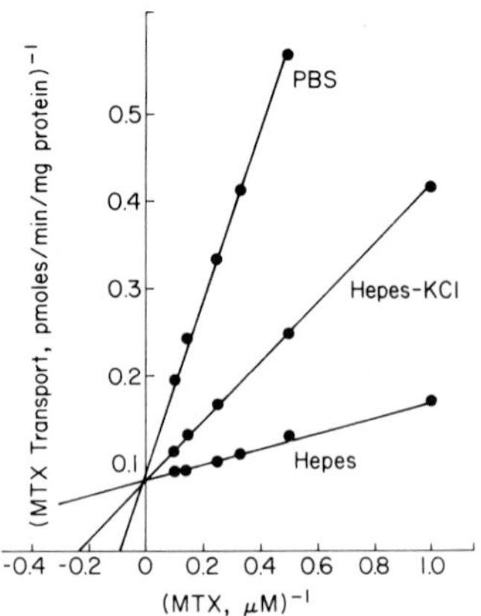

Fig. 8. Double reciprocal plot of MTX transport rate as a function of MTX concentration in HEPES, HEPES-KCl, and PBS. For a description of buffers see Fig. 7. From Henderson and Zevely (25).

TABLE III

Inhibition of Methotrexate Transport in L1210 Cells by Various Anions[a]

Anion	K_i (μM)
Chloride	46,000
Phosphate	870
Sulfate	810
Arsenate	890
Pyrophosphate	400
Molybdate	300
Glucose 6-phosphate	1,200
AMP	74
ADP	26
ATP	18
Thiamine pyrophosphate	2.3

[a] Experimental procedure as in Fig. 9.

anions (12,25,30,31). Such a mechanism would be consistent with the broad specificity of the system for negatively charged compounds (Table III). The driving force for this exchange would be a concentration gradient ($C_{in} > C_{out}$) of anions. Phosphate may be the anion that fulfills this function under physiological conditions (25,30), since L1210 cells possess a Na^+-dependent phosphate trans-

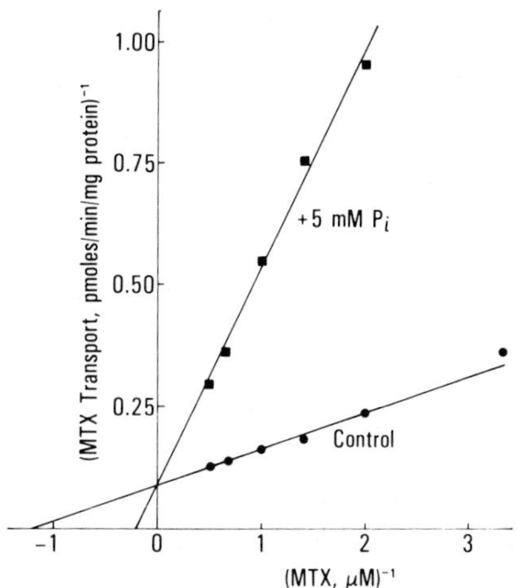

Fig. 9. Double reciprocal plot of MTX transport rate as a function of MTX concentration in the absence and presence of 5 mM inorganic phosphate (P_i). For a description of procedures see Fig. 5 in Henderson and Zevely (30).

port system (K_t= 0.3 mM) that could serve to return the anion and maintain the high intracellular concentration (unpublished observations from this laboratory).

III. Transport of Folate in L1210 Cells

In contrast to the efficiency with which reduced folates and MTX are taken up by L1210 cells (as indicated by K_t values in the range of 1–5 μM), folate itself appears to be a poor substrate. Various laboratories have reported K_t values in excess of 100 μM for folate [see Table IV in Huennekens *et al.* (6)], and several lines of evidence [reviewed in Huennekens *et al.* (6)] suggested that the oxidized vitamin was not transported by the 5-methyltetrahydrofolate–MTX system. Accordingly, a search was made for some other system that might be used uniquely, or shared, by folate. Adenine was found to be a potent competitive inhibitor of folate transport (32), and the correspondence between the K_i (20 μM) for adenine inhibition of folate transport and the K_t (17 μM) for adenine transport itself led to the conclusion that folate entered the cells via an adenine transport system.

During the course of these studies, it was observed that the K_t and V_{max} values for folate transport showed considerable variation in separate determinations. This raised the possibility that a contaminant in the commercially available [^{3}H]folate was responsible for at least a portion of the uptake ascribed to folate. Analysis of the [^{3}H]folate by thin-layer chromatography showed that, in addition to the parent compound, two other radioactive components comprising about 5% of the total material were present. One of these components [detected previously by Caston and Kamen (33) in commercial [^{3}H]folate] was *p*-aminobenzoylglutamate, but it was transported poorly by L1210 cells. The second component, a mixture of fluorescent pteridines, was taken up rapidly and efficiently by the cells, and uptake was strongly inhibited by adenine.

The pteridine fraction was resolved by high-pressure liquid chromatography into a number of radioactive and/or 254-nm absorbing peaks (Fig. 10A). By comparison with authentic standards (Fig. 10B), 6-carboxypterin and 6-hydroxymethylpterin were identified in this fraction. It is not yet clear, however, whether one or both of these pterins can be transported by the adenine system. [^{3}H]Folate from which these contaminants had been removed was transported much less efficiently than reported previously by various groups, and only a small fraction (10–20%) of the uptake was inhibited by adenine (Fig. 11). Conversely, transport of purified folate was inhibited extensively (80–90%) by pCMS or MTX, suggesting that its uptake occurred primarily via the 5-methyltetrahydrofolate–MTX system. In summary, L1210 cells prefer to transport reduced folate compounds, but their growth requirement can be met by uptake of the oxidized form of the vitamin. The reduced folate transport system

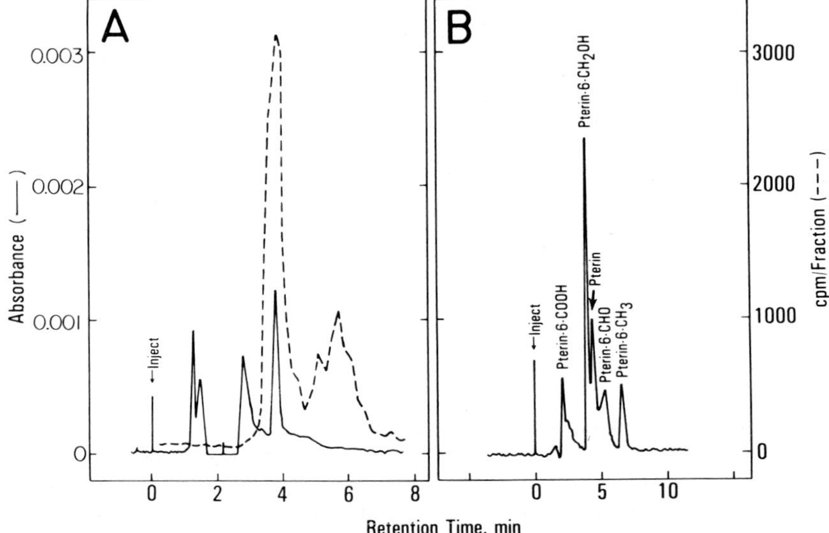

Fig. 10. Separation of pteridine compounds by high-pressure liquid chromatography. (A) Pteridine fraction isolated from [^{3}H]folate. [^{3}H]Folate was subjected to thin-layer chromatography using 0.1 *M* HEPES, pH 7.4, as the solvent system. The fluorescent band ($R_f = 0.4$) was eluted and chromatographed on a C_8 column using 15% methanol as the mobile phase. (B) Pteridine standards.

(and, to a lesser extent, the adenine system) is utilized for this purpose, but in both instances folate is a poor substrate.

IV. Conclusions

Transport of folate compounds in L1210 cells is accomplished by means of a mechanism whose broad outlines are now visible. How the substrates actually traverse the membrane should become more evident when the putative binding

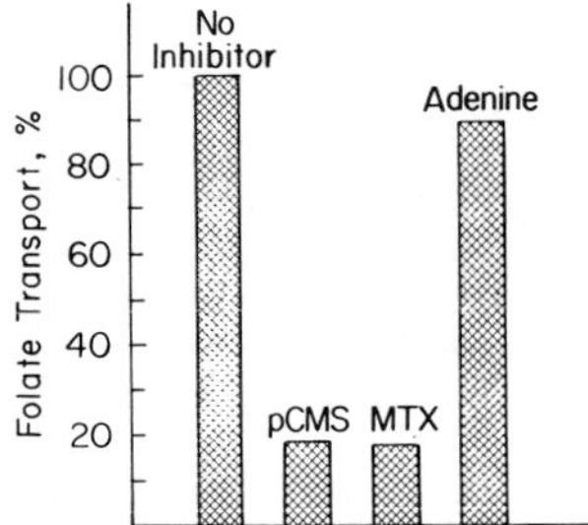

Fig. 11. Inhibition of folate transport by various compounds. Uptake of [^{3}H]folate (100 μM) was measured in HEPES-KCl buffer [as described in Henderson and Zevely (25)]. Inhibitors were each present at 100 μM.

protein has been isolated and characterized and when the energy-coupling aspects are better understood. Calculations indicate that each folate molecule requires at least several seconds to be internalized, and it would be desirable to be able to measure what fraction of this time is consumed by each of the three formal phases of a transport process (binding, translocation, and release of the substrate). There is also a need to determine (1) the spatial relationships between the binding protein and fixed elements of the membrane during transit of the substrate, and (2) whether energy (in addition to that required to create gradients or potentials) is utilized elsewhere in the mechanism, e.g., to facilitate conformational changes in the binding protein.

Fundamental information about the transport of folate compounds in eukaryotes should be useful in designing new types of chemotherapeutic regimens for the destruction of malignant cells. Two separate approaches can be envisioned. The first would make use of chemically synthesized analogues, which have the potential for blocking the uptake of naturally occurring forms of the vitamin and causing cell death via folate starvation. This is similar in principle to the utilization of an extracellular agent, carboxypeptidase G_1, to interdict the supply of folates (34). As an alternate approach, analogues of MTX might be prepared that are transported more efficiently than the parent compound into cells whose resistance to the drug is due to an altered transport system. Both of these objectives could of course be pursued in the traditional manner by synthesizing and testing a large number of analogs A more rational approach would involve the isolation of folate-binding proteins from various cells; this would allow a study to be made of the binding site and its interaction with the substrate. Recent success in obtaining the three-dimensional structures of dihydrofolate reductases by X-ray diffraction (35) has revealed a wealth of detail about the binding of MTX to this enzyme, and it would be highly desirable to have a similar degree of understanding in the case of the transport proteins. This will require, however, crystallization of the latter—a somewhat difficult feat, at present, for these hydrophobic membrane proteins.

Acknowledgment

The authors are indebted to Mr. E. Zevely for expert technical assistance.

Experimental work described in this chapter was supported by grants from the National Cancer Institute (CA-06522, CA-16600, and CA-23970), the American Cancer Society (CH-31), and the National Science Foundation (PCM77-23414). M.R.S. is the recipient of a Junior Fellowship from the California Division, American Cancer Society.

References

1. F. M. Huennekens, R. B. Dunlap, J. H. Freisheim, L. E. Gundersen, N. G. L. Harding, S. A. Levison, and G. P. Mell, *Ann. N.Y. Acad. Sci.* **186,** 85 (1971).

2. R. L. Blakley, "The Biochemistry of Folic Acid and Related Pteridines," Chapter 5. North-Holland Publ., Amsterdam, 1969.
3. F. M. Huennekens, *in* "Biological Oxidations" (T. P. Singer, ed.), p. 439. Wiley (Interscience), New York, 1968.
4. V. Herbert, A. R. Larrabee, and J. Buchanan, *J. Clin. Invest.* **41,** 1134 (1962).
5. O. D. Bird, V. M. McGlohon, and J. W. Vaitkus, *Anal. Biochem.* **12,** 18 (1965).
6. F. M. Huennekens, K. S. Vitols, and G. B. Henderson, *Adv. Enzymol.* **47,** 313 (1978).
7. F. M. Huennekens, P. M. DiGirolamo, K. Fujii, D. W. Jacobsen, and K. S. Vitols, *Adv. Enzyme Regul.* **14,** 187 (1976).
8. A. Nahas, P. F. Nixon, and J. R. Bertino, *Cancer Res.* **32,** 1416 (1972).
9. J. P. Groff and R. L. Blakley, *Cancer Res.* **38,** 3847 (1978).
10. K. Fujii, T. Nagasaki, and F. M. Huennekens, *in* "Vitamin B_{12} and Intrinsic Factor" (B. Zagalak, ed.) p. 1127. Walter de Gruyter, Berlin, 1979.
11. S. D. Balk, D. LeStourgeon, and R. S. Mitchell, *Cancer Res.* **38,** 3966 (1978).
12. I. D. Goldman, *Ann. N.Y. Acad. Sci.* **186,** 400 (1971).
13. F. M. Sirotnak, P. L. Chello, and R. W. Brockman, *Methods Cancer Res.* **16,** 381 (1979).
14. J. I. Rader, D. Niethammer, and F. M. Huennekens, *Biochem. Pharmacol.* **23,** 2057 (1974).
15. I. D. Goldman, *J. Biol. Chem.* **244,** 3779 (1969).
16. G. B. Henderson, M. R. Suresh, E. M. Zevely, K. S. Vitols, and F. M. Huennekens, *Cancer Res.* (submitted for publication).
17. G. B. Henderson, E. M. Zevely, and F. M. Huennekens, *Cancer Res.* **38,** 359 (1978).
18. G. B. Henderson and F. M. Huennekens, *Arch. Biochem. Biophys.* **164,** 722 (1974).
19. G. B. Henderson, E. M. Zevely, and F. M. Huennekens, *Biochem. Biophys. Res. Commun.* **68,** 712 (1976).
20. G. B. Henderson, E. M. Zevely, R. J. Kadner, and F. M. Huennekens, *J. Supramol. Struct.* **6,** 239 (1977).
21. G. B. Henderson, E. M. Zevely, and F. M. Huennekens, *J. Bacteriol.* **139,** 552 (1979).
22. G. B. Henderson, E. M. Zevely, and F. M. Huennekens, *J. Biol. Chem.* **252,** 3760 (1977).
23. G. B. Henderson, E. M. Zevely, and F. M. Huennekens, *J. Bacteriol.* **137,** 1308 (1979).
24. G. B. Henderson, B. Grzelakowska-Sztabert, E. M. Zevely, and W. B. Dandliker, *Fed. Proc. Fed. Am. Soc. Exp. Biol.* **38,** 624 (1979).
25. G. B. Henderson and E. M. Zevely, *Arch. Biochem. Biophys.* **200,** 149 (1980).
26. V. Chowdry and F. Westheimer, *Annu. Rev. Biochem.* **48,** 293 (1979).
27. H. Bayley and J. R. Knowles, *in* "Methods in Enzymology" (W. B. Jakoby and M. Wilchek, eds.), Vol. 46, p. 69. Academic Press, New York, 1977.
28. G. B. Henderson, E. M. Zevely, and F. M. Huennekens, *J. Biol. Chem.* **254,** 9973 (1979).
29. G. B. Henderson, E. M. Zevely, and F. M. Huennekens, *J. Biol. Chem.* **255,** 4829 (1980).
30. G. B. Henderson and E. M. Zevely, *in* "Chemistry and Biology of Pteridines" (R. Kisliuk and G. Brown, eds.), p. 549. Am Elsevier, New York, 1979.
31. I. D. Goldman, *Adv. Exp. Med. Biol.* **84,** 85 (1977).
32. M. R. Suresh, G. B. Henderson, and F. M. Huennekens, *Biochem. Biophys. Res. Commun.* **87,** 135 (1979).
33. J. D. Caston and B. A. Kamen, *in* "Chemistry and Biology of Pteridines" (R. Kisliuk and G. Brown, eds.), p. 515. Am Elsevier, New York, 1979.
34. J. R. Bertino, P. O'Brien, and J. McCullough, *Science* **172,** 161 (1971).
35. D. A. Matthews, R. A. Alden, J. T. Bolin, D. J. Filman, S. T. Freer, N. Xuong, *in* "Chemistry and Biology of Pteridines" (R. Kisliuk and G. Brown, eds.), p. 465. Am. Elsevier, New York, 1979.

17

Membrane Transport and the Molecular Basis for Selective Antitumor Action of Folate Analogs

F. M. SIROTNAK, P. L. CHELLO, J. I. DEGRAW, J. R. PIPER, AND J. A. MONTGOMERY

I. Introduction

Extensive evidence for a critical role of membrane transport in the cytotoxic action of folate analogs has been provided by studies with a variety of mammalian cell types (reviewed in references 1–4 and in Section III A). Related studies

MOLECULAR ACTIONS AND TARGETS FOR CANCER CHEMOTHERAPEUTIC AGENTS

ISBN 0-12-619280-4

from our laboratory (reviewed in references 3 and 4 and in Section III, C) have more specifically addressed the question of the selectivity of antitumor action of this general category of agents. These studies, which were done with murine tumor models, have revealed differences in the membrane transport of folate analogs among various proliferative tissues, both normal and tumorous. Most important, these differences appear to account for the selective action observed in responsive tumor models, since in these cases they favor the accumulation and maintenance of pharmacologically effective levels of the analogs in tumors more so than in normal proliferative tissue. While the work to be described has been carried out in animal models, based on the nature of the experimental evidence and the predictiveness of these models, our results appear to have important implications for a more effective use of these agents in the treatment of human cancer.

The mediated transport of anticancer drugs, as well as other pharmacologically active agents, represents a xenobiotic phenomenom. That is, mediation of entry of these artificial substrates occurs by a mechanism already functioning for the accumulation of naturally occurring substrates. A large number of different transport systems have been found to exist in the cytoplasmic membrane of living cells [reviewed in (5–7)]. These systems provide a means by which the internal nutrient and osmotic environment of the cell is maintained relatively constant. For pharmacological agents which are analogs of existing nutrients, the appropriate mechanism (or mechanisms) are more readily identified and studies involving transport of these agents are more easily pursued. In the case of folate analogs transport of these agents in a variety of mammalian cells involves, at least during influx, the carrier system mediating the accumulation of folate coenzymes (see Section II).

In this chapter we will briefly review the current literature on the membrane transport of the entire group of folate compounds and consider the biochemical and pharmacokinetic evidence generated in our laboratory by companion *in vitro* and *in vivo* studies which bear on the question of selective antitumor action of folate analogs. We will also review some of our most recent studies on the structural specificity of membrane transport of folate compounds in support of our contention that differences in this property represent the molecular basis of the tissue-specific differences in transport observed during our studies. Finally, we will present data relating to new analogs which represent an attempt to exploit our studies for the design of more effective clinical entities.

II. Mammalian Systems Transporting Folate Analogs

A. General Properties

Since the folate analog methotrexate appears to share at least one of the carrier systems for natural folates in mammalian cells and, under conditions in which short-term transport measurements are made, is essentially metabolically inert (two forms of metabolic alterations of folate analogs will be discussed in Section V), it has been used in our laboratory and by others as a model compound for many studies of transport of both synthetic and natural folate derivatives. Its transport in murine tumor cells is primarily carrier-mediated and apparently "active." Influx shows Michealis–Menten saturation kinetics in L1210 leukemia cells (8–14). Influx is also saturable in P288 and P388 lymphoidal, Ehrlich carcinoma, and Sarcoma 180 (S180) cells (13). Saturability of influx in L5178Y cells has also been reported (15). Saturation kinetics for methotrexate influx have also been demonstrated in human leukemia cells (16), rabbit reticulocytes (17), and isolated epithelial cells from mouse small intestine (18,19). The murine and human tumor cell systems show a low capacity but exhibit a fairly high affinity for methotrexate, with measured values for K_m in the range of 3–11 μM. Based on earlier (11,12) and more recent (18,20) results with L1210 cells, all 2,4-diamino folate analogs appear to share, at least during influx, the same transport carrier, but have different affinities for the system depending upon the analog and the cell type. In all the tumor cells examined, competitive inhibition of methotrexate influx by folic acid, 5-formyltetrahydrofolate, and 5-methyltetrahydrofolate has also been demonstrated. The affinity for both 5-substituted reduced folates, as inferred from the values for K_i, is comparable to that exhibited for methotrexate and other 2,4-diamino folate analogs, but the affinity for folate is approximately two orders of magnitude lower (10,13,20–23). The efflux kinetics of methotrexate for L1210, P288, P388, Ehrlich, and S180 cells are apparently first-order (11–14). However, data suggestive of a "saturable" efflux of methotrexate in L1210 cells were reported in an earlier study (10). In all the tumor cells examined, both influx (10,13,24) and efflux (13) were highly temperature-dependent, with Q_{10} (27°–37°C) values between 6 and 8. The transport system in L1210 cells appears also to be capable of exchange diffusion, since both countertransport (10,25) and heterologous (but not homologous) transconcentration effects (26) could be demonstrated. In the latter case, preloading cells with folate, 5-formyltetrahydrofolate, and 5-methyltetrahydrofolate accelerated influx of methotrexate. During studies in our laboratory (23), preloading of isolated membrane vesicles from L1210 cells with 5-methyltetrahydrofolate also resulted in an acceleration of methotrexate influx.

In L1210 cells influx of methotrexate (24,10,27) and 5-substituted reduced folates (27), but not folate (27), was inhibited by sulfhydryl inhibitors. These results suggest the importance of sulfhydryl groups on the carrier for effective binding of methotrexate and the 5-substituted reduced derivatives. They also were interpreted as evidence for the existence of a second carrier for folic acid which was not shared by 5-substituted reduced folates or methotrexate (27). Other studies have provided supporting evidence (28). In these studies, resistant L1210 cells showed a reduced uptake of methotrexate and 5-methyltetrahydrofolate, but folate uptake was unaffected. Similar findings have been reported for W1-L2 human lymphoblastoid cells (29). Very recently, evidence was reported showing that transport of folic acid was mediated by a system whose primary substrate was adenine (30). Folic acid uptake was inhibited competitively by adenine. The value for K_i derived (17 μM) was similar to the K_m derived (21 μM) for adenine uptake. Also, the K_m for folic acid transport was essentially identical (430–450 μM) to the K_i for folic acid inhibition of adenine uptake.

B. Kinetics and Energetics of Folate Analog Transport

Unusual kinetics for methotrexate transport were described in an early report by Hakala (31,32) in a S180 cell line established in culture. Methotrexate influx in these cells was extremely slow and did not exhibit saturation kinetics. However, since some competition with a natural folate and a high-temperature coefficient (Q_{10} = 6–7) could be demonstrated, influx of methotrexate most likely occurred by a carrier mechanism exhibiting a very high K_m. Alternative explanations, however, have not been entirely excluded by the data. The reason for the marked differences in the influx kinetics described in our laboratory (13) for another S180 cell line are unexplained. However, they may relate to the fact that the natural history of each subline was quite different. The studies on the S180 subline reported by Hakala (31,32) are of further interest from the aspect of the energetics of methotrexate transport. The finding that the addition of dinitrophenol to the system resulted in an increase in the steady-state intracellular level of methotrexate suggested an active efflux mechanism in this cell line.

Some energetic properties for methotrexate transport in L1210 cells have been elaborately documented by Goldman (26,33). Transport by this system is neither sodium-dependent nor inhibited by ouabain, an inhibitor of Na,K-ATPase in the membrane. However, the steady-state intracellular level of exchangeable drug is markedly increased by the addition of NaN_3. This effect was explained by observations showing a minimal effect on influx but a pronounced reduction of efflux produced by the inhibitor, which is reversed by exogenous glucose. These workers also demonstrated some reduction in influx by the presence of extracellular organic phosphates. A model was described proposing a balance between energy for influx produced by a downhill counterflow of organic phosphate ions out of the cell and reaction coupling to provide energy for efflux (22).

Based on a mathematical analysis of the kinetics of methotrexate transport in our laboratory, an asymmetric model for folate analog transport in L1210 cells has been proposed which incorporates the notion that influx and efflux of methotrexate occur by separate carriers (14). Properties of the system which form the basis of this notion include the following: (1) influx is saturable; (2) approach to steady-state during uptake is exponential; (3) half-time for methotrexate uptake is independent of external concentration of drug and equal to the half-time for efflux; (4) efflux is first-order; and, (5) transport of methotrexate is concentrative at low external concentrations, whereas the reverse is true at high external concentrations. Three lines of biochemical evidence derived in our laboratory support the conclusion obtained from the kinetic data. First, there is a drastically different structural specificity for influx versus efflux that is difficult to explain solely as a random property of the same carrier species (12,20). Second, during growth in culture, the influx and efflux capacities fluctuate in an inverse and nonstoichiometric manner with respect to each other (34). That is, when influx is highest (mid-logarithmic phase) efflux is lowest, and when influx is lowest (early logarithmic and stationary phases) efflux is highest. Also, the amplitude of the change in influx is threefold, while the change in efflux is only twofold. Third, during studies on transport in L1210 cell membrane vesicles (23,35), transstimulation of [^{3}H]methotrexate influx by folate coenzymes (heteroexchange diffusion) could be demonstrated, but not transstimulation by physiological concentrations of nonradioactive methotrexate (homoexchange diffusion). Similar evidence for heteroexchange but not homoexchange diffusion of [^{3}H]methotrexate influx using intact L1210 cells was reported earlier by Goldman (26). Overall, these studies strongly suggest that efflux of methotrexate preferentially takes place by a carrier system different from the system for folate coenzymes. We have limited the present discussion to systems transporting folate analogues in tumor cells. In addition, some details have been provided concerning similar systems in rabbit reticulocytes (17) and in isolated murine intestinal epithelial cells (18,19). Further details pertaining to the epithelial cell system will be provided below. It should also be pointed out that systems for folate analog transport, with some properties resembling those described in tumor cells, have also been described in rat hepatocytes (36), rabbit (37,38) and hog (39) choroid plexus and rabbit kidney cortical tissue (40), and both normal and leukemic human leukocytes (41).

III. Role of Membrane Transport in the Pharmacological Action of Folate Analogs

A. Correlates of Antifolate Transport and Cytotoxicity

Folate analogs mediate their cytotoxic effects through the inhibition of dihydrofolate reductase (reviewed in references 42,43). The inhibition results in depletion of the tetrahydrofolate pool, with a consequent cessation in dTMP synthesis and, ultimately, purine nucleotide and amino acid synthesis. The magnitude of the cytotoxicity observed in each tissue is a function of both the extent and duration of the inhibition of DNA synthesis (44–50), the primary metabolic effect of the drug–enzyme interaction. The period during which complete inhibition of dihydrofolate reductase is sustained appears to reflect the properties of the transport system in each tissue, since the accumulation of exchangeable levels of antifolate, i.e., unbound to dihydrofolate reductase, appear necessary to initiate and sustain inhibition of DNA synthesis. This was inferred from studies *in vivo* showing the rapidly reversible nature of the drug-induced inhibition of DNA snythesis in mouse small intestine (44,45) and an extracellular concentration dependence for resumption of [^{3}H]deoxyuridine ([^{3}H]UdR) incorporation in L1210 cells, small intestine, and bone marrow (47). Our *in vivo* studies (46,48,49) provided direct evidence associating the decrease in intracellular exchangeable methotrexate with a resumption in DNA synthesis in both small intestine and tumor cells. Related studies *in vitro* with resting cell suspensions also provide evidence for a relationship between the level of intracellular exchangeable methotrexate and the extent of supression of DNA, RNA, and tetrahydrofolate synthesis (48,51,52). Exchangeable levels of intracellular antifolate appear to be necessary in order to saturate dihydrofolate reductase fully (48,51,52), even though the enzyme-binding constant is orders of magnitude below the concentration of methotrexate required to inhibit tetrahydrofolate synthesis in the cell. This seems to be related (48,51,52) to the partially reversible nature of the binding of antifolate to this enzyme [first described by Werkheiser (42)], to the increased competition for reversible binding of antifolate (52) resulting from the accumulation of dihydrofolate during dTMP synthesis, and to other observations (48,53) showing that L1210 cells, and probably other mammalian cells, are capable of synthesizing appreciably more dihydrofolate reductase than is actually needed to maintain DNA synthesis normally. In agreement with the theoretical considerations of Goldman (1), we also concluded from our experimental evidence (13,46,48,49) that the critical determinant of cytotoxicity of antifolates is the intracellular level of exchangeable drug.

B. Membrane Transport and Acquired Drug Resistance

Carrier-mediated membrane transport systems are under gene control in very much the same way as enzymatic mechanisms. Structural genes for transport proteins in bacteria have been identified, and in some cases regulatory models which explain the coordinate fluctuation in related transport and enzyme capacities have been proposed. Excellent reviews on this aspect of transport in bacteria have been published (54,55). "Transport" mutants are a major class of drug-resistant phenotypes which have been found, at least in bacteria and most likely in mammalian cells, to originate from gene mutation. In a manner similar to that seen with enzymatic properties, mutational effects on transport may lead to the modification of one or more of the kinetic parameters of transport (56,57). A functional deletion of the transport system is also theoretically possible. However, in view of the obligatory role of transport systems in accumulating and maintaining intracellular levels of the natural substrate (nutrient), it is unlikely that such a deletion would be permissive, that is, occur without some detriment to cell survival. Likewise, a marked reduction in transport capacity (reduced influx V_{max}) would also impair not only the influx of drug but the influx of the natural substrate as well. Consequently, the frequency of occurrence of this resistance phenotype (complete absence or marked reduction in transport capacity) in the case of any particular transport activity would depend upon how limiting on growth rate influx of the essential nutrient was in the parental (wild-type) drug-sensitive cell. Moreover, the influx V_{max}, which would reflect the number of carriers present and the rate of carrier translocation (or orientation) from outside to inside for a specific transport system, would most likely depend upon regulatory interrelationships common to many transport systems in the cell (reviewed in references 6,54,58). For this reason, a mutational effect involving these aspects of transport could have profound effects highly detrimental to overall membrane function. On the other hand, a modification of the binding site on the carrier, resulting in an increase in the influx K_m, should require only a simple mutation (one base pair substitution determining a change in one amino acid) in the corresponding structural gene (56,57,59,60). Since the structural basis of binding of the analog may be different than for the natural nutrient (see Section IV, A for a discussion of this aspect in connection with folate compounds), such a mutational effect may or may not affect the transport of the natural substrate. Finally, a mutational effect on transport which would increase efflux of drug is also theoretically possible, bearing in mind that the same limitations in regard to concomitant effects on the transport of natural nutrients, which were already indicated for influx, would also apply.

The association of a reduced rate of methotrexate influx with required resistance in mammalian cells was first reported in an L5178Y murine cell line (61). A similar observation in another resistant variant of the same cell line was made later by other workers (15). In other earlier studies, resistance of L1210 and P288 murine lymphomas (62) to methotrexate and resistance of Yoshida rat sarcoma (63,64) to aminopterin were associated with a reduced rate of uptake of the drug. Unfortunately, an analysis of the data which might have discriminated between the possible kinetic bases of the differences observed were not carried out in any of these studies. In work reported from our laboratory (8,9), a comparison of methotrexate transport in drug-sensitive and -resistant L1210 cells revealed a reduction in the influx of drug in the resistant cells. A kinetic analysis showed a very small difference ($<50\%$) in the values for the influx V_{max} but revealed a fourfold increase in the value for the influx K_m, which appeared to explain the difference in the transport properties observed in both cell types. Measurements of efflux were not carried out at that time. However, a comparison of individual values for the steady-state level of exchangeable methotrexate obtained during these experiments showed a difference between cell lines equal to the difference in values for the influx K_m (9). This implies a similarity in the efflux rate constants in these cell lines based on the kinetic interrelationships subsequently reported from our laboratory for the same parental line (14). The kinetic differences in transport observed correlate closely with the relative responsiveness of these two cell lines during therapy with methotrexate. [Mice bearing the resistant cell line exhibit a fourfold lower response to a regimen of therapy (3–6 mg/kg every 2 days $\times 10$, which increases the life span of mice bearing the parental sensitive line L1210V about 150% (F. M. Sirotnak, unpublished results).] The increase in the influx K_m of this system virtually eliminates the antitumor effect of this agent. More recent reports have presented evidence for a similar change involving the value for the influx K_m for antifolate transport in another methotrexate-resistant L1210 cell line (28) and in a resistant W1-L2 human lymphoblastoid cell line (29). The value for the influx V_{max} (in resistant and sensitive cells) was unaltered in the L1210 cell line but was reduced in the W1-L2 cell line. These workers also observed a decrease in the rate of accumulation of 5-methyltetrahydrofolate in the resistant cell line as compared to the parental drug-sensitive cell line, but no difference was observed in the rate of accumulation of folate by the two cell lines.

C. Relative Responsiveness and Selective Antitumor Action

A general correlation between the extent of uptake of methotrexate by a group of murine leukemias *in vitro* and their therapeutic responsiveness *in vivo* was first reported by Kessel and co-workers (62). These workers found a linear relationship over a fourfold range between the extent of uptake of methotrexate and the response of these tumors to a standard therapeutic regimen. While the data reported did not provide a kinetic basis for the differences in uptake observed, nor information on the steady-state levels in these tumors, the results were highly suggestive of a role for membrane transport as a determinant of response. The same correlation applied to cell lines with natural or acquired resistance to methotrexate.

Observations similar to those reported for murine tumors (62) were also made for a group of human leukemias by the same group of workers (41). Responders in both the acute lymphocytic leukemia group and acute myelocytic leukemia group were generally associated with higher rates of methotrexate uptake *in vitro,* while nonresponders in each group were not. This was an extremely important finding, since it strongly supported the notion that similar evidence derived in predictive murine tumor models would have some relevance to human cancer.

More recently, we reported on coordinated *in vitro* (13,18) and *in vivo* (46,49,50) studies in our laboratory which extended the earlier observations of

Kessel *et al.* (62) and correlated specific differences in kinetic parameters for the transport of methotrexate and related folate analogs by a group of lymphoidal and nonlymphoidal murine tumors with their relative responsiveness to this agent. Similar differences were found in the transport of these antifolates by responsive murine tumors and proliferative tissue in small intestine, the drug-limiting organ, which explained the selective antitumor action of these agents in mice.

Our initial observations *in vivo* (46) were made during the course of tissue pharmacokinetic experiments with L1210 leukemia, a murine tumor highly responsive to methotrexate. In these studies, we documented (see Fig. 1) a markedly greater persistence of levels of exchangeable intracellular methotrexate in tumor cells as compared to small intestine following administration of a therapeutic dose. The difference in persistence correlated with a greater duration of

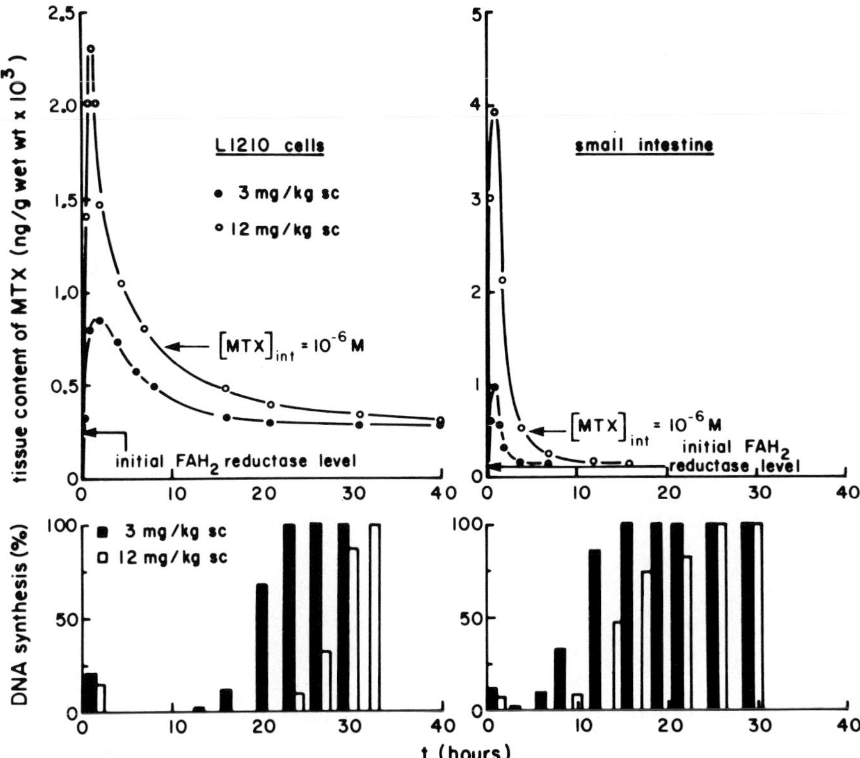

Fig. 1. Accumulation and retention of methotrexate (MTX) *in vivo* in L1210 cells and in the intracellular compartment of mouse small intestine and the relationship to effects on DNA synthesis. Average values derived for two to four animals in three replicate experiments (SD $\leqslant \pm 30\%$). See text for further details. FAH_2, Dihydrofolate.

inhibition of [^{3}H]UdR incorporation into DNA of the tumor cells. There was a similar accumulation of drug initially and a similar time course for onset of inhibition of [^{3}H]UdR incorporation in each tissue until inhibition was essentially complete. As the level of exchangeable drug within intracellular water decreased and approached the level equivalent to drug bound to dihydrofolate reductase, the incorporation of [^{3}H]UdR into DNA resumed. However, the rate of decrease in exchangeable drug was lower and the resumption of [^{3}H]UdR incorporation far more delayed in the tumor cells. Both the extent of persistence and the duration of inhibition of [^{3}H]UdR incorporation L1210 cells at different doses correlated with the difference in increased life span obtained in each case (46). Although the dosage relationships were different, a similar correlation had already been shown for drug persistence and duration of inhibition of [^{3}H]UdR incorporation in mouse small intestine, on the one hand, and lethal toxicity (44,45). From these studies, we tentatively concluded the following: (1) greater persistence of methotrexate and longer duration of inhibition of DNA synthesis in tumor cells compared to small intestine appears to account for the selective antitumor action observed in this tumor model; (2) the pharmacokinetics for exchangeable drug in each tissue most likely reflect the properties of the membrane transport system in each case; (3) the critical role of the transport system is to sustain exchangeable drug levels in the face of rapidly falling plasma levels of drug; and (4) differences in the persistence of exchangeable drug in tumor versus small intestine probably reflect a difference in some kinetic property of the transport system in each case.

Our *in vivo* studies were extended to include a number of other murine tumor models differing in responsiveness to antifolates (49,50). We confirmed our initial observation by showing the same differences in the persistence of exchangeable methotrexate and the duration of inhibition of DNA synthesis between small intestine and other responsive murine tumors. We also showed a similar correlation between these two parameters in each tumor, and between these parameters and the responsiveness of these tumors during therapy. The pharmacokinetics for exchangeable drug in these tumors and small intestine are shown in Fig. 2 for a subcutaneously administered dose of 3 mg/kg. The half-time for the net loss of exchangeable drug was proportional to the increase in survival time obtained when this dosage was employed against tumor-bearing mice on a standard regimen. In another series of experiments, the same dosage of methotrexate was given intraperitoneally, and the net loss of exchangeable drug with time compared to the time course for onset and duration of inhibition of [^{3}H]UdR incorporation also measured in each tissue. Again, the half-time for net loss of exchangeable drug was proportional (Fig. 3) to the increase in survival time obtained during therapy *in vivo*. Also, the time required for intracellular exchangeable levels of drug to approach the binding equivalence for dihydrofolate reductase, without exception, correlated (Fig. 4) with the time required for the resumption of [^{3}H]UdR incorporation. It should also be mentioned that only

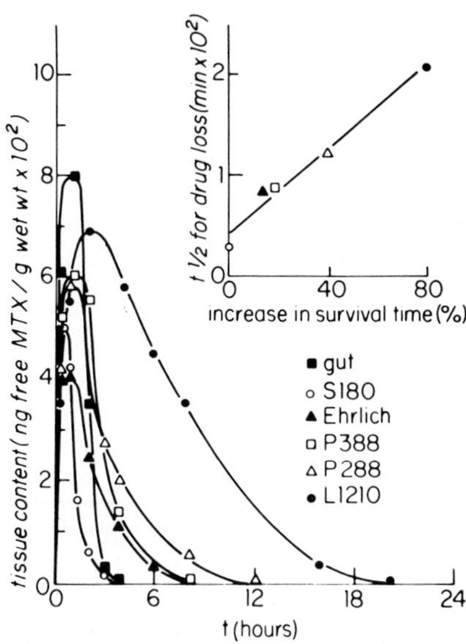

Fig. 2. Time course for accumulation and retention of exchangeable methotrexate (MTX) *in vivo* in different murine tumor cells and in the intracellular compartment of mouse small intestine following a single subcutaneous dose of 3 mg/kg. The inset shows the relationship between the half-time for drug loss and the increase in survival time. Average values derived for two to four mice in two separate experiments (SD $\leqslant \pm 30\%$). Data on average survival time were obtained in two separate experiments with 10 mice in each control and treated group (SD $\leqslant \pm 15\%$). See text for further details.

small differences in the dihydrofolate reductase content were found among these (49,13) and other (65) tumor cells and that these differences did not correlate with the relative responsiveness of the tumors (13,49,65).

In other studies (18,49,50), we associated differences in the lethal potency of 10-ethylaminopterin, methotrexate, aminopterin, and two quinazoline analogues, methasquin and 5-chlorodeazaaminopterin (relative potency = 16:14:1 for the pteridine analogs and 5:0.3 for the quinazoline analogues) with differences in the persistence of exchangeable levels of each in the intracellular compartment of small intestine (Fig. 5). After a dose of 3 mg/kg given subcutaneously or intraperitoneally persistence was in the order 5-chlorodeazaaminopterin > aminopterin > methasquin > methotrexate ≃ 10-ethylaminopterin. A similar correlation was derived (49,50; see also Fig. 6) for these agents when given at equitoxic doses. Moreover, differences in the therapeutic index for these five agents against L1210 leukemia reflected (18,49,50; see also Fig. 6) the relationship in the persistence of each agent at maximum tolerated doses and also the duration of inhibition of [^{3}H]UdR incorporation into DNA in tumor cells vis-à-vis small intestine. From these studies, we are now able to explain, at

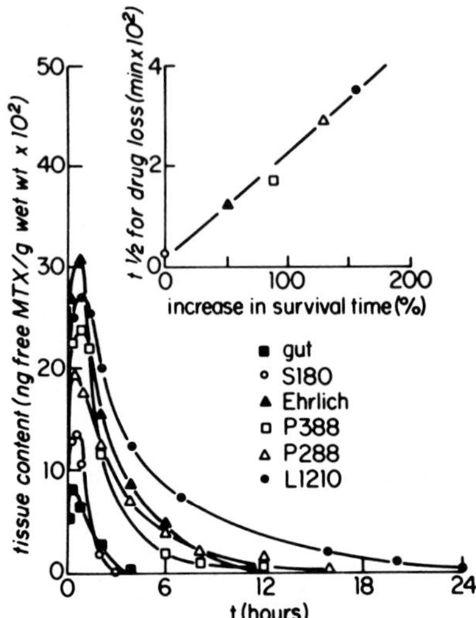

Fig. 3. Time course for accumulation and retention of exchangeable methotrexate (MTX) *in vivo* in different murine tumor cells and in the intracellular compartment of mouse small intestine following a single intraperitoneal dose of 3 mg/kg. The inset shows the relationship between the half-time for drug loss and the increase in survival time. Average values derived for two to three mice in two separate experiments (SD $\leq \pm 30\%$). Data on average survival time were obtained in two separate experiments with 10 mice in each control and each treated group (SD $\leq \pm 18\%$). Data shown in Figs. 3 and 4 were obtained in the same experiment. See text for further details.

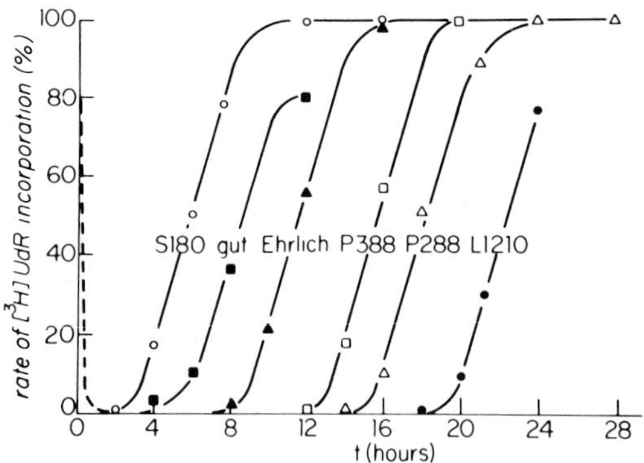

Fig. 4. The incorporation of [^{3}H]UdR into DNA *in vivo* in mouse small intestine and in different tumor cells at various times after a single intraperitoneal dose of 3 mg/kg methotrexate. Data are expressed as percentage of control rates of incorporation in two to four mice in two separate experiments (SD $\leq \pm 30\%$). Data shown in Figs. 3 and 4 were obtained in the same experiment.

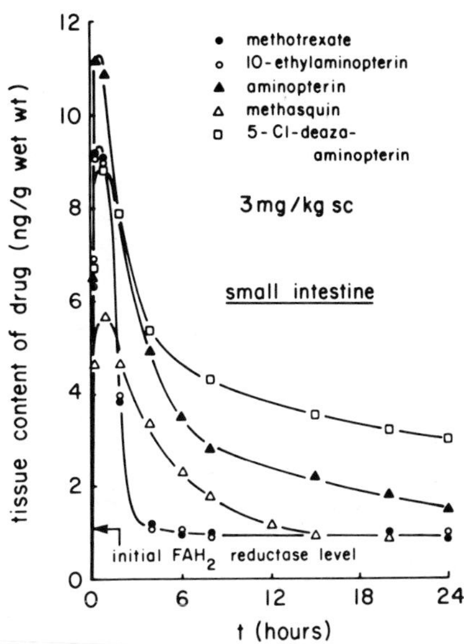

Fig. 5. Time course for accumulation and retention of different folate analogues *in vivo* in mouse small intestine. The analogues were administered subcutaneously as a single dose of 3 mg/kg. Average values were derived for drug content of the intracellular compartment of small intestine from three to four animals in three replicate experiments. (SD $\leqslant \pm 30\%$). See text for further details. FAH_2, Dihydrofolate.

least in mice, the greater lethal potency of aminopterin and these two quinazoline analogs and the higher therapeutic index observed for methotrexate and 10-ethylaminopterin compared to the other agents.

In more recent *in vivo* studies (66), we examined the pharmacokinetics of methotrexate in mouse bone marrow in an attempt to explain the basis of the greater tolerance in mice (67) of this major host proliferative population in comparison to that of renewal sites in small intestine. Following subcutaneous administration of varying doses of methotrexate (12–400 mg/kg) to mice, accumulation and persistence of drug in marrow were markedly reduced in comparison to that seen in small intestine (Fig. 7). In addition, the lower persistence of exchangeable drug in marrow versus small intestine correlated with a substantially shorter duration of inhibition of DNA synthesis in the former. Earlier recovery of DNA synthesis as a consequence of more rapid loss of exchangeable drug appears to explain the large difference in sensitivity of these two major proliferative populations to the effects of this agent. These results and those of prior studies in our laboratory (46,48–50) and elsewhere (47) are consistent with the observed differences in the cytotoxicity of methotrexate in various tissues in the order tumor $\geqslant\geqslant$ small intestine $\geqslant$ marrow for responsive tumor models such as L1210, P288, and P388 leukemias.

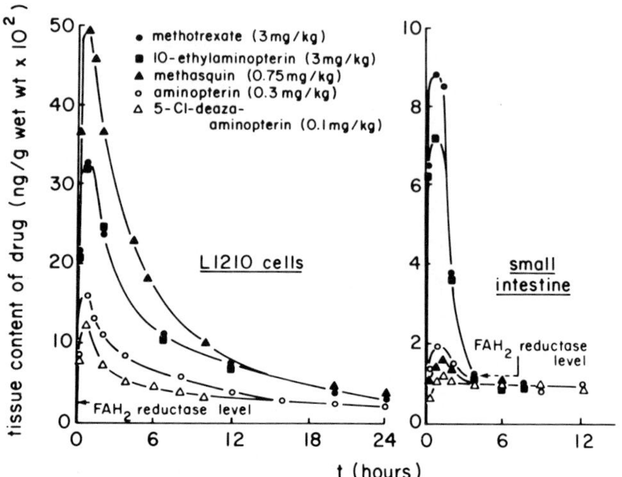

Fig. 6. Time course for accumulation and retention of different folate analogues *in vivo* in L1210 leukemia cells and mouse small intestine. The analogs were administered subcutaneously as a single dose which was shown to be equitoxic (LD_{10}) on a therapeutic schedule of once every 2 days ×10. Average values were derived for drug content of tumor cells and the intracellular compartment of small intestine from three to four animals in three replicate experiments (SD ≤ ±30%). See text for further details. FAH_2, Dihydrofolate.

During more recent studies *in vitro* (13,18), we provided direct evidence which confirmed the predictions derived from our pharmacokinetic data (46,49,50) regarding the role of membrane transport in both the relative responsiveness among tumors and the selective antitumor action obtained with antifolates. We identified the influx K_m for methotrexate, rather than the influx V_{max} or the efflux rate constant, as the parameter of the transport system for antifolates which had the highest correlation with relative therapeutic responsivenss (13). Both the relatively unresponsive tumors (S180 and Ehrlich carcinoma) and the responsive tumors (L1210, P288, and P388 leukemias) appeared to possess transport systems for methotrexate with similar properties (13). Relative responsiveness among this group of tumors as determined from the increased life span (%ILS) *in vivo* following treatment with methotrexate showed (Fig. 8) a linear relationship with the steady-state level of exchangeable (osmotically active) drug over a fourfold range. Although some differences were observed in the individual values for V_{max}, they were relatively small (<50%) and might merely reflect differences in cell size (13). In any event, these small differences in V_{max} alone showed no correlation with relative responsiveness in these tumors. The relationship between steady-state levels of exchangeable drug and relative responsiveness, with one exception (P388), could be explained entirely by a difference in saturability of influx among these tumors (variation in K_m = 3.13–11.3 μM),

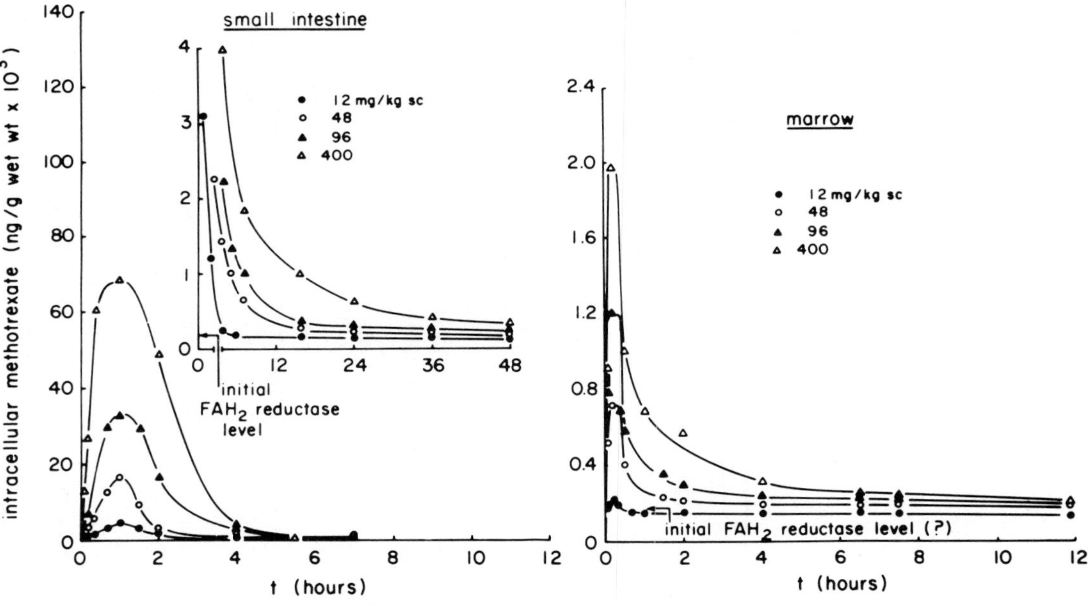

Fig. 7. Methotrexate pharmacokinetics in bone marrow and small intestine in non-tumor-bearing mice. Drug was administered subcutaneously. Values shown were derived in triplicate experiments done on different days employing two or three mice for each determination. Standard deviation did not exceed ±26% of mean values. FAH_2, Dihydrofolate.

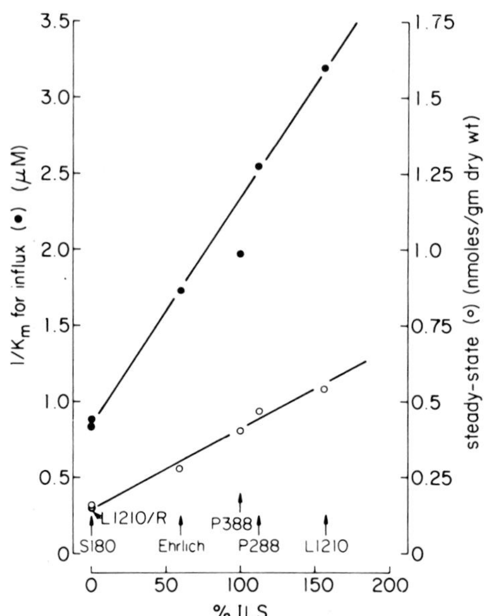

Fig. 8. The relationship between parameters for methotrexate transport *in vitro* and relative therapeutic responsiveness of murine tumors *in vivo*. $[MTX]_{ext} = 0.44\ \mu M$; ILS, increased life span obtained when tumor-bearing mice were treated every other day with 3 mg/kg intraperitoneal methotrexate (three separate experiments; SD $< \pm 24\%$).

which was also shown (Fig. 8) to correlate with relative responsiveness. The single exception could be explained by a difference in the value for the efflux rate constant in the same tumor (13). Although the differences in responsiveness observed in this study were explained largely by the differences in the value for the influx K_m, it should be emphasized that it is not these differences per se which account for relative responsiveness but the net effect of these differences on the accumulation of free drug in each tumor. It was also of interest to note during these studies that the quantitative relationship between the values of specific kinetic parameters for transport (K_m or steady state) and relative responsiveness shown for the poorly responsive S180 and Ehrlich tumors approximated the same relationship shown (9 and Fig. 8) or inferred (62) for L1210 cell lines with acquired resistance to methotrexate.

The question concerning the role of membrane transport in the selective antitumor action of folate analogues in murine tumor models was also addressed via a series of *in vitro* experiments reported recently from our laboratory (18). Epithelial cell populations were isolated from mouse small intestine, the site of drug-limiting toxicity in these animals. These suspensions, consisting of approximately equal numbers of immature crypt and mature villar epithelial cells (18), rapidly accumulated folate analogs by carrier mediation in a manner similar to that observed for tumor cells (13). The kinetic analysis of influx delineated only a single saturable component with a value for apparent K_m of approximately 90 μM. A difference between isolated epithelial cells and L1210 cells was observed in all the kinetic parameters examined (Table I). The V_{max} (2-fold) and the efflux rate constant (3-fold) were lower in the epithelial cell suspensions. However, the influx K_m for epithelial cells was approximately 25-fold higher than the value derived with L1210 cells. The same kinetic data were also derived (18; also Table I) for two other analogs, aminopterin and 10-ethylaminopterin, which compete with methotrexate. Values for the efflux rate constant and the influx V_{max} in each tissue were similar for all three analogs. In each cell type, the alkyl substitution resulted in a decrease in the value for influx K_m. However, the decrease was 4-fold greater in the case of epithelial cells. The relative cytotoxic consequences anticipated from these kinetic differences can be derived from calculated values for steady state, which are shown for a concentration of 1 μM in Table I. At this concentration, values derived for steady-state levels of exchangeable drug in L1210 cells versus epithelial cells are only 2-fold higher for aminopterin, but 12-fold higher for the two alkyl-substituted analogs. The correlation between the individual kinetic values and calculated values for steady-state level shown in Table I and the actual pharmacokinetic data derived from earlier (18,49,50; also Figs. 1–6) and companion studies *in vivo* is striking. The results of these *in vitro* studies appear to substantiate the role of transport in the selective antitumor action of this class of compounds in murine tumor models. They also identify, as well, a difference in specificity of transport systems of tumor and epithelial cells from the drug-limiting organ for N-10 substituents as the molecular basis of the differences observed in each cell type.

IV. Interrelationships in Structural Specificity of Relevance to Pharmacological Action of Anticancer Drugs—Transport versus Intracellular Targets

A. Some Theoretical Considerations

The interaction of substrate with a carrier-mediated transport system appears to involve the complexing of substrate to a recognition site on the carrier in very much the same way documented for substrate binding to enzyme molecules. The difference essentially relates to the consequence of the binding in each case, that is, translocation of substrate with no alteration (excluding the special case of group translocation reactions; see ref. 3) for the carrier–substrate interaction and chemical alteration of substrate for enzyme–substrate interaction. The best examples of detailed studies on the molecular aspects of substrate binding to carrier molecules were derived in the case of sugars (reviewed in reference 68) and amino acids (reviewed in reference 6). These studies will not be reviewed in

TABLE I

Values for Individual Kinetic Parameters of Folate Analog Transport by L1210 Cells and by Isolated Murine Intestinal Epithelial Cells[a]

Cell type	Analog	K_m (μM)	V_{max} (nmoles/minute/gm dry wt)	K ($minute^{-1}$)[b]	Calculated steady state	
					nmoles/gm dry wt)[c]	μM[d]
L1210	Aminopterin	1.22 ± 0.10	3.27 ± 1.1	0.25 ± 0.03	5.94	1.73
	Methotrexate	3.52 ± 0.53	4.55 ± 1.4	0.25 ± 0.07	4.01	1.21
	10-Ethyl-aminopterin	3.30 ± 0.83	4.32 ± 1.5	0.23 ± 0.02	4.29	1.18
Intestinal epithelium	Aminopterin	7.23 ± 3.64	1.74 ± 0.48	0.084 ± 0.01	2.52	0.83
	Methotrexate	87.06 ± 6.34	2.41 ± 0.31	0.077 ± 0.02	0.34	0.11
	10-Ethyl-aminopterin	123.77 ± 17.90	2.56 ± 0.56	0.067 ± 0.01	0.31	0.10

[a] Average value ± SD (n = 3–5 separate determinations on different days).

[b] $K = \ln 2/t_{1/2}$.

[c] $C_\infty = V_{max}[\text{drug}]/(K_m + [\text{drug}])\,K$; [drug] = 1 μM.

[d] Calculated from values of intracellular water per gram dry weight of 3.67 ml ± 0.54 (L1210 cells) and 2.98 ± 0.3 (epithelial cells). See text for related methodology.

detail here, but some generalities applicable to the transport of folate compounds will be considered.

Normally there is a minimum set of structural requirements for any particular category of transport systems, that is, specified regions necessary for recognition by the appropriate carrier-binding site. These structural requirements usually imply the necessity for some type of bond formation between regions of the substrate molecule and contact amino acids within the binding site. In addition, there is almost always a certain geometric consideration (stereochemical specificity). That is, the substrate molecule must exhibit a specific conformation compatible with the distribution of contact points which reflect the conformation of the binding site itself. For any particular carrier (or enzyme), one can also identify additional (unspecified) regions on the substrate molecule where further modification will either reduce (low tolerance) or have no effect (high tolerance) on binding. In addition, separate regions on the molecule may also exist where further modification may in fact enhance binding. It should also be pointed out that the change in chemical reactivity resulting from the modification itself may contribute profoundly to the overall effect on binding in either a positive or negative way. The actual effect of modification in any one of these "nonspecified" regions will depend upon the particular carrier (or enzyme) in question. This of course explains the differences in specificity that have been observed in many related transport systems and enzymes.

For anticancer agents requiring carrier mediation for effective penetration into the cell, there are at least two separate structural requirements which must be satisfied before a cytotoxic effect is obtained—one for the carrier and one for an intracellular binding site. The latter may be a target enzyme (as in the case of folate analogues and dihydrofolate reductase) or a macromolecule (as in the case of anthracyclines and DNA). In addition, there may be a third structural requirement, e.g., for an activating enzyme (nucleoside kinase) or inactivating enzyme (nucleoside deaminase). As is often the case for naturally occurring substrates, the specificity of the carrier and the intracellular binding site(s) for a group of related analogs may be distinctly different. In fact, for folate analogues (Section IV, B), such differences have already been well documented in murine tumor and proliferative epithelial cells. Therefore, for a fruitful approach to the design of more effective analogs, it seems that an analysis of structure-activity relationships should focus on the specificity of transport in addition to the intracellular binding interactions more directly associated with the biochemical mode of cytotoxic action.

B. Aspects of the Structural Specificity of Folate and Folate Analog Transport and Binding to Dihydrofolate Reductase

A meaningful analysis of the structural specificity of systems transporting folate compounds requires an evaluation of individual naturally occurring folates and folate analogs in terms of both influx and efflux properties of the system. It is also important from the point of view of eventual therapeutic exploitation to relate this information to similar data on the structural specificity for binding to dihydrofolate reductase. Knowledge of the structural basis of effective analog interaction at both transport and target enzyme sites permits a more balanced approach to the design of new analogues and a greater probability for the rational design of an agent with greater therapeutic effectiveness. The evidence derived so far suggests (reviewed in references 42,69–72) that there are relatively few differences in the structural specificity of dihydrofolate reductase from different mammalian tissues. On the other hand, transport of folates (and folate analogs) in some tissues (13,18) appears to show a wide variation in structural specificity. In tissues where a comparison between transport and target enzyme binding has been made, there are some similarities, but also distinct differences, in the requirements for effective analog interaction in each case. It should also be noted that binding of 2,4-diamino analogs to dihydrofolate reductase is as much as six orders of magnitude greater than that recorded for binding to components of the transport system during influx. A summary of the data available from our studies on the L1210 cell and epithelial cell system are given in Fig. 9.

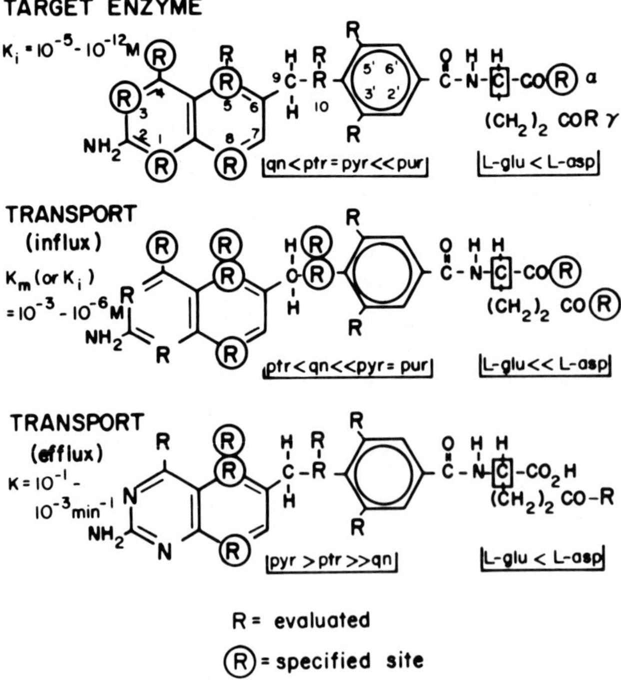

Fig. 9. Structure–activity relationships in L1210 cells for dihydrofolate reductase inhibition and transport of folate analogs.

Quantitative details on the extent of the interaction at enzyme and transport sites in various murine tumor cells and epithelial cells are given in Tables II–VI.

Two structural features of the folate molecule are of paramount importance to effective enzyme binding and influx by the transport system in L1210 cells (Table II). These include the type of substituent at position 4 of the pteridine ring and the number or location of free carboxyl groups on the glutamyl moiety. Substitution of an amino group for the oxo group at position 4 increases binding on the enzyme by at least six orders of magnitude. (Folic acid is a competitive inhibitor of this enzyme from L1210 cells when dihydrofolate is used as a substrate at pH 7.4. However, at pH 6.0–6.5, folate can also serve as a substrate for this enyzme.) Also, only a free α-carboxyl group is necessary for effective binding. [Amide or peptide bond formation at the α-carboxyl group but not at the γ-carboxyl group virtually eliminates binding to this enzyme (20).] In regard to transport, the same substitution at position 4 increases influx by two orders of magnitude (the effect of this substitution on efflux has not been determined). Also, influx is decreased if there is only one free carboxyl group.

An interesting difference in the structural specificity of dihydrofolate reductase and the folate transport system involves both the N-10 position and the γ-carboxyl group. Both sites appear to be regions of high tolerance for enzyme binding but not transport. A variety of modifications of these positions (see Table II) have no effect on enzyme binding. The high tolerance observed for the γ-carboxyl group is also consistent with the X-ray diffraction model proposed for the complex between methotrexate and dihydrofolate reductase from *Escherichia coli* (73). Peptide bond formation involving the attachment of a second amino acid or amidization (20) of the γ-carboxyl group markedly increases the influx K_m but has little or no effect on efflux. Also, the presence of a methyl or ethyl substituent at N-10 increases the influx K_m 3- to 4-fold (12,18). Replacement of nitrogen with carbon at positions 1 and 3 decreased enzyme binding. At position 8, the same replacement increased binding. Halogenation at position 3′ or 5′ on the benzene ring (data not shown) had no effect on enzyme binding. Substitution at the α-carboxyl group reduced binding approximately 200-fold. There was little effect on influx by a replacement of nitrogen with carbon at position 1 or 3, by a replacement of nitrogen with oxygen at position 10, or halogenation of the benzene ring at position 3′ or 5′ (data not shown). However, influx was increased by a replacement of nitrogen with carbon at position 8 and decreased by alkyl substitution at position 10. Substitution at either the α- or γ-carboxyl group reduced influx in a substituent-specific manner. Efflux was unaffected by replacement of nitrogen with oxygen, or alkyl substitution at position 10. Also, halogenation at position 3′ or 5′ had no effect on efflux (data not shown). With the exception of the γ-amine derivative, none of the other amines or peptide derivatives evaluated had an altered efflux.

Differences in the specificity of dihydrofolate reductase and the folate transport system are also observed (Table III) among analogues having different

TABLE II

Structure-Activity Relationships for L1210 Cell Dihydrofolate Reductase Inhibition and Membrane Transport Involving Pteridine Folate Analogs[a]

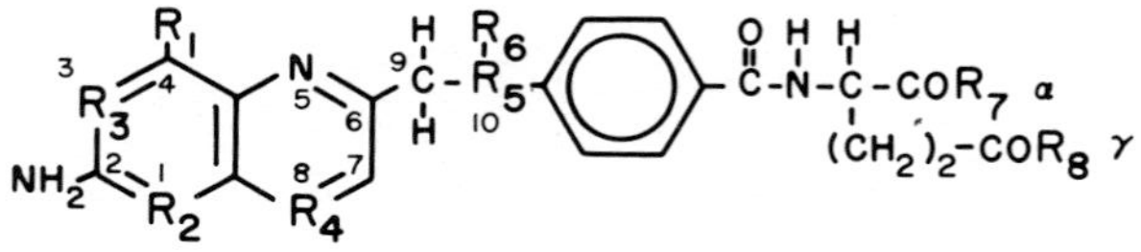

R_1	R_2	R_3	R_4	R_5	R_6	R_7	R_8	FAH_2 reductase inhibition, K_i (nM)	Transport: Influx K_m (μM)	Transport: Influx K_i (μM)	Transport: Efflux k ($minute^{-1}$)
OH	N	N	N	N	H	OH	OH	1982.0		228.0	
OH	N	N	CH	N	H	OH	OH	1207.30		51.9	
NH_2	N	N	N	N	H	OH	OH	0.0032	1.2	1.4	0.24

NH_2	N	N	N	N	CH_3	OH	OH	0.0043	3.3	3.5	0.23
NH_2	N	N	N	N	C_2H_5	OH	OH	0.0039	3.8		0.25
NH_2	CH	N	N	N	CH_3	OH	OH	338.50		1.9	
NH_2	N	CH	N	N	CH_3	OH	OH	31.10		3.5	0.21
NH_2	N	N	N	O		OH	OH	[b]	3.28	3.5	0.23
NH_2	N	N	N	N	H	OH	Glu	0.0041	18.9		0.24
NH_2	N	N	N	N	CH_3	OH	Glu	0.0037	49.3		0.22
NH_2	N	N	N	N	CH_3	OH	NH_2	0.0027	9.4	8.4	0.15
NH_2	N	N	N	N	CH_3	OH	$NHCH_3$	0.0027	27.6		0.21
NH_2	N	N	N	N	CH_3	OH	$NH(CH_3)_2$	0.0039	48.4		0.26
NH_2	N	N	N	N	CH_3	OH	$NH(C_5H_{11})$	0.0035	16.9	16.8	0.26
NH_2	N	N	N	N	CH_3	OH	$NHCH_2\phi$	0.0036	3.9	3.8	0.19
NH_2	N	N	N	N	CH_3	OH	Asp	0.0028	>300.0		
NH_2	N	N	N	N	CH_3	OH	Gly	0.0029	3.9		0.21
NH_2	N	N	N	N	CH_3	Glu	OH	170.1		61.0	
NH_2	N	N	N	N	CH_3	Asp	OH	208.4		146.2	
NH_2	N	N	N	N	CH_3	Gly	OH	208.2		66.6	

[a] See Table III, footnotes *a*–*c*.
[b] $\simeq$ Methotrexate (estimated from intracellular binding).

TABLE III

Structure-Activity Relationships for L1210 Cell Dihydrofolate Reductase Inhibition and Membrane Transport Involving 2,4-Diamino Folate Analogs

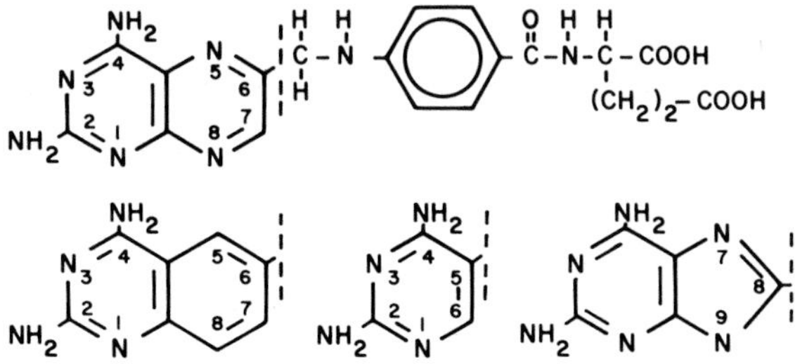

Primary ring system	FAH_2 reductase inhibition, K_i (n*M*)[a]	Influx[b] K_m (μM)	Influx[b] K_i (μM)[c]	Efflux, *k* ($minute^{-1}$)
Pteridine	0.0032	1.22	1.41	0.249
Quinazoline	0.0006	5.65	4.86	0.034
Pyrimidine	0.0041	102.0	78.2	0.147
Purine	10,100		132.8	

[a] Method of G. B. Henderson [*Biochem. J.* **135,** 101-107 (1973)] for titration inhibitors, otherwise from Lineweaver-Burk or Dixon plots). SD $\leqslant$ 33% (n = 3-5).

[b] Values for V_{max} are identical, since these are competing analogs. For the same reason $K_m \cong K_i$. SD $\leqslant$ 22% (*n* = 3-5).

[c] K_i determined from Lineweaver-Burk or Dixon plots during measurements of competitive inhibition of [^{3}H]methotrexate uptake.

primary ring systems. Both pteridine and pyrimidine analogues are bound effectively and to about the same extent by the enzyme. However, binding of the corresponding quinazoline analog is somewhat better. The purine analog , on the other hand, is bound very poorly. Influx by the transport system is most effective for the pteridine analog and somewhat less effective (four- to fivefold greater K_m) for the quinazoline analog , while influx of the pyrimidine and purine analogs is much less effective. On the other hand, the relationship observed for efflux is quite different. The rate is greatest for the pyrimidine analogue and decreases in the order pyrimidine > pteridine > quinazoline. No data are available for the purine analog.

The availability of a series of quinazoline derivatives allowed an analysis (12,20) of the effect of a variety of additional structural modifications on binding to dihydrofolate reductase and transport (Table IV). As was the case for folic acid, quinazoline analogs with a 2-amino-4-hydroxypyrimidine configuration were poor inhibitors of this enzyme. The L-glutamyl derivatives were the best overall inhibitors of dihydrofolate reductase. Binding of a 5-methyl derivative was greater, and of a 5-chloro derivative much greater, than that of the unsubstituted analog. The L-aspartyl analog was bound considerably less than the L-glutamyl analog However, substitution at position 5 with a methyl or chloro group increased. binding to a level comparable to that of corresponding 5-substituted glutamyl derivatives. Both D-glutamyl and D-aspartyl analogs were bound considerably less than the corresponding L forms.

Again, as in the case of folate, the 2-amino-4-hydroxy derivatives were poor substrates for this transport mechanism, since they did not compete effectively with [^{3}H]methotrexate for influx by the transport mechanism. Of the 2,4-diamino derivatives, influx was greatest for the L-glutamyl analogs. Influx was more rapid for the 5-methyl analogs and two- to threefold more rapid for the 5-chloro analog. The converse was true for efflux. The rate was reduced by the presence of a 5-substituent. The L-aspartyl analogs as a group were relatively

TABLE IV

Structure-Activity Relationships for L1210 Cell Dihydrofolate Reductase Inhibition and Membrane Transport Involving Quinazoline Folate Analogs[a]

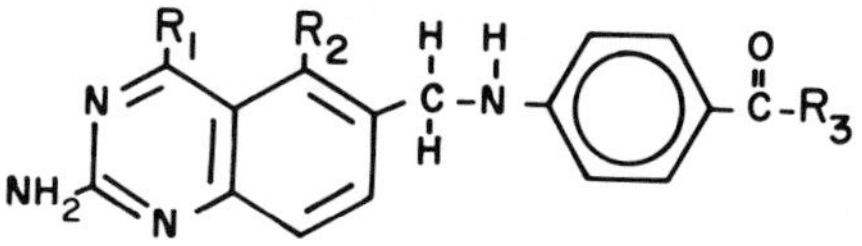

				Transport		
				Influx		
R_1	R_2	R_3	FAH_2 reductase inhibition, K_i (nM)	K_m (μM)	K_i (μM)	Efflux, k (minute^{-1})
OH	H	L-Glu	>100.0		>20.0	
NH_2	H	L-Glu	0.0006	5.65	4.8	0.034
NH_2	CH_3	L-Glu	0.0004	4.76		0.027
NH_2	C1	L-Glu	0.0001	2.23		0.011
NH_2	H	D-Glu	0.0314	45.70		0.047
NH_2	H	L-Asp	0.0132	30.70		0.019
NH_2	CH_3	L-Asp	0.0009	21.82	23.9	0.017
NH_2	C1	L-Asp	0.0003	18.74		0.018
NH_2	H	D-Asp	0.0423	6.13		0.053

[a] See Table III, footnotes *a*–*c*.

more inert. Influx was reduced an average of sixfold compared to that of the corresponding glutamyl derivatives, but increased influx was obtained by substitution of a methyl or chloro group at position 5. Efflux of the aspartyl analogues did not depend upon the presence of a 5-substituent but occurred at a rate less than that observed for the unsubstituted glutamyl analog. A most surprising result was obtained with the D-glutamyl and D-aspartyl analogs. Influx of the D-glutamyl derivative was ninefold lower than for the corresponding L form. However, influx of the D-aspartyl derivative was fivefold greater than that of the corresponding L form. In other words, influx of the D-aspartyl analog was approximately equal to that of the L-glutamyl analog. Efflux of both D forms was equal to or greater than that of any of the L forms studied. These quinazoline analogs have been shown to be considerably more toxic than the pteridine analogs (74). This could be explained by the reduced rate of efflux associated with this group, with consequent increased retention of drug by host tissues (49,50). Also, there are relatively low rates of plasma clearance associated with certain derivatives in this series (45).

Although there appear to be rather substantial differences in the transport of 2,4-diaminopteridine analogs in different murine tumor cells, transport of naturally occurring folate derivatives is similar. The influx K_m for methotrexate (Table V) differs by as much as fourfold and in a manner which correlates with the relative responsiveness of these tumors during therapy (13). Binding of methotrexate by dihydrofolate reductase from these tumors (49) and the efflux kinetics (13), with one exception (P388 cells), are also quite similar. Moreover, there is a good correlation between the steady-state level of exchangeable methotrexate *in vitro* and relative responsiveness for all the cell types (Fig. 8). In sharp contrast to these results with methotrexate, the transport of folate and 5-methyl- and 5-formyltetrahydrofolate showed little difference among the various tumor cell types.

Additional data on the structural specificity of the system transporting folate analogs and folate coenzymes in L1210 cells and murine intestinal epithelial cells are shown in Table VI. The system in L1210 cells exhibits the lowest affinity for folic acid. The affinity increases as a consequence of both reduction and methylation. A similar effect of these modifications of folic acid were shown for the epithelial cell system. However, this system shows a much lower affinity overall for natural folates. A similar effect of reduction and methylation was observed, but the magnitude of the net effect of both modifications was less (10-fold) than that seen for the system (100- to 200-fold) in L1210 cells. It was also found that the system in L1210 cells (75) (Table VI) and other murine tumor cells (75) exhibited a relatively low affinity for the unnatural isomer of the formylated reduced derivative, thus providing evidence for stereochemical specificity at the 6 position in these tumor cell systems.

TABLE V

Structure–Activity Relationships for Folate and Folate Analog Transport in Different Murine Tumor Cells

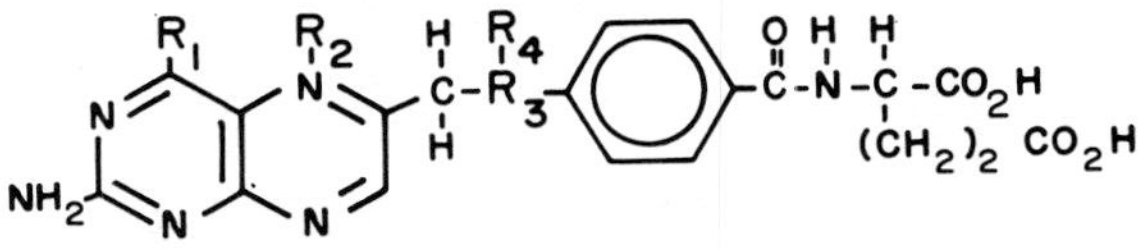

				Influx kinetics[a]									
				S180		Ehrlich		P388		P288		L1210	
R_1	R_2	R_3	R_4	K_m (μM)	K_i (μM)	K_m (μM)	K_i (μM)	K_m (μM)	K_i (μM)	K_m (μM)	K_i (μM)	K_m (μM)	K_i (μM)
OH	H	N	H		216.0		253.0		176.0		188.0		228.0
OH	CH_3[b]	N	H		1.1		1.5		1.4		0.9		0.9
OH	CHO[b]	N	H		1.7		3.7		1.6		1.6		2.2
NH_2	H	N	CH_3	11.20		5.80		6.1		3.92		3.13	

[a] Values for V_{max} are similar (13) for the different tumors. Values for $K_m \simeq K_i$, since K_i values were determined during competition for [^{3}H]methotrexate influx. Reduced derivatives with additional hydrogen atoms at positions 6, 7, and 8. $K_i = [I]/(K_p/K_m - 1)$, where $K_p = K_m$ in the presence of inhibitor [I].

[b] Reduced derivatives with additional hydrogen atoms at positions 6, 7, and 8. Values shown for each tumor cell type are expressed as concentration of the natural diastereoisomer.

TABLE VI

Structure-Activity Relationships for Transport of Natural Folate Derivatives by L1210 Cells and Murine Intestinal Epithelial Cells

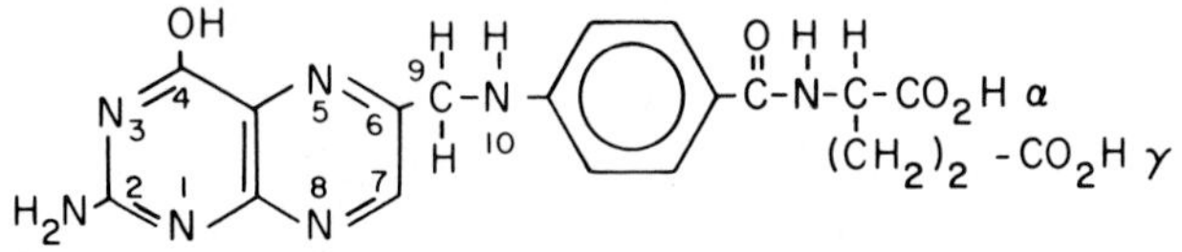

	Substituent position				Influx kinetics[a]	
Isomer	5′	6′	7′	8′	L1210 cells, K_i (μM)	Epithelial cells, K_i (μM)
					228.0	1769.0
			H	H	91.8	
1	H	H	H	H	13.9	
1	CH_3	H	H	H	0.9	164.0
1	CHO	H	H	H	2.1	159.0
d	CHO	H	H	H	39.2	

[a] Values for $K_m \cong K_i$ which were determined during competition for [^{3}H]methotrexate influx. $K_i = [I]/(K_p/K_m - 1)$, where $K_p = K_m$ in the presence of inhibitor [I] when determined graphically.

C. Exploitation of Knowledge of the Specificity of Folate and Folate Analog Transport for New Drug Design

We have reviewed studies in our laboratory which provide pharmacokinetic and biochemical evidence implicating membrane transport of folate analogs as the major determinant of relative responsiveness and selective antitumor action of this class of agents in a group of well-known murine tumor models. These studies extend previous findings in our laboratory and elsewhere showing that the exchangeable level of intracellular antifolate is the critical determinant of cytotoxicity and that limitations on these levels in different tissues are an expression of the individual membrane transport mechanism in each case. Our studies have also provided a kinetic basis for the tissue-specific differences in membrane transport observed. As an obvious approach to achieving preferentially and maintaining greater levels of antifolate accumulation in tumor cells, one would hope to identify new analogs which would interact with transport systems in tumor cells more effectively with regard to net intracellular accumulation than in drug-limiting proliferative normal tissue. This approach seems to have a sound conceptual basis in view of our studies, which have clearly revealed differences in the structural specificity of transport systems for influx which apparently favor greater levels of accumulation and retention of certain analogs in some tumor tissues. A more favorable differential interaction for a new analog at the level of transport, which has as its consequence an increase in accumulation in tumor tissue, could occur as a result of increased influx or decreased efflux in tumor or, alternatively, by decreased influx or increased efflux in normal tissue. Differences in both these parameters have already been well documented for a number of analogs during earlier studies in our laboratory (11,12). The studies of structural specificity of both influx and efflux parameters of tumor cell transport systems vis-à-vis target enzyme binding, which were just described, sought a systematic kinetic evaluation of a large number of available analogs for the purpose of identifying regions on the folate molecule where structural modification would have an effect which was potentially favorable to transport but would be compatible with effective binding by dihydrofolate reductase. Although our current emphasis has been confined to a few tumor cells and epithelial cells, we are currently expanding these studies to include an evaluation of these analogs in a larger number of cell types. The results of these studies to date have confirmed our initial findings in regard to the importance of the N-10 position and have led to the development of a new analogue, 10-deazaaminopterin, with potential clinical importance, primarily because of its apparent broader spectrum of activity in murine tumor models (76). Some relevant information on the transport of this new analog is summarized in Table VII. Whereas the value of the influx K_m for methotrexate varies as much as fourfold among the three tumor cell types, the value derived for aminopterin and 10-deazaaminopterin is essentially the same for the three cell types. The efflux and inhibition of dihydrofolate

TABLE VII

Structure-Activity Relationships for Folate Analog Transport in Various Murine Tumor Cells

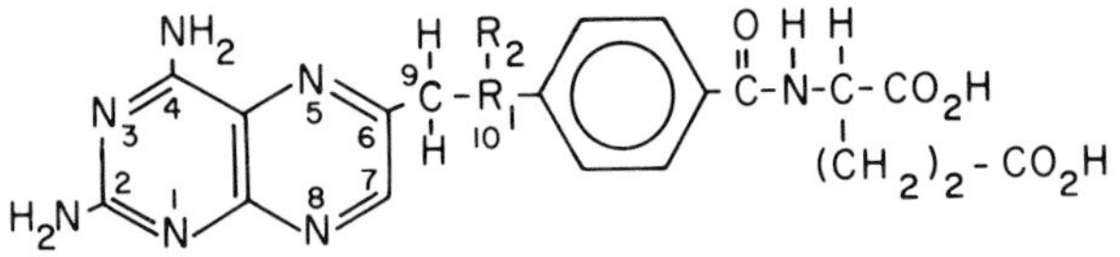

		Influx[a]		
R_1	R_2	L1210, K_m (μM)	Ehrlich, K_m (μM)	S180, K_m (μM)
N	H	1.1	1.9	1.6
N	CH_3	3.3	6.1	11.2
CH	H	1.1	0.9	1.4

[a] Values for V_{max} are similar (13) for the different tumors. Also, values for efflux of all three analogues are similar in each cell type.

reductase for both analogues in each cell type are identical (76). These data on the influx K_m would imply a greater therapeutic potential for 10-deazaaminopterin, particularly in the case of S180 and Ehrlich tumors, if it could also be shown that transport and toxicity in the drug-limiting host proliferative cell population were at least comparable. Subsequent studies *in vitro* (20) and *in vivo* (76) did in fact show that this was the case, and evidence (77) was generated in these and other tumor models which document the therapeutic superiority of 10-deazaaminopterin compared to methotrexate. Some of this evidence is summarized in Fig. 10. In experiments comparing these analogs on a schedule of subcutaneous administration of every other day ×5 at the LD_{10} dosage (12 mg/kg for methotrexate, 9 mg/kg for 10-deazaaminopterin, and 0.25 mg/kg for aminopterin), the relative increase in life span was two- to threefold greater with 10-deazaaminopterin for three out of the five tumors (S180, Ehrlich, Taper). Activity against the other two tumors (L1210 and P815) was marginally better. Aminopterin was the least effective of the three analogs against all the tumors studied. These studies are continuing, and a number of new N-10 analogs with even more favorable transport properties are now under evaluation. In addition,

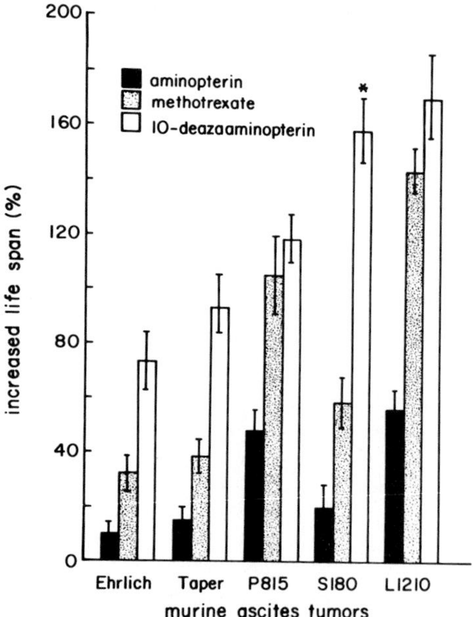

Fig. 10. Relative antitumor efficacy of 10-deazaaminopterin, methotrexate, and aminopterin. Therapy was administered subcutaneously at the LD_{10} dosage (12 mg/kg, methotrexate; 9 mg/kg, 10-deazaaminopterin; 0.25 mg/kg aminopterin) on a schedule of once every other day for a total of five doses beginning 1 day after tumor implantation (10^6 cells) intraperitoneally. Asterisk indicates 60-day survivors.

our studies have also demonstrated that new analogs with modifications at N-5 and/or the γ-carboxyl group may also have potential for improved therapeutic action.

V. Conclusions and Future Goals

The overall significance of these findings for folate analog pharmacology are severalfold. They establish the same pharmacokinetic basis for differences in the recovery of normal proliferative tissues and various tumor tissues following antifolate therapy. Moreover, the degree of documentation provided in these studies now allows us to propose, with some degree of confidence, that the property of accumulating and maintaining pharmacologically effective intracellular levels of folate analogs is different in all proliferative tissues of the mouse, and probably, in all mammals. These findings also delineate a concept for the basis of selective action in the case of responsive tumor models, which takes into consideration antiproliferative effects against tumor within the context of limiting effects against both major host renewal sites. In so doing, further validity is derived for extrapolation of a concept elucidated in animal models to patients where antifolate effects in bone marrow are as serious as in gastrointestinal tissue.

Although the relative responsiveness and selective antitumor action observed during folate analogue therapy of these murine tumor models appear to be explained largely within the framework of current knowledge of carrier-mediated membrane transport, we only tentatively suggest that there may be a similar basis for related observations in other tumor models or in patients. Certainly, the possibility must be considered that factors other than those related to membrane transport per se may play a contributing, if not a determining, role in specific cases. For instance, differences in the extent of methotrexate inhibition have been reported for dihydrofolate reductase isolated from different rodent and human tumor cell lines, which show some correlation with growth inhibition of these cell lines *in vitro* (78). However, it will be necessary to provide some documentation for the existence of these differences *in situ* and evidence for their therapeutic significance at a pharmacological level. Some correlation has also been shown (79–81) between the relative oxidation rates of folate analogs to the 7-hydroxy derivative by liver aldehyde oxidase and toxicity in different animal species. Any relevance to the difference in toxicity of these two agents in rodents and humans, however, is doubtful, since the overall level of activity of these enzymes is so low. Last, enzyme-mediated polyglutamation may enhance the toxicity of methotrexate, or other folate analogs, in some tissues more than in others because of greater retention and/or inhibitory effects of these derivatives on other folate-utilizing enzymes. In regard to the former, our studies of the γ-glutamyl peptide of methotrexate suggest a rate of loss of this peptide derivative from L1210 cells equal to that of methotrexate itself (20,82). Although the metabolism of folate analogs of the sort described above is well documented for a variety of mammalian tissues, no evidence has been reported so far for direct involvement in the selective antitumor action of these agents in animal models or patients.

The importance of membrane transport to the question of therapeutic responsiveness and selective antitumor action of various categories of anticancer agents for the most part remains to be elucidated. Although much evidence now exists for a determining role of transport in the case of folate analogs, essentially all the evidence has been derived in murine tumor models. The study by Kessel and Hall (24) is a singular exception and provides (Section III, C) evidence for a role of folate analogue transport in the responsiveness of a group of human leukemias. In the interim, any useful extrapolation of data derived in tumor models to a clinical level must necessarily rely on the appropriateness of these models in predicting the responsiveness of specific human cancers. Evidence associating alterations in transport with acquired resistance to some nucleoside analogs (83–85), alkylating agents (86–88), vinca alkaloids (89), and anthracycline antibiotics (90) is suggestive of a role for transport in the therapeutic action of these categories of agents. These observations considered in the light of detailed evidence available with respect to the folate analogs appear to justify further studies on transport as a fruitful approach to more effective therapy with a variety of categories of agents. Findings showing a difference in structural specificity of transport systems for folate analogs in tumor versus drug-limiting normal proliferative tissue, which favors greater accumulation and retention of folate analogs in tumor, are of special importance in this regard. These findings give a clear indication of diversity in the properties of specific transport systems in different tissues, which is nor ordinarily seen for enzyme targets. It is reasonable to assume that a similar tissue-specific qualitative diversity may exist in the case of other transport systems.

Further documentation of the role of membrane transport in the effective therapeutic action of agents other than folate analogues will require the development (or application) of experimental systems which isolate the transport process from subsequent intracellular metabolism and/or binding to macromolecules characteristic of these agents. This will allow the detailed rate measurements and kinetic analyses necessary for meaningful studies of comparative structural specificity. Such systems might include the use of inhibitors or conditions in a manner already suggested by other workers (91), which selectively suppress complicating intracellular interactions. Another promising approach involves the study of drug transport in isolated plasma membrane vesicles. This methodology (5,60,92) has already been effectively applied in the study of a variety of systems transporting natural substrates. We have used similar methodology for a study of antifolate transport in plasma membrane vesicles isolated from L1210 leukemia cells (23). This type of approach not only eliminates the complications of intracellular metabolism and macromolecular binding but also could be readily applied in the study of transport in solid tumor models and in human cancer tissue. With this type of methodology, repetitive examination of clinical material under stable biochemical conditions is possible, and questions relating to transport and responsiveness prior to treatment or in the event of relapse can be meaningfully addressed. The successful outcome of this biochemical approach in animal models will also require its application to tumor and proliferative normal cell populations which have pharmacological relevance, so that any data derived will have therapeutic significance, at least with respect to predictive tumor models, if not in patients.

Another approach to more preferential accumulation of antifolates in tumor cells compared to normal drug-limiting tissue is an attempt to manipulate transport systems selectively by agents which might interfere with their energetics or regulatory control. The ultimate success of such an approach will require further investigation of these aspects of transport in both tumor cells and normal proliferative tissues. Of considerable interest in this regard are the *in vitro* studies in murine (93,94) and human (16) tumor cells showing augmentation of net accumulation of intracellular methotrexate by the vinca alkaloids vincristine and vinblastine. The effect observed appears to be related to a pronounced inhibition of the efflux of methotrexate (94). Although vincristine was incorporated in some clinical protocols using high-dose methotrexate (95,96), pharmacokinetic evidence for augmentation of methotrexate accumulation in tumor cells *in vivo* is lacking. Our studies with the L1210 murine tumor model gave no evidence of augmentation *in vivo* (97) and, contrary to prior reports (93), we could not demonstrate therapeutic synergism of simultaneous, or near simultaneous, administration of both agents. Interestingly, however, rather substantial synergism was observed in this tumor model when vincristine administration was delayed 24 or 32 hours after methotrexate (97,98). Also, these studies provided evidence for a selective augmentation by vincristine *in vitro* of the net accumulation of methotrexate in isolated suspensions of L1210 cells but not in isolated epithelial cells (97). Although the clinical potential for the use of this combination of agents is uncertain, these data suggest that some form of selective intervention *in vivo* at the level of membrane transport, which will render antifolate therapy more effective, may eventually be possible.

Acknowledgments

The studies carried out in the authors' laboratory were supported in part by grants from the National Cancer Institute, Department of Health, Education and Welfare, USPHS, and the American Cancer Society.

References

1. I. D. Goldman, *Cancer Treat. Rep.* **61,** 51 (1975).
2. I. D. Goldman, *Cancer Treat. Rep.* **61,** 549 (1977).
3. F. M. Sirotnak, *Pharmacol. Ther.* **8,** 71 (1980).
4. F. M. Sirotnak, P. L. Chello, and R. W. Brockman, *Methods Cancer Res.* **16,** 381 (1979).
5. J. Hochstadt, *Crit. Rev. Biochem.* **2,** 259 (1974).
6. H. N. Christensen, "Biological Transport." Benjamin, Reading, Massachusetts, 1975.
7. A. Kotyk and K. Janacek, "Cell Membrane Transport." Plenum, New York, 1975.
8. F. M. Sirotnak, S. Kurita, M. G. Sargent, D. J. Robinson, and D. J. Hutchison, *Nature (London)* **216,** 1236 (1967).
9. F. M. Sirotnak, S. Kurita, and D. J. Hutchison, *Cancer Res.* **28,** 75 (1968).
10. I. D. Goldman, N. S. Lichtenstein, and V. T. Oliverio, *J. Biol. Chem.* **243,** 5007 (1968).
11. F. M. Sirotnak and R. C. Donsbach, *Cancer Res.* **32,** 2120 (1972).
12. F. M. Sirotnak and R. C. Donsbach, *Cancer Res.* **34,** 371 (1974).
13. F. M. Sirotnak and R. C. Donsbach, *Cancer Res.* **36,** 1151 (1976).
14. M. Dembo and F. M. Sirotnak, *Biochim. Biophys. Acta* **448,** 505 (1976).
15. K. R. Harrap, B. T. Hall, M. E. Furness, and L. I. Hart, *Ann. N.Y. Acad Sci.* **186,** 312 (1971).
16. R. A. Bender, W. A. Bleyer, S. A. Frisby, and V. T. Oliverio, *Cancer Res.* **35,** 1305 (1975).
17. W. F. Bobzien and I. D. Goldman, *J. Clin. Invest.* **51,** 1688 (1972).
18. P. L. Chello, F. M. Sirotnak, and R. C. Donsbach, *Cancer Res.* **37,** 4297 (1977).
19. P. L. Chello, F. M. Sirotnak, D. M. Dorick, and J. Gura, *In* "Chemistry and Biology of Pteridines" (R. Kisliuk and G. Brown, eds.), p. 521. Am. Elsevier, New York, 1979.
20. F. M. Sirotnak, P. L. Chello, J. P. Piper, J. A. Montgomery, and J. I. DeGraw, *In* "Chemistry and Biology of Pteridines" (R. Kisliuk and G. Brown, eds.), p. 597. Am. Elsevier, New York, 1979.
21. N. S. Lichtenstein, V. T. Oliverio, and I. D. Goldman, *Biochim. Biophys. Acta* **193,** 456 (1969).
22. I. D. Goldman, *Ann. N.Y. Acad. Sci.* **186,** 400 (1971).
23. C. H. Yang, R. H. F. Peterson, F. M. Sirotnak, and P. L. Chello, *J. Biol. Chem.* **25,** 1402 (1979).
24. D. Kessel and T. C. Hall, *Cancer Res.* **27,** 1539 (1967).
25. A. Nahas, P. F. Nixon, and J. R. Bertino, *Cancer Res.* **32,** 1416 (1972).
26. I. D. Goldman, *Biochim. Biophys Acta* **233,** 624 (1971).
27. J. F. Rader, D. Niethammer, and F. M. Huennekens, *Biochem. Pharmacol.* **23,** 2057 (1974).
28. R. C. Jackson, D. Niethammer, and F. M. Huennekens, *Cancer Biochem. Biophys.* **1,** 151 (1975).
29. D. Niethammer and R. C. Jackson, *Eur. J. Cancer* **11,** 845 (1975).
30. M. R. Suresh, G. B. Henderson, and F. M. Huennekens, *Biochem. Biophys. Res. Commun.* **87,** 135 (1979).
31. M. T. Hakala, *Biochim. Biophys Acta* **102,** 198 (1965).
32. M. T. Hakala, *Biochim. Biophys Acta* **102,** 210 (1965).
33. I. D. Goldman, *J. Biol. Chem.* **244,** 3729 (1969).
34. P. L. Chello, F. M. Sirotnak, and R. C. Donsbach, *Pharmacologist* **19,** 207 (1977).
35. C. H. Yang and F. M. Sirotnak, *Fed. Proc., Fed. Am. Soc. Exp. Biol.* **38,** 247 (1979).
36. D. W. Horne, W. T. Briggs, and C. Wagner, *Biochem. Biophys. Res. Commun.* **68,** 70 (1976).
37. R. C. Rubin, E. Owens, and D. Rall, *Cancer Res.* **28,** 689 (1968).
38. R. Spector and A. V. Lorenzo, *Science* **187,** 540 (1975).
39. C. P. Chen and C. Wagner, *Life Sci.* **16,** 1571 (1975).
40. R. C. Rubin, E. S. Henderson, E. S. Owens, and D. P. Rall, *Cancer Res.* **27,** 553 (1967).

41. D. Kessel, T. C. Hall, and D. Roberts, *Cancer Res.* **28,** 564 (1968).
42. W. C. Werkheiser, *Cancer Res.* **23,** 1277 (1963).
43. J. R. Bertino, *Cancer Res.* **23,** 1286 (1963).
44. S. Margolis, F. S. Philips, and S. S. Sternberg, *Cancer Res.* **31,** 2037 (1971).
45. F. S. Philips, F. M. Sirotnak, J. E. Sodergren, and D. J. Hutchison, *Cancer Res.* **33,** 153 (1973).
46. F. M. Sirotnak and R. C. Donsbach, *Cancer Res.* **33,** 1290 (1973).
47. B. A. Chabner and R. C. Young, *Clin. Invest.* **52,** 1804 (1973).
48. F. M. Sirotnak and R. C. Donsbach, *Cancer Res.* **34,** 3332 (1974).
49. F. M. Sirotnak and R. C. Donsbach, *Cancer Res.* **35,** 1737 (1975).
50. F. M. Sirotnak and R. C. Donsbach, *Biochem. Pharmacol.* **24,** 156 (1975).
51. I. D. Goldman and M. J. Fyfe, *Mol. Pharmacol.* **10,** 275 (1974).
52. J. C. White and I. D. Goldman, *Mol. Pharmacol.* **12,** 711 (1976).
53. R. C. Jackson and K. R. Harrap, *Arch. Biochem. Biophys.* **158,** 827 (1973).
54. D. L. Oxender, *Annu. Rev. Biochem.* **41,** 777 (1972).
55. Y. S. Halpern, *Annu. Rev. Genet.* **8,** 103 (1974).
56. F. M. Sirotnak, M. G. Sargent, and D. J. Hutchison, *J. Bacteriol.* **93,** 309 (1967).
57. F. M. Sirotnak, M. G. Sargent, and D. J. Hutchison, *J. Bacteriol.* **93,** 315 (1967).
58. H. R. Kaback, *Annu. Rev. Biochem.* **39,** 562 (1970).
59. R. Benveniste and J. Davis, *Annu. Rev. Biochem.* **42,** 471 (1973).
60. F. M. Sirotnak, *Antibiot. Chemother.* (*Basel*) **20,** 67 (1976).
61. G. A. Fisher, *Biochem. Pharmacol.* **11,** 1233 (1962).
62. D. Kessel, T. C. Hall, D. Roberts, and I. Wodinsky, *Science* **150,** 752 (1965).
63. B. M. Braganca, A. Y. Divekar, and N. R. Vaidya, *Biochim. Biophys. Acta* **135,** 937 (1967).
64. A. Y. Divekar, N. R. Vaidya, and B. M. Braganca, *Biochim. Biophys. Acta* **135,** 927 (1967).
65. D. Roberts, I. Wodinsky, and T. C. Hall, *Cancer Res.* **25,** 1899 (1965).
66. F. M. Sirotnak and D. M. Moccio, *Cancer Res.* **40,** 1230 (1979).
67. F. C. Ferguson, Jr., J. B. Thiersch, and F. S. Philips, *J. Pharmacol. Exp. Ther.* **98,** 293 (1950).
68. W. D. Stein, "The Movement Across Cell Membranes." Academic Press, New York, 1967.
69. J. R. Bertino and R. T. Skeel. In "*Pharmacological* Basis of Cancer Chemotherapy," M. D. Anderson Hospital and Tumor Institute at Houston, pp. 681–689. Williams and Wilkons, Co., Baltimore, Maryland, 1975.
70. B. R. Baker, "Design of Active-Site Directed Irreversible Enzyme Inhibitors." Wiley, New York, 1967.
71. R. L. Blakley, "The Biochemistry of Folic Acid and Related Pteridines." North-Holland Publ., Amsterdam, 1969.
72. R. W. Brockman, *in* "Handbuch der Experimentellan Pharmakologie" (A. Sartorelli and D. Johns, eds.), Vol. 38 p. 352. Springer-Verlag, Berlin and New York, 1974.
73. D. A. Mathews, R. A. Alden, J. T. Bolin, S. T. Freer, R. Hamlin, N. Xuong, J. Kraut, M. Poe, M. Williams, and K. Hoogsteen, *Science* **197,** 452 (1977).
74. D. J. Hutchison, *Cancer Treat. Rep.* **52,** 697 (1968).
75. F. M. Sirotnak, P. L. Chello, D. M. Moccio, R. L. Kisliuk, G. Combepine, Y, Gaumont, and J. A Montgomery, *Biochem. Pharmacol.* **28,** 2993 (1979).
76. F. M. Sirotnak, J. I. DeGraw, and P. L. Chello, *Curr. Chemother.* **1,** 1128 (1978).
77. F. M. Sirotnak, J. I. DeGraw, D. M. Moccio, and D. M. Dorick, *Cancer Treat. Rep.* **62,** 1047 (1978).
78. R. C. Jackson, L. I. Hart, and K. R. Harrap, *Cancer Res.* **36,** 1991 (1976).
79. H. M. Redetzki, J. E. Redetzki, and A. L. Ellis, *Pharmacologist* **7,** 180 (1965).
80. D. J. Johns, A. T. Ionatti, A. C. Sartorelli, and J. R. Bertino, *Biochem. Pharmacol.* **15,** 555 (1965).

81. D. J. Johns, A. T. Ionatti, A. C. Sartorelli, B. A. Booth, and J. R. Bertino, *Biochem. Biophys. Acta* **105,** 380 (1965).
82. F. M. Sirotnak, P. L. Chello, J. R. Piper, and J. A. Montgomery, *Biochem. Pharmacol.* **27,** 1821 (1978).
83. R. E. Breslow and R. A. Goldsby, *Exp. Cell Res.* **55,** 339 (1969).
84. J. J. Freed and I. M. Hames, *Exp. Cell Res.* **99,** 126 (1976).
85. T. P. Lynch, C. E. Cass and A. R. P. Paterson, *J. Supramol. Struct.* **6,** 363 (1977).
86. G. J. Goldenberg, C. L. Vanstone, and I. Bihler, *Science* **172,** 1148 (1971).
87. G. J. Goldenberg, H. B. Land, and D. V. Cormack, *Cancer Res.* **34,** 3274 (1974).
88. M. K. Wolpert and R. W. Ruddon, *Cancer Res.* **29,** 873 (1969).
89. W. A. Bleyer, S. A. Freiberg, and V. T. Oliverio, *Biochem. Pharmacol.* **24,** 633 (1975).
90. K. Danø, *Biochim. Biophys. Acta* **323,** 466 (1973).
91. P. G. W. Plagemann and D. P. Richey, *Biochim. Biophys. Acta* **344,** 263 (1974).
92. H. R. Kaback, *Science* **186,** 882 (1974).
93. R. F. Zager, S. A. Frisby, and V. T. Oliverio, *Cancer Res.* **33,** 1670 (1973).
94. M. J. Fyfe and I. D. Goldman, *J. Biol. Chem.* **248,** 5067 (1973).
95. G. Rosen, F. Ghavini, and R. Venucci, *J. Am. Med. Assoc.* **230,** 1149 (1974).
96. E. Frei, III, N. Jaffe, M. H. N. Tattersall, S. Pitman, and L. Parker, *N. Engl. J. Med.* **292,** 846 (1975).
97. P. L. Chello, F. M. Sirotnak, and D. M. Dorick, *Cancer Res.* **39,** 2106 (1979).
98. P. L. Chello, F. M. Sirotnak, D. M. Dorick, and D. M. Moccio, *Cancer Treat. Rep.* **63,** 1889 (1979).

18

Cellular Mechanisms of Resistance to Methotrexate

J. R. BERTINO, B. J. DOLNICK, R. J. BERENSON, D. I. SCHEER, AND B. A. KAMEN

I. Introduction

Drug resistance of bacterial, protozoan, and neoplastic diseases of humans continues to be a difficult and challenging problem. An important approach to the study of the biology and biochemistry of drug resistance has been the isolation and characterization of drug-resistant subpopulations.

Cell lines highly resistant to methotrexate (MTX) have been particularly useful in the study of drug resistance, and several different mechanisms by which cells become resistant to this drug have been elucidated. The status of these studies is briefly reviewed in this chapter with particular emphasis on cell lines resistant to MTX by virtue of an increased level of dihydrofolate reductase (DHFR).

ISBN 0-12-619280-4

II. A Brief Description of Methotrexate Action and Natural or Intrinsic Resistance to This Drug

Methotrexate is an effective inhibitor of DNA synthesis and consequently cell replication when (1) intracellular levels of this compound are achieved that exceed the binding capacity of DHFR (1–7), and (2) these levels are present for a sufficient time during S phase so as to result in a series of irreversible events that prove lethal to the cell. Cell death occurs rapidly when a "thymineless" state exists (3,4); if RNA and protein synthesis are also inhibited, the cell kill by MTX is less rapid (3,4). Cells which accumulate MTX poorly, either because of a slow influx or a rapid efflux, or that synthesize DHFR at a relatively rapid rate, may be less sensitive than cells that accumulate the drug rapidly or have a slow rate of synthesis of DHFR (8).

Another consideration, more recently emphasized, is that MTX binding by DHFR is maximal only in the presence of NADPH (9–12); thus intracellular DHFR without associated NADPH would not necessarily be stoichiometrically inhibited by MTX, as has been assumed in the past. Since it has been shown that there is polymorphism of cellular DHFR, in part based upon the presence or absence of NADPH or folates (13), it is significant to note that current work in our laboratory, using [^{3}H]MTX and [^{3}H]dihydrofolic acid in radioassays to separate DHFR binding and enzyme activity (11,14), has demonstrated that, while NADH can substitute for NADPH as an enzymatic cofactor, this pyridine nucleotide does not enhance binding of MTX. Therefore, with NADH as cofactor, even in the presence of excess MTX, tetrahydrofolate synthesis occurs when there would otherwise be no detectable enzyme activity if NADPH were the sole cofactor (12). This enzyme polymorphism and use of an alternate pyridine nucleotide could in part explain the need for MTX to accumulate in the cell above the apparent DHFR concentration to be optimally effective, as previously noted (6,7).

Another factor related to the rate at which a cell can synthesize new DHFR and thus overcome MTX-induced blockage is a phenomenon called enzyme "induction" (8,15,16). The mechanism of the DHFR increase after MTX treatment was found to be due not to an increase in the rate of synthesis of this enzyme but to protection of DHFR from degradation by MTX, leading to an increase in the intracellular steady-state level of this enzyme (mostly bound to MTX) (17). This resultant increase in the enzyme level may allow cells to survive MTX treatment since, once efflux of drug occurs from the cell, a small amount of MTX dissociating from this increased amount of enzyme may allow resumption of tetrahydrofolate biosynthesis, especially in the presence of elevated levels of dihydrofolate (16). This is possible because thymidylate synthetase rather than DHFR is the rate-limiting enzyme in thymidylate biosynthesis. These considerations also provide an explanation for the apparently disproportionate degree of resistance noted when mutant cell lines emerge with an elevated DHFR level. For example, cells with a 200-fold increase in DHFR may be resistant to concentrations of MTX 100,000-fold greater than that necessary to inhibit parent cell line growth 50%.

III. Acquired Resistance to Methotrexate

Acquired resistance to MTX develops when cells are exposed to low concentrations of this drug, and the surviving cells are exposed to gradually increasing concentrations of the folate analogue in a stepwise fashion. The most common mechanism of resistance that occurs is an elevated intracellular level of DHFR, and cell lines with levels of DHFR 200- to 400-fold higher than that of the parent line have been described (18–24). Less commonly found are cell lines resistant by virtue of impaired transport of MTX or of an altered DHFR exhibiting a decrease in affinity for this drug (25–29).

Cell lines have been described in which a high level of resistance to MTX is conferred via two mechanisms; for example, we have isolated a mutant of L1210 leukemia with an elevated level of DHFR (35-fold) together with decreased ability to transport the drug (28). In addition, Flintoff *et al.* (29) have described a Chinese hamster cell line with an elevated DHFR level, which also has a decreased affinity for MTX.

When resistant murine lines are obtained by treatment of transplanted tumors propagated *in vivo,* they are almost always found to contain elevated levels of DHFR. Lines obtained in this manner exhibiting altered DHFR or impaired transport are less common.

During the past few years, the genetic mechanism by which cells are able to synthesize high levels of DHFR has been elucidated, particularly in the laboratory of Schimke (30–33). Several mammalian cell lines with an increased level of DHFR have been found to have a corresponding increase in the rate of synthesis of this enzyme, which corresponds in turn to an increase in the amount of mRNA for DHFR (24,32–34). An unexpected finding was the manner in which these mutant cells increased DHFR synthesis, namely, by a proportionate increase in the number of genes coding for this enzyme (24,33,34). Several mouse and Chinese hamster lines have now been shown to have increases in gene copies of DHFR proportionate to the increase in enzyme activity, rate of enzyme synthesis, and mRNA content of this enzyme (Table I) (24,30,32,35,35a). The mechanism by which a cell can amplify the genes coding for a specific protein is not yet clear. One observation that is of interest in this regard is the reversion of some resistant cell lines, cultured in the absence of MTX, to partial loss of resistance with a corresponding decrease in both DHFR activity and gene copies of this enzyme (22,23).

A powerful tool for the study of cell populations with different levels of DHFR

TABLE I

Relative Dihydrofolate Reductase Activity, mRNA Level, and Gene Dosage Level in Methotrexate-Sensitive and -Resistant Cell Lines

Cell line	Relative DHFR activity	Rate of synthesis[a]	Relative level of DHFR mRNA[b]	Relative DHFR gene dosage[b]	Reference
Sarcoma 180					(30,32)
S-3	1	ND	1	1	
AT3000	250	5.9	220	180	
L1210 leukemia					(32)
S	1	ND	1	1	
RR	35	2.2	35	45	
L5178Y lymphoma					
S	1	0–0.1	1	1	(24)
R	300	10–12	300	300	
Chinese hamster ovary					
K1	1	0.2		1	(35)
MK42	240	4.1		150	
3T6-R1		3.3	30	35	(35a)
3T6-R2		10.4	>90	100	

[a] Percentage of total protein synthesis immunoprecipitable material as DHFR in an *in vitro* rabbit reticulocyte translation assay.
[b] Relative to parent sensitive cell line.

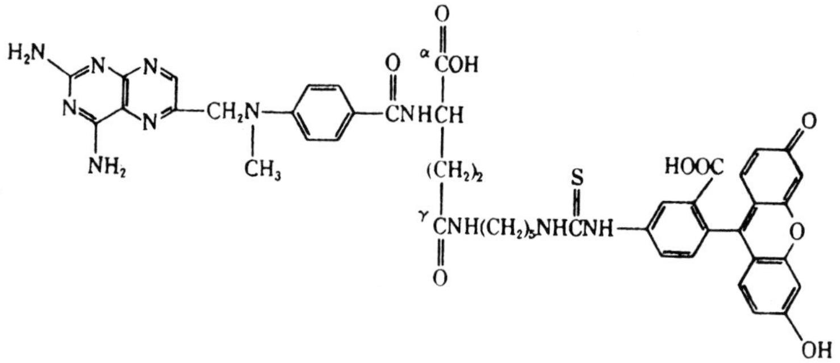

Fig. 1. Structure of fluorescein-labeled MTX.

is the use of fluoroscein-labeled MTX, with analysis by a fluorescence-activated cell sorter (36). The structure of fluorescein-labeled MTX is shown in Fig. 1. This compound, synthesized initially by Gapski *et al.* (37), is a tight-binding inhibitor of DHFR, and under appropriate conditions the amount of drug bound intracellularly is proportional to the DHFR content of the cell. When Sarcoma-180 cells were analyzed after growth in the absence of MTX for 8 generations, before reversion to a lower level of DHFR had taken place, it was found that the resistant Sarcoma-180 line was composed of a heterogeneous population with a wide distribution of DHFR levels and DHFR genes (36). After continued culture in the absence of MTX for 400 generations, a new stable state was reached, characterized by a relatively homogeneous population of cells containing a 7- to 10-fold increase in the level of DHFR. Thus cells with a lower gene copy number are capable of replicating more rapidly than high-level mutants and, in the absence of the selective pressure exerted by MTX, eventually become the dominant cell type. This technique has great promise for the further study of events involved in the selective multiplication and loss of DHFR genes. We plan to employ this technique to study population changes in human neoplastic cells during the emergence of resistance to MTX.

A. Location of the Amplified Dihydrofolate Reductase Genes

The question of the chromosomal location of the amplified genes has been answered using *in situ* hybridization techniques. Previous reports by Biedler and Spengler (38,39) indicated that a specific chromosomal abnormality in a Chinese hamster lung cell line was associated with MTX resistance and elevated levels of DHFR. These resistant cells contained a homogeneously staining region (HSR) when stained by the trypsin–Giemsa method. Of interest was the finding that this region decreased in size as the cells lost resistance to MTX. Studies on a resistant Chinese hamster ovary line, using a [^{3}H]cDNA probe prepared against the DHFR mRNA from an amplified Sarcoma-180 MTX-resistant line, have shown by *in situ* hybridization techniques that all or most of the amplified genes are located on chromosome 2 (35). Studies carried out in our laboratory (24) have shown that MTX-resistant L5178Y murine lymphoma cells contain a HSR in chromosome 2 and that this HSR contains DHFR genes, as measured by *in situ* hybridization (Figs. 2 and 3). In both cases, a rough estimate of DNA content present in this

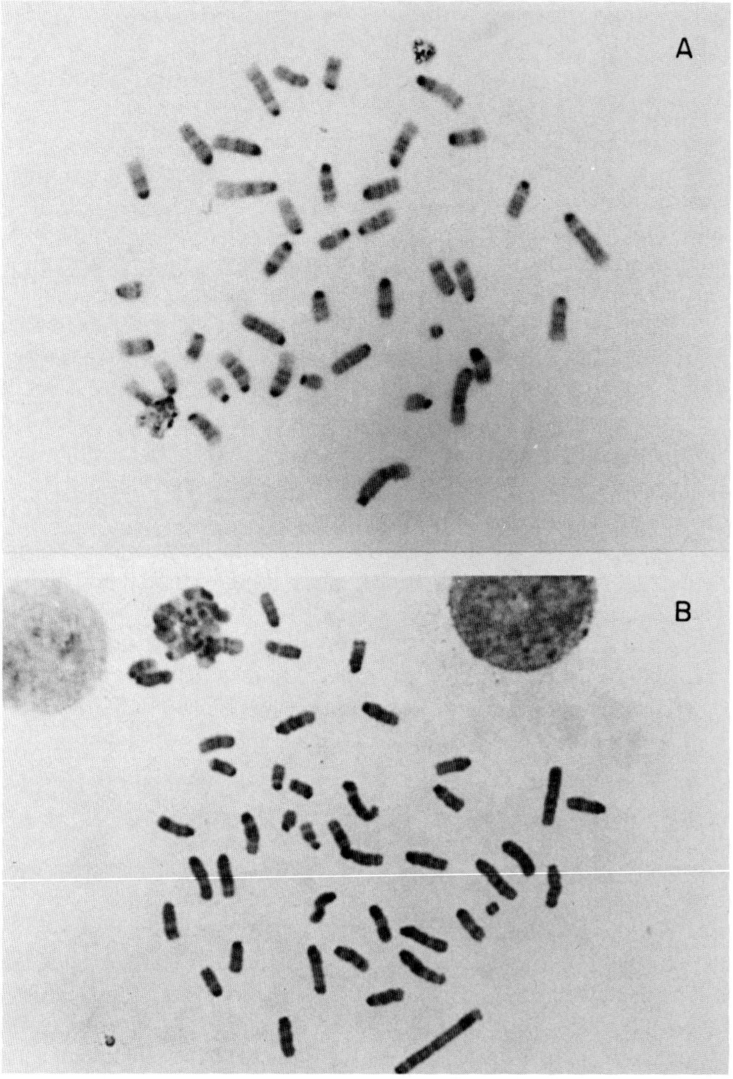

Fig. 2. Giemsa-trypsin-stained metaphase chromosome spreads. (A) MTX-sensitive L5178Y cells (B) MTX-resistant L5178YR cells. Note HSR in large chromosome at bottom of (B). Reprinted with permission of *The Journal of Cell Biology* (24).

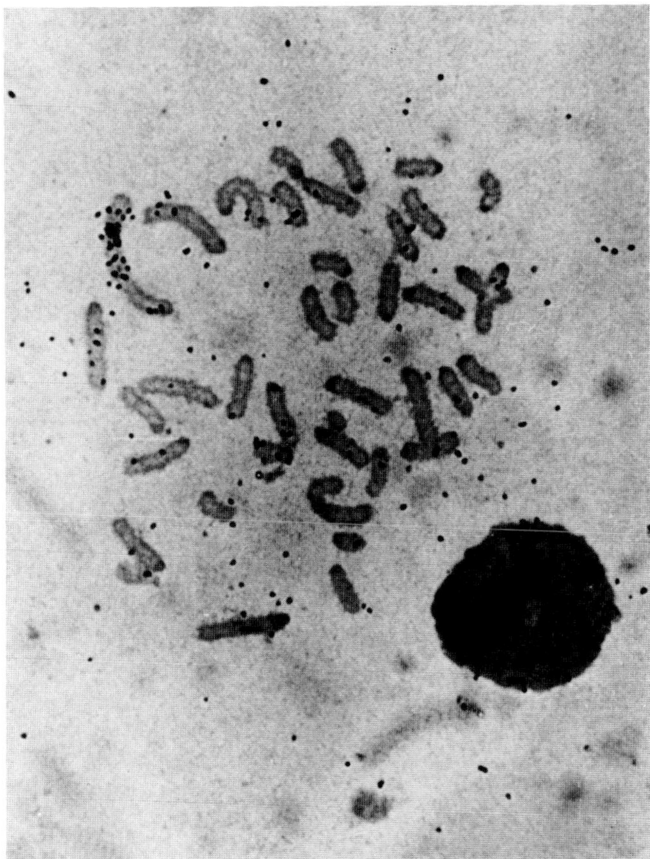

Fig. 3. *In situ* molecular hybridization of MTX-resistant L5178YR cells. Note accumulation of grains, corresponding to DHFR coding sequences, over large chromosome. Reprinted with permission of *The Journal of Cell Biology* (24).

region is about 3–5% of the total DNA. This is equivalent to 2.3×10^8 bp in the HSR. Each repeat unit is approximately 800 kbp in size; thus each unit contains considerably more DNA than is necessary to code for the DHFR mRNA. What information is represented in the other sequences within the amplified unit, as well as the possible function of these sequences, awaits further study. It is also possible, as suggested by Wahl *et al.* (40), that insertion-like sequences mediate gene amplification. Preliminary work from Schimke's laboratory, as well as from our own, indicates that the DHFR gene most likely contains at least five intervening sequences and that the RNA transcript produced must be processed in a manner similar to the processing that occurs from mRNA for hemoglobin, ovalbumin, and immunolglobulins (41–47).

B. Organization of the Dihydrofolate Reductase Gene

The DHFR gene is organized according to a now classic picture, as seen for several genes of higher eukaryotes [for review see Crick (48)]. Evidence suggesting that there are multiple intervening sequences within the DHFR gene is depicted in Fig. 4. Since the probe pDHFR 21 contains no internal restriction cleavage sites for the enzymes *Eco*RI, *Bam*HI, and *Pst*I, the appearance of multiple hybrid fragments in a Southern blot suggests a complex intervening sequence structure for the DHFR gene. Based on mapping information derived from overlapping double and single digests, as well as partial *Pst*I cleavage, the gene can be shown to contain five intervening sequences. A representative blotting experiment is shown in Fig. 4, containing comparative data for a cloned subline of L5178YR, the heterogeneous line, and human placenta. Definitive information awaits the characterization of cloned genomic DHFR fragments.

C. Dihydrofolate Reductase mRNA Processing

The evidence for processing of mRNA for DHFR derives from experiments in which RNA from the MTX-resistant L5178YR cell line was fractionated by agarose gel electrophoresis and then transferred to diazobenzoxymethylated paper (49). RNA species containing structural sequences for DHFR were screened by hybridization with a ^{32}P-labeled nick-translated cDNA probe (50). As Fig. 5 indicates, there appear to be at least nine distinct species present in the L5178YR MTX-resistant cell line. Most of these species are poladenylated, indicating that discrete cleavage occurs in the 5′-portion of the RNAs. Whether each of these species represents mature message, processing intermediates of mRNA, or degradation remains to be determined.

IV. Discussion

Gene amplification as a mechanism of resistance is not unique to MTX. Resistance of bacteria to chloramphenicol and penicillin occurs via an amplification of genes resident on episomal elements such as plasmids that confer the characteristic phenotype (51,52). Resistance of insects to malathion may also derive from a mechanism involving gene amplification (53). In mammalian cells, amplification of the gene coding for the multienzyme complex of carbamyl phosphate synthetase, asparate transcarbamylase, and dihydroorotase (CAD) has been observed in cell lines highly resistant to N-(phosphonacetyl)-L-aspartate (54). Although the mechanism of resistance has not been elucidated, an increase in enzyme activity has been observed to accompany an increase in resistance to several other drugs as well, i.e., hydroxyurea (ribonucleotide reductase) (55), pyrazofurin (orotidylate decarboxylase) (56), and methylornithine (ornithine decarboxylase) (57).

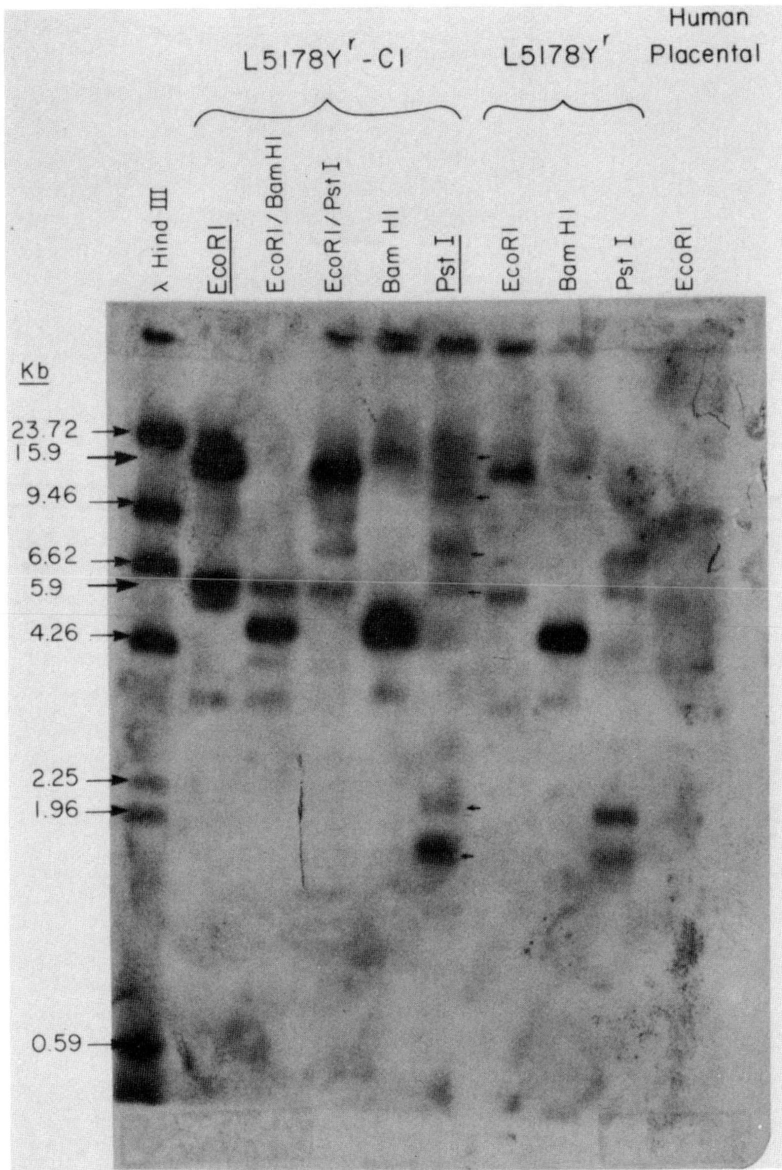

Fig. 4. Restriction cleavage of the DHFR gene from MTX-resistant L5178YR cells, as well as human placenta. DNA was cleaved with the indicated restriction endonucleases and electrophoresed in 0.8% agarose, and the resulting fragments were transferred to DBM-paper according to the procedure of Wahl *et al.* (40). Molecular-weight marker fragments were obtained by labeling *Hind*III-restricted phage lambda DNA with ^{32}P by a modified use of nick translation, catalyzed by the large fragment of DNA polymerase I (Klenow fragment) at 0°C. Following transfer, the filter was hybridized with a ^{32}P-labeled, cloned cDNA probe (pDHFR 21) derived from mouse DHFR mRNA (kindly provided by R. Schimke).

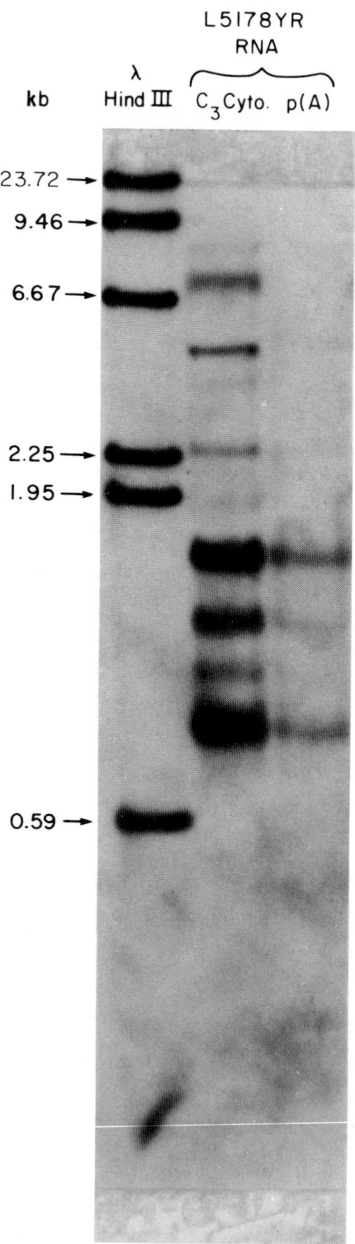

Fig. 5. Analysis of DHFR coding RNAs from a MTX-resistant L5178YR (3 subcloned). Cells were harvested at mid-log phase (5×10^5 cells/ml), and cytoplasmic RNA and poly(A)-containing RNA prepared as described previously (24). RNA was subject to electrophoresis through 1.5% agarose containing 5 m*M* methylmercury hydroxide, transferred to diazotized paper, and hybridized with ^{32}P-labeled nick-translated pDHFR 21 (49,50). RNA appeared undegraded as determined by the appearance of 28 and 18S rRNA upon ethidium bromide staining of gels.

Studies on the mechanisms of resistance to antifolates have provided fertile ground for gaining insights into fundamental cellular processes. It can be seen that the manner in which cells exhibit resistance to agents such as MTX reflects a complex range of events including transport, fluctuation in gene dosage, and gene sequence divergence. Historically, pharmacologists have had little difficulty in comprehending the resistance phenotype in terms of impaired drug transport. However, changes in gene dosage and in gene sequence divergence have led to a more startling view of storage and transfer of genetic information. The ability of certain drugs to select for cells with amplified gene sequences has led to a "revisionist" formulation for the organization of the eukaryotic gene. Dispensing with the previous dogma that genes coding for proteins are only present as single-copy sequences, one can now describe a stochastic process of gene dosage fluctuation which is obvious only under conditions providing selective pressure. Under normal circumstances, the net "flux" in such a system (i.e., the net change in gene dosage) is generally undetectable. This is a reflection of the fact that the frequency of these events is quite low. However, the drug exerts its effect by selecting for such rare events, driving the process to an apparent net positive flux. Clearly, the existence of ongoing gene dosage fluctuation within sensitive cell populations supports this view of drug resistance. The use of sophisticated fluorescence-activated cell-sorting techniques may make it possible to correlate the stages of drug resistance with corresponding enzyme fluctuations. That the system possesses the capacity to undergo a net negative flux in gene dosage is seen as a logical interpretation of the abundant data on reversion in unstable resistant cell lines. As a result, use of the term "fluctuation" is invoked to account for the reversibility in these cells. Drug resistance therefore has clearly provided a vehicle for studies leading to a novel depiction of gene and chromosome organization and function.

Acknowledgment

This work was supported by grants CA-08010 and CA-08341 from the USPHS.

References

1. J. R. Bertino, B. L. Hillcoat, and D. G. Johns, *Fed. Proc., Fed. Am. Soc. Exp. Biol.* **26,** 893 (1967).
2. D. Roberts and I. Wodinsky, *Cancer Res.* **28,** 1955 (1968).
3. J. Borsa and G. F. Whitmore, *Mol. Pharmacol.* **5,** 303 (1969).
4. J. Borsa and G. F. Whitmore, *Mol. Pharmacol.* **5,** 318 (1969).
5. S. Margolis, F. S. Phillips, and S. S. Sternberg, *Cancer Res.* **31,** 2037 (1971).
6. F. M. Sirotnak and R. C. Doorsbach, *Cancer Res.* **33,** 1290 (1973).
7. I. D., Goldman, *Cancer Chemother. Rep.* **7,** 51 (1975).

8. J. R. Bertino, W. L. Sawicki, A. R. Cashmore, E. C. Cadman, and R. T. Skeel, *Cancer Treat.* Rep. **61,** 667 (1977).
9. J. P. Perkins and J. R. Bertino, *Biochemistry* **5,** 1005 (1966).
10. F. Otting and F. M. Huennekens, *Arch. Biochem. Biophys.* **152,** 429 (1972).
11. B. A. Kamen, P. L. Takach, R. V. Vater, and J. D. Caston, *Anal. Biochem.* **20,** 54 (1976).
12. B. A. Kamen and J. R. Bertino, *Blood* **52,** 287 (1978).
13. L. E. Gunderson, R. B. Dunlap, F. Otting, and F. M. Huennekens, *Biochem.* **11,** 1018 (1972).
14. R. Hayman, R. McGready, and M. B. Vander Weyden, *Anal. Biochem.* **87,** 460 (1978).
15. J. R. Bertino, D. M. Donohue, B. Simmons, B. W. Gabrio, R. Silber, and F. M. Huennekens, *J. Clin. Invest.* **42,** 466 (1963).
16. J. R. Bertino, A. R. Cashmore, M. Fink, P. Calabrisi, and E. Lefkowitz, *Clin. Pharmacol. Ther.* **6,** 763 (1965).
17. B. L. Hillcoat, V. Swett, and J. R. Bertino, *Proc. Natl. Acad. Sci. U.S.A.* **58,** 1632 (1967).
18. G. A. Fischer, *Biochem. Pharmacol.* **7,** 75 (1961).
19. M. Friedkin, E. J. Crawford, S. R. Humphreys, and H. Goldin, *Cancer Res.* **22,** 600 (1962).
20. M. T. Hakala, S. F. Zakrezewski, and C. A. Nichol, *J. Biol. Chem.* **236,** 952 (1961).
21. J. W. Littlefield, *Proc. Natl. Acad. Sci. U.S.A.* **62,** 88 (1969).
22. J. P. Perkins, B. L. Hillcoat, and J. R. Bertino, *J. Biol. Chem.* **242,** 4771 (1967).
23. R. E. Kellems, V. B. Morhenn, E. A. Pfendt, F. W. Alt, and R. T. Schimke, *J. Biol. Chem.* **254,** 309 (1979).
24. B. J. Dolnick, R. J. Berenson, J. R. Bertino, R. J. Kaufman, J. H. Nunberg, and R. T. Schimke, *J. Cell Biol.* **83,** 394 (1979).
25. A. M. Albrecht, J. L. Biedler, and D. J. Hutchinson, *Cancer Res.* **32,** 1539 (1972).
26. G. Blumenthal and D. M. Greenberg, *Oncology* **24,** 223 (1970).
27. J. R. Bertino and R. T. Skeel, *in* "Pharmacological Basis of Cancer Chemotherapy," pp. 681–689. Williams & Wilkins, Baltimore, Maryland, 1975.
28. C. Lindquist, "Characterization of a New Murine Leukemia, L1210RR and Comparative Studies of Human Dihydrofolate Reductase Enzymes." Yale U. Sch. Med., PhD Thesis. 1979.
29. W. F. Flintoff, S. V. Davidson, and L. Siminovitch, *Somatic Cell Genet.* **2,** 245 (1976).
30. F. W. Alt, R. E. Kellems, J. R. Bertino, and R. T. Schimke, *J. Biol. Chem.* **251,** 3063 (1976).
31. R. E. Kellems, F. W. Alt, and R. J. Schimke, *J. Biol. Chem.* **251,** 6987 (1976).
32. F. W. Alt, R. E. Kellems, J. R. Bertino, and R. T. Schimke, *J. Biol. Chem.* **253,** 1357 (1978).
33. R. T. Schimke, R. J. Kaufman, F. W. Alt, and R. E. Kellems, *Science* **202,** 1051 (1978).
34. U. K. Hanggi and J. W. Littlefield, *J. Biol. Chem.* **251,** 3075 (1976).
35. J. H. Nunberg, R. J. Kaufman, R. T. Schimke, G. Urlaub, and L. A. Chasin, *Proc. Natl. Acad. Sci. U.S.A.* **75,** 5553 (1978).
35a. R. E. Kellems, V. B. Morhenn, E. A. Pfendt, F. W. Alt, and R. T. Schimke, *J. Biol. Chem.* **254,** 309 (1979).
36. R. J. Kaufman, J. R. Bertino, and R. T. Schimke, *J. Biol. Chem.* **253,** 5852 (1978).
37. G. R. Gapski, J. M. Whitely, J. I. Rader, P. L. Cramer, G. B. Henderson, V. Neef, and F. M. Huennekens, *J. Med. Chem.* **18,** 526 (1975).
38. J. L. Biedler and B. A. Spengler, *J. Cell Biol.* **70,** 2,Part 2, 117a (1976).
39. J. L. Biedler and B. A. Spengler, *Science* **191,** 185 (1976).
40. G. M. Wahl, R. A. Radgett, and G. R. Stark, *J. Biol. Chem.* **254,** 8679 (1979).
41. S. M. Tilghman, D. C. Tiemeier, J. G. Seidman, B. M. Peterlin, M. Sullivan, J. V. Maizel, and P. Leder, *Proc. Natl. Acad. Sci. U.S.A.* **75,** 725 (1978).
42. J. van den Berg, A. van Ooyen, N. Mantei, A. Schambock, G. Grosveld, R. A. Klavell, and C. Weissman, *Nature* (*London*) **276,** 37 (1978).
43. R. Breathnack, J. L. Mandel, and P. Chambon, *Nature* (*London*) **270,** 314 (1977).
44. R. Weinstock, R. Sweet, M. Weiss, H. Cedar, and R. Axel, *Proc. Natl. Acad. Sci. U.S.A.* **75,** 1299 (1978).

45. E. C. Lai, S. L. C. Woo, A. Dugaiczyk, J. F. Catterall, and B. W. O'Malley, *Proc. Natl. Acad. Sci. U.S.A.* **75,** 2205 (1978).
46. N. Hozumi and S. Tonegewa, *Proc. Natl. Acad. Sci. U.S.A.* **73,** 3628 (1976).
47. T. H. Rabbits and A. Forster, *Cell* **13,** 319 (1978).
48. F. H. C. Crick, *Science* **204,** *264 (1979).*
49. J. C. Alwine, D. J. Kemp, and G. R. Stark, *Proc. Natl. Acad. Sci. U.S.A.* **74,** 5350 (1977).
50. A. C. Y. Chang, J. H. Nunberg, R. J. Kaufman, H. A. Erlich, R. T. Schimke, and S. N. Cohen, *Nature (London)* **275,** 617 (1979).
51. D. Perlman and R. H. Rownd, *J. Bacteriol.* **123,** 1913 (1975).
52. S. Normark, T. Edlund, T. Grundstrom, S. Bergstrom, and H. W. Wolfwatz, *J. Bacteriol.* **132,** 912 (1977).
53. C. R. Walker and L. C. Terriere, *Entomol. Exp. Appl.* **13,** 264 (1970).
54. G. M. Wahl, R. A. Padgett, and G. R. Stark, *J. Biol. Chem.* **254,** 8679–8689 (1979).
55. W. H. Lewis, B. A. Kuzin, and J. A. Wright, *J. Cell Physiol.* **94,** 287 (1978).
56. D. P. Suttle and G. R. Stark, *J. Biol. Chem.* **254,** 4602 (1979).
57. P. S. Mamont, M. C. Duchesne, J. Grove, and C. Tardif, *Exp. Cell Res.* **115,** 387 (1978).

PART V

Radiation Sensitizers

19

Hypoxia-Dependent Radiation Sensitizers and Chemotherapeutic Agents

G. E. ADAMS and I. J. STRATFORD

I. Introduction

Hypoxic cells occur in most solid tumors in experimental animals and probably in most human tumors also. According to a model first proposed in 1955 by Thomlinson and Gray (1), they arise as a result of tumor growth essentially outstripping the blood supply.

Viable cells that line or are near to a microcapillary in a tumor are fairly well-oxygenated by the oxygen delivered to the tumor by the blood supply. Provided the oxygen tension suffices for the requirements of the cell, division

MOLECULAR ACTIONS AND TARGETS FOR CANCER CHEMOTHERAPEUTIC AGENTS

ISBN 0-12-619280-4

can occur. However, as one progresses away from the capillary beds, the oxygen tension decreases and eventually falls to a level below that required for cell viability. Cells that are sufficiently distant from a blood vessel eventually die, resulting in necrotic areas that are usually seen about 150–200 μm from the nearest capillary. Hypoxic cells are believed to occur in the interface region between the well-oxygenated tumor tissue and the necrotic areas.

In general, relative to oxygenated cells, hypoxic cells of all types are resistant to radiation, and it has long been thought that these hypoxic tumor cells may be an obstacle to successful local tumor control by radiation. In an untreated tumor, hypoxic cells would eventually die. However, if regression occurs either during or after radiation treatment, some of the hypoxic cells may reoxygenate, enter the cell cycle, and cause tumor regrowth.

The possibility that hypoxic cells may be relatively resistant to chemotherapy has received much less consideration. Hypoxic cells may influence drug action in several ways. Cells with a low oxygen status may reduce their rate of progression through the cell cycle or may be arrested altogether. They would be less sensitive, therefore, to cycle-specific drugs. Furthermore, since hypoxic cells are usually located some distance from the nearest blood vessel, drug accessibility may be a problem.

This article discusses some of the advances made in the development of drugs aimed at overcoming hypoxic cell radiation resistance in tumors and considers also the general question of whether hypoxic cells are a significant factor in the response of solid tumors to chemotherapy.

II. Hypoxic Cells in Radiotherapy

A. Radiation Resistance of Hypoxic Cells

The cellular response to radiation is usually an exponential function of dose, although cellular survival curves may show an initial shoulder region. In mammalian cells, the oxygen enhancement ratio (OER), defined as the slope ratio of the oxic and hypoxic survival curves, is usually about three. Relatively small amounts of oxygen are required to give a significant oxygen effect, and most normal tissues contain enough oxygen for radiation sensitivity to be at or near the maximum value. In tumors also, most of the cells will be sufficiently oxygenated to be radiation-sensitive. However, the consequence of an OER of three is that even a small proportion of hypoxic cells profoundly affects the overall tumor radiation sensitivity.

At low doses of radiation, the response of the more numerous oxic cells predominates. However, following a dose sufficient to kill all oxic cells, some of the original hypoxic cells will survive. In clinical practice, tumors are treated by multiple fractions of radiation rather than single doses, since experience has long since shown that such methods give better results. It is believed that this effect is due partly to the phenomenon of reoxygenation of hypoxic cells that can occur during treatment. Reoxygenation is probably one of the main reasons that some human tumors respond very well to radiation. Nevertheless, tumors can vary widely in their radiation sensitivity, and it is possible that those neoplasms that respond badly are the ones that reoxygenate very poorly, if at all, or do so over a time scale different from that of the treatment schedules usually given.

Several methods aimed at overcoming the hypoxia problem have been investigated clinically. Various trials have been carried out using unconventional fractionation regimens. While some of these studies have been empirical in design, any influence of radiation scheduling on the proportion of hypoxic cells could theoretically affect tumor radiation sensitivity.

Radiation treatment in high pressure oxygen chambers is another approach that has been under study for many years. The rationale here is that the concentration of free oxygen in the blood should increase and thereby extend the diffusion gradient of oxygen sufficiently to reoxygenate hypoxic cells. A few trials have shown some limited benefit, but practical problems limit the usefulness of this technique.

Part of the rationale behind a third approach, heavy particle radiotherapy (which includes neutrons), is that the oxygen effect decreases with increasing ionization density of the radiation. This decrease means that the adverse protective effect of tumor hypoxia is reduced. Trials are in progress and may show some benefit, but it remains true that this approach requires specialized, expensive hardware, and that, while the oxygen effect is reduced, it is not completely eliminated.

A fourth method, the use of drugs that specifically sensitize hypoxic cells to radiation, appears to be the preferred approach on the grounds of economy and simplicity. The development of such agents is briefly discussed in the next section.

B. Development of Hypoxic Cell Sensitizers

Radiobiological studies have shown that many chemical compounds are able to increase the radiation sensitivity of hypoxic cells of various types without affecting the radiation response of oxygenated cells. By far the largest group comprises the electron-affinic agents, so called because the efficiency of sensitization is related directly to the electron affinities or reduction potentials of the various compounds (2–5).

Early studies showed simple conjugate diketones and quinones, ketoesters, aromatic ketones, and various other structures containing conjugate electrophors to be active sensitizers in hypoxic bacteria (2) or bacterial spores (6, 7), but few of these compounds showed any activity in mammalian cells *in vitro*. However, substantial sensitizing activity was found with nitro-containing aromatic compounds, including paranitroacetophenone (PNAP) (8, 9) and its derivatives (10–12). Of particular significance at the time was the finding that some nitrofurans were also active sensitizers *in vitro* (13), since several of these compounds were already in clinical use as antibiotics. However, numerous *in vivo* studies with nitrofurans showed little sensitization, since the drugs are fairly toxic at the levels necessary for appreciable sensitization and generally do not possess favorable pharmacokinetic properties.

At present, only a small minority of known sensitizers show significant sensitization *in vivo,* mainly because of the difficulties in penetration into the regions of tumors where hypoxic cells occur. A series of compounds, the substituted nitroimidazoles, seem suitable in this respect. In 1973, it was reported that the 5-nitroimidazole, metronidazole or Flagyl, was able to sensitize both hypoxic bacterial and mammalian cells (13, 14). Numerous studies have shown significant sensitization by metronidazole of the response of various mouse tumors to radiation (15). Furthermore, some clinical evidence exists for sensitizing activity in human glioblastomas (16).

C. Misonidazole

Successful demonstration of *in vivo* sensitization by metronidazole led to the search for more active compounds in the nitroimidazole series. Electron affinity considerations led naturally to investigations of 2-nitroimidazoles. With these compounds, the greater interaction of the 2-nitro group with the electron system of the ring should lead to enhanced activity; this was demonstrated with a series of compounds in studies *in vitro* (17). One such compound, Ro-07-0582 or misonidazole (Fig. 1), has been found to be an efficient sensitizer in various radiation studies both *in vitro* and in experimental tumor systems of various kinds.

Figure 2 illustrates the sensitizing action of misonidazole in Chinese hamster cells irradiated *in vitro* (5). In oxygen, misonidazole shows no sensitization, whereas in the absence of oxygen, sensitization is marked, and at 10 m*M*, the enhancement ratio is near to that of oxygen.

Numerous studies have been reported on sensitization of experimental tumors in mice by misonidazole using clonogenic cell assay and lung colony assay, with regrowth delay and tumor cure as endpoints (see refs (15) and (18) for collected data). As an example, Fig. 3 shows typical results of radiation sensitization by misonidazole, using tumor cure as the endpoint (19).

Large sensitization factors (defined as the ratios of TCD_{50}, the radiation doses required for 50% tumor control) are observed, even for relatively low drug doses. Although large enhancement ratios are usually observed in tumors of various

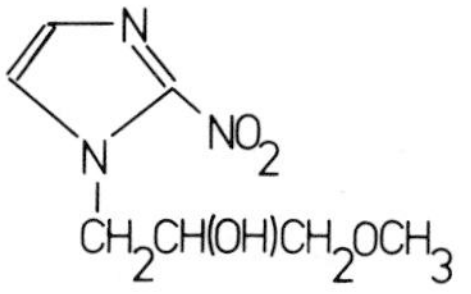

N
N NO_2
$CH_2CH(OH)CH_2OCH_3$

Fig. 1. Structure of misonidazole.

types irradiated with *single* radiation doses, lower values are often found when the radiation is given in multiple small fractions. These lower values almost certainly reflect the influence of reoxygenation, which reduces hypoxic cell fractions (20).

Clinical studies with misonidazole, including prospective randomized controlled trials, are in progress in several countries. In general, drug tolerance is fairly good, as is tumor penetration in most cases (21–23). However, drug dosage is limited to levels below those required for maximum sensitization by

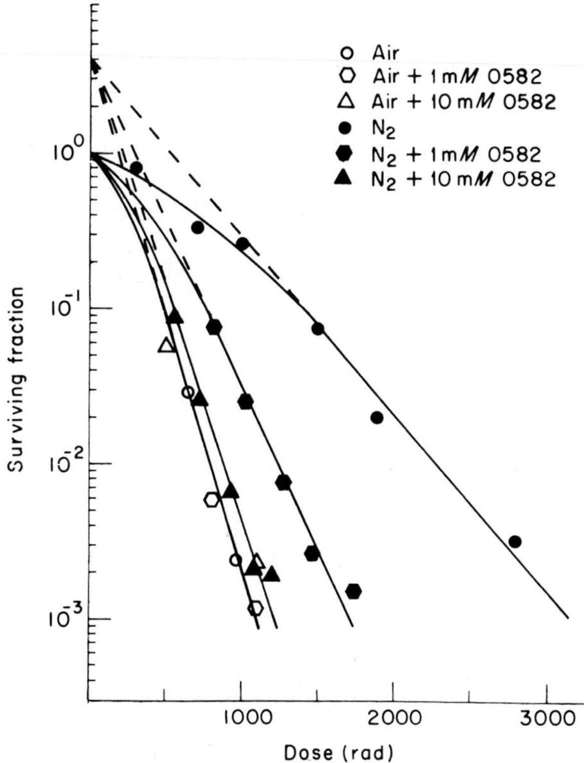

Fig. 2. Dose ln-survival curves showing radiation sensitization of hypoxic Chinese hamster cells by misonidazole (5).

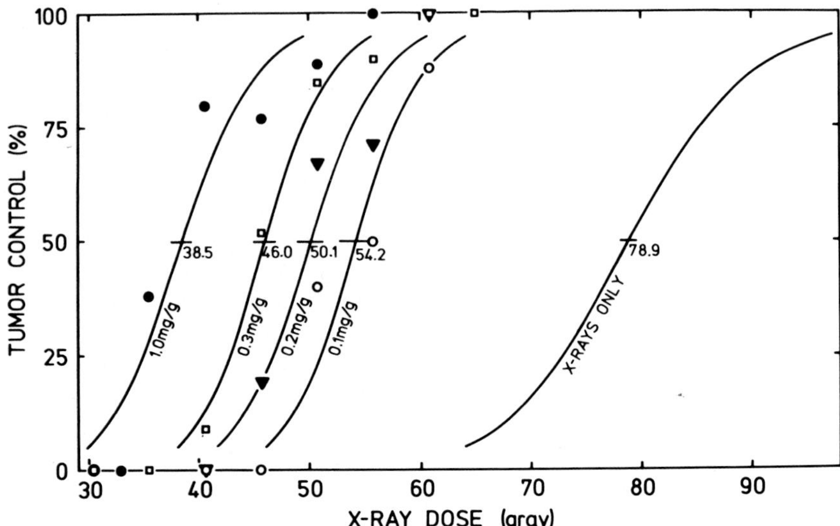

Fig. 3. Radiation sensitization of mouse MT tumors by misonidazole. ●, 1 mg/g; □, 0.3 mg/g; ▼, 0.2 mg/g; ○, 0.1 mg/g. [redrawn (19)].

peripheral neurotoxicity. At present, it is recommended (21) that the maximum *total* dose should not exceed 12 g/m^2. Since the dose given will clearly depend on the total number of fractions given, choice of fractionation regimens is important in clinical trials. Not surprisingly, options are being kept open, and the drug is being investigated with a range of fractionation regimens (8, 24).

D. The Search for More Active Radiosensitizers

The toxicity limitations of misonidazole have stimulated the search for new drugs. The most important factor influencing sensitizing efficiency is the "electron affinity." Relative electron affinities are closely related to relative one-electron reduction potentials, which can be determined under equilibrium conditions by pulse radiolysis techniques (5, and earlier references quoted therein). Figure 4 shows data for mammalian cells, indicating the relationship between reversible one-electron reduction potential and sensitization efficiency, defined as the concentration required for a fixed degree of sensitization (enhancement ratio of 1.6). The relationship appears to hold over a wide range of sensitizing efficiencies and includes compounds that are more efficient than misonidazole.

The electron affinity correlation has helped considerably in identifying new sensitizing compounds. However, structure–activity relationships derived from studies of this type will be considerably more valuable in developing new clinical agents when more information is available on the structural, chemical, and

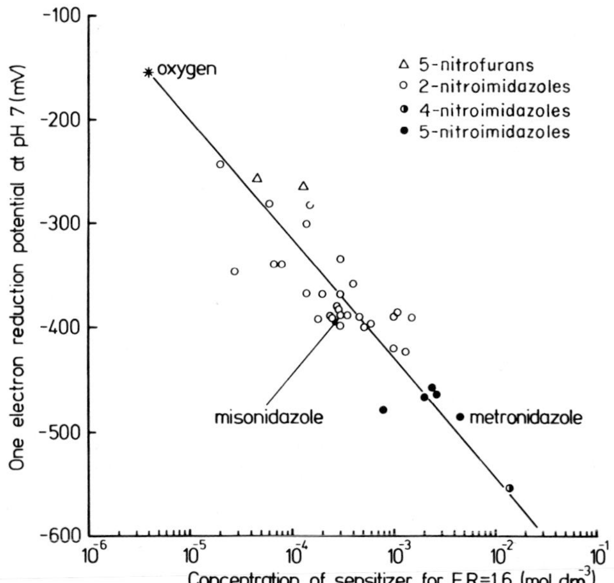

Fig. 4. Correlation of sensitizing efficiency [concentration required for enhancement ratio of 1.6 ($C_{1.6}$)] with one-electron reduction potential (5, 64).

physical factors that relate to the unwanted neurotoxic properties. Much current effort is devoted to experimental investigations in this area (24).

Although redox potential is clearly an important or perhaps the major influence on sensitization efficiency, other factors can contribute. Some results have been published recently on the sensitizing properties in vitro of a variety of 2-nitroimidazoles of the type shown in Fig. 5, where *n* ranges from 1 to 11 and *X* is a nitrogenous base (25). When *X* = morpholine, compounds of varying *n* showed a fairly constant one-electron reduction potential (−379 mV to −403 mV). However, the sensitizing efficiencies ($C_{1.6}$) ranged from $1.5 \times 10^{-3} M$ to $0.05 \times 10^{-3} M$, showing a maximum efficiency (minimum $C_{1.6}$) for the C_4 and C_5 compounds. In contrast, the cytotoxicities against aerobic cells increased progressively as *n* increased.

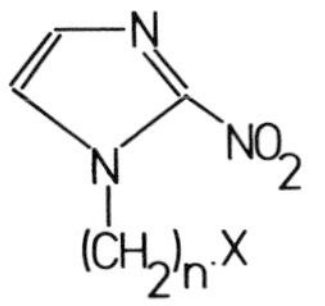

N
NO_2
N
$(CH_2)_n \cdot X$

Fig. 5. Structure of a series of 2-nitroimidazoles substituted at N1; *n* is the number of methylene groups in the side-chain and *X* the terminating group.

The ratio of the toxicity to sensitizing efficiency is a measure of "sensitizer effectiveness," and is a term analogous to the therapeutic ratio concept applicable *in vivo*. Figure 6A shows the "effectiveness" as a function of *n*. The apparently smooth parabola shows that the effectiveness varies overall by a factor of about 20 and shows a maximum for $n = 5$. Although the compounds show variation in partition coefficient and pKa, these variations are not responsible for the shape of the curve in Fig. 6A. Further results that differ only in the nature of the basic function *X* have been obtained for some other nitroimidazoles, including five piperidino compounds with *n* values of 2,3,4,6, and 8, and three pyrrolidino derivatives with *n* values of 2,4, and 8. Sensitizer "effectiveness" data obtained from measurements of sensitizing efficiencies ($C_{1.6}$) and aerobic toxicities are shown in Fig. 6B. Both types of compound show the same chain length/effectiveness-dependence as the morpholino compounds. Interestingly,

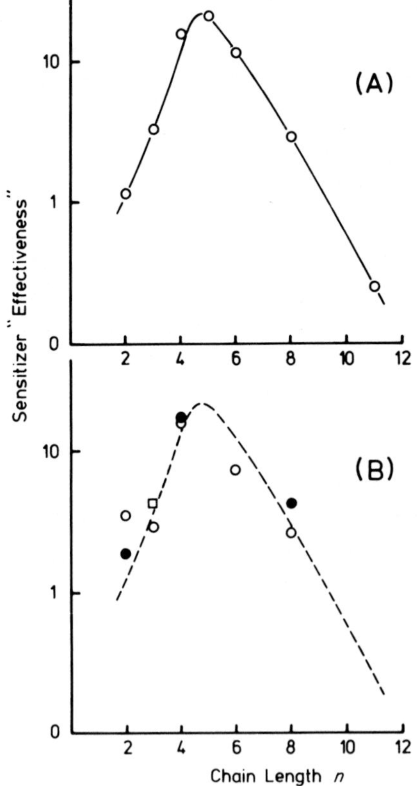

Fig. 6. Sensitizer effectiveness as a function of chain length *n*. *A*, morpholine series; *B*, piperidine series, ○; pyrrolidine series, ●; misonidazole, □. dotted line taken from Fig. 6A (25)

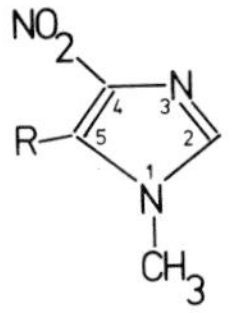

Fig. 7. General structure of 5-substituted-4-nitroimidazoles.

data for misonidazole, which has a 3-carbon side-chain, also falls on the plot. This marked dependence of sensitizer effectiveness on side-chain structure indicates that factors in addition to electron affinity can affect sensitization. However, it remains to be seen whether such factors are relevant in the design of drugs with better therapeutic ratio *in vivo*.

Some other compounds of particular interest are the 5-substituted 4-nitroimidazoles, a structural group that again illustrates the influence in some cases of factors other than redox potential in radiosensitization. Usually, 4- or 5-nitroimidazoles are much less efficient as sensitizers than are 2-nitroimidazoles, owing to the generally lower electron affinities. However, there is a group of 4-nitroimidazoles that shows unexpectedly high efficiencies; these are compounds containing sulfonamide or sulfonate groups in the 5-position (Fig. 7). The electrophilic groups in this position increase the electron affinities of the compounds, as would be expected. However, the sensitizing efficiencies are much greater than would be predicted on the basis of the electron affinity correlation. Previously, an abnormal sensitization efficiency had been observed for a related 4-nitroimidazole, 5-chloro-1-methyl-4-nitroimidazole (26). Figure 8 shows a plot of the enhancement ratios for Chinese hamster cells irradiated in the presence of the compound NSC 38087 (25). The sensitizing

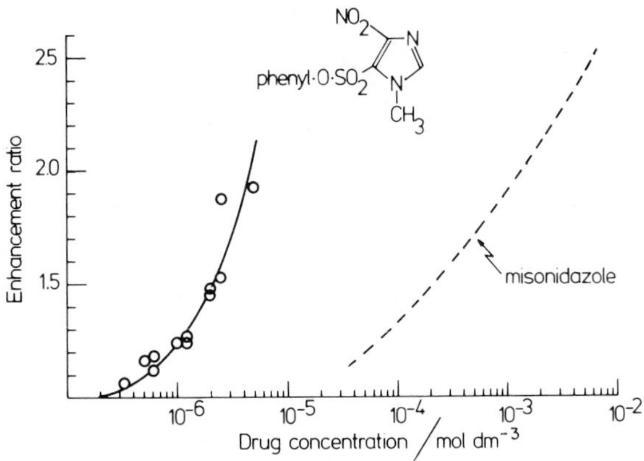

Fig. 8 Dependence of enhancement ratio for hypoxic Chinese hamster cells irradiated in the presence of various concentrations of NSC 38087 (27).

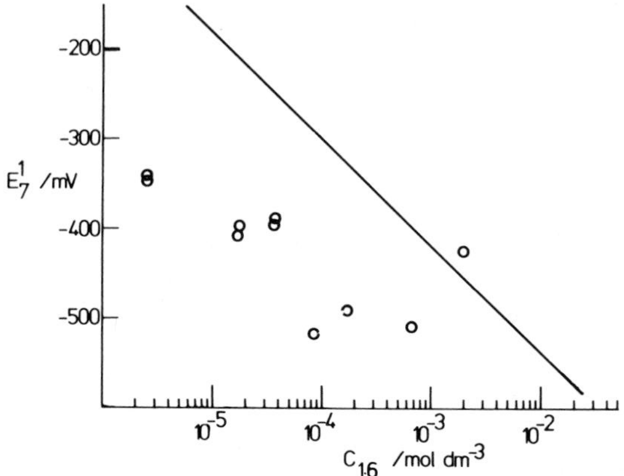

Fig. 9. Variation of sensitizing efficiency for some 5-substituted-4-nitroimidazoles with one-electron reduction potential (solid line taken from Fig. 4) (7).

efficiency of this compound is comparable to that of oxygen and is one of the highest yet observed for mammalian cells in vitro. The dashed line in the figure shows the concentration dependence of enhancement ratios for misonidazole in the same mammalian cell line. Clearly, the sensitization efficiency of NSC 38087 is about 100 times greater than that of misonidazole, even though the slightly higher reduction potential of the compound (−342 mV, compared to −385 mV for misonidazole) would predict only a small increase in sensitizer efficiency.

Studies with other 4-nitroimidazoles containing electron-withdrawing sulfur-containing groups in the 5-position have shown unusually high sensitizing efficiencies, and Fig. 9 shows values of sensitizing efficiency ($C_{1.6}$) plotted as a function of one-electron reduction potential for a number of such compounds (27). The data show that generally, as electron affinity increases, sensitization efficiency increases. However, with one exception, the data points lie well to the left of the line correlating reduction potential with sensitizing efficiency (taken from Fig. 4). The reasons for this enhanced activity are not known and it whether compounds of this type will be clinically useful remains to be seen.

III. Hypoxic Cells in Chemotherapy

A. Hypoxic Cell Resistance

As mentioned earlier, there are sound theoretical reasons for anticipating that hypoxic tumor cells might be relatively resistant to some chemotherapeutic agents. Indeed, there is some supporting evidence from studies in which cells are exposed to various drugs in vitro. Exponentially growing cells in culture that are rendered chronically hypoxic show more resistance than do proliferating aerobic cells to bleomycin (28), actinomycin D (29), arabinosylcytosine, 5-fluorouracil, and vincristine (30). Further, adriamycin, a drug commonly used in the treatment of solid neoplasms, has been shown to be less effective when killing cells in EMT6 spheroids than with monolayer cells in exponential or plateau phase growth (31). One reason for this difference was that only the peripheral cells of the spheroids took up cytotoxic concentrations of the drug. Also, cells from dissociated spheroids took up more drug than did those from intact spheroids, which is further indication of the existence of a diffusion barrier. In these studies, it was shown that the innermost cells of the spheroids were the most drug-resistant. It was concluded, therefore, that this resistance was not due to differences in the cell cycle state, since it was found that cells in both exponential and plateau phase monolayers were about equally sensitive when the surviving fraction was plotted against *absorbed* drug concentrations. Hence, other factors related to the metabolic state of the cells or to the microenvironment were believed to be involved (31).

Other studies (30) have shown directly that prolonged exposure to hypoxia alone can produce resistance to adriamycin in Chinese hamster cells (Fig. 10). The resistance is dependent upon the time the cells are maintained under hypoxic

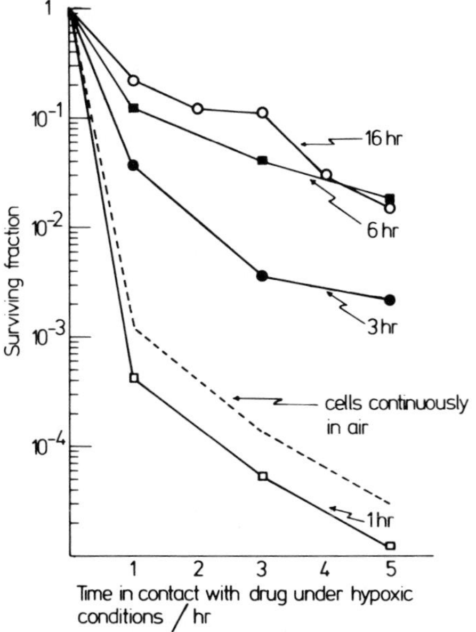

Fig. 10. Effect of time in hypoxia 1, 3, 6, and 16 hours prior to exposure of exponentially growing mammalian cells to 5 μg/ml adriamycin (30).

conditions; further, when chronically hypoxic cells are reoxygenated, these cells retain the resistance for a period exceeding the generation time of the cells.

Such evidence indicates the need to identify drugs that can be used in combination therapy and will preferentially destroy hypoxic cells. The remainder of this article discusses the cytotoxic effects of some compounds that may satisfy these criteria.

B. Drugs Preferentially Cytotoxic to Hypoxic Cells

In 1972, Tannock and co-workers (32) attempted to sterilize selectively the hypoxic cells in a C3H mouse mammary carcinoma, using the alkylating agent triethylene melamine. The aim of this approach was to exploit the biochemical status of the hypoxic cell, which is dependent on anaerobic glycolysis as a source of energy; the production of lactic acid under these conditions probably leads to a low pH in the immediate environment of these cells. Triethylene melamine was chosen because it was thought to be more active at an acidic pH. However, no selective killing of hypoxic cells could be demonstrated.

The fact that hypoxic cells depend mainly on glucose and glycolysis as an energy source was subsequently exploited in studies showing that 5-thio-D-glucose was preferentially toxic towards hypoxic cells in vitro (33–35). This compound is a competitive inhibitor of the active transport of D-glucose and interferes with the formation of D-glucose-6-phosphate in glycolysis. The toxic action of this analog was enhanced by hyperthermia (35), and recent studies in vivo have shown that tumors treated with radiation, heat (41°C for 2 hours), and 5-thio-D-glucose, respond significantly better than those tumors given only radiation and heat (36).

A significant development was the hypothesis, put forward by Sartorelli and colleagues in 1972 (37), that hypoxia might be exploited by developing chemotherapeutic agents that become cytotoxic after reductive activation. At present, there are two broad classes of compound that satisfy this criterion. The first group includes quinone bioreductive alkylating agents, e.g., mitomycin C. It is believed that these compounds are activated under hypoxia to form a quinone methide intermediate that can alkylate DNA. The second group includes some nitroaromatic and nitroheterocyclic hypoxic cell radiosensitizers that demonstrate selective hypoxic cell toxicity.

C. The Cytotoxicity of Nitro Compounds

Using the in vitro spheroid system, Sutherland (38) noted that metronidazole was more toxic to hypoxic cells than to aerobic cells. Preferential toxicity to hypoxic cells was also found for a range of other nitroheterocyclic radiosensitizers (39–44). The difference in toxicity of misonidazole to hypoxic and aerobic cells is shown in Fig. 11. Under hypoxic conditions, 5 m*M* misonidazole reduces survival to 10^{-3} in 5 hours, whereas aerobic cells are not reduced to this level of survival until after 4 days of exposure to 5 m*M* misonizadole. The hypoxic cell cytotoxicity of misonidazole and other nitro-containing radiosensitizers has been determined with regard to drug concentration and incubation time (41–44), oxygen concentration (41,45), temperature (42,46), cell age distribution (47,48), and cell type (41,49).

The efficiency of these compounds as cytotoxic agents has been correlated with electron affinity (44), with those compounds of highest electron affinity producing the greatest toxicity. This effect is similar to the dependence of radiosensitization efficiency on electron affinity, but it does not necessarily imply that the mechanisms for sensitization and toxicity are similar. Indeed, there is good evidence that they are different. Toxicity varies from cell line to cell line and is dependent on temperature and on the presence of different additives in the medium, including serum (50) and ascorbic acid (51,52). In contrast, sensitization efficiency in vitro shows little or no dependence on the cell line employed, the temperature, or in most cases the nature of the irradiation medium.

The dependence of cytotoxicity on the redox properties of the nitro compounds is indicative of the involvement of reductive reactions in the toxic process (44).

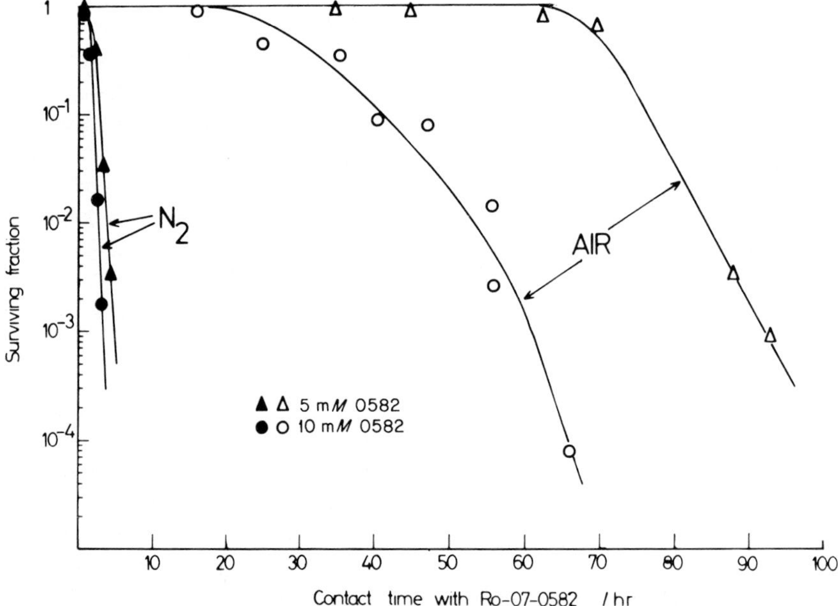

Fig. 11. Cytotoxicity of misonidazole (Ro-07-0582) to oxic and hypoxic Chinese hamster cells at 37°C.

Vitamin C and hyperthermia both increase the toxic effect of misonidazole, probably by increasing the rate and/or the extent of reduction. It would follow, therefore, that the potentiating action of heat or vitamin C on the toxicity of nitro compounds should be dependent on their electron affinities, with those of lowest affinity being most affected. This premise was confirmed by comparing the effects of hyperthermia and vitamin C on the cytotoxicity of metronidazole, misonidazole, and nitrofurantoin (53,54).

There is now good evidence to suggest that the toxicity of misonidazole to hypoxic cells is a consequence of the reductive metabolism of the drug (55,56). Products found, after incubation of misonidazole, with dense cell suspensions under hypoxic conditions are identical to those formed by chemical reduction of the drug (55), and the amine derivative of misonidazole has been determined as a metabolic product in man (57). Wong *et al.* (56) observed that the products of chemical reduction of misonidazole were toxic to both hypoxic and aerobic cells. These observations lead to the attractive hypothesis that a toxin formed in the hypoxic regions in tumors can not only kill hypoxic cells but may also kill neighboring oxic tumor cells if it is diffusible. The requirement of tumor hypoxia for generation of the cytotoxic effect would be a rare example of tumor specificity. Evidence of support of this hypothesis has come from the work of Brown (58) and of Sutherland and co-workers (59). The latter authors used EMT6 spheroids and EMT6 tumors to examine the cytotoxic effects of the nitroimidazoles misonidazole, Ro-05-9963, and SR2508. For each sensitizer, they found that under appropriate conditions, the number of clonogenic cells could be reduced by up to 50% in the spheroids and 90% in the tumors. Interestingly, the same authors noted that in spite of the degree of cell kill, little change was seen in the growth rate of the tumors. This lack of change was attributed to rapid repopulation and increased growth fraction after cytotoxic treatment (59). It is likely that for the cytotoxic effects of these compounds to be expressed fully in vivo, they would have to be used in combination with agents that are more effective against *proliferating* aerobic cells.

The use of nitroaromatic compounds in combination with other chemotherapeutic agents has been examined *in vivo* by a number of groups (60–62). The cytotoxic action of cyclophosphamide, melphalan, a *cis*-platinum(II) complex, and 5-fluorouracil were all found to be potentiated by misonidazole. Data from Rose *et al.* (61) are shown in Fig. 12. In this experiment, mice bearing the Lewis lung carcinoma were treated with misonidazole 30 minutes prior to exposure to varying concentrations of melphalan. Twenty four hours after this treatment, animals were sacrificed and survival of tumor cells assayed in vitro. Misonidazole alone had no apparent effect on the number of clonogenic cells per tumor; however, in combination with melphalan, there was a marked enhancement of tumor cell kill with a dose modification factor of 2.0. Some *in vitro* data that are relevant to these results have been obtained (63).

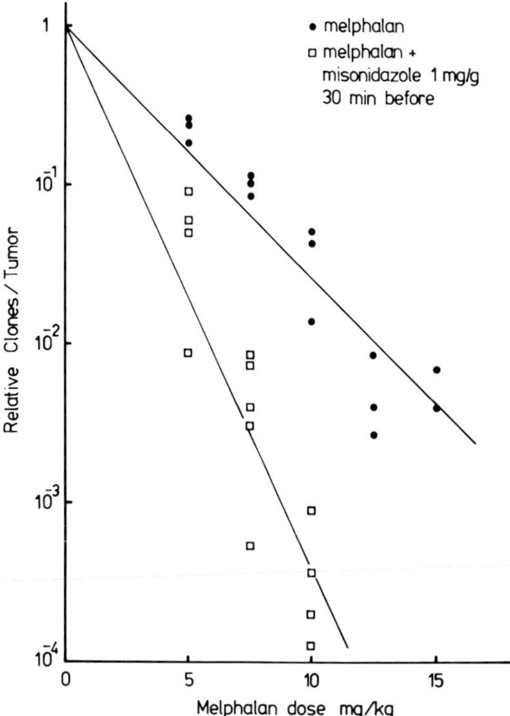

Fig. 12. Dose-survival curves for Lewis lung carcinoma treated with melphalan alone or with melphalan and 1 mg/g misonidazole (61).

Figure 13 shows a survival curve for hypoxic Chinese hamster cells exposed to 5 m*M* misonidazole (1 mg/milliliter). After an initial lag period, survival decreases exponentially with time. The pre-exponential portion of the survival curve may be due to the buildup of some toxic metabolite of misonidazole and/or the accumulation of sublethal damage. Experiments have been carried out in which cells were exposed to misonidazole for a time sufficient to bring cells just off the shoulder of the survival curve. The cells were then treated with varying concentrations of other chemotherapeutic agents.

Data for cells pretreated with misonidazole under hypoxic conditions, then exposed to melphalan in air, are given in Fig. 14. The surviving fraction of the cells pretreated with misonidazole was 0.4, but when these pretreated cells were exposed to melphalan, they were considerably more sensitive than cells exposed to melphalan without misonidazole pretreatment. The cytotoxic action of mustine and cis-dichlorodiammine platinum (II) on aerobic cells is also potentiated if the cells are pretreated with misonidazole under hypoxic conditions. No potentiation is observed if the pretreatment is carried out in aerobic cultures. In addition,

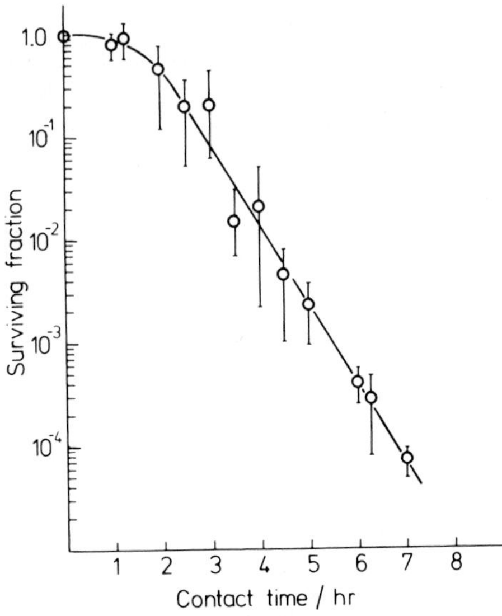

Fig. 13. Toxicity of 5 m*M* misonidazole to hypoxic Chinese hamster cells. Results taken from 15 separate experiments. Error bars indicate standard deviations (63).

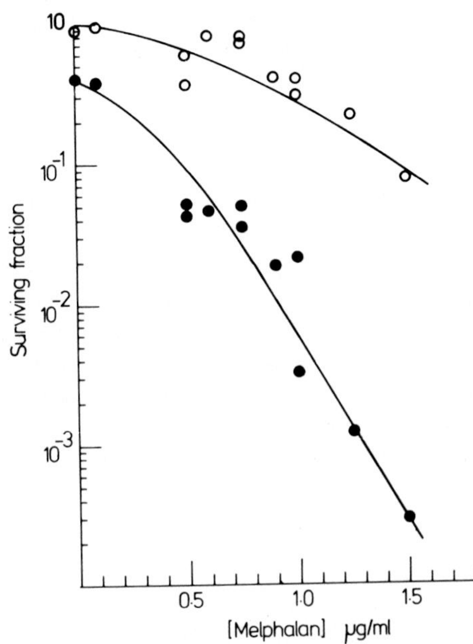

Fig. 14. Effect of pretreating hypoxic Chinese hamster cells with 5 m*M* (1 mg/g) misonidazole for 2 hr at 37°C on their responses to melphalan. Cells were reoxygenated and exposed to melphalan for 1 hr. ○, melphalan alone; ●, misonidazole pretreated (63).

some of the cytotoxic effects of hyperthermia and radiation can also be potentiated by this pretreatment (63).

In summary, both in vitro and in vivo results suggest that under hypoxic conditions, misonidazole causes additional damage that is expressed only when the cells are exposed to another agent. The mechanism involved in this effect is unknown and clearly requires much further work. However, the fact that the action of one drug can be potentiated by another agent in a mechanism that requires a physiological property of a tumor (hypoxia) for its expression is an attractive prospect in chemotherapy. Whether this prospect can be realized with misonidazole or related but less toxic drugs remains to be seen.

References

1. R. H. Thomlinson and L. H. Gray, *Br. J. Cancer* **9,** 539 (1955).
2. G. E. Adams and M. S. Cooke, *Int. J. Radiat. Biol.* **15,** 457 (1969).
3. J. A. Raleigh, J. D. Chapman, J. Borsa, S. W. Kremer, and A. P. Reuvers, *Int. J. Radiat. Biol.* **23,** 377 (1977).
4. M. Simic and E. L. Powers, *Int. J. Radiat. Biol.* **26,** 87 (1974).
5. G. E. Adams, I. R. Flockhart, C. E. Smithen, I. J. Stratford, P. Wardman, and M. E. Watts, *Radiat. Res.* **67,** 9 (1976).
6. A. Tallentire, N. L. Schiller, and E. L. Powers, *Int. J. Radiat. Biol.* **14,** 397 (1968).
7. A. Tallentire, A. B. Jones, and G. P. Jacobs, *Isr. J. Chem.* **10,** 1185 (1972).
8. J. D. Chapman, R. G. Webb, and J. Borsa, *Int. J. Radiat. Biol.* **19,** 561 (1971).
9. G. E. Adams, J. C. Asquith, D. L. Dewey, J. L. Foster, B. D. Michael, and R. L. Willson, *Int. J. Radiat. Biol.* **19,** 575 (1971).
10. J. D. Chapman, J. A. Raleigh, J. Borsa, R. G. Webb, and R. Whitehouse, *Int. J. Radiat. Biol.* **21,** 475 (1972).
11. G. E. Adams, J. C. Asquith, M. E. Watts, and C. E. Smithen, *Nature (London)* **239,** 23 (1972).
12. G. F. Whitmore, S. Gulyas, and A. J. Varghese, *Radiat. Res.* **61,** 325 (1974).
13. J. D. Chapman, A. P. Reuvers, J. Borsa, A. Petkau, and D. R. McCalla, *Cancer Res.* **32,** 2616 (1972).
14. J. L. Foster and R. L. Willson, *Br. J. Radiol.* **6,** 234 (1973).
15. J. F. Fowler and J. D. Denekamp, *Pharmacol. 8 Ther., Part C* **7.**
16. R. C. Urtasun, J. D. Chapman, M. C. Feldstein, R. P. Band, H. R. Rabin, A. F. Wilson, B. Marynowski, E. Starreveld, and T. Shnitha, *Br. J. Cancer* **37,** Suppl.III, 271 (1978).
17. J. C. Asquith, G. E. Adams, M. E. Watts, K. Patel, C. E. Smithen, and *Radiat. Res.* **60,** 108 (1974).
18. Collected papers, *in* "Hypoxic Cell Sensitizers in Radiobiology and Radiotherapy" (G. E. Adams, J. F. Fowler and P. Wardman, eds.), *Br. J. Cancer* **37,** Suppl.III (1978).
19. P. W. Sheldon and S. A. Hill, *Br. J. Cancer* **35,** 795 (1977).
20. P. W. Sheldon and J. F. Fowler, *Br. J. Cancer* **37,** Suppl.III, 242 (1978).
21. S. Dische, M. I. Saunders, M. E. Lee, G. E. Adams, and I. R. Flockhart, *Br. J. Cancer* **35,** 567 (1977).
22. D. V. Ash, M. R. Smith, and R. D. Bugden, *Br. J. Cancer* **39,** 503 (1979).
23. T. H. Wassermann, T. L. Phillips, R. J. Johnson, C. J. Gomer, G. A. Lawrence, W. Sadee, R. A. Marques, V. A. Levin, and G. Van Raalt, *Int. J. Radiat. Oncol. Biol. Phys.* **5,** 775 (1979).
24. Collected papers, *in* "Proceedings of Conference on Combined Modality Cancer Treatment: Radiosensitizers and Radioprotectors" (L. W. Brady, ed.), Masson, New York, in press.

25. G. E. Adams, I. A. Ahmed, E. M. Fielden, P. O'Neill, and I. J. Stratford and C. Williamson, *Cancer Clin. Trials* **3,** 37 (in press).
26. M. E. Watts and R. S. Jacobs, *Br. J. Cancer* **37,** Suppl. III, 80 (1978).
27. G. E. Adams, E. M. Fielden, B. C. Millar, P. O'Neill, I. J. Stratford, and C. Williamson, *Int. J. Radiat. Biol.* (in press).
28. L. Roizin-Towle and E. J. Hall, *Br. J. Cancer* **37,** 254 (1978).
29. G. E. Adams, K. B. Dawson, and I. J. Stratford, *in* "Proceedings of the International Meeting for Radio-Oncology" (K. H. Kärcher, H. D. Kogelnik, and K. Meyer, eds.). Thieme, Stuttgart, 1980.
30. E. Smith, I. J. Stratford, and G. E. Adams, *Br. J. Cancer* **40,** 316 (1979).
31. R. M. Sutherland, H. A. Eddy, B. Bareham, K. Reich, and D. Vanantwerp, *Int. J. Radiat. Oncol. Biol. Phys.* **5,** 1225 (1979).
32. I. F. Tannock, N. Marshall, and L. M. Van Putten, *Eur. J. Cancer* **8,** 501 (1972).
33. C. W. Song, J. J. Clement, and S. H. Levitt, *J. Natl. Cancer Inst.* **57,** 603 (1976).
34. C. W. Song, J. J. Clement, and S. H. Levitt, *Cancer Res.* **38,** 4499 (1978).
35. S. H. Kim, J. H. Kim, and E. W. Hahn, *Cancer Res.* **38,** 2935 (1978).
36. C. W. Song and S. H. Levitt, *Cancer Clin. Trials* (in press).
37. A. J. Lin, L. A. Cosby, C. W. Shansky, and A. C. Sartorelli, *J. Med. Chem.* **15,** 1247 (1972).
38. R. M. Sutherland, *Cancer Res.* **34,** 3501 (1974).
39. E. J. Hall and L. Roizin-Towle, *Radiology* **117,** 453 (1975).
40. B. A. Moore, B. Palcic, and L. D. Skarsgard, *Radiat. Res.* **67,** 459 (1976).
41. J. K. Mohindra and A. M. Rauth, *Cancer Res.* **36,** 930 (1976).
42. I. J. Stratford and G. E. Adams, *Br. J. Cancer* **35,** 307 (1977).
43. I. J. Stratford, M. E. Watts, and G. E. Adams, *in* "Cancer Therapy by Hyperthermia and Radiation" (C. Streffer, ed.), p. 267. Urban & Schwarzenberg, Munich, 1978.
44. G. E. Adams, I. J. Stratford, R. G. Wallace, P. Wardman, and M. E. Watts, *J. Natl. Cancer Inst.* **64,** 555 (1980).
45. I. J. Stratford, *Br. J. Cancer* **38,** 130 (1978).
46. E. J. Hall, M. Astor, C. Geard, and J. Biaglow, *Br. J. Cancer* **35,** 809 (1977).
47. E. J. Hall and J. Biaglow, *Int. J. Radiat. Oncol. Biol. Phys.* **2,** 521 (1977).
48. G. F. Whitmore and S. Gulyas, *Cancer Clin. Trials* (in press).
49. Y. C. Taylor and A. M. Rauth, *Cancer Res.* **38,** 2745 (1978).
50. I. J. Stratford and P. Gray, *Br. J. Cancer* **37,** Suppl.III 129 (1978).
51. P. D. Josephy, B. Palcic, and L. D. Skarsgard, *Nature (London)* **271,** 370 (1978).
52. C. J. Koch, R. L. Howell, and J. E. Biaglow, *Br. J. Cancer* **39,** 321 (1979).
53. M. R. Horsman, I. J. Stratford, and G. E. Adams, unpublished observations.
54. S. Rajaratnam, C. Clarke, I. J. Stratford, and G. E. Adams, unpublished observations.
55. A. J. Varghese, S. Gulyas, and J. K. Mohindra, *Cancer Res.* **36,** 3761 (1976).
56. T. W. Wong, G. F. Whitmore, and S. Gulyas, *Radiat. Res.* **75,** 541 (1978).
57. I. R. Flockhart, P. Large, D. Troup, S. L. Malcolm, and T. R. Marten, *Xenobiotica* **8,** 97 (1978).
58. J. M. Brown, *Radiat. Res.* **72,** 469 (1977).
59. R. M. Sutherland, B. J. Bareham, and K. A. Reich, *Cancer Clin. Trials* (in press).
60. I. F. Tannock, *Br. J. Cancer* (in press).
61. C. M. Rose, J. L. Millar, J. H. Peacock, T. A. Phelps, and T. C. Stephens, *Cancer Clin. Trials* (in press).
62. I. Wodinsky, R. K. Johnson, and J. J. Clement, *Proc. Am. Assoc. Cancer Res.* **20,** 230 (1979).
63. I. J. Stratford, G. E. Adams, M. R. Horsman, S. Kandayia, S. Rajaratnam, E. Smith, and C. Williamson, *Cancer Clin. Trials* **3,** 231.
64. G. E. Adams, E. D. Clarke, I. R. Flockhart, R. S. Jacobs, D. S. Sehmi, I. J. Stratford, P. Wardman, and M. E. Watts, *Int. J. Radiat. Biol.* **35,** 133 (1979).

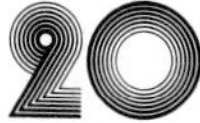

Mechanistic and Pharmacological Considerations in the Design and Use of Hypoxic Cell Radiosensitizers

J. D. CHAPMAN, J. NGAN-LEE, AND B. E. MEEKER

I. Introduction

Ionizing radiation is used in the treatment of almost 50% of the cancers diagnosed in North America. In fact, radiation is the treatment modality of choice for several cancers, including carcinoma of the cervix where, when properly applied, it can yield an overall cure rate of 62% (1). A study by Bush *et al.* (1) also showed that anemia (hemoglobin levels of <12 gm %) at the time of treatment was associated with a significantly higher rate of local recurrence in patients with advanced disease. This observation is consistent with the thesis that hypoxia controls the radiocurability of some human cancers (2,3).

Mammalian cells irradiated under aerobic conditions are killed at a rate 2.5–3.0 times greater than if they are irradiated in the absence of oxygen. Consequently, radioresistant hypoxic cells constitute a physiologically distinct component of solid tumors for which methods of selective killing might be devised.

ISBN 0-12-619280-4

A recent rationale which addresses this problem is the use of drugs which can mimic the radiosensitizing effectiveness of molecular oxygen and can diffuse readily into the hypoxic regions of solid tumors (4,5). Figure 1 schematically depicts a histological section of a tumor nodule and the expected distribution of molecular oxygen and a hypoxic cell radiosensitizer throughout. Enhanced killing of hypoxic cells by radiation effected by the sensitizing drug could result in improved therapy for cancers where hypoxia is known to control radiocurability. Selective radiosensitization of tumor cells would be equivalent to an increase in the effective radiation dose to the tumor and result in an improved chance for cure. This principle of radiation oncology is easily verified with experimental animal tumor models (6), and some clinical data suggest that it is equally true for human cancer (7–9). The maximum radiation dose used in cancer treatment protocols is determined by the detrimental effects in normal tissues adjacent to the tumor which invariably are exposed during treatment. The therapeutic ratio of ionizing radiation is defined as the ratio of tumor response to normal tissue complication, usually for a specific radiation dose. Hypoxic cell sensitizers whose action is selective for a resistant population of tumor cells would consequently be expected to produce a higher therapeutic ratio and increased radiocures as shown in Fig. 2.

Criteria for the selection of an effective radiosensitizing drug for clinical application have been defined (10,11) and include: (1) an activity selective for hypoxic cells, (2) acceptable toxicity at radiosensitizing concentrations, (3) activity against both slowly proliferating and nonproliferating hypoxic cells, (4) good diffusability to facilitate the rapid penetration of large solid tumors, coupled with (5) a relatively low chemical and biochemical reactivity to facilitate delivery of the active drug to the target cells which are several cell layers removed from the capillaries.

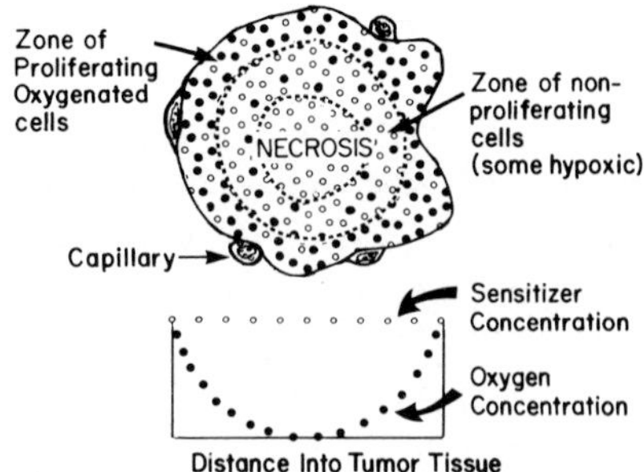

Fig. 1. Schematic of a section of a tumor nodule showing a zone of proliferating oxygenated cells adjacent to the vasculature, a central zone of necrosis, and an intermediate zone of nonproliferating cells (some of which could be hypoxic). The solid circles represent oxygen, and the open circles represent sensitizer molecules. The lower figure indicates the relative concentrations of oxygen and sensitizer throughout the tumor.

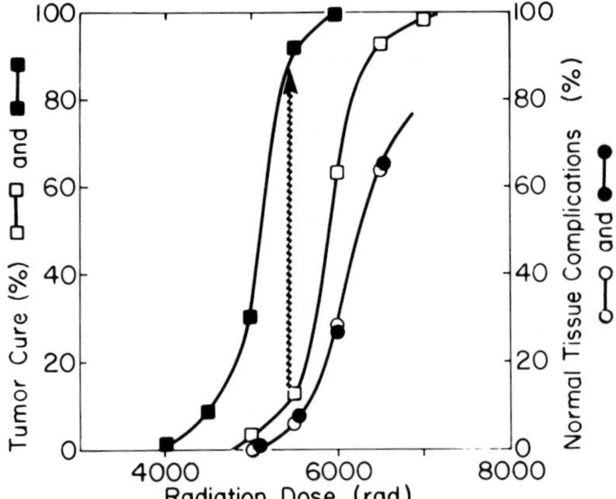

Fig. 2. Schematic showing the potential increase in therapeutic ratio expected for a tumor whose radiocurability is controlled by hypoxic cells. The tumor response with sensitizer is shifted to lower doses by a sensitizer enhancement ratio of 1.15, where no radiosensitization of the limiting normal tissues is assumed. With a 5400-rad total dose (a treatment which produces normal tissue complications in 5% of the patients) tumor cure probability can be increased from 12 to 90% with this modest radiosensitizing effect. Open symbols, Without sensitizer; Solid symbols, with sensitizer.

Several studies were performed to relate chemical structure and properties to radiosensitizing activity (12–17) and to suitable pharmacological properties (5,18–20). These structure-activity relationships are reviewed in Section II with reference to the criteria for sensitizer selection stated above.

The mechanisms by which electrophilic radiosensitizers act have also been studied (21–25). Section III describes at least two mechanisms by which misonidazole can act in radiosensitizing cells, and the relevance of these mechanisms to current clinical practice with this drug is discussed.

II. Structure-Activity Considerations in Sensitizer Design

The most important chemical property in the selection and design of ‘‘oxygen-mimicking’’ radiosensitizers has been electrophilicity. Adams and Cooke (26) suggested that electron affinity was the dominant property that conferred radiosensitizing potential on chemicals. Electron affinity had previously been invoked in a mechanism proposed to explain the radiosensitizing effect of molecular oxygen (27). Chapman *et al.* (12) showed that a threshold in electron affinity near that of nitrobenzene (half-wave reduction potential of −0.46 V) existed for the radiosensitization of hypoxic Chinese hamster lung fibroblasts growing *in vitro*. This observation led to a systematic study of the radiosensitizing activity of several substituted nitrobenzenes and resulted in the first experimental confirmation that sensitizing activity correlated strongly with electrophilicity (14). It was then recognized that several nitroheterocyclic drugs in current clinical use should have good radiosensitizing activity. This was quickly confirmed when nitrofurazone, nitrofurantoin, and nifuroxime (28,29) were shown to have good radiosensitizing activity in hypoxic cells *in vitro* and metronidazole and niridazole (15) somewhat less effectiveness. The discovery of radiosensitizing activity in an approved drug generated hope that early clinical investigations might be possible and stimulated new interest in the pharmacology and toxicity of these drugs.

Adams and co-workers at the Gray Laboratory in Northwood, England, exploited the principle of electron affinity in selection of the radiosensitizing drug misonidazole (Ro-07-0582) (30). Adams *et al.* (16,31) used a pulse radiolysis technique for measuring the one-electron reduction potential of several nitroheterocyclic compounds and demonstrated that, for several different ring structures and for molecular oxygen itself this chemical property was correlated with hypoxic cell-radiosensitizing activity. The principle of electrophilicity in predicting sensitizer activity has thus been clearly established. Several clinical investigations are in progress to determine if misonidazole can be combined with various radiation therapies for various cancers to effect an improved response (32).

The water solubility of a sensitizing drug is of importance, especially when applications in animals or humans are considered. It appears that concentrations of at least 0.1 m*M* sensitizing drug are required in hypoxic tumor cells at the time of irradiation to effect significant radiosensitization. This relatively high concentration of a drug will likely be distributed systemically after oral or intravenous administration. Consequently, dosages of 1 gm or more must be administered to a patient of average weight so that radiosensitizing concentrations can be established in hypoxic tumor cells. Water solubilities of at least 10 mg/ml are therefore required to promote rapid absorption from the gastrointestinal tract if given orally or to limit the volume of concentrated drug solutions given intravenously.

Lipophilicity or lipid solubility of nitroaromatic drugs did not correlate with either toxicity or sensitizing effectiveness in studies with mammalian cells growing *in vitro* (12,14,16). On the other hand, early studies on the pharmacokinetics and distribution of sensitizers in mice (5) indicated that lipid solubility could be an important factor. Recent studies by Brown *et al.* (18) and Brown and Lee (19) on a series of 2-nitroimidazole compounds of similar electron affinity but varying lipophilicity clearly show that lipophilicity is an important chemical property for determining drug concentrations in brain and other nervous tissues. As the lipid–water partition coefficient (P) decreased from values of 0.4 to 0.01 the concentrations of sensitizer in brain tissue relative to serum decreased from 1.0 to 0.03. For the same compounds, the concentration of sensitizer in tumor tissue relative to serum remained near 1.0 except for the most hydrophilic compound ($P = 0.014$) tested. In this series of 2-nitroimidazoles, compounds with partition coefficients between 0.4 and 0.02 might have improved therapeutic ratios, since sensitizer concentrations in tumor tissue relative to brain and nervous tissue (presumably related to the limiting neurotoxicity) increase from 1.0 to 30. Three drugs from this series are currently being developed for clinical testing, and the *O*-demethylated derivative of misonidazole is in a phase-1 clinical study by the Radiation Therapy Oncology Group (Philadelphia).

The ionization constant of a sensitizing compound is of importance, since charged drugs do not freely diffuse through cell membranes and can become ionically bound to cellular molecules. Analogues of nitrobenzene which were negatively charged at neutral pH were less effective in radiosensitizing hypoxic cells, presumably because of poor diffusion to the sites of the radiation targets within cells (14). Positively charged compounds, on the other hand, often showed enhanced radiosensitizing effect, possibly because of their ability to bind to intracellular molecules and/or their ability to concentrate within cells (13,14). The drugs under current study as clinical sensitizers are not charged at neutral pH, and consequently the complications associated with charged chemicals have been avoided.

III. Mechanisms of Radiosensitizer Action

The radiobiological target within a mammalian cell most readily linked with its reproductive death is the nucleoprotein. Radiation induces numerous lesions in cellular nucleoprotein including single-strand and double-strand breaks, specific base damage, covalent cross-links to adjacent molecules, and ultimately chromosome aberrations evidenced at mitosis. It is the lack of fidelity in the assortment of nucleoprotein to daughter cells at mitosis that results in the eventual inability of irradiated cells to proliferate indefinitely. The molecular lesions most likely to contribute to this misassortment of nucleoprotein are unrepaired DNA strand breaks and DNA cross-links.

Several studies on the mechanisms of chemical radiosensitization by nitroaromatic drugs show characteristics with strong similarities to the sensitizing action of molecular oxygen. For example, both oxygen and several nitroaromatic drugs enhance the rate of radiation-induced DNA strand breakage in hypoxic cells by factors proportional to the radiosensitizing enhancement ratios measured for cell survival (33,34). Also, both oxygen and nitroaromatic drugs rapidly and efficiently oxidize free radicals generated in DNA by radiation (35,36). This process of target radical oxidation by electron-affinic chemicals competes within cells with a process of target radical reduction by endogenous reducing species (23,37). This radiation-chemical mechanism in the action of nitroaromatic drugs is similar to the "oxygen fixation hypothesis" (38–40), which attributes the radiosensitizing effect of molecular oxygen to its ability to bind to and fix free radicals in vital cellular molecules, a process in competition with free-radical repair by hydrogen donation from endogenous sulfhydryl groups. A major component of hypoxic cell radiosensitization involves interaction of the sensitizing drug with transient free-radical species, and consequently for effect the drug must be present at the time of irradiation. This radiation-chemical process of direct radiosensitization by a specific drug is readily estimated by irradiating cell cultures at room temperature or immediately after addition of the drug to hypoxic cells at 37°C. Most of the structure–activity studies with nitroaromatic drugs have used such experimental procedures (12,14,16).

When mammalian cells are exposed to metronidazole or misonidazole at 37°C for prolonged times, a cytotoxicity selective for hypoxic cells is observed (41,42). Figure 3 shows the extent of killing of hypoxic Chinese hamster lung fibroblasts effected at various times by various concentrations of misonidazole. No killing was observed in parallel experiments with cells incubated under aerobic conditions for 6 hours in the presence of 5 m*M* misonidazole. This selective cytotoxic action of sensitizers could play a role in the chemotherapy of solid human tumors if used in combination with other agents effective on the cycling oxygenated cells. Wong *et al.* (43) reported that the effectiveness of misonidazole in radiosensitizing hypoxic Chinese hamster ovary (CHO) cells increased if the cells were incubated in the presence of the drug for 3 hours prior

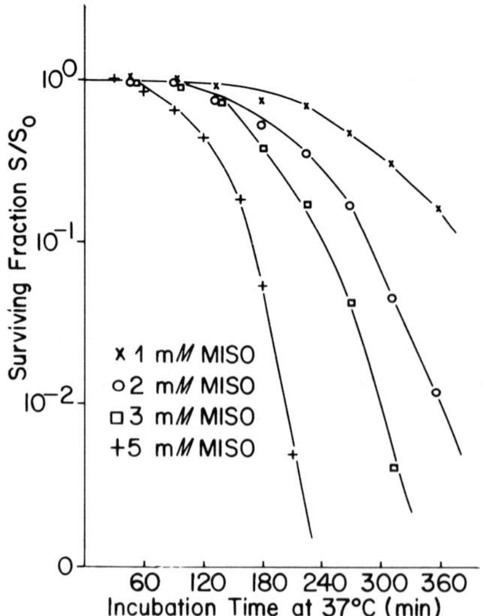

Fig. 3. Survival of Chinese hamster cells after exposure in complete medium to various concentrations of misonidazole (MISO) under hypoxia at 37°C.

to irradiation. This metabolism-related mechanism of sensitization was described as a loss of shoulder from the survival curve observed when cells were irradiated 15 minutes after exposure to misonidazole. Similar radiation experiments have been performed with Chinese hamster V79 cells which are more resistant to the cytotoxic action of misonidazole (see Fig. 3) than CHO cells. Figures 4 and 5 show complete radiation survival curves for cells irradiated in the presence of 1 and 2 m*M* misonidazole, respectively, after 1- and 3-hour preirradiation incubation times. The radiosensitivities of the same cell population under aerobic and hypoxic conditions are shown in each case. The plating efficiency of these cells, incubated for 3 hours under hypoxic conditions in the presence of these drug concentrations, was at least 90% of that of the untreated control cells, indicating that the additional radiosensitizing effect was not simply an additive chemical cytotoxicity. The metabolism-related mechanism of misonidazole radiosensitization is much more pronounced for these Chinese hamster V79 cells than for CHO cells as measured by Wong *et al.* (43). Furthermore, the effect shown in Figs. 4 and 5 cannot be described as simply a loss of shoulder from the survival curve, although the effect may be slightly larger at a low radiation dose than at a high radiation dose. A new additional feature of these data is that a nontoxic exposure to misonidazole (2 m*M* for 3 hours prior to irradiation) results in a cell radiosensitivity greater than that of cells irradiated under aerobic conditions. The ability of a chemical to radiosensitize cells beyond the effect of oxygen is reminiscent of the effect observed with diamide and *N*-ethylmaleimide, compounds known to

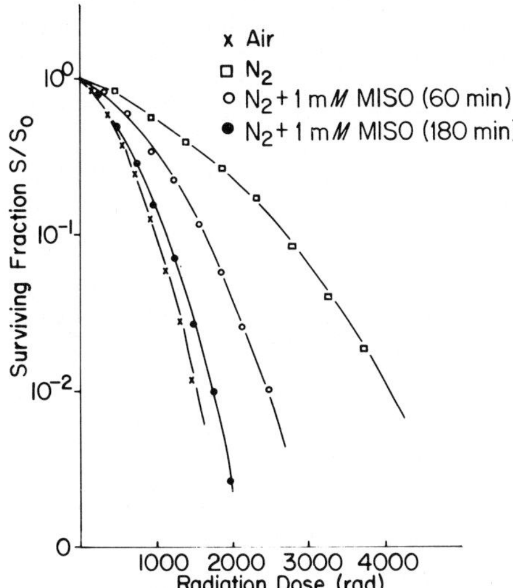

Fig. 4. Survival of Chinese hamster cells after irradiation under aerobic conditions, under hypoxia, and under hypoxia and preincubated with 1 m*M* misonidazole (MISO) for 1 and 3 hours.

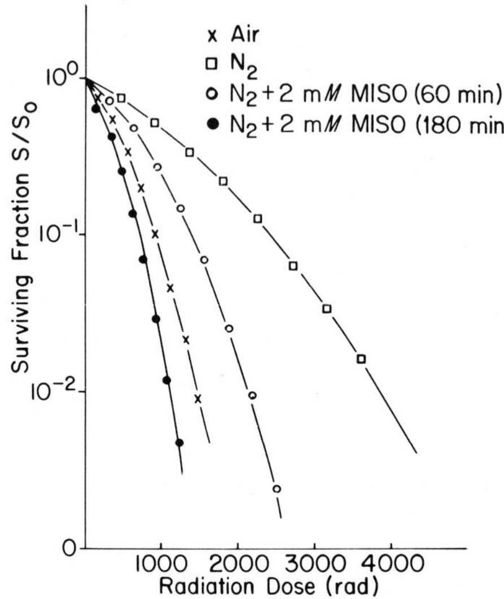

Fig. 5. Survival of Chinese hamster cells after irradiation under aerobic conditions, under hypoxia, and under hypoxia and preincubated with 2 m*M* misonidazole (MISO) for 1 and 3 hours.

oxidize cellular reducing species chemically (23). Metabolism-related radiosensitization by misonidazole differs from that observed with diamide and *N*-ethylmaleimide in that it is selective for hypoxic cells and consequently could be an extremely important mechanism for exploitation in cancer radiotherapy.

Experiments similar to those shown in Figs. 4 and 5 were performed at 24° and 10°C. Very little or no increase in radiosensitizing effectiveness was observed at the longer exposure time, and the extents of radiosensitization were much smaller than those measured at 37°C. Table I gives the sensitizing enhancement ratios (ratios of doses under hypoxia alone and hypoxia plus sensitizer required to produce 90% cell kill) observed with this cell line for the radiation-chemical mechanism (low-temperature effect) and the metabolism-related mechanism (high temperature effect/low temperature effect) for various incubation times. It is apparent that the metabolism-related mechanism observed with 1 m*M* misonidazole is the dominant mechanism at incubation times of 2 hours or more. The limited data with 2 m*M* misonidazole show a similar result. This metabolism-related radiosensitizing effect has not been extensively studied with other nitroaromatic drugs, and consequently the chemical properties of importance for this mechanism are not known.

Wong *et al.* (43) have associated this time-dependent mechanism of chemical radiosensitization with toxic products produced when misonidazole is metabolized in hypoxic cells. Other mechanisms which must be considered include the production of sublethal lesions in cellular radiation targets, such as DNA strand breaks (44), which can interact with radiation-induced sublesions to effect enhanced radiosensitivity. It is also known that electrophilic agents can bind cellular reducing equivalents, such as glutathione, and indirectly enhance the effectiveness of intracellular oxidizing species in target free-radical reactions (45). Such a radiosensitizing mechanism has been proposed for compounds which can chemically oxidize cell reducing species and for some nitroaromatic drugs (15).

The fact that this metabolism-related radiosensitizing effect is selective for hypoxic cells is important in cancer therapy. Preliminary experiments have shown that Chinese hamster V79 cells preconditioned by hypoxic incubation in the presence of 1 m*M* misonidazole are sensitized to killing by cyclophosphamide as well as by radiation. Consequently, experimental protocols which attempt to combine the effects of nitroaromatic drugs with radiation or chemotherapeutic agents should attempt to guarantee exposure of the hypoxic cells to the sensitizer for possibly 4 hours or more prior to treatment with the principal modality. This could mean that in experimental radiotherapy protocols the radiation treatment should be given 8–10 hours after oral administration of the drug to maximize the potential effectiveness of the sensitizer on hypoxic tumor cells, instead of 4–6 hours after administration as is the current practice.

In conclusion, misonidazole and other electrophilic sensitizers can potentially contribute to cancer treatment in at least three ways. The first benefit of these drugs is direct radiation sensitization of resistant hypoxic tumor cells, the initial rationale for drug selection. A second potential benefit arises from the selective cytotoxic action of the drugs against hypoxic cells which are often resistant to

TABLE I

Radiosensitizer Enhancement Ratios for Misonidazole at 10° and 37°C and Various Times of Exposure under Hypoxia[a]

Misonidazole concentration	Time (hours)	Sensitizer enhancement ratio (SER)		
		10°C	37°C	37°C/10°C
1 m*M*	1	1.3	1.6	1.2
	2	1.3	1.9	1.5
	3	1.4	2.3	1.6
	4	1.4	2.6	1.9
2 m*M*	1	1.6	1.9	1.2
	3	1.8	3.6	2.0

[a] The radiation-chemical component of sensitizer action is defined as that observed at 10°C. The metabolism-induced component of sensitizer action is defined as $SER_{37°C}/SER_{10°C}$.

current chemotherapies. A third potential benefit involves a sublethal conditioning of hypoxic cells, which makes them significantly more sensitive to subsequent treatments with radiation or with alkylating agents.

IV. Summary

The chemical property of electrophilicity (or electron affinity) has been the most important factor in the selection of compounds which can mimic molecular oxygen in sensitizing cells to the lethal action of ionizing radiation. Properties of secondary importance include water solubility, lipophilicity, and ionization constant (p*K*). For example, the partitioning of nitroheterocyclic sensitizers into brain and other nervous tissues relative to tumor tissue has been shown to depend upon lipid–water partition coefficients. This principle could prove to be useful in the design of new sensitizers which are less neurotoxic, the limiting toxicity of misonidazole in humans.

Hypoxic cell radiosensitizers are considered to act as dose-modifying agents. Recent studies indicate that the radiosensitizing effectiveness of some compounds, including misonidazole, results from at least two mechanisms which can be distinguished by time and temperature. A component of sensitizer action involves the fixation of target radicals produced by both direct and indirect effects of radiation within cells. This process of target radical oxidation competes within the cell with a repair process involving target radical reduction by normal cellular reducing species. Another mechanism of misonidazole radiosensitization requires minutes to hours of incubation of cells in the absence of oxygen at 37°C for expression. This second mechanism could involve the biochemical oxidation of cellular reducing equivalents prior to irradiation treatment and thereby enhance the radiosensitizing effectiveness of the radical oxidizing species within cells at the time of irradiation.

Acknowledgments

The experiments described in this manuscript were supported by the Alberta Heritage Savings and Trust Fund—Applied Cancer Research. The skillful assistance of Shirley Dawson and Karl Liesner in preparing the manuscript for this chapter is appreciated.

References

1. R. S. Bush, R. D. T. Jenkin, W. E. C. Alt, F. A. Beale, H. Bean, A. J. Dembo, and J. F. Pringle, *Br. J. Cancer* **37,** Suppl. III, 302 (1978).
2. R. H. Thomlinson and L. H. Gray, *Br. J. Cancer* **9,** 539 (1955).

3. I. F. Tannock, *Br. J. Cancer* **22,** 258 (1968).
4. G. E. Adams, *Br. Med. Bull.* **29,** 48 (1973).
5. J. D. Chapman, A. P. Reuvers, J. Borsa, J. S. Henderson, and R. D. Migliore, *Cancer Chemother. Rep., Part 1* **58,** 559 (1974).
6. H. D. Suit, *in* "Textbook of Radiotherapy" (G. H. Fletcher, ed.), 2nd ed., p. 75. Lea & Febiger, Philadelphia, Pennsylvania, 1973.
7. L. J. Shukovsky, *Am. J. Roentgenol., Radium Ther. Nucl. Med.* [N.S.] **108,** 27 (1970).
8. G. H. Fletcher, *Br. J. Radiol.* **46,** 1 (1973).
9. G. H. Fletcher and L. J. Shukovsky, *J. Radiol., Electrol., Med. Nucl.* **56,** 383 (1975).
10. G. E. Adams, J. C. Asquith, D. L. Dewey, J. L. Foster, B. D. Michael, and R. L. Wilson, *Int. J. Radiat. Biol.* **19,** 575 (1971).
11. J. D. Chapman, *Curr. Top. Radiat. Res. Q.* **7,** 286 (1972).
12. J. D. Chapman, J. A. Raleigh, J. Borsa, R. G. Webb, and R. Whitehouse, *Int. J. Radiat. Biol.* **21,** 475 (1972).
13. G. E. Adams, J. C. Asquith, M. E. Watts, and C. E. Smithen, *Nature (London), New Biol.* **239,** 23 (1972).
14. J. A. Raleigh, J. D. Chapman, J. Borsa, W. Kremers, and A. P. Reuvers, *Int. J. Radiat. Biol.* **23,** 377 (1973).
15. J. D. Chapman, A. P. Reuvers, and J. Borsa, *Br. J. Radiol.* **46,** 623 (1973).
16. G. E. Adams, I. R. Flockhart, C. E. Smithen, I. J. Stratford, P. Wardman, and M. E. Watts, *Radiat. Res.* **67,** 9 (1976).
17. J. A. Raleigh, J. D. Chapman, A. P. Reuvers, J. E. Biaglow, R. E. Durand, and A. M. Rauth, *Br. J. Cancer* **37,** Suppl. III, 6 (1978).
18. J. M. Brown, N. Y. Yu, and P. Workman, *Br. J. Cancer* **39,** 310 (1979).
19. J. M. Brown and W. W. Lee, *Cancer Clin. Trials* (in press).
20. R. A. White, J. M. Brown, and P. Workman, *Cancer Clin. Trials* (in press).
21. G. E. Adams, *in* "Radiation Protection and Sensitization" (H. L. Moroson and M. Quitiliani, eds.), p. 3. Taylor & Francis, London, 1970.
22. J. L. Redpath and R. L. Willson, *Int. J. Radiat. Biol.* **23,** 51 (1973).
23. J. D. Chapman, A. P. Reuvers, J. Borsa, and C. L. Greenstock, *Radiat. Res.* **56,** 291 (1973).
24. G. E. Adams, B. D. Michael, J. C. Asquith, M. A. Shenoy, M. E. Watts, and D. W. Whillans, *in* "Radiation Research: Biomedical, Chemical and Physical Perspectives" (O. F. Nygaard, H. I. Adler, and W. K. Sinclair, eds.), p. 478. Academic Press, New York, 1976.
25. J. D. Chapman, D. L. Dugle, A. P. Reuvers, C. J. Gillespie, and J. Borsa, *in* "Radiation Research: Biomedical, Chemical and Physical Perspectives" (O. F. Nygaard, H. I. Adler, and W. K. Sinclair, eds.), p. 752. Academic Press, New York, 1976.
26. G. E. Adams and M. S. Cooke, *Int. J. Radiat. Biol.* **15,** 457 (1969).
27. G. E. Adams and D. L. Dewey, *Biochem. Biophys. Res. Commun.* **12,** 473 (1963).
28. A. P. Reuvers, J. D. Chapman, and J. Borsa, *Nature (London)* **237,** 402 (1972).
29. J. D. Chapman, A. P. Reuvers, J. Borsa, A. Petkau, and G. R. McCalla, *Cancer Res.* **32,** 2616 (1972).
30. J. C. Asquith, M. E. Watts, K. Patel, C. E. Smithen, and G. E. Adams, *Radiat. Res.* **60,** 108 (1974).
31. G. E. Adams, E. D. Clarke, I. R. Flockhart, R. J. Jacobs, D. S. Sehmi, I. J. Stratford, P. Wardman, J. Parrish, R. G. Wallace, and C. E. Smithen, *Int. J. Radiat. Biol.* **35,** 133 (1979).
32. J. D. Chapman, *N. Engl. J. Med.* **301,** 1429 (1979).
33. D. L. Dugle, J. D. Chapman, C. J. Gillespie, J. Borsa, R. G. Webb, B. E. Meeker, and A. P. Reuvers, *Int. J. Radiat. Biol.* **22,** 545 (1972).
34. B. Palcic and L. D. Skarsgard, *Int. J. Radiat. Biol.* **21,** 417 (1972).
35. R. L. Willson, *Int. J. Radiat. Biol.* **17,** 349 (1970).

36. J. D. Chapman, C. L. Greenstock, A. P. Reuvers, E. McDonald, and I. Dunlop, *Radiat. Res.* **53,** 190 (1973).
37. J. C. Asquith, J. L. Foster, R. L. Willson, R. Ings, and J. A. McFadzean, *Br. J. Radiol.* **47,** 474 (1974).
38. T. Alper, *Radiat. Res.* **5,** 573 (1956).
39. P. Howard-Flanders, *Adv. Biol. Med. Phys.* **5,** 533 (1958).
40. P. Alexander, *Trans. N.Y. Acad. Sci.* [2] **24,** 966 (1962).
41. R. M. Sutherland, *Cancer Res.* **34,** 3501 (1974).
42. E. J. Hall and L. Riozin-Towle, *Radiology* **117,** 453 (1975).
43. T. W. Wong, G. F. Whitmore, and S. Gulyas, *Radiat. Res.* **75,** 541 (1978).
44. P. L. Olive and D. R. McCalla, *Cancer Res.* **35,** 781 (1975).
45. L. F. Chasseaud, *Adv. Cancer Res.* **29,** 175 (1979).

PART VI

Membrane Targets

21

Plasma Membranes as Targets and Mediators in Tumor Chemotherapy

DONALD F. HOELZL WALLACH, ROSS B. MIKKELSEN, AND LESTER KWOCK

I. Introduction

Drugs used in tumor chemotherapy may act at the plasma membrane or at intracellular loci. Drugs that act intracellularly must penetrate the plasma mem-

MOLECULAR ACTIONS AND TARGETS FOR CANCER CHEMOTHERAPEUTIC AGENTS

ISBN 0-12-619280-4

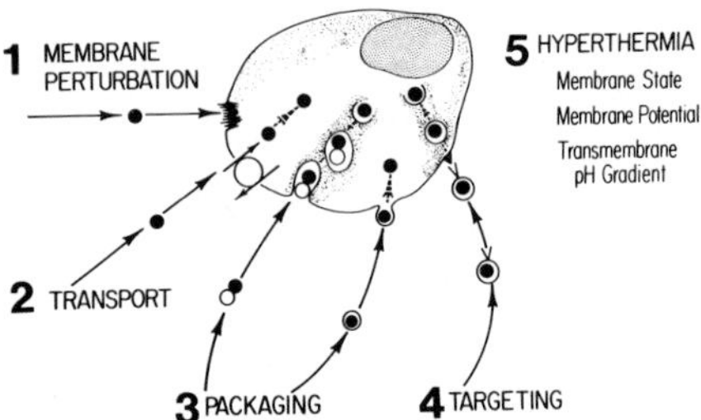

Fig. 1. Schematic view of plasma membrane participation in tumor chemotherapy.

branes of target cells by diffusion, endocytosis, or some carrier mechanism. The effectiveness of many antitumor drugs is limited by their relative membrane impermeability and thereby their exclusion from critical sites of action. Moreoever, carrier-deficient or poorly permeant variants may be selected from a tumor cell population during chemotherapy, leading to drug resistance.

We will present a brief review of the roles of plasma membranes as targets and mediators in tumor chemotherapy (Fig. 1). We will further introduce arguments indicating how moderate hyperthermia might serve as a general adjunct to tumor chemotherapy.

II. Plasma Membrane-Active Drugs

A. Polyene Antibiotics

Polyene antibiotics are macrolide ring molecules, each including a conjugated polyene sequence linked to a polyhydroxyl chain. The separation of polar and apolar segments in these compounds creates an unusual amphipathic character. Polyene antibiotics act pharmacologically on membranes containing 3-β-hydroxyl sterols, i.e., primarily the plasma membranes of animal and fungal cells (1). Such sterols are thought to "buffer" the fluidity of phospholipid acyl chains, to lower the cooperativity of phospholipid phase transitions, and to promote mixing of dissimilar membrane lipids (2). Interference, by polyene antibiotics, with normal membrane sterol functions can thus be expected to alter plasma membrane properties that depend on the lipid state. Polyene antibiotics can also be expected to modify the accumulation of drugs that enter cells by processes other than active or facilitated transport.

The polyene antibiotics filipin and amphotericin B interact differently with phospholipid vesicles. The initial rate of reaction of filipin with sterol-free lecithin vesicles is 50–100 times slower than with cholesterol–lecithin vesicles under identical conditions (3). In contrast, the reaction rate of amphotericin B with cholesterol–lecithin vesicles is slower than that of filipin and slower than with sterol-free vesicles (4). This suggests that filipin reacts only with sterol but that amphotericin B interacts also (or primarily) with phospholipids. Moreover, Chen and Bittman (4) found that the rate of association of amphotericin B with lecithin vesicles varied with the nature of the acyl chains. The shorter the chains of saturated lecithins or the greater the number of double bonds in unsaturated lecithins—i.e., the looser the chain packing—the greater the initial rate. Also, Bunow and Levin (5) have shown, for lecithin cholesterol–amphotericin B liposomes, that the nature of the sterol–antibiotic interaction, as measured by Raman spectroscopy, depends strongly on the order of the phospholipid acyl chains; that is, it varies with the lecithin gel ↔ liquid crystal transition. Present information thus indicates that the association of amphotericin B with phospholipid vesicles does not require the presence of sterols and that it depends upon the relative strengths of lipid–lipid and amphotericin B–lipid interactions. The weaker the lipid–lipid interaction, the faster the rate of association.

The association rate of amphotericin B with sterol–lecithin vesicles varies with the sterol (4). With sterol–dimyristoyl lecithin, at a molar ratio of ½ and a 1 mM total lipid concentration, the initial rate constants are: no sterol, 0.78 μM/sec; thiocholesterol, 0.48 μM/sec; androst-5-en-3β-ol,0.42 μM/sec; epicholesterol, 0.34 μM/sec; ergosterol, 0.13 μM/sec; and cholesterol, 0.084 μM/sec.

Findelstein and associates (6–8) have presented evidence suggesting that polyene antibiotics form complexes with membrane sterols and that these complexes aggregate to form transmembrane hydrophilic channels. However, this model cannot apply simply to amphotericin B, which associates strongly with phospholipid molecules. Chen and Bittman (4) therefore suggest that membrane sterols increase the order of membrane acyl chains in the liquid crystalline state, favoring orientation of amphotericin B molecules parallel to membrane acyl chains and perpendicular to the membrane plane. This would increase the probability of alignment of antibiotic molecules in apposed halves of the bilayer, allowing two "half-pores" to form a transmembrane channel.

Polyene antibiotics cause abnormal proton (and potassium) permeability of renal tubular membranes and are therefore nephrotoxic (9–11). They can thus be therapeutically valuable only if the target cells' sterol, their phospholipid–phospholipid, and their sterol–phospholipid interactions favor association of the antibiotics with their membranes rather than those of host cell systems.

Several workers have explored the possible value of amphotericin B in tumor therapy, exploiting the ergosterol affinity of this antibiotic and the fact that membrane sterols can be readily exchanged (12,13). Thus Schiffman and Klein (14) have conferred amphotericin B sensitivity on mouse L1210 leukemia cells (normally resistant) by preincubating these cells with lecithin–ergosterol liposomes to exchange cholesterol for ergosterol. Hahn *et al.* (15) have shown that amphotericin B inactivates HA1 cells *in vitro* at 43°C but not at 41°C, and that amphotericin B is damaging to EMT6 mouse mammary carcinoma *in vivo* when the tumors are locally heated to 43°C. Nystatin, a molecule with a slightly lower affinity for cholesterol than amphotericin B ($K_a = 7 \times 10^5\ M^{-1}$ versus 2–6 × $10^6\ M,^{-1}$ respectively), does not show the thermosensitivity of amphotericin B. The difference between amphotericin B and nystatin may relate to the different thermal properties of the transmembrane channels formed by these antibiotics (6–8). The conductances of these channels are extraordinarily temperature-sensitive, and that of nystatin channels reversibly decreases by $\sim 10^4$ for each 10°C rise in temperature in the physiological range. Amphotericin B shows a different thermal response, and the conductance decrement caused by a temperature increase is not reversible.

The data of Schiffman and Klein (14) and Hahn *et al.* (15) point out some features of amphotericin B resistance in tumor cells. Additional data (16–18) indicate that the amphotericin B resistance of fibroblasts neoplastically transformed by simian virus 40 (SV40) is under cellular genetic control. Resistance is not expressed upon neoplastic transformation by polyoma or murine sarcoma virus and does not involve diminished binding of amphotericin B. This suggests that the organization of cholesterol is abnormal in the membranes of SV40-transformed cells. The same conclusion has been reached independently by Verma *et al.* (19) to explain the less cooperative lipid-phase transitions of the plasma membranes from SV40-transformed hamster lymphocytes compared with those of membranes from normal cells.

B. Streptolysin O

Membrane sterols that contain an (equatorial) 3-β-hydroxyl group on the steroid nucleus and interact with polyene antibiotics also react with streptolysin O, a 68,000-dalton protein from *streptococcus pyogenes*. Present evidence, reviewed by Alouf (20), suggests that this protein binds to cholesterol with high affinity via the 3-β-hydroxyl group, as well as at another site. The toxin contains one or more intrachain disulfides which are required for binding to membranes. Binding proceeds rapidly in the cold, but membrane lysis requires warming to 37°C. Whether streptolysin O has any potential for tumor therapy remains to be established.

C. Tubulin and Drugs Acting on Tubulin

Cellular tubulin is primarily in the form of microtubules. Microtubules are long, 20 to 25-nm-diameter cylinders composed predominantly of tubulin, a protein with a 55,000-dalton monomer molecular mass that normally exists either as a 110,000-dalton dimer or a polymer of such dimers (i.e., a microtubule). The conditions for the *in vitro* assembly and disassembly of microtubules have been well characterized and suggest that assembly requires certain nontubulin ancillary proteins, e.g., τ protein (21).

The assembly and stability of tubulin can be modulated by colchicine and related drugs (e.g., vincristine). The action of colchicine on microtubules is fairly well understood (22). The drug forms 1:1 molar complexes with the tubulin dimer. Added to a polymerizing tubulin mixture, tubulin–colchicine complexes terminate microtubule assembly at the growing end of a microtubule (in a "capping" step). The polymer–dimer equilibrium, which normally favors the polymer, in the presence of colchicine leads to the formation of short segments capped with colchicine rather than with native tubulin. Accordingly, microtubule disassembly following exposure of cells to colchicine occurs only when microtubules are in an active steady state of assembly–disassembly in the absence of the drug. Differences between cells in sensitivity to colchicine and related drugs may reflect different assembly–disassembly steady states of different microtubule populations.

The status of tubulin as a target for chemotherapeutic agents is treated by Horwitz (23) elsewhere in this volume. What we wish to stress here is the fact that some cellular tubulin is membrane-associated. This suggests the possibility that some chemotherapeutic agents that act on tubulin may modify plasma membrane structure and function. Bhattacharyya and Wolff (24) have collected highly purified synaptic membranes from guinea pigs injected with [^{3}H]leucine and isolated tritiated tubulin therefrom, achieving constant specific activity after three cycles of polymerization and depolymerization in nonionic detergent. These authors' careful control experiments rule out the possibility that the tubulin represents contaminating soluble tubulin. Zenner and Pfeuffer (25) have shown that pigeon erythrocyte membrane proteins solubilized in 2% sodium cholate compete with ^{125}I-labeled bovine brain tubulin in radioimmunoassays using antibody against brain tubulin. The presence of tubulin in the membranes was further verified by affinity chromatography. Intact pigeon erythrocytes were bound to colchicine–Sepharose beads at 37°C, a process which could be blocked by free colchicine (5 m*M*) or incubation at 0°C. Complexes of Sepharose with lumicolchicine (which does not cap tubulin) did not bind to the erythrocytes. The reaction of the membranes was much too great to be accounted for by cytoplasmic tubulin.

The above experiments point to the presence on some plasma membrane of tubulin or closely related proteins. However, other studies indicate that the action of colchicine, thought to be tubulin-specific, and related drugs may not be limited to tubulin. Thus Wunderlich *et al.* (26) have shown that colchicine impairs the temperature-induced translational mobility of intramembranous particles in *Tetrahymena* alveolar membranes; these structures are not associated with microtubules, and *Tetrahymena* microtubules are not disassembled under the conditions used by these authors. Also, Furcht and Scott (27) have demonstrated that the distribution of intramembranous particles of fibroblast plasma membranes can be modified by lumicolchicine, as well as colchicine, although the former drug does not affect microtubules. These authors also found that the distribution of fibroblast intramembranous particles was modulated by colchicine at levels as low as 10^{-9} M (28).

III. Drug Transport

A. Introduction

Most cancer chemotherapeutic drugs act intracellularly but depend on plasma membrane permeability, some by specific transport processes, to reach their sites of action. Plasma membrane properties thus influence chemotherapeutic efficiency. Concordantly, drug resistance is often due to the emergence of neoplastic cell populations which lack the permeability or transport mechanisms that normally allow drug uptake.

B. Active Transport

Nitrogen mustards are agents known to be actively transported by a carrier system for choline (29–31). In nitrogen mustard-insensitive malignant cell strains, drug resistance has been shown to involve impaired transport (30–35). Transport of nitrogen mustards is not competitively inhibited by other alkylating agents, including cyclophosphamide (35,36). Moreover, uptake of the latter drug, which occurs by facilitated diffusion, is not affected by nitrogen mustard, melphalan, or chlorambucil.

In various strains of Yoshida sarcoma, nitrogen mustard sensitivity correlates well with drug uptake (33), and impaired alkylating agent binding to DNA in resistant lines can be restored to the levels found in sensitive lines by increasing membrane permeability (34). Similar results have been obtained with alkylating agent-resistant strains of Ehrlich ascites carcinoma (32). Finally, Tween 80, a nonionic detergent, has been shown to sensitize rat hepatoma cells to nitrogen mustard (37).

Melphalan, a phenylalanine mustard, is accumulated in L5178 lymphoblasts by carrier-mediated transport (38,39). At low concentrations, drug accumulates via both the Na^+-independent L system of amino acid transport and a Na^+-dependent system resembling ASC (alanine, serine, cysteine) transport; at high drug concentrations the L system predominates. Uptake is not influenced by inhibitors of sugar transport. Nitrogen mustard, chlorambucil, and cyclophosphamide are also not inhibitory. Melphalan transport clearly occurs by processes distinct from the mechanisms known to be involved in the uptake of other alkylating agents.

Arrhenius plots of melphalan uptake are linear between 0° and 37°C, but other data indicate enhanced uptake above 37°C. Melphalan has been reported to be clinically more effective when combined with 39°–40°C local hyperthermia (40). Also, the work of Goss and Parsons (41) on the survival of human fibroblast strains and melanoma cell lines treated with melphalan at varying temperatures *in vitro* suggests that the permeation of the drug is temperature-sensitive. In addition, human fibroblasts and melanoma cells exhibit about equivalent drug sensitivity at 16°C; however, the response of melanoma cells to phenylalanine mustard increases dramatically between 36° and 44°C, while that of the fibroblasts is stable between 42° and 44°C. Sharp thermal responses, such as those described for melphalan (and below for other drugs), may be due to thermotropic transitions of membrane state and function.

As also discussed in this volume by Sirotnak (42) and Huennekens (43), the effectiveness of folate analogues in tumor therapy depends on the membrane properties of target neoplastic (and normal) cells. Folate analogues, such as aminopterin, methotrexate, and 10-ethylaminopterin, are accumulated by a carrier-mediated active transport (44,45). However, evidence suggests that the influx and efflux of methotrexate occurs either by different carriers or slowly interconverting species of the same protein (46). Either mechanism, if appropriately modified in tumor cells, could make these cells more susceptible than their normal counterparts. On the other hand, the emergence of rapid-efflux variants would lead to drug resistance.

Chello *et al.* (45) have explored the possibility that differences in the transport of folate analogues by normal and tumor cells might be exploited to maximize antitumor action, as well as to reduce damage to dividing normal cells. They measured the transport of three folate analogues by murine intestinal epithelial cells and L1210 leukemia cells. The uptake affinity of the L1210 transport system was much greater than that of the epithelial cells for the three drugs studied, aminopterin, methotrexate, and 10-ethylaminopterin. Differences between the two cell types in terms of maximum uptake velocity were small, and efflux of drug from epithelial cells was in all cases about three times slower than from tumor cells. Importantly, substitution of a methyl or ethyl residue at the 10-position of aminopterin decreased the affinity for the tumor system about 3-fold, but reduced that for the epithelial cells by 12- and 17-fold, respectively. The known preferential antitumor action of folate analogues may thus derive from the relatively greater affinity of the tumor cell transport system for the drugs.

In methotrexate-insensitive tumor strains (47,48), drug resistance may derive from deficient transport of the drug into the cells. In L1210 mouse leukemia, methotrexate uptake can be increased by corticosteroids and vinca alkaloids, with marked enhancement of therapeutic efficiency (49). Moreover, Herman *et al.* (50) found that 43°C hyperthermia for 1 hour could overcome the high methotrexate resistance of Chinese hamster ovary cells. A cell kill of 50% occurred with 1 μg/ml of methotrexate after exposure for 1 hour at 43°C. This is in contrast to exposure at 37°C, where 500 μg/ml of methotrexate for 13 hours did not affect cell survival.

In clinical situations, methotrexate is often administered in high doses so as to induce responses in previously refractory or poorly responsive solid tumors (51–53). The mechanism suggested for the often observed high-dose sensitization is that at high doses methotrexate penetrates by an energy-independent process, whereas uptake at conventional doses is via active transport. While high doses of methotrexate may prove cytocidal to otherwise unresponsive tumor cells, such high drug concentrations also may be highly toxic to normal cells. Better therapeutic ratios may, however, be achieved locally by perfusion (40) or by hyperthermic targeting (54).

C. Energy-Independent Drug Uptake

Membrane permeation appears to limit the action of several anticancer agents including adriamycin, bleomycin, actinomycin D, daunorubicin, and vincristine, agents which enter cells by processes not requiring metabolic energy and apparently not involving specific carriers (55–58). Recent evidence suggests that resistance of tumor cells to adriamycin or daunorubicin is due less to low uptake of these drugs by refractory cells than to high active efflux. Thus omission of glucose or addition of inhibitors of glycolysis (e.g., azide or iodoacetamide) enhances the accumulation of adriamycin in resistant cells (55–57).

Since uptake of these drugs does not involve metabolically driven specific carriers, it can be influenced by agents that tend to increase membrane permeability nonspecifically. For example, treatment of Chinese hamster ovary cells with Tween 80, a nonionic detergent, overcomes their resistance to actinomycin D and daunorubicin, presumably by increasing plasma membrane permeability (59). Related work has shown that amphotericin B, another membrane-active agent (Section II,A), potentiates the cytotoxic effects of actinomycin D, adriamycin, and vincristine on AKR leukemia cells resistant to these drugs (60). Finally, a clinical study by Presant *et al.* (61) suggests that inclusion of amphotericin B in an adriamycin chemotherapeutic regimen can reverse adriamycin resistance in some tumors.

The uptake of adriamycin and bleomycin can be markedly enhanced, in the case of Chinese hamster HA1 cells, by raising the temperature to 42°–43°C (62). This thermal effect, as well as that observed with phenylalanine mustard (41), and possibly the increased cytotoxicity of solvents such as dimethyl sulfoxide and dimethylformamide at temperatures >41°C (63), suggests a membrane permeability change at high fever temperatures.

While presenting barriers to the passage of adriamycin, the plasma membranes of some cells may not be inert to the action of this drug. Thus Myers *et al.* (64)

found that the cardiac toxicity following administration of adriamycin to mice was associated with extensive peroxidation of cardiac lipids. Both cardiac toxicity and lipid peroxidation could be diminished by preadministration of a free-radical scavenger without altering the antitumor action of adriamycin. It appears that adriamycin acts on tissues not only through binding to DNA but also via peroxidation of unsaturated lipids.

IV. Drug Packaging

A. Introduction

Numerous studies have explored the effects of the charge, hydrophobicity, carrier affinity, and other properties of drugs acting on intracellular targets to achieve superior membrane penetration without compromising therapeutic efficiency. Similar approaches have been employed to overcome drug resistance in tumor cell populations when refractoriness to chemotherapeutic agents is due to inadequate drug uptake.

B. "Lysosomotropism"

Drugs are made lysosomotropic (65) by the use of carriers that are endocytosed or phagocytosed by target cells. Fusion of the internalized, drug-bearing vesicles with primary lysosomes produces secondary lysosomes in which the carriers are hydrolyzed and the active drug is released into the cell.

Several lysosomotropic drugs have been tested in tumor therapy. Daunorubicin, introduced parenterally as noncovalent complexes with DNA, was tested first, with somewhat ambiguous results in screens against animal leukemias (66). A preliminary trial on human leukemias (67) suggested that daunorubicin complexed to DNA might be more effective and less toxic than the free drug. The noncovalent complex of adriamycin with DNA, tested more recently (68), appears less toxic than the free drug, and therapeutically more effective against L1210 leukemia. Cytotoxic drugs have also been coupled, covalently or noncovalently, to proteins or polypeptides without impairing biological potency (69–71). Moreover, screening against mouse leukemia systems of a variety of drugs linked covalently or noncovalently to a diversity of carriers (70), suggests that complexation generally lowers toxicity and often increases therapeutic efficiency. Also, methotrexate bound covalently to bovine serum albumin controls metastases from transplanted Lewis lung carcinomas more effectively and with less toxicity than free methotrexate, at the same time lowering the growth rate of the primary tumor (72).

C. Liposomes

Another strategy for the introduction of drugs and other agents into target cells has been to entrap them in phospholipid spherules or liposomes (73,74). Initially, liposomes were employed for the treatment of enzyme storage diseases, and this area is under investigation. Moreover, considerable progress has been achieved in the formation and manipulation of liposomes (e.g., 75), even to the point of allowing encapsulation of poliovirus (76) and stabilization of interferon against degradation (77). Enzyme entrapment within erythrocyte plasma membrane vesicles (78) and "resealed" erythrocytes (79) has also proven feasible. Concerning the fate of liposomes *in vivo,* Hwang and Mauk (80) prepared lecithin vesicles containing complexes of $^{111}In^{3+}$ and nitrilotriacetic acid. Within the vesicles the complexes tumble rapidly, but released complexes dissociate, allowing the tracer to bind to macromolecules. This decreases the tumbling rate of the tracer. The fate of vesicles can therefore be determined by γ-ray perturbed correlation, and the vesicles located by combining this technique with scanning. Model studies on mice revealed the presence of intact dipalmitoyl lecithin-cholesterol vesicles in liver, kidney, spleen, skin, and blood for up to 13 hours after intraperitoneal injection.

Three mechanisms make entrapment of antitumor agents in liposomes an attractive approach. The first is protection of the entrapped agent against enzymatic degradation (77) or immunological inactivation (76). The second is that liposomes delivered intravenously may act as lysosomotropic agents, i.e., are phagocytosed and taken up into lysosomes. The third is that, given a suitable lipid composition of the liposome wall (81), it will fuse with the plasma membrane of the target cell, discharging its contents into the cell (76, 81–85). This third process has allowed introduction of poliovirus into virus-resistant cells (76) and introduction of enzymes into cells incapable of phagocytosis (85). Moreover, the ability of liposomes containing macrophage-activating factor (MAF), to stimulate mouse macrophages cytotoxic for tumor cells *in vitro* is enhanced over that of free MAF (86). The liposomal MAF, unlike free MAF, also stimulates protease-treated macrophages. This finding suggests that MAF is released into the macrophages by fusion of the liposome wall with the macrophage plasma membrane.

In the area of tumor chemotherapy, initial reports indicated that entrapment of actinomycin D improved the action of this drug on mouse tumors (74,87). More recently, Kimelberg *et al.* (88) studied the effect of methotrexate entrapment in positively charged liposomes in terms of drug distribution and liposome charge and size. The results indicate that (1) whether drugs entrapped in liposomes act as lysosomotropic agents or via fusion depends upon liposome composition and dispersion; (2) sonically dispersed, positively charged liposomes allow the highest plasma drug maintenance level; and (3) drug entrapment decreases renal and gastrointestinal toxicity. However, it remains to be determined whether these factors will improve therapeutic efficacy per se or whether this will require development of liposome targeting to tumor cells (73,74), possibly by linking them to lectins or to antitumor antibodies.

Many tumor cells appear insensitive to actinomycin D. However, Papahadjopoulos *et al.* (89), comparing the action of free actinomycin D with that of drug encapsulated in unilamellar cholesterol or lecithin liposomes on actinomycin D-resistant DC-3F/ADX Chinese hamster tumor cells, noted that entrapment reduced by a factor of 200 the drug concentration required to inhibit RNA synthesis *in vitro* and produced a 120-fold reduction of the dose needed for 50% growth inhibition. These findings suggest that drug resistance arises from the inability of cells to take up actinomycin D and that this can be overcome *in vitro* by liposome entrapment of the drug. Success has also been reported *in vitro* and *in vivo* with liposome-entrapped arabinosylcytosine (90).

V. Drug Targeting

Approaches to specific drug targeting have been recently reviewed by Gregoriadis (73), with emphasis on the use of specific antibodies as "homing" agents. One such approach is of considerable interest in tumor therapy (91). Diphtheria toxin, which is cytotoxic at doses of >50 molecules per cell, was coupled to specific antibodies for targeting. Prophylactic effects only were obtained using SV40-transformed hamster sarcoma cells and diphtheria toxin–anti-SV40 surface antigen conjugates, but regressions were frequent with a SV40-induced lymphoma. Penetration of toxin presumably occurred by endocytosis.

Specific antibody-mediated targeting may be of limited value in cancer therapy, because most tumors do not elicit strong humoral immunity and those that do tend to produce antibodies specific for a given tumor only. Therefore strategies using less specific carriers may be preferable; one such approach has been published by Kitao and Hattori (71). These workers coupled daunorubicin covalently via its sugar moiety to concanavalin A (2–3 moles of drug per mole of lectin) in the anticipation then the complex would bind to tumor cell plasma membranes, be endocytosed and cleaved in the lysosomes, and release the drug. Kitao and Hattori (71) report that the drug–lectin conjugate was more effective than free drug against both mouse L1210 leukemia and Ehrlich ascites carcinoma.

Liposomes release encapsulated drugs 10 times more rapidly at or above the gel ↔ liquid crystal transition temperature of the phospholipid walls than below (54), 100 times more rapidly in the presence of serum. This observation forms the basis of an interesting targeting proposal for the chemotherapy of localized tumors (54). Drug is encapsulated in liposomes with a transition temperature in the moderate fever range (e.g., 42°C). The liposomes are injected into the circulation of a tumor-bearing individual whose tumor is heated locally to or above the transition temperature. This achieves a high concentration of released drug in the tumor and may also produce optimal and targeted conditions for liposome–tumor membrane fusion. If the approach suggested in Yatvin *et al.* (54) merely achieves high localized concentration of drug, it may not constitute a significant improvement over hyperthermic drug perfusion (40). Increased fusion-mediated drug uptake could, however, yield an important therapeutic advantage.

VI. Hyperthermia as an Adjunct to Chemotherapy

A. Introduction

As recounted above, some drugs used in tumor chemotherapy appear more effective at temperatures >37°C. Extensive evidence further suggests that many tumor cells are damaged by heat under conditions innocuous for normal cells (92). Accordingly, several clinical trials have been initiated combining chemotherapy with local or whole-body hyperthermia. An early study, utilizing local hyperthermia and local melphalan infusion in the treatment of melanoma appears encouraging (40). Concerning disseminated disease, a recent study (93) combining repetitive ~40.5°C whole-body hyperthermia with multidrug chemotherapy demonstrates the feasibility of this approach and suggests increased therapeutic benefit for some types of pulmonary carcinoma.

The following findings lead one to suspect that cellular membranes, particularly plasma membranes, may be targets for thermotherapy: (1) Drug can permeate through lipid bilayers, provided they are in the proper physical state, and this state may be highly temperature-dependent. (2) Membrane proteins are known to undergo state changes in the 39°–43°C range, and these changes can influence membrane permeability and membrane electrochemical potential. (3) Much active membrane transport depends on membrane electrochemical potential. (4) Many tumors produce more lactic acid than normal (94); the lactate is exported from the cells together with H^+, producing extracellular acidification and thereby changing membrane electrochemical potential (92,94). (5) Some tumor cell membranes have enhanced thermosensitivity.

We will now comment briefly on mechanisms possibly involved.

B. Membrane Lipids

Small changes in temperature or ionic conditions can bring about large alterations in the structure of lipid assemblies, e.g., bilayers, without modifying covalent linkages. Pure glycerophospholipids or sphingolipids in bilayer arrays can exist in two temperature-dependent types of physical state: (1) gel phases, where the polar groups and acyl chains are in ordered two-dimensional crystalline arrays, and (2) liquid crystalline phases, where the polar groups are in two-dimensional crystalline arrays but the hydrocarbon chains form a disordered, liquid (fluid) continua. In pure systems gel ↔ liquid crystal phase transitions can be brought about by very small temperature shifts. This is because such transitions are highly cooperative; a state change in one acyl chain markedly facilitates that in other chains. The critical transition temperature T_c depends on the nature of the acyl chain, e.g., length and unsaturation, as well as on the nature of the polar group, the charge in particular. Phospholipids with charged polar groups exhibit T_c values well below those characterizing uncharged but otherwise identical phospholipids. For such lipids, a phase transition brought about under given ionic conditions (e.g., pH, Ca^{2+}) by a temperature shift can be induced isothermally by an appropriate change in ionic environment.

The behavior of homogeneous lipid bilayers does not properly represent that of biomembranes for the following reasons: First, biomembrane lipids are heterogeneous in acyl chain and head group composition. In mixtures of lipids with sufficiently dissimilar hydrocarbon and/or polar residues, one class of lipid may form a liquid crystalline phase under given conditions and the other a gel phase. Molecules of the second class will then segregate to form solid islands in a liquid crystalline continuum (or vice versa). Second, plasma membranes contain cholesterol, which modifies phase changes. Cholesterol makes phase transitions less cooperative, maintains an intermediate state of acyl chain "fluidity" above and below a normally sharp T_c, and can allow chain mixing. Cholesterol thus "buffers" cooperativity as well as fluidity and may allow formation of a single phase out of a lipid mixture which might otherwise segregate into separate phases. Third, penetrating membrane proteins can influence the gel ↔ liquid crystal transitions of lipids, producing a shift, usually upward, in T_c and generally broadening the transitions. These effects are due to the influence of penetrating proteins on surrounding acyl chains. Surface-located proteins may also alter lipid-phase behavior.

Various physical techniques have been employed to detect lipid-phase changes in mammalian cell plasma membranes (95–99). Available data indicate that phase changes can occur, but at temperatures below 30°C. This implies that membrane lipid, free to undergo phase changes, is in a fluid state above 30°C, and that hyperthermia, i.e., shifting temperature to >37°C, is unlikely to exert effects related to the state of bulk lipid. Accordingly, pure lipid domains of biomembranes are unlikely to increase their permeability to drugs between 30° and 50°C. It is conceivable, however, that some drug permeation proceeds at lipid-protein boundaries and that this permeation is enhanced by changes in membrane protein state induced by hyperthermia.

C. Membrane Proteins

Several physical methods, Raman spectroscopy in particular, have shown that membrane proteins of erythrocytes and lymphoid cells can undergo temperature- and pH-sensitive state changes above 38°C (19,95–102). Typically, no thermotropic changes are observed between 0° and 38°C at neutral pH, but a large change in amino acid environment occurs between 38° and 45°C. This is generally irreversible above 42°C. When the pH is dropped from 7.0 to 6.5, the protein transition shifts to lower temperatures (by as much as 15°C) (100). The data suggest that membrane proteins, like soluble proteins, unfold more readily in response to a temperature shift at reduced pH than at physiological pH. However, to lower the mean transition temperature of a soluble protein, e.g., RNase, by 20°C requires a change in H^+ more than 10^4 greater than that needed for an equivalent effect in erythrocyte membrane proteins (96, 98, 100). This implies that small modifications in electrostatic interactions may destabilize membrane proteins more readily than proteins dissolved in aqueous media. The pH sensitivity of the membrane proteins may also relate to the discovery that protein modifications similar to the pH-dependent, thermotropic changes described can be induced isothermally by imposition of alkali cation gradients across the walls of sealed membrane vesicles (101). The data suggest that hyperthermic effects on membrane–drug interactions or drug permeation through membranes most likely involve membrane proteins or protein–lipid boundaries (103).

D. Membrane Electrochemical Potential

Two aspects of membrane structure and function that directly relate to drug uptake are the transmembrane electrochemical potential and one of its components, the transmembrane pH gradient. All intact cells exhibit a negative transmembrane electrical potential; i.e., the cytoplasmic surface of the membrane is electrically negative relative to the extracellular surface. However, several studies suggest that rapidly dividing cells, including cancer cells, are characterized by a "depolarized" membrane potential (i.e., interior less negative) relative to quiescent control cells (104,105). For example, in the case of SV40-transformed hamster GD248 lymphocytes, the transmembrane potential is −35 mV compared to −48 mV for normal hamster splenocytes.

Another characteristic of many fast-growing tumors is a high rate of aerobic glycolysis and a concomitant high rate of lactic acid efflux (92,94). Coupled lactate–proton export leads to pericellular acidification. The interstitial fluid pH of glycolyzing tumors can therefore be lower by 0.1–0.4 pH units than normal extracellular pH (e.g., see 106). Since intracellular pH remains near neutrality, because of lactate efflux (e.g., see 107), a transmembrane pH gradient is established.

Many drugs of importance in tumor chemotherapy are organic anions or cations with appreciable lipophilic character. Of immediate interest therefore is the fact that the transmembrane distributions of lipophilic cations or anions are in part dependent on the cell membrane potential. Indeed, measurements of such ion distributions have been used to quantitate the membrane potential of diverse cells (e.g., see 108). The membrane potential E_m is related to the distribution of the cation triphenylmethylphosphonium (TPMP), for example, according to the equation

$$E_m \text{ (mV)} = -58 \log ([\text{TPMP}_{in}]/[\text{TPMP}_{ex}]) \tag{1}$$

and of the anion thiocyanate (SCN) according to the equation

$$E_m \text{ (mV)} = -58 \log ([\text{SCN}_{ex}]/[\text{SCN}_{in}]) \tag{2}$$

As the membrane potential becomes more negative (hyperpolarized), the intracellular TPMP concentration will increase and the intracellular SCN concentration will decrease. Lipophilic cationic or anionic drugs should also distribute across the cell membrane according to the transmembrane potential.

Lipophilic weak acids (e.g., acetate) and bases (e.g., methylamine) have also been used to measure pH gradients across the plasma membranes of cells (109) and isolated membrane vesicles (110). As shown in Fig. 2, weak acids will concentrate in alkaline compartments, whereas weak bases will localize in an acid environment. Lipophilic weak-acid drugs (e.g., aspirin and chlorambucil) and weak-base drugs (e.g., mechlorethanine) will also distribute according to the direction of transmembrane pH gradients.

The above considerations provide a rationale for the movement of some drugs across cell membranes. Of more significance to an eventual clinical application is that the membrane potentials of normal and tumor cells respond differently to temperatures in the hyperthermic range (105,111,112). Figure 3 compares the membrane potential of SV40-transformed GD248 lymphocytes with that of nor-

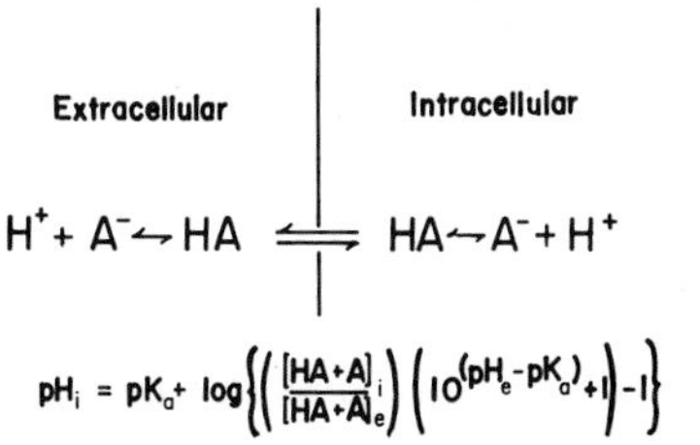

Extracellular | **Intracellular**

$$H^+ + A^- \leftrightarrows HA \rightleftharpoons HA \leftrightarrows A^- + H^+$$

$$pH_i = pK_a + \log\left\{\left(\frac{[HA+A]_i}{[HA+A]_e}\right)\left(10^{(pH_e - pK_a)} + 1\right) - 1\right\}$$

Fig. 2. Measurement of intracellular pH with weak acids. Theory and experimental details are described in Mikkelsen *et al.* [110]. The basic premise of the technique is that the conjugate base (A^-) is impermeable to the membrane, whereas the acid (HA) as an uncharged lipophilic agent is permeable. Thus the transmembrane distribution of A ($HA + A^-$) will depend on the transmembrane pH according to the Henderson-Hasselbalch equation. pH_i = intracellular pH; pH_e = extracellular pH; pK_a = association constant of weak acid.

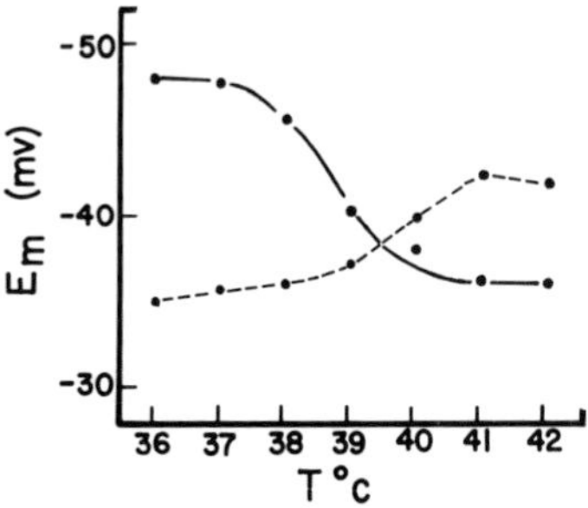

Fig. 3. Thermosensitivity of membrane potential of normal and SV40-transformed hamster lymphocytes. Cells were incubated at designated temperatures for 60 minutes at 10^7 cells/ml in the presence of 2.6×10^{-6} *M* [^{3}H]-triphenylmethylphosphonium. At the end of incubation, 0.2 ml of cell suspension was layered over 500 μl of SF1250 silicone oil (General Electric Company) and centrifuged for 1 minute at 12,000 *g*. Radioactivity in the pellet and supernatent solution was determined by scintillation counting. Extracellular and intracellular water volumes were measured with [^{3}H]polyethylene glycol (MW 4000) and ^3H_2O in parallel experiments. Solid line, splenocytes; dashed line, GD248 lymphocytes.

mal hamster splenocytes, using TPMP as a probe of potential. As the temperature is increased from 37° to 40°C, depolarization of the splenocyte membrane potential occurs, in contrast to hyperpolarization of the tumor cell membrane potential. In terms of TPMP distribution, the depolarization of normal cells corresponds to a decrease in the ratio $[\mathrm{TPMP}]_{in}/[\mathrm{TPMP}]_{ex}$ from 7 to 4, whereas hyperpolarization of tumor cells reflects a 1.5-fold enhancement in intracellular TPMP concentration. If an anticancer drug behaves in a manner similar to TPMP, the effect of hyperthermia combined with drug treatment would be an enhanced therapeutic effectiveness together with lesser toxicity for normal cells.

The *in vivo* situation is of course considerably more complicated, since the membrane potentials of different cells may not respond identically to heat. However, both T- and B-cell components of the immune system depolarize in the fever range (105), and with one other normal cell type, the human erythrocyte, fever temperatures also induce membrane depolarization (111).

No direct information is available concerning the effect of hyperthermia on transmembrane pH gradients of tumor cells. However, Poole *et al.* (113), studying glycolyzing Ehrlich ascites carcinoma cells, found that intracellular pH increased and extracellular pH fell as a function of lactate production. Lactate production and export can therefore increase transmembrane ΔpH. Moreover, several studies (cf. 92) indicate that, at hyperthermic temperatures, tumor cell respiration is depressed, whereas aerobic glycolysis is stable and with some tumor cells increased. These results suggest that the relative therapeutic effectiveness of some weak-acid antitumor drugs (e.g., chlorambucil) might be enhanced by hyperthermia on the basis of the elevated lactate production of many tumor cells and its further relative enhancement by hyperthermia.

To date, no experimental evidence has demonstrated that specific drugs respond to the membrane potential of pH gradients of cells by increased or decreased uptake. However, tumor and normal cells differ in these plasma membrane functional parameters, and several drugs exist that have physicochemical properties responsive to the membrane potential and/or pH gradients.

E. Facilitated Glucose Diffusion

5-Thio-D-glucose (5TDG) inhibits transport of D-glucose by competing with the natural sugar in the hexokinase reaction. It can therefore kill tumor cells that derive metabolic energy solely from glycolysis (114,115). Moreover, 40°–42.5°C hyperthermia potentiates tumor cell killing by 5TDG, possibly because of increased drug entry (116). A regimen in adriamycin- and/or daunorubicin-resistant tumor cells which includes hyperthermia and 5TDG might prove beneficial in overcoming drug resistance in certain instances.

References

1. A. W. Norman, A. M. Spielvogel, and R. G. Wong, *Adv. Lipid Res.* **14,** 127 (1976).
2. D. F. H. Wallach, "Membrane Molecular Biology of Neoplastic Cells," Chapter I. Elsevier, Amsterdam, 1975.
3. L. Blau and R. Bittman, *Biochemistry* **16,** 4139 (1977).
4. W. C. Chen and R. Bittman, *Biochemistry* **16,** 4145 (1977).
5. M. Bunow and I. W. Levin, *Biochim. Biophys. Acta* **464,** 202 (1977).
6. A. Cass, A. Finkelstein, and V. Krespi, *J. Gen. Physiol.* **56,** 125 (1970).
7. R. Holz and A. Finkelstein, *J. Gen. Physiol.* **56,** 125 (1970).
8. A. Finkelstein and R. Holz, *in* "Membranes: Lipid Bilayers and Antibiotics" (G. Eisenman, ed.) p. 378. Dekker, New York, 1973.
9. T. H. Gouge and V. T. Andriole, *J. Lab. Clin. Med.* **78,** 713 (1971).
10. P. R. Steinmetz, Q. Al-Aquate, and W. D. Lawton, *Am. J. Med. Sci.* **271,** 40 (1976).
11. J. T. Finn, L. H. Cohen, and P. R. Steinmetz, *Kidney Int.* **11,** 261 (1977).
12. Y. Lange and J. S. D'Alessandro, *Biochemistry* **16,** 4439 (1977).
13. Y. Lange, G. M. Cohen, and M. J. Poznansky, *Proc. Natl. Acad. Sci. U.S.A.* **74,** 1538 (1977).
14. F. J. Schiffman and I. Klein, *Nature (London)* **269,** 65 (1977).
15. G. M. Hahn, G. C. Li, and E. Shiu, *Cancer Res.* **37,** 761 (1977).
16. D. Amati and C. Lago, *Nature (London)* **247,** 466 (1974).
17. D. Amati and C. Lago, *Cold Spring Harbor Symp. Quant. Biol.* **39,** 371 (1975).
18. C. Lago, B. Sartorius, D. Framontano, and P. Amati, *J. Cell. Physiol.* **92,** 265 (1977).
19. S. P. Verma, R. Schmidt-Ullrich, W. S. Thompson, and D. F. H. Wallach, *Cancer Res.* **37,** 3490 (1977).
20. J. E. Alouf, *in* "The Specificity and Action of Animal Bacterial and Plant Toxins" (P. Cuatrecasas, ed.) p. 221. Chapman & Hall, London, 1977.
21. J. Connolly, V. I. Kalnins, D. W. Cleveland, and M. W. Kirschner, *Proc. Natl. Acad. Sci. U.S.A.* **74,** 2437 (1977).
22. R. L. Margolis and L. Wilson, *Proc. Natl. Acad. Sci. U.S.A.* **74,** 3466 (1977).

23. S. B. Horwitz, *in* "Molecular Actions and Targets for Cancer Chemotherapy" (A. C. Sartorelli, J. S. Lazo, and J. R. Bertino, eds.). Academic Press, New York, 1980.
24. B. Bhattacharyya and J. Wolff, *Nature* (*London*) **264,** 576 (1977).
25. H. P. Zenner and F. Pfeuffer, *Eur. J. Biochem.* **71,** 177 (1976).
26. F. Wunderlich, R. Miller, and V. Speth, *Science* **182,** 1136 (1973).
27. L. Furcht and R. E. Scott, *Exp. Cell Res.* **96,** 271 (1975).
28. L. T. Furcht, R. E. Scott, and P. B. Maercklein, *Cancer Res.* **36,** 4584 (1977).
29. G. J. Goldenberg, C. L. Vanstone, I. G. Israils, D. Ilse, and I. Bihler, *Cancer Res.* **30,** 2285 (1970).
30. G. J. Goldenberg, C. L. Vanstone, and I. Bihler, *Science* **172,** 1148 (1971).
31. G. J. Goldenberg, R. M. Lyons, J. A. Lepp, and C. L. Vanstone, *Cancer Res.* **31,** 1616 (1971).
32. M. K. Wolpert and R. W. Ruddon, *Cancer Res.* **29,** 873 (1969).
33. M. Inaba and Y. Sakurai, *Int. J. Cancer* **7,** 430 (1971).
34. M. Inaba, A. Morwaki, and Y. Sakurai, *Int. J. Cancer* **10,** 411 (1972).
35. G. J. Goldenberg, *Cancer Res.* **35,** 1687 (1975).
36. G. J. Goldenberg, H. B. Land, and D. V. Mormeck, *Cancer Res.* **34,** 3274 (1974).
37. K. M. Yamada, S. S. Yamada, and I. Pastan, *J. Cell Biol.* **74,** 649 (1977).
38. G. J. Goldenberg, M. Lee, H.-Y. P. Lam, and A. Begleiter, *Cancer Res.* **37,** 755 (1977).
39. A. Begleiter, H.-Y. P. Lam, J. Grover, E. Froese, and G. J. Goldenberg, *Cancer Res.* **39,** 353 (1979).
40. J. S. Stehlin, B. C. Giovanella, P. D. Delpoly, R. L. Munez, and B. A. Anderson, *Surg., Gynecol. Obstet.* **140,** 339 (1975).
41. P. Goss and P. G. Parsons, *Cancer Res.* **37,** 152 (1977).
42. F. M. Sirotnak, *in* "Molecular Actions and Targets for Cancer Chemotherapy" (A. C. Sartorelli, J. S. Lazo, and J. R. Bertino, eds.). Academic Press, New York, 1980.
43. F. M. Huennekens, *in* "Molecular Actions and Targets for Cancer Chemotherapy" (A. C. Sartorelli, J. S. Lazo, and J. R. Bertino, eds.). Academic Press, New York, 1980.
44. I. D. Goldman, N. S. Lichtenstein, and V. T. Oliviero, *J. Biol. Chem.* **243,** 5007 (1968).
45. P. T. Chello, F. M. Sirotnak, D. M. Dovick, and R. C. Donsbach, *Cancer Res.* **37,** 4297 (1977).
46. M. Dembo and F. M. Sirotnak, *Biochim. Biophys. Acta* **448,** 505 (1976).
47. G. A. Fischer, *Biochem. Pharmacol.* **11,** 1233 (1962).
48. F. M. Sirotnak and R. C. Donsbach, *Cancer Res.* **33,** 1290 (1973).
49. R. F. Zager, S. A. Frisby, and V. T. Oliviero, *Cancer Res.* **33,** 1670 (1973).
50. T. S. Herman, A. E. Cress, and E. W. Gerner, *Proc. Am. Assoc. Cancer Res.* **19,** 66 (1978).
51. N. Jaffe, E. Frei, and D. Traggis, *N. Engl. J. Med.* **291,** 994 (1974).
52. I. Djerassi, C. J. Rominger, and J. S. Kim, *Cancer* **30,** 22 (1972).
53. M. S. Mitchell, N. W. Wawso, and R. C. DeConti, *Cancer Res.* **28,** 1088 (1968).
54. M. E. Yatvin, J. N. Weinstein, W. H. Dennis, and R. Blumenthal, *Science* **202,** 1290 (1978).
55. T. Skovsgaard, *Cancer Res.* **38,** 1785 (1978).
56. T. Skovsgaard, *Cancer Res.* **38,** 4722 (1978).
57. D. Bowen and I. D. Goldman, *Cancer Res.* **35,** 3054 (1975).
58. Y. P. See, S. A. Carlsen, J. E. Till, and V. Ling, *Biochim. Biophys. Acta* **373,** 242 (1974).
59. H. Riehm and J. L. Biedler, *Cancer Res.* **32,** 1195 (1972).
60. F. Valeriote, G. Medoff, and J. Dieckman, *Cancer Res.* **39,** 2041 (1979).
61. C. A. Presant, C. Klahr, and R. Santala, *Cancer Res.* **36,** 2988 (1976).
62. G. M. Hahn, J. Braun, and I. Har-Kedar, *Proc. Natl. Acad. Sci. U.S.A.* **72,** 937 (1975).
63. G. C. Li, G. M. Hahn, and E. C. Shiu, *J. Cell. Physiol.* **93,** 331 (1977).

64. C. E. Myers, W. P. McGuire, R. H. Liss, I. Iprim, K. Grotzinger, and R. C. Young, *Science* **197,** 165 (1977).
65. C. DeDuve, T. DeBarsy, B. Poole, A. Trouet, P. Tulkens, and F. Van Hoof, *Biochim. Pharmacol.* **23,** 2495 (1974).
66. A. Trouet, D. Deprez-De Campaneere, and C. DeDuve, *Nature (London)* **239,** 110 (1972).
67. G. Sokol, A. Trouet, J. L. Michaux, and B. Cornu, *Eur. J. Cancer* **9,** 391 (1973).
68. G. Atassi, H. J. Tagnow, F. Bournonville, and M. Wyands, *Eur. J. Cancer* **10,** 399 (1974).
69. E. Hurwitz, R. Levy, R. Maron, M. Wilchek, R. Arnon, and M. Sela, *Cancer Res.* **35,** 1175 (1975).
70. M. Szekerke and J. S. Driscoll, *Eur. J. Cancer* **13,** 529 (1977).
71. T. Kitao and K. Hattori, *Nature (London)* **265,** 81 (1977).
72. B. C. F. Chu and J. M. Whiteley, *J. Natl. Cancer Inst.* **62,** 79 (1979).
73. G. Gregoriadis, *Nature (London)* **265,** 407 (1977).
74. J. H. Fendler and A. Romeo, *Life Sci.* **20,** 1109 (1977).
75. J. M. H. Kremer and J. W. J. Esker, *Biochemistry* **16,** 392 (1977).
76. T. Wilson, D. Papahadjopoulos, and R. Taber, *Proc. Natl. Acad. Sci. U.S.A.* **74,** 3560 (1977).
77. C. LaBonnardiere, *FEBS Lett.* **77,** 191 (1977).
78. S. R. Thorpe, M. B. Fiddler, and R. J. Desnick, *Pediatr. Res.* **9,** 908 (1975).
79. G. L. Dale, D. G. Villacorte, and E. Beutler, *Biochem. Med.* **18,** 220 (1977).
80. K. J. Hwang and M. R. Mauk, *Proc. Natl. Acad. Sci. U.S.A.* **74,** 4991 (1977).
81. L. Huang, K. Ozata, and R. E. Pagano, *Membr. Biochem.* **1,** 1 (1977).
82. R. E. Pagano and L. Huang, *J. Cell Biol.* **67** (1975).
83. F. J. Martin and R. C. MacDonald, *J. Cell Biol.* **70,** 494 (1976).
84. F. J. Martin and R. C. MacDonald, *J. Cell Biol.* **70,** 560 (1976).
85. G. Weissman, C. Cohen, and S. Hoffstein, *Biochim. Biophys. Acta* **498,** 375 (1979).
86. G. Poste, R. Kirsch, W. E. Fogler, and I. J. Fidler, *Cancer Res.* **39,** 881 (1979).
87. G. Gregoriadis and E. D. Neerjun, *Res. Commun. Chem. Pathol. Pharmacol.* **10,** 351 (1975).
88. H. K. Kimelberg, T. F. Tracy, S. M. Biddlecome, and R. S. Bourke, *Cancer Res.* **36,** 2949 (1976).
89. D. Papahadjopoulos, G. Poste, W. J. Vail, and J. L. Biedler, *Cancer Res.* **36,** 2988 (1976).
90. E. Mayhew, D. Papahadjopoulos, Y. M. Rustum, and C. Dane, *Cancer Res.* **36,** 4406 (1976).
91. F. L. Moolten, N. J. Capparell, S. H. Zajdel, and S. R. Cooperband, *J. Natl. Cancer Inst.* **55,** 473 (1975).
92. D. F. H. Wallach, *J. Mol. Med.* **2,** 381 (1977).
93. H. A. Fabricius, H. Neuman, R. Stahn, W. Henklebein, and R. Engelhardt, unpublished observations.
94. P. L. Pedersen, *Prog. Exp. Tumor Res.* **22,** 190 (1978).
95. M. P. Sheetz and S. T. Chen, *Biochemistry* **11,** 548 (1972).
96. V. G. Bieri and D. F. H. Wallach, *Biochim. Biophys. Acta* **406,** 415 (1975).
97. S. P. Verma and D. F. H. Wallach, *Biochim. Biophys. Acta* **436,** 307 (1976).
98. B. Sato, K. Nishikida, L. T. Samuels, and F. H. Tyler, *J. Clin. Invest.* **61,** 251 (1978).
99. S. P. Verma, R. Schmidt-Ullrich, and D. F. H. Wallach, *J. Recept. Res.* **1,** 1 (1980).
100. S. P. Verma and D. F. H. Wallach, *Proc. Natl. Acad. Sci. U.S.A.* **73,** 3558 (1976b).
101. R. B. Mikkelsen, S. P. Verma, and D. F. H. Wallach, *Proc. Natl. Acad. Sci. U.S.A.* **75,** 5478 (1978).
102. E. A. Nigg and R. J. Cherry, *Biochemistry* **18,** 3457 (1979).
103. D. F. H. Wallach, "Plasma Membranes and Disease," Vol. II, Chapter 1 (in press).
104. C. D. Cone, *J. Theor. Biol.* **30,** 151 (1971).
105. R. B. Mikkelsen and B. Koch, *Cancer Res.* (in press).

106. P. M. Guillino, F. H. Franthan, S. H. Smith, and A. C. Haggerty, *J. Natl. Cancer Inst.* **34,** 857 (1965).
107. T. L. Spencer and A. L. Lehninger, *Biochem. J.* **154,** 405 (1976).
108. C. J. Deutsch, A. Holian, J. K. Holian, R. P. Daniele, and D. F. Wilson, *J. Cell. Physiol.* **99,** 79 (1979).
109. A. Roos, *Respir. Physiol.* **33,** 27 (1978).
110. R. B. Mikkelsen, R. Schmidt-Ullrich, and D. F. H. Wallach, *J. Cell Physiol.* **102,** 113 (1980).
111. R. B. Mikkelsen and D. F. H. Wallach, *Cell Biol. Int. Rep.* **1,** 51 (1977).
112. R. B. Mikkelsen, S. P. Verma, and D. F. H. Wallach, *in* "Cancer Therapy by Hyperthermia and Radiation" (C. Streffer, ed.), Urban and Schwarzenberg, Munich, p. 160. 1978.
113. D. T. Poole, T. C. Butler, and W. J. Waddell, *J. Natl. Cancer Inst.* **32,** 939 (1964).
114. M. Chen and R. L. Whistler, *Arch. Biochem. Biophys.* **165,** 392 (1975).
115. R. Whistler and W. C. Lake, *Biochem. J.* **130,** 919 (1972).
116. S. H. Kim, J. H. Kim, and E. W. Hahn, *Cancer Res.* **38,** 2935 (1978).

22

Altered Plasma Membrane Glycoconjugates of Chinese Hamster Cells with Acquired Resistance to Actinomycin D, Daunorubicin, and Vincristine

JUNE L. BIEDLER AND ROBERT H. F. PETERSON

I. Introduction

The basic mechanisms whereby cells acquire resistance to cancer chemotherapeutic agents such as the antibiotic actinomycin D, the anthracycline

MOLECULAR ACTIONS AND TARGETS FOR CANCER CHEMOTHERAPEUTIC AGENTS

ISBN 0-12-619280-4

antibiotics adriamycin and daunorubicin, and various plant alkaloids like vincristine and vinblastine are not well understood despite considerable need of such knowledge for the clinical management of cancer. A variety of *in vivo* and *in vitro* studies have indicated that, for this group of agents, reduced plasma membrane permeability to the drug may be an important determinant of resistance. Alterations of the plasma membrane affecting permeability could have diverse effects on membrane-mediated processes. Therefore identification of the presumably altered membrane component(s) of resistant cells could help in understanding observed resistance-related phenomena as well as mechanisms of resistance development per se. Another important question in regard to this group of agents is whether there are cellular changes, in addition to membrane alterations, which also contribute significantly to expression of the resistant phenotype.

Studies in our laboratory have been directed toward identifying cellular alterations that are concomitants of acquired resistance to actinomycin D, daunorubicin, and vincristine. Our initial approach in these studies has been the experimental development *in vitro* of cells with very high levels of resistance by growing Chinese hamster lung fibroblasts with stepwise increases in drug concentration over a 1- to 2-year period. The rationale for the use of high, nonpharmacological concentrations of drug for the selection of resistant cells is to magnify the cellular changes occurring during resistance development in order to identify them more readily and to facilitate the sorting out of cellular and molecular alterations that are relevant and important in expression of the resistant phenotype from those that are relatively unimportant, inconsistent, or coincidental. Table I lists the cell lines used in the studies to be described.

In this chapter we will briefly survey the literature dealing with mechanisms of resistance to three agents (actinomycin D, daunorubicin, and vincristine) as

TABLE I

Drug-Resistant Chinese Hamster Cell Lines

Cell line	Selective agent	Selective concentration (μg/ml)	ED_{50} (μg/ml)[a]	Increase in resistance
DC-3F	None		0.0024	1
DC-3F/AD II	Actinomycin D	0.1	0.20	81
DC-3F/AD IV	Actinomycin D	1.0	0.91	376
DC-3F/AD X	Actinomycin D	10.0	5.94	2450
DC-3F/DM XX	Daunorubicin	10.0	20.3	883
DC-3F/VCRd	Vincristine	10.0	13	650

[a] ED_{50} is the dose effective in inhibiting cellular proliferation by 50% at the end of a 3-day period of drug exposure.

related to our own observations. We will review our recent findings on altered plasma membrane glycoconjugates of actinomycin D-resistant cells and present new results with cells selected with daunorubicin and vincristine (Table I). Finally, we will describe a newly observed feature of vincristine-resistant cells suggesting that there may be cellular alterations in addition to changes in membrane composition that are specifically involved in the development of resistance to the vinca compound.

II. Evidence of More Efficient Permeability Barriers to Drug Uptake in Drug-Resistant Cells

A. Cross-Resistance Studies

An informative approach to understanding the mechanism of resistance to a particular agent has been assessment of cross-resistance patterns [reviewed in Hutchison *et al.* (1,2)]. Cross-resistance of actinomycin D-resistant cells to puromycin (3,4) and of vinca alkaloid-resistant cells to actinomycin D and daunorubicin (5,6) has been demonstrated for a variety of mammalian cell types, both *in vitro* and *in vivo*. This approach was extended in our laboratory in studies on Chinese hamster sublines with acquired resistance to actinomycin D (7). One subline, DC-3F/AD IV, which exhibited a 376-fold increase in resistance to the antibiotic (Table I), was found to be cross-resistant to mithramycin, vinblastine, vincristine, puromycin, daunorubicin, and Colcemid, in declining order. The data indicated not only a reduced sensitivity of actinomycin D-resistant cells to a wide variety of chemical agents but also a clear correspondence between degree of cross-resistance to an agent and its molecular weight. Furthermore, the higher the resistance level of a subline selected with actinomycin D, the proportionately greater its cross-resistance to daunorubicin and vincristine. These findings suggested that the specific cellular determinant(s) of resistance to actinomycin D also determined response to the other agents which are unrelated in chemical structure and/or mechanism of action. The most likely explanation, based on these and other observations with the Chinese hamster system (Sections II,B and C), as well as on earlier findings of uptake differences in actinomycin D-resistant human cells (8), was that the plasma membrane of the resistant cell had increased efficiency as a barrier to drug entry. Cross-resistance among actinomycin D, drugs of the anthracycline class, and vinca alkaloids is now well documented (9–11).

We have recently assessed cross-resistance characteristics of a vincristine-resistant subline, DC-3F/VCRd (Table I), which was selected *in vitro* from the same Chinese hamster fibroblast cell population giving rise to the actinomycin D-resistant cells, as a first step in the characterization of cells exhibiting a high

TABLE II

Relative Responses of Vincristine-Resistant DC-3F/VCRd Cells to Chemical Agents

Agent	Molecular weight	ED_{50} (μg/ml)	Increase in resistance[a]
Vincristine sulfate	923	13	650
Vinblastine sulfate	930	2.2	512
Mithramycin	1089	30	441
Colchicine	399	7.0	350
VP-16-213	588	7.9	139
Daunorubicin	528	2.1	131
Actinomycin D	1256	0.30	125
Puromycin	471	155	105
Ethidium bromide	394	20	67
Colcemid	371	0.36	28
Hydroxyurea	76	12	5.9
6-Thioguanine	167	0.091	2.1
Arabinosylcytosine	243	0.076	1.9
Methotrexate	454	0.012	1.8
1,3-Bis (2-chloroethyl)-1-nitrosourea	214	2.4	1.3

[a] Ratio of ED_{50} for DC-3F/VCRd to ED_{50} for DC-3F.

level of resistance to a vinca compound (Table II). Results indicate that DC-3F/VCRd cells are cross-resistant to the same agents to which DC-3F/AD IV exhibits increased resistance (7). Although in general, the higher the molecular weight of an agent, the greater the cross-resistance of the vincristine-resistant cells, correlations are somewhat less exact than for the actinomycin D-resistant subline (7). One major exception is actinomycin D itself, to which DC-3F/VCRd cells show only a 125-fold increase in resistance. Whether this result is indicative of an important difference between the two cell lines with respect to resistance mechanisms remains to be elucidated.

Another drug-resistant cell line included in our current investigations is DC-3F/DM XX (Table I). This subline was selected with daunorubicin and is cross-resistant to adriamycin and actinomycin D, the only agents tested (9).

Cross-resistance patterns of cells selected with plant alkaloids, such as colchicine and maytansine, have also been described (12–16). Since these sublines exhibit increased resistance to actinomycin D, vinca alkaloids, and/or anthracyclines, certain features of these cells will be discussed along with our own findings.

B. Drug Uptake and Efflux

A major function of the plasma membrane is to modulate permeability to extracellular molecules. It is not surprising therefore that the membrane acts as a natural barrier to foreign molecules such as antibiotics and plant alkaloids and that enhancement of exclusion efficiency may be advantageous to cells exposed to these agents. The observations of cross-resistance to these widely differing types of agents suggest that alteration of the same cellular attribute(s) controls response to actinomycin D, daunorubicin, and vincristine. Markedly reduced uptake of actinomycin D by highly resistant HeLa cells was demonstrated by Goldstein *et al.* (8) by both autoradiographic and scintillation-counting techniques. Initially, contrasting results were obtained by Simard and Cassingena (17), who suggested that the acquired resistance of Syrian hamster cells in culture was due to a new degradative enzyme and/or alternative pathways for synthesis of nucleolar RNA. This view, however, was later changed in favor of permeability alteration (18). Likewise, Cremisi *et al.* (19), working with the same cell line, concluded that resistance was indeed due to decreased permeability to the antibiotic. Kessel and Wodinsky (6), working with mouse leukemia cells, postulated that resistance was due to lack of retention of the drug. It was subsequently reported by Kessel (20), however, that membrane permeability barriers could account for resistance to actinomycin D as well as to daunorubicin and vinca alkaloids.

Experimental evidence obtained in our laboratory in a series of studies on actinomycin D- and daunorubicin-resistant Chinese hamster sublines (7,9,21–23) has led us to conclude that the primary determinant of resistance of these cells is altered plasma membrane permeability to the drug. In an autoradiographic study of several sublines, the mean number of grains per nucleus for cells exposed to tritiated actinomycin D was inversely proportional to the degree of resistance or cross-resistance to the antibiotic (7). This observation was confirmed by the use of scintillation-counting techniques (22,23); there was an inverse proportionality between drug uptake and degree of resistance to actinomycin for all the sublines listed in Table I. Vincristine- and daunorubicin-resistant cells showed a reduced uptake of actinomycin D corresponding to their degree of cross-resistance to this antibiotic. Autoradiographic determinations with tritiated daunorubicin gave direct evidence of reduced uptake of this agent by both daunorubicin- and actinomycin D-resistant cells (9); actinomycin D-resistant cells, moreover, showed reduced uptake of isotopically labeled puromycin comparable to the degree of cross-resistance to it (22).

The resistance and cross-resistance patterns exhibited by vincristine-resistant DC-3F/VCRd cells likewise indicate a reduced capacity for transport of vinca compounds (Fig. 1). Comparisons of vincristine and vinblastine data with those obtained with actinomycin D, however, are informative. A similar degree of increase in resistance is associated with a relatively lesser decrease in uptake of vincristine than of actinomycin D (Fig. 1), suggesting that the membrane barrier to drug entry may be a somewhat less crucial determinant of resistance to vincristine than to actinomycin D. Our interest in this possibility will become evident from a description of a novel attribute of DC-3F/VCRd cells (Section

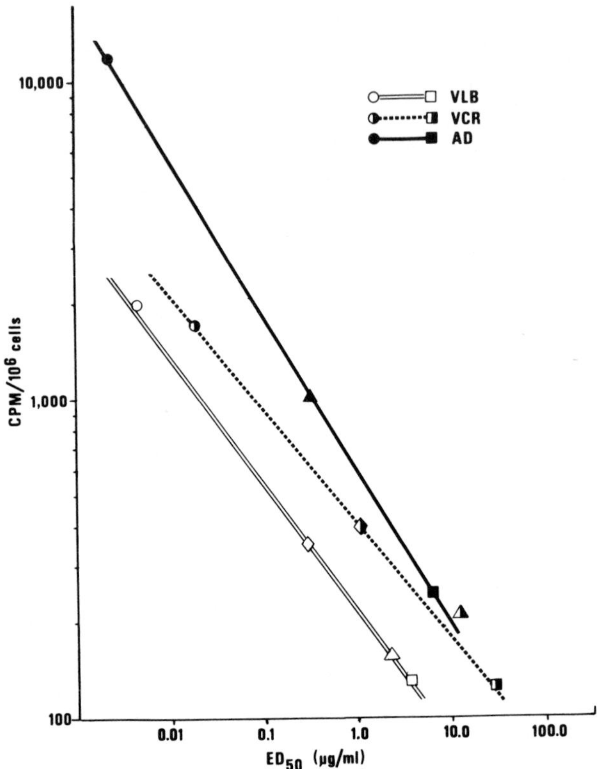

Fig. 1. Relationship between uptake of isotopically labeled drugs and degree of resistance in terms of ED_{50} (see Table I). Uptake was measured in 1-hour experiments as previously described (23). Exponentially growing cells were exposed to 2 μg/ml of actinomycin D (AD) (1.3 Ci/mmole), vincristine (VCR) (0.46 Ci/mmole), and vinblastine (VLB) (0.093 Ci/mmole). Cell lines were DC-3F (○ ◑ ●), Dc-3F/AD X (□ ◨ ■), DC-3F/VCRd (△ ◭ ▲), and the re-revertant clone VCRd-5-U (◇ ◈).

IV). In any event, the delineation of similarities and differences in cellular resistance mechanisms for the pharmacologically heterogeneous group of agents is of potential usefulness in cancer therapy.

Understanding of transport characteristics of sensitive and resistant cells in regard to the group of compounds under consideration is relevant to identification of molecular alterations mediating drug resistance. However, the mode of entry of the various antibiotics and plant alkaloids into cells with acquired resistance to these agents and into tumor cells never exposed to the drug has been investigated in only a few different systems. It was concluded in two independent studies (24,25) that the transport of vincristine and several anthracycline antibiotics was carrier-mediated; there was, however, no indication of an active mechanism. For actinomycin D, likewise, evidence of an active transport system has not been found (22,26,27). Results of studies on colchicine-resistant cells, on the other hand, are compatible with an unmediated diffusion mode (28). It is obvious that much remains to be learned about molecular determinants of drug influx.

A series of recent investigations has emphasized the importance of a somewhat different cellular response to cytotoxic agents. For mouse leukemia P388 cells selected with daunorubicin or adriamycin, resistance to these compounds and cross-resistance to actinomycin D, vincristine, and vinblastine is due primarily to an impaired ability to retain the drug (29–33); results suggest the possibility of a common efflux mechanism. Nevertheless, as pointed out by Johnson *et al.* (31), diminished drug uptake may also play a role in the acquired resistance of P388 cells. Danø (34) has demonstrated the presence of an active outward transport mechanism in daunorubicin-resistant Ehrlich ascites cells. Skovsgaard (35,36) has obtained data indicating that, in Ehrlich ascites cells, resistance to daunorubicin and cross-resistance between this agent and vincristine may be the result of at least two different mechanisms: an energy-dependent drug extrusion mechanism shared by the two agents, and a nonspecific change(s) in the plasma membrane that reduces the influx of both agents. Further knowledge of the efflux mechanism would be useful in understanding and identifying molecular alterations of the plasma membrane involved in resistance associated with decreased drug retention.

Results of our studies on drug-resistant Chinese hamster fibroblasts point to an altered drug uptake mechanism as an important determinant of resistance and are in accord with results obtained with colchicine-resistant Chinese hamster ovary cells, namely, the operation of a more efficient, energy-dependent permeability barrier (13,37,38). In addition to substantiating the involvement of the plasma membrane in resistance development, the biological consequences to the cell of the plasma membrane alterations we have delineated are far-reaching (Section II,C). Observations of different mechanisms of resistance to any one drug are commonplace, however. Differences may stem from inherent differences in cell systems, such as species or tissue type, or from differences in mode of selection. *In vitro* selection procedures, where exposure to drug is apt to be continuous and where high drug levels can be attained, in contrast to intermittent, low-dose treatment schedules more representative of the *in vivo* selection method, appear to favor the kind of membrane changes characterizing the actinomycin D-, daunorubicin-, and vincristine-resistant cells described here.

C. Alterations in Cell Morphology and Oncogenic Potential: Phenotypic Reversion

A unique aspect of our drug-resistant system is the marked alteration in cell morphology and growth characteristics *in vitro* and diminution in oncogenic potential *in vivo* accompanying the development of resistance to all three agents under consideration: actinomycin D, daunorubicin, and vincristine (23). Drug-sensitive control DC-3F cells were established in culture from normal Chinese hamster lung tissue (7). By several criteria, DC-3F cells are spontaneously transformed. They are highly tumorigenic when inoculated into the cheek pouch of immunosuppressed Syrian hamsters (23) and regularly produce tumors in nude (athymic) mice. Their morphology is characteristic of malignant cells *in vitro;* DC-3F cells grow in a loose, disordered network and, as cultures age, form large, discrete aggregates loosely attached to the substrate (22,23). During the course of development of the resistant sublines, we began to note transformations in cell morphology and growth patterns. Cells became progressively more oriented and/or flattened, and there was an apparent increase in cell–cell and cell–substrate adhesiveness. When drug-resistant sublines were tested in the Syrian hamster heterotransplant system, all sublines were found to be reduced in oncogenic potential (23). Furthermore, there was a positive correlation between increase in resistance and decrease in tumorigenicity (Table III); highly actinomycin D-resistant DC-3F/AD X cells were nontumorigenic in this heterotransplant system and in nude mice as well. In order to test the relationship between these two parameters, the DC-3F/AD X subline was maintained for a prolonged period in drug-free medium and assessed periodically for resistance and tumor-producing capacity. The DC-3F/AD X-U cells ("U" for untreated) gradually declined in both resistance and tumorigenicity (Table III) and also regained some of the morphological characteristics of control DC-3F cells (23),

TABLE III

Tumorigenic Capacity of Drug-Resistant Chinese Hamster Cell Lines

Cell line	Increase in resistance	Tumor frequency (%)[a]
DC-3F	1	82
DC-3F/AD II	81	27
DC-3F/AD IV	376	18
DC-3F/AD X	2,450	0
DC-3F/AD X-U[b]	54	42
DC-3F/DM XX	883	10
DC-3F/VCRd	650	7
DC-3F/A3[c]	108,400	89

[a] Cells were inoculated at 1×10^6 cells per cheek pouch in 19–44 individual pouches for each cell line (23).

[b] After 3 years of growth in drug-free medium, the ED_{50} was 0.13 μg/ml of actinomycin D.

[c] DC-3F/A3 cells were selected with methotrexate (see Table VI).

thus substantiating the observed correlations between resistance, oncogenicity, and morphology.

An important question is whether or not the triumvirate of phenotypic changes observed for Chinese hamster cells is somehow unique to drug-resistant sublines derived from spontaneously transformed cells of this species. To test the generality of the phenotypic reversion phenomenon, cells established in culture from a hydrocarbon-induced mouse tumor were cloned and selected with actinomycin D, ethidium bromide, and vincristine. The drug-resistant murine lines likewise manifested striking morphological alteration and reduction in oncogenic potential (39,40). Like the drug-resistant Chinese hamster cells, resistant sublines derived from several different clones (EPO, MAZ, QUA) showed a reduced capacity for uptake of actinomycin D correlated with their degree of resistance or cross-resistance to the antibiotic (Table IV). These findings with tumor-derived cells indicate the generality of the phenomenon: Development of high levels of resistance associated with impaired drug uptake regularly leads to suppression of the malignant phenotype.

The Chinese hamster as well as mouse cells with acquired resistance to chemotherapeutic agents in the molecular-weight range of about 350–1250, and exhibiting reduced uptake of actinomycin D, puromycin, daunorubicin, vincristine, and/or vinblastine, may be classified as permeability variants or mutants without inference, much less knowledge, as to origin. Because of their manifested reversion to more normal (less malignant) phenotypes, they may also be classified as revertants without implication of any particular mechanism or pathway. (In this context the DC-3F/AD X-U subline that partially regained certain features of progenitor control cells, such as drug sensitivity and oncogenicity, will of necessity be referred to as a re-revertant.)

In other laboratories means have been devised for selecting cells with reduced tumorigenicity from transformed or tumor-derived cells in culture and from transplantable tumors as well. For example, back-variants or revertants with lowered tumorigenicity, increased growth control in culture, and a more normal morphology were indirectly selected with 5-fluoro-2′-deoxyuridine from SV40 transformants as reported by Pollack *et al.* (41). Rabinowitz and Sachs (42,43) described revertants derived from hamster cell clones transformed by polyomavirus and by dimethylnitrosamine, and Stephenson *et al.* (44) characterized revertants of mammalian cells transformed by avian and murine sarcoma viruses. Loss of tumorigenicity was frequently accompanied by detectable changes in cell surface properties, such as loss of transplantation antigens (45,46) and a decrease in resistance to agglutination by various plant lectins (47,48). Mondal *et al.* (49) found that less malignant variants of chemically transformed cells were deficient in cell surface antigen(s) capable of evoking humoral and cell-mediated immune responses in syngeneic mice. In contrast, Silagi *et al.*

TABLE IV

Drug Resistance, Actinomycin D Uptake, and Tumorigenicity of C57BL/6 Mouse Cell Lines

Cell line	Selective agent	Selective concentration (μg/ml)	Increase in resistance	[^{3}H]-labeled AD uptake (cpm/10^6 cells)[a]	Tumor frequency (%)[b]	
					2×10^5-cell inoculum	2×10^6-cell inoculum
EPO	None		1	31,860	93	100
EPO/ADj	Actinomycin D	0.02	9.7	7,710	11	0
MAZ	None		1	44,220	100	
MAZ/ADs-4	Actinomycin D	0.5	236	1,390	0	0
MAZ/VCR	Vincristine	5.0	308	4,130	10	90
QUA	None		1	32,330	100	
QUA/ADsx	Actinomycin D	1.0	1290	1,770	0	11
QUA/ADj	Actinomycin D	2.0	1548	450	0	50
QUA/EB8	Ethidium bromide	50	867	3,720	25	100

[a] Cells in exponential growth phase were exposed for 1 hour to a total external concentration of 2 μg/ml of actinomycin D (AD) including 2 μCi/ml of tritiated drug (23).

[b] Cells were tested in 10–30 syngeneic mice at each inoculum size. Only progressively growing tumors were scored as positive.

(50,51) found that 5-bromodeoxyuridine-induced suppression of malignancy was linked to increased immunogenicity of mouse melanoma cells owing to enhanced virus production.

Considerable emphasis has been placed on changes in immunogenic potential of drug-treated or drug-resistant cells. Investigations concerning the antigenic status of mouse leukemia cells exposed to and/or resistant to chemotherapeutic agents have yielded somewhat disparate results. There are reports of altered antigenic properties suggestive of new or stronger antigen expression by drug-treated cells associated with their lowered oncogenic potential (52–54). Schmid and Hutchison (55) found that continual exposure of L1210 cells to triazenes resulted in lower growth rates and tumor takes in the mouse; heterotransplantation tests suggested that cells were intrinsically less tumorigenic. On the other hand, Nicolin *et al.* (56,57) demonstrated an increased immune response to triazene-treated cells. From studies on actinomycin D-resistant L1210 cells (58,59), the observed reduction in tumorigenicity appeared related to the budding and release of virus. Nevertheless, the resistant cells showed lowered agglutinability with concanavalin A (Section II,D) and altered surface morphology. These resistant leukemia cells, like the actinomycin D-resistant Chinese hamster cells, appeared to have drug-associated plasma membrane alterations.

Findings of immunogenic changes in other drug-treated cells raise a similar question about our phenotypically revertant drug-resistant cells. Is the reduced tumorigenicity exhibited by drug-resistant Chinese hamster and mouse cells due to increases in cellular immunogenicity? All the data obtained so far indicate that this is not the case. Chinese hamster cells were tested in Syrian hamsters receiving cortisone acetate (23). Thus cells were inoculated at a permissive site in immunosuppressed hosts. In addition. actinomycin D-resistant DC-3F/AD X cells produced no tumors in nude mice even at very high inoculum levels. It could be anticipated that the drug-resistant mouse sublines were even more likely to have undergone drug-induced antigenic change, since the drug-sensitive progenitor cells are known to possess a unique tumor-associated transplantation antigen (40). An enhanced immunogenic capacity could have led to the rejection of resistant cells inoculated into syngeneic hosts. However, transplantation tests on drug-resistant mouse sublines in immunosuppressed hamsters in our laboratory and elsewhere (40), as well as tests on irradiated (40) and rabbit antimouse thymocyte serum-treated syngeneic mice, showed no differences in tumor take or tumor growth from that occurring in untreated animals (Table IV). These results substantiate indications of an inherently lowered oncogenic potential for the permeability variant Chinese hamster and mouse cells with acquired resistance and cross-resistance to actinomycin D.

Results obtained in other laboratories have supported our experimental findings. Wicker *et al.* (60), utilizing a different Chinese hamster cell system (17), observed that both tumorigenicity and ability to grow in soft agar were strongly reduced in actinomycin D-resistant as compared to control cells. Tumorigenic potential of cloned cell hybrids between DC-3F and actinomycin D-resistant DC-3F/AD X cells was tested by Blanchard *et al.* (61) in an independent study. Among clones, resistance was usually associated with reduced or nonexpressed tumorigenicity, whereas drug sensitivity was linked to high malignancy. Also using our Chinese hamster cells, Imbert *et al.* (62) noted an inverse correlation between resistance to actinomycin D and tumorigenicity.

D. Additional Evidence and Summary

Several lines of evidence indicating that altered plasma membrane structure and/or composition most likely accounts for the high levels of resistance exhibited by Chinese hamster cells exposed to actinomycin D, an anthracycline, and a vinca alkaloid were discussed in the foregoing sections and are summarized here. Additional data obtained by several different experimental approaches also implicate cell membrane alteration and provide further understanding of the nature of such alterations and their biological consequences to the cell.

1. *Evidence for Membrane Change*

1. Cross-resistance to a variety of agents unrelated in chemical structure and/or cytotoxic action.

2. Correlations between degree of cross-resistance to a drug and its molecular weight.

3. Reduced cellular uptake of isotopically labeled drugs in proportion to degree of resistance.

4. Potentiation of drug uptake by Tween 80. As reported earlier (21,22), uptake and cytotoxic effect of actinomycin D and daunorubicin are enhanced by the presence of the nonionic detergent Tween 80. In later studies on cells resistant to colchicine and Colcemid, other examples of permeability variant cells, similar results were obtained (28,63,64). It is of interest to note that use of Tween 80 and liposome-encapsulated actinomycin D (see item 6) did not reverse the resistance of adriamycin-resistant P388 cells (29), supporting evidence that for these cells resistance is not due to membrane change.

5. Altered susceptibility to a plant lectin. Actinomycin D-resistant and primary Chinese hamster embryo cells showed low agglutinability in the presence of concanavalin A, in contrast to the high agglutinability of control DC-3F cells and several SV40-transformed Chinese hamster lines (65).

6. Increased cytotoxicity following introduction of lipid vesicle-encapsulated actinomycin D into resistant cells. Papahadjopoulos *et al.* (66) demonstrated that vesicle-mediated uptake of the antibiotic resulted in a 200-fold reduction in the concentration of drug required to inhibit RNA synthesis (22) in the highly resistant DC-3F/AD X cells. These results strongly support the hypothesis that resistance to actinomycin D is due to reduced permeability to the drug.

2. *Nature of Membrane Change and Consequences to the Cell*

1. Marked alterations in cell shape, *in vitro* growth behavior, and cell adhesiveness. These changes are perhaps also indicative of cytoskeletal (possibly membrane-associated) protein changes.
2. Reduced oncogenic potential related to the degree of resistance.
3. Dominant expression of the membrane-related resistant phenotype in hybridized cells. Intraspecific cell hybrids between actinomycin D-resistant cells (DC-3F/AD IV) and a methotrexate-resistant subline (DC-3F/A3) were almost as resistant to actinomycin D, as demonstrated by autoradiographic determinations of drug uptake, as the DC-3F/AD IV input cells (67). Thus the altered membrane property of the actinomycin D-resistant parent appeared to govern permeability to antibiotic for the cell hybrid. A similar result was obtained by Ling and Baker (68) in a study of their colchicine-resistant permeability mutants.

III. Alterations in Plasma Membrane Components

A. Glycoproteins

As summarized in Section II,A–D, a variety of observations and experimental findings strongly indicate that drug-resistant cells have altered plasma membrane permeability properties and suggest that differences in plasma membrane composition in drug-sensitive cells and permeability variants might account for the constellation of phenotypic changes observed, namely, increased resistance, decreased oncogenic potential, and more normal cell morphology and *in vitro* growth behavior.

An obvious course of investigation, when dealing with membrane-related phenomena, is analysis of membrane proteins and glycoproteins. Surface membrane proteins represent structural, enzymatic, and receptor molecules responsible for many functional properties of cells such as cell recognition, cell motility, antigenicity, growth regulation, and maintenance of structure. Considerable emphasis has been placed on glycoproteins, particularly in attempts to discern and understand differences between normal cells and their malignant counterparts (see 69–71 for recent reviews). Our malignant, drug-sensitive Chinese hamster cells and drug-resistant derivatives exhibiting a suppressed tumor phenotype can be considered in this context. However, although we observed clearly defined glycopeptide differences between tumorigenic DC-3F cells and the phenotypic revertants selected by the chemotherapeutic agents under study, we have gained no understanding of how these differences may relate to the observed differences in oncogenic potential.

For investigation of possible differences in plasma membrane glycoprotein composition, we isolated plasma membranes of cells metabolically labeled with

[^{3}H]glucosamine by the method of Atkinson and Summers (72), modified in our laboratory for substrate-attached cells. Membranes were purified on two cycles of discontinuous sucrose gradients and analyzed by sodium dodecyl sulfate polyacrylamide gel electrophoresis (SDS-PAGE) according to the procedure of Laemmli (73). These analyses showed that sensitive control DC-3F cells displayed a prominent glycoprotein peak with an apparent molecular weight of 100,000, whereas the predominant glycoprotein species of highly actinomycin D-resistant DC-3F/AD X cells had a molecular weight of 150,000 (74). We have now extended these observations. The re-revertant DC-3F/AD X-U cells, grown in the absence of drug for over 3 years and exhibiting only a low level of resistance to actinomycin D (Table III), regained the 100K glycopeptide component as the most prominent membrane species (Fig. 2). The daunorubicin- and

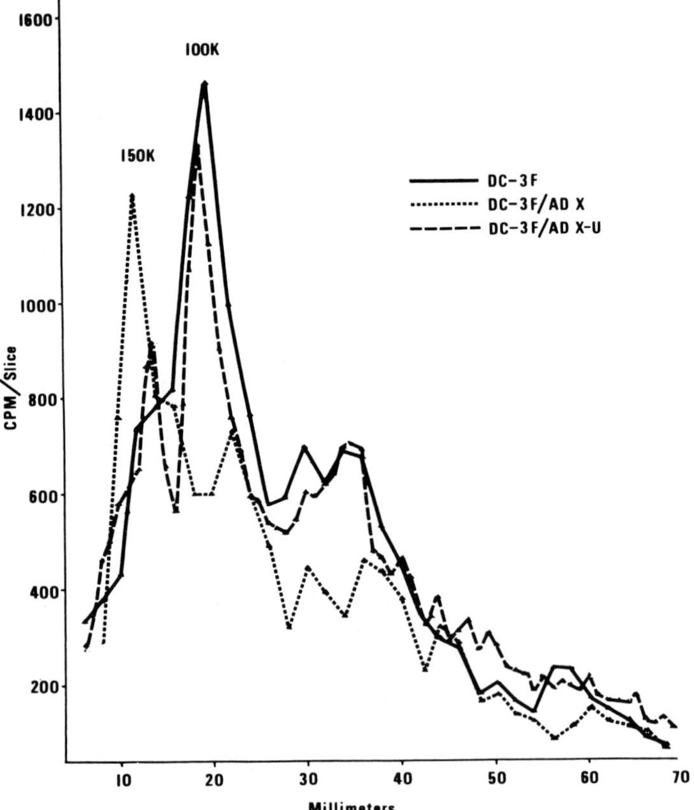

Fig. 2. Glycopeptide profiles obtained by SDS-PAGE of plasma membranes isolated from control and actinomycin D-resistant cells metabolically labeled with 0.2 μCi/ml of [^{3}H]-glucosamine as described previously (74). Molecular weights were determined from markers run on replicate 10% gels stained with Coomassie blue.

vincristine-resistant sublines were similarly examined; a representative comparison of parental DC-3F and resistant DC-3F/VCRd cells is shown in Fig. 3. These sublines display relatively more of the 150K glycoprotein component than the DC-3F control.

Quantitative assessments of the most abundant plasma membrane glycopeptides, based on a large series of independent experiments, indicate that all the resistant sublines express the 150K peptides as a major component, whereas control and re-revertant DC-3F/AD X-U cells have a relative abundance of the 100K component and little of the 150K component (Table V). Furthermore, the only consistent differences between control and resistant cells is in these polypeptides (Fig. 4). These data also provide evidence of a relationship between the degree of drug resistance and the relative amount of the 150K component; this

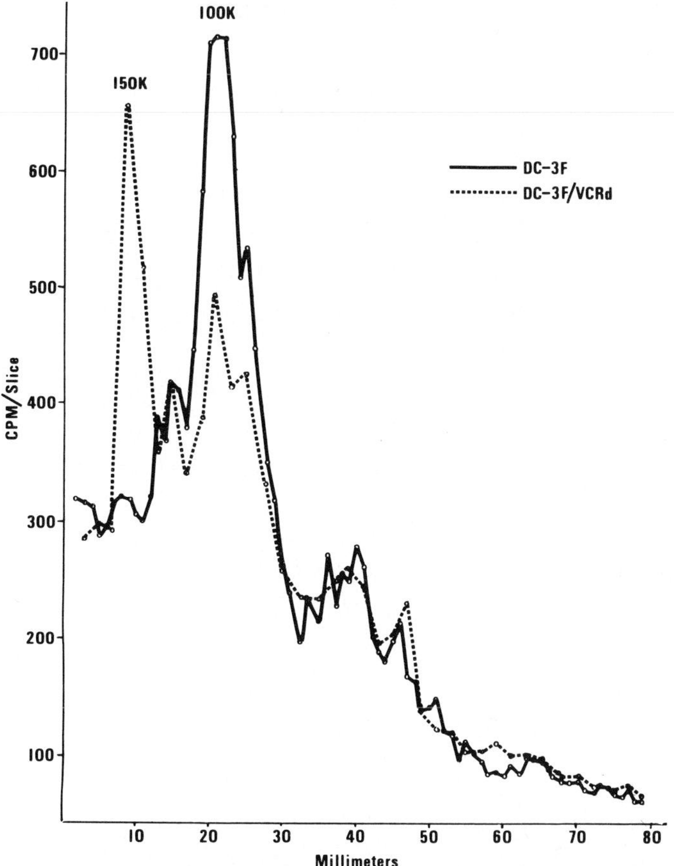

Fig. 3. SDS-PAGE of DC-3F control and vincristine-resistant cells. (See legend for Fig. 2.)

TABLE V

Distribution of Plasma Membrane Glycopeptides of Drug-Sensitive DC-3F Cells and Drug-Resistant Sublines

Cell line	Increase in resistance or cross-resistance to actinomycin D	Number of membrane isolates	Percent ± SEM[a]					
			170K	150K	130K	100K	90K	75K–20K
DC-3F	1	6	7 ± 3	9 ± 2	15 ± 2	30 ± 2	10 ± 2	29 ± 3
DC-3F/AD IV	376	4		21 ± 4	16 ± 2	21 ± 3	12 ± 1	30 ± 3
DC-3F/AD X	2450	8	6 ± 1	26 ± 2	14 ± 1	15 ± 1	8 ± 3	31 ± 2
DC-3F/AD X-U	54	2	3	8	15	24	9	41
DC-3F/DM XX	279	7	7 ± 2	16 ± 2	17 ± 4	21 ± 5	11 ± 1	28 ± 2
DC-3F/VCRd	125	8	8 ± 1	14 ± 2	13 ± 1	22 ± 2	11 ± 2	32 ± 3

[a] The percent distribution of glycopeptides was derived from estimates of area under the most prominent peaks in profiles obtained after SDS-PAGE analysis (see, for example, Figs. 2 and 3). The 75K–20K regions comprise five to eight small peaks.

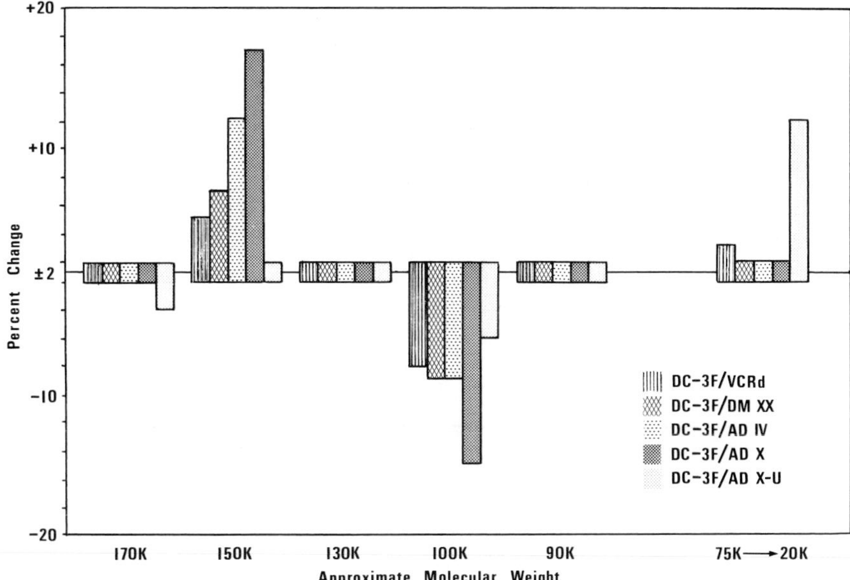

Fig. 4. Difference in relative amounts of glucosamine-labeled polypeptides in drug-resistant sublines and the re-revertant DC-3F/AD X-U cell line grown in drug-free medium, as compared to control DC-3F cells (see Table V). In each molecular weight set resistant sublines are arranged in increasing order of resistance to actinomycin D.

correlation is particularly close when based on the degree of resistance or cross-resistance to actinomycin D itself (Table V and Fig. 4). In cells with the highest level of resistance, the 150K species constitutes about 26% of the total membrane glycoprotein.

The results indicate clearly that quantitative alteration in plasma membrane glycoprotein components is a concomitant of resistance development in these cell lines and that a similar set of alterations apparently occurs in cells with acquired resistance to the three different agents, actinomycin D, daunorubicin, and vincristine.

In earlier studies on mouse leukemia L5178Y cells sensitive and resistant to actinomycin D, Kessel and Bosmann (75) found that alterations in glycoproteins accompanied the resistant state. Bosmann (76) reported a greatly enhanced synthesis of glycoprotein for DC-3F/AD X cells, based on increased incorporation of radioactive precursors into plasma membrane glycoprotein, as well as on the finding of increased glycosyltransferase activities as compared to that in the DC-3F control. Results obtained in studies on colchicine-resistant Chinese hamster ovary cells (13,15), however, more closely parallel our own; the resistant cells showed reduced drug uptake and were cross-resistant to a wide spectrum of chemical agents correlating strongly with reduced permeability to the drug. Surface labeling via the galactose oxidase–borohydride technique and metabolic labeling with glucosamine followed by membrane isolation and SDS-PAGE analysis revealed the presence of a 170,000-molecular-weight surface carbohydrate-containing component in resistant cells but not in the drug-sensitive progenitors (77). Furthermore, the relative amount of this glycoprotein was correlated with the degree of resistance for a number of independently derived resistant sublines and a revertant clone (78). In contrast, the two major peaks in control Chinese hamster ovary cells corresponded to apparent molecular weights of 139,000 and 95,000–100,000. A similar analysis of actinomycin D-resistant Syrian hamster cells (17,18) likewise demonstrated a high-molecular-weight component present in resistant cells and not in controls (78). Despite these apparent similarities between our resistant variants and the membrane-altered colchicine-resistant cells of Juliano *et al.* (77,78), these workers did not observe changes in other phenotypic characteristics such as morphology and *in vitro* growth behavior. Possibly the comparatively low level of resistance, a 184-fold increase at most, precludes the sorts of phenotypic changes we have observed. A recent report by Beck *et al.* (79), on the other hand, describes cultured human leukemia cells, highly resistant to vinblastine, that showed a resistance-related increase in a high-molecular-weight surface membrane glycoprotein and an increased tendency to form aggregates during the stationary-growth phase. From such studies as these and from our own findings of glycoprotein alteration associated with resistance to the various antibiotics and alkaloids, we may propose that plasma membrane glycoproteins somehow modulate passage of these drug molecules into the cell and that increased synthesis of a high-molecular-weight species renders the cell less permeable to the drug. Perhaps purification of these high-molecular-weight glycopeptides, such as that recently reported by Riordan and Ling (80), will permit informative experiments in this regard.

The literature concerned with the question of glycoprotein differences in normal cells is vast and varied and often of necessarily questionable relevance to our somewhat unique drug-resistant cell system. Nevertheless, several recent observations lend further support to the possibility that the specific plasma membrane glycoproteins distinguishing tumorigenic control (DC-3F) cells from drug-resistant cells with lowered tumorigenicity either may mediate expression of malignancy or serve as markers for malignancy and normalcy. Bramwell and Harris (81,82) reported that the glycosylation pattern, as indicated by lectin-binding experiments, of a 100,000-molecular-weight membrane glycoprotein was preferentially altered in many different types of tumor cells. That this glycoprotein is analogous to the 100K glycopeptide species associated with the malignant phenotype in our cell system is a tenuous but intriguing possibility. In another recent report, Koyama *et al.* (83) describe phenotypic revertant cells, i.e., variant clones of rat tumor cells with extremely low tumorigenicity; these cells showed pronounced differences from tumorigenic cells in the extent of glycosylation of a 150K glycoprotein(s). Whether the differential glycosamine-labeling patterns of the 100K and 150K glycopeptides of our malignant DC-3F cells and the drug-resistant revertants reflect the kinds of glycoprotein alterations described by these workers (81–83) has not been investigated. In any event, their studies and our emphasize the possibility that plasma membrane glycoprotein expression may mark, if not mediate, malignant expression.

B. Gangliosides

Gangliosides, acidic glycosphingolipids that contain sialic acid, are well-defined components of the membrane (reviewed in 84,85). There is now considerable evidence that gangliosides are involved in a number of membrane-related phenomena. They appear to act as membrane receptors for various substances such as glycoprotein hormones, interferon, and toxins (85); G_{M1}, for example, is a highly specific receptor for cholera toxin. Gangliosides also appear to be altered during malignant transformation. The most frequent finding, for cell lines transformed by tumor viruses, tumor cells both *in vivo* and *in vitro,* and spontaneously transformed cells in culture, has been that of simplification in ganglioside expression. The extensive series of investigations dealing with the role of ganglioside alteration in malignancy (reviewed in 86,87), coupled with our own observations of malignancy suppression in drug-resistant permeability variants (Section IIC), impelled us to investigate the possible involvement of ganglioside alteration in resistance development.

In initial studies in our laboratory, we examined the ganglioside content of control DC-3F cells and the highly actinomycin D-resistant DC-3F/AD X cells (88). For this purpose cultures were grown for 4–5 days in the presence of [^{14}C]glucosamine, and gangliosides were extracted (89) and separated by thin-layer chromatography. Analyses showed that DC-3F cells expressed a full complement of gangliosides from hematosides to disialogangliosides (Fig. 5), hematosides (G_{M3}) being the least abundant species by far. DC-3F/AD X cells, in contrast, exhibited only hematosides (G_{M3}). To determine whether or not the pattern of ganglioside synthesis exhibited by control cells was influenced by cell culture and environment, we also analyzed tumors produced in athymic (nude) mice by DC-3F cells and found no differences in ganglioside expression. That growth conditions may indeed alter patterns of ganglioside synthesis is exemplified by the studies of Yogeeswaran *et al.* (90); mouse melanoma lines in culture exhibited a simple ganglioside pattern consisting primarily of G_{M3} with traces of G_{D1a}, whereas the same lines grown in the mouse contained the full G_{M3}, G_{M2}, G_{M1}, and G_{D1a} complement. It should be emphasized that the ganglioside composition of the drug-sensitive DC-3F cells, which are tumorigenic and have morphological characteristics of malignant cells (Section II,C), is opposite that of the majority of transformed and tumor-derived cell lines

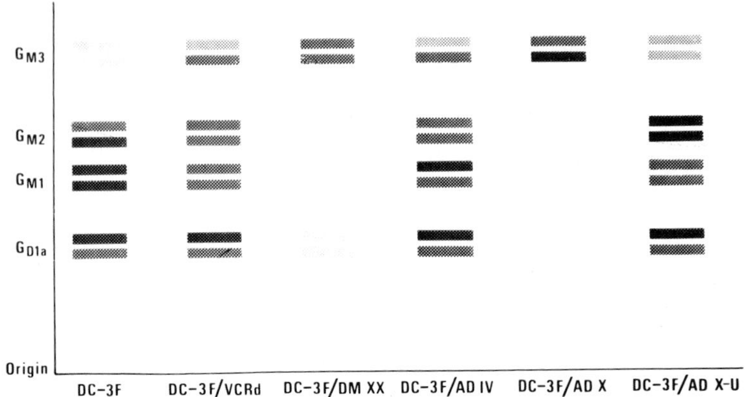

Fig. 5. Diagrammatic representation of ganglioside patterns displayed by control DC-3F, drug-resistant, and re-revertant DC-3F/AD X-U cells. Relative amounts of gangliosides were estimated from radioautograms of gangliosides separated by thin-layer chromatography (88).

that have been described (86,87). However, it should be noted also that there are a variety of exceptions to this general finding (e.g., 90–93). We therefore centered our attention on possible differences in ganglioside composition, as related to type and degree of acquired resistance to the drug, for the various sublines under study.

In view of the striking dissimilarities between DC-3F and DC-3F/AD X cells with respect to ganglioside pattern, it was of interest to examine the re-revertant DC-3F/AD X-U population. The untreated cell line, which underwent a 45-fold decrease in resistance (Table III), regained the full ganglioside complement characteristic of the control cells (88) while retaining a considerable amount of hematosides. Quantitative assessments of the ganglioside composition of several other drug-resistant sublines are now in progress, and initial results are represented diagrammatically in Fig. 5. The ganglioside pattern of the 883-fold resistant DC-3F/DM XX cells is similar to that of DC-3F/AD X cells; i.e., there is a blockage in synthesis of the higher gangliosides with the exception that the daunorubicin-resistant subline synthesizes trace amounts of G_{D1a}. (Trisialogangliosides have not been detected in any of the Chinese hamster lines.) Vincristine-resistant DC-3F/VCRd cells, like the DC-3F control, express a full complement with, however, minor quantitative differences from the control pattern (Fig. 5). Vincristine-resistant cells and the 400-fold resistant DC-3F/AD IV cells appear to synthesize relatively more hematosides (G_{M3}) than DC-3F. The quantitative differences in ganglioside expression between sublines (DC-3F/AD X-U, DC-3F/AD IV, DC-3F/VCRd) with lower levels of resistance and control cells, in contrast to the qualitative differences exhibited by sublines (DC-3F/DM XX, DC-3F/AD X) with higher resistance levels, suggest that ganglioside expression in this system is a resistance-related phenomenon. There appears to be a threshold effect: Cells with increases in resistance greater than about 1000-fold have simplified ganglioside patterns. Further insight may be gained by analysis of newly developed cell lines with a higher level of resistance to vincristine than is characteristic of DC-3F/VCRd cells. It must be stated once again, however, that the possibility that the changes in ganglioside composition, like the glycoprotein alterations (Section III,A), are secondary phenomena related more to the tumorigenicity alterations of the drug-resistant revertant cells than to the resistance-related permeability alterations per se cannot be excluded at this time. We are aware of only one other study on ganglioside patterns in drug-resistant cells. Like our resistant cells, however, the actinomycin D-resistant Syrian hamster cells (17) investigated by Nigam *et al.* (94) underwent phenotypic reversion, and the relationship between change in ganglioside pattern and permeability alteration is thus inconclusive with regard to the possible relationships between drug resistance development and plasma membrane ganglioside altera tion.

IV. Homogeneously Staining Metaphase Chromosome Region in Cells Resistant to Vincristine

Results obtained in investigations of plasma membrane components of the variously resistant sublines suggest a close link between somewhat nonspecific alteration of the membrane and manifestation of altered membrane permeability. However, it is difficult to determine whether the extent of permeability decrease is sufficient to account for the degree of resistance measured. In fact, the results of Papahadjopoulos *et al.* (66) with vesicle-encapsulated actinomycin D suggest that there may be resistance mechanisms in addition to permeability change that contribute to the high level of resistance exhibited by the actinomycin D-resistant DC-3F/AD X subline. Another indication of additional resistance mechanisms, possibly differing for one drug as compared to another, was noted earlier (Section II,B); uptake data suggest that permeability alteration may be a less important factor in resistance to vincristine than in resistance to actinomycin D in our cell system. It is reasonable that prolonged exposure to drug, a multistep selection process, and attainment of high levels of resistance would result in or permit a variety of cellular alterations effecting, in different degrees, the resistant phenotype.

The recent finding of a homogeneously staining region (HSR), as revealed by trypsin–Giemsa banding analysis, on a metaphase chromosome of vincristine-resistant DC-3F/VCRd cells (Fig. 6), but not in DC-3F/AD X or DC-3F/DM XX cells, further emphasizes the possibility of a unique mode of resistance specific for perhaps each of the drugs (actinomycin D, daunorubicin, and vin-

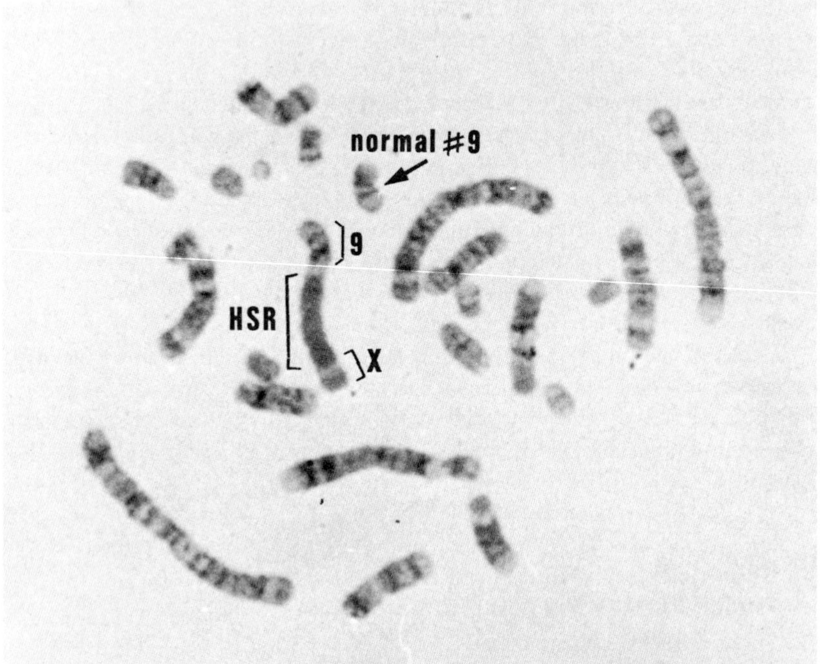

Fig. 6. Giemsa-banded metaphase cell of the vincristine-resistant DC-3F/VCRd subline characterized by one HSR per cell. The HSR-bearing chromosome consists of an apparently entire chromosome 9 followed by an unidentifiable G-negative band at the terminus of the short arm, the HSR, and the distal portion of the late-replicating long arm of an X chromosome joined to the HSR at a point just proximal to the secondary constriction of the X.

cristine), in addition to comparatively nonspecific plasma membrane permeability alteration.

These regions were first detected and described in our laboratory in antifolate-resistant Chinese hamster sublines (95,96) derived from the same cells (DC-3F) giving rise to the permeability variant lines under consideration here. Since HSRs were present only in sublines with the highest increases in target enzyme dihydrofolate reductase, and because of the extreme length (relative to a normal chromosome band) as well as the staining homogeneity of these abnormal regions, we hypothesized that they represented regions of DNA sequence amplification involved in enzyme overproduction. Dihydrofolate reductase gene amplification was subsequently reported by Alt *et al.* (97) and localized to an HSR-like region of Chinese hamster ovary cells by Nunberg *et al.* (98). Evidence of increases in dihydrofolate reductase-specific mRNA and in the number of genes coding for the enzyme in our DC-3F-derived methotrexate- and methasquin-resistant sublines has been obtained in a series of recent studies (99,100); direct confirmation that the HSRs of our antifolate-resistant sublines contain dihydrofolate reductase genes is attendant upon planned *in situ* hybridization experiments utilizing a DNA probe originating from a 650-bp insert cloned from cDNAs prepared as reverse transcripts of dihydrofolate reductase-specific mRNA. There are now several different cell systems where methotrexate-resistant sublines are characterized by overproduction of dihydrofolate reductase and the presence of consistent metaphase chromosomes with expanded regions (96,98,101–103). From these various studies it is clear that HSRs of antifolate-resistant cells signal the location of transcriptionally active genes and that the gene product is the target enzyme dihydrofolate reductase.

Increasing knowledge of the prevalence, properties, and function of the HSRs in methotrexate-resistant cells enables us to evaluate, in specific ways, the HSRs of DC-3F/VCRd cells. It should be stated at the outset that the vincristine-resistant cells do not overproduce dihydrofolate reductase. In overproducing cells, this enzyme is readily visualized by SDS-PAGE analysis of the cytosol fraction, as displayed on Coomassie blue-stained slab gels (99,104). Efforts to identify, by a similar approach, the putative protein product(s) associated with the HSR of vincristine-resistant cells have not, however, yielded definitive results. Nevertheless, several similarities and differences between the HSRs of the two different drug-resistant populations derived from the same control line are intriguing.

1. *Chromosomal Location*

In a large series of DC-3F-derived antifolate-resistant sublines, HSRs were preferentially localized to the long arm of chromosome 2 (96,105). The HSR of DC-3F/VCRd cells is part of a structurally abnormal chromosome consisting of chromosome 9, the HSR, and part of the long arm of an X chromosome (Fig. 6). We can draw no conclusions about chromosomal locations of HSRs in vincristine-resistant cells on the basis of one cell line. However, at least for this subline, the HSR is not on chromosome 2.

2. *DNA Replication Characteristics*

For several antifolate-resistant sublines, we have determined that the DNA of HSRs is replicated before the midpoint of S phase (96,106). The HSR of DC-3F/VCRd cells is likewise replicated in the first half of S phase. It is clearly not late-replicating and thereby readily distinguishable from the late-replicating X chromosome segment adjoining the HSR (Fig. 6). Early replication of the HSR, in both drug-resistant systems, is consistent with possible transcriptional activity.

3. *Reversion of Resistance and Homogeneously Staining Region Length*

When cell clones isolated from antifolate-resistant sublines were grown in drug-free medium over a 2-year period, resistance, dihydrofolate reductase levels, and the mean length of the HSR declined in parallel (105,107). The quantitative relationship among these three parameters provided strong circumstantial evidence of a relationship between the size of the HSR and the degree of enzyme overproduction.

We have isolated clones designated VCRd-1 and VCRd-5 from the DC-3F/VCRd cell line and have grown them in vincristine-free medium for over a year (Fig. 7). Resistance of VCRd-5 cells has declined progressively with time. The mean length of the HSR in DC-3F/VCRd cells and in the clone before and after growth in drug-free medium was determined in a sample of 15–25 cells (Table

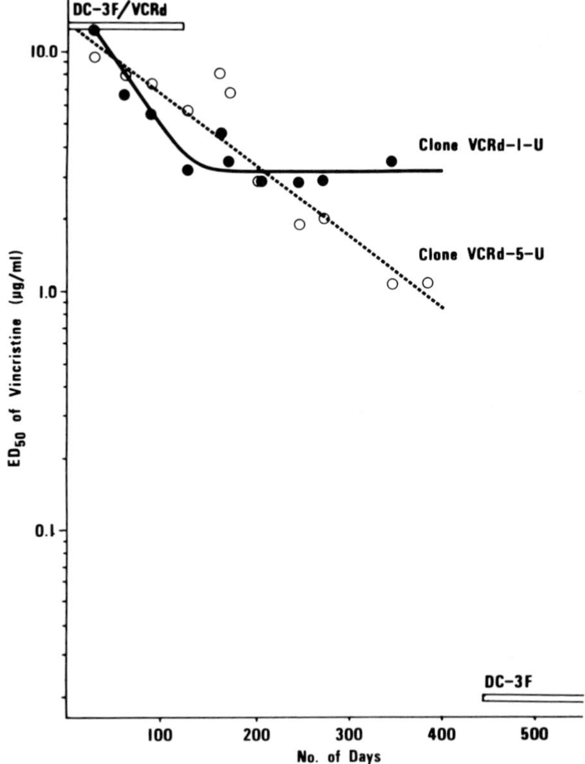

Fig. 7. Decrease in resistance to vincristine, in terms of the ED_{50}, with time in drug-free medium for two clones isolated from the vincristine-resistant DC-3F/VCRd subline. ED_{50} values for the resistant and control sublines are indicated by horizontal bars (see Table I).

TABLE VI

Relative Length of the Homogeneously Staining Region in Cell Lines Resistant to Vincristine or Antifolate and in Clones Grown in Drug-Free Medium

Cell line	Increase in resistance	HSR length ± SEM: Relative to chromosome 2p	HSR length ± SEM: Percent of complement	Number of gene copies[a]
DC-3F/VCRd	650	0.58 ± 0.045	2.7 ± 0.27	
Clone VCRd-5	500	0.68 ± 0.028		
VCRd-5-U[b]	55	0.043 ± 0.017		
DC-3F/MQ19[c]	1,585	1.1 ± 0.029	4.9 ± 0.23	120
DC-3F/A3[c]	108,400	0.97 ± 0.025	3.9 ± 0.11	53
A3-P-U[c]	179	0		7

[a] Dihydrofolate reductase gene copy number was determined by comparing $C_0t_{\frac{1}{2}}$ values, obtained with use of a cDNA probe specific for dihydrofolate reductase mRNA, with the $C_0t_{\frac{1}{2}}$ value established for DC-3F which is considered to represent a single gene equivalent (100).

[b] Resistance was measured when cells had been grown for 324 days in drug-free medium (see Fig. 7). At this time 9/15 cells were HSR-negative.

[c] The sublines resistant to methasquin (MQ) and methotrexate (A) are described elsewhere (105). A3-P-U is a clonal derivative of the DC-3F/A3 subline maintained in methotrexate-free medium for about 2 years, which showed a marked decrease in resistance and target enzyme dihydrofolate reductase activity (105,107).

VI) as described for antifolate-resistant cells (105). A 9-fold decrease in resistance was accompanied by a 16-fold decrease in the mean length of the HSR; about 60% of the cells were HSR-negative after 11 months. These findings indicate a positive correlation between degree of resistance to the vinca compound and HSR length and suggest that in this system, as for antifolate-resistant cells, the HSR is a consequence of the selection pressure imposed by vincristine.

The similarities in cytological and behavioral properties of the HSRs in the two different drug-resistant systems are strong. The reversion properties of the VCRd clone in the presence and absence of drug are highly suggestive of DNA sequence amplification and loss in these cells, as in antifolate-resistant cells. As noted earlier, a major step in gaining understanding of the HSR phenomenon exhibited by the vincristine-resistant cell lines would be identification of a protein overproduced in resistant cells as compared to controls.

Long-term untreated VCRd-5-U cells now have a morphology that is intermediate between that of DC-3F and their resistant parent cells, as was also observed for the re-revertant DC-3F/AD X-U cells (23); tumorigenicity has not been assessed. Drug uptake studies, however, indicated a decrease in the permeability impairment manifested by the highly resistant DC-3F/VCRd subline

(Fig. 1). Although it is by no means excluded that an increased synthesis of some plasma membrane component, such as the 150K glycoprotein species described in Section III,A, is related to HSR formation in vincristine-resistant cells, the absence of HSRs in the actinomycin D- and daunorubicin-resistant sublines makes this an unlikely explanation. Overproduction, in vincristine-resistant cells specifically, of other membrane-associated proteins such as fibronectin and collagen is to be considered. However, if HSR formation is associated with increases in these proteins, it appears unlikely that they would mediate drug permeability to a significant extent only in (HSR-containing) vincristine-resistant cells. Correlations between drug uptake and resistance (Fig. 1) are suggestive of membrane alteration common to all three antibiotic- and alkaloid-resistant lines, whereas the HSR is found in only the latter. Other candidate proteins include tubulin and microtubule-associated proteins because of known interactions of vinca alkaloids with tubulin (108); studies to assess these possibilities are in progress in our laboratory. Of possible relevance in this regard is the report by Ling *et al.* (109) that Colcemid-resistant cells appear to synthesize selectively a tubulin with altered drug-binding properties. Assuming that there is indeed a protein product encoded by amplified genes contained in the HSR of the vincristine-resistant cells, and assuming that gene size and/or size of the amplification unit [calculably larger, for example, than the dihydrofolate reductase gene itself (98)] are similar in magnitude in the two cell systems, we can estimate the degree of increase in the putative gene product. Using mean HSR length relative to average gene copy number in two antifolate-resistant sublines, we arrive at the necessarily crude estimate of a 59-fold increase in a protein(s) in clonal VCRd-5 cells (Table VI).

The gene amplification phenomena of antifolate-resistant cells and the amplification of genes coding for a multifunctional protein with aspartate transcarbamylase activity in *N*-(phosphonacetyl)-L-aspartate (PALA)-resistant cells (110) are now well established. Whether the HSR-containing vincristine cells represent a third example of selective gene amplification in a drug-resistant cell system awaits clarification.

V. Summary and Overview

In the foregoing sections we have described our studies on the development of resistance to three different cancer chemotherapeutic agents. As mentioned at the outset, very high drug concentrations and an *in vitro* cell system were utilized in a deliberate attempt to attain maximal drug exposure and high levels of resistance and thereby to amplify determinants of drug response in resistant cells. The phenotype of the drug-resistant sublines, derived from spontaneously transformed Chinese hamster fibroblasts, obtained by this approach comprises three essential, interrelated elements: reduced plasma membrane permeability to the drug, morphological change toward a more normal cell type, and reduced oncogenic potential. The association of these elements in the resistant phenotype is a reproducible phenomenon; resistant sublines derived from mouse tumor cells by similar selection procedures displayed the same pattern.

All the data obtained in direct assessments of malignancy in animal hosts have indicated that the drug-resistant permeability variants are intrinsically more normal (less malignant), rather than more immunogenic, than their drug-sensitive counterparts. Since this means of suppressing the tumor phenotype is of theoretical as well as of practical interest in cancer therapy, we are proceding in attempts to identify molecular determinants of the resistant phenotype. Several components of the plasma membrane have been selected as candidate molecules. Comparisons of membrane glycopeptides and gangliosides of cells sensitive and resistant to actinomycin D, daunorubicin, and vincristine have revealed alterations in these glycoconjugates. In all resistant sublines examined, there is a relative increase in a 150K and decrease in a 100K glycopeptide species quantitatively related to the degree of drug resistance. The most resistant sublines, irrespective of the selective agent, also show a blockage in the synthesis of higher gangliosides, in marked contrast to the somewhat exceptional display of a full hematoside to disialoganglioside complement of the tumorigenic control cells. These findings of similar alterations in the expression of membrane glycoconjugates in sublines with acquired resistance to three agents unrelated in chemical structure or mechanism of action are consistent with results obtained in cross-resistance and drug uptake experiments. Thus it appears that these permeability variants share similar membrane attributes, quantitatively altered according to resistance level and determining degree of cross-resistance to other agents.

Relationships between the closely associated phenotypic alterations exhibited by the drug-resistant cells need to be clarified in both molecular and genetic terms. We do not know whether the specific differences observed in glycopeptide composition, for example, mediate drug uptake or reduced tumorigenicity. An interesting possibility is that these are not separable phenomena, that the same group of membrane molecules is involved in the expression of both drug resistance and malignancy. As yet we have no information about how the observed alterations in glycoprotein and ganglioside patterns may be related to each other. An obvious possibility is that the two glycoconjugates share one or more biosynthetic enzymes; this question may be approached experimentally. It is also difficult at this time, despite the advanced state of knowledge of membrane structure and function, to reconcile the observed correlation between drug molecular weight and cross-resistance suggestive of a nonspecific sieving mechanism with the (nonspecific) alterations in membrane glycoconjugates. Perhaps the latter are involved in configurational changes that impede the passage of drug molecules through the plasma membrane. Finally, we do not know to what extent, and for which of the drugs, there are important determinants of resistance in addition to membrane determinants. The observation of an HSR in vincristine-resistant cells underscores the intriguing possibility that a transcribed product of selectively amplified genes may contribute to expression of the resistant phenotype. Identification of molecules determining phenotypic expression will be facilitated. However, even if the process of DNA sequence amplification (and loss) observed in these resistant cells is not related to excessive synthesis of a cellular product, the phenomenon promises to be informative. The presence of an HSR in this permeability variant line, coupled with currently expanding knowledge of the genetics of methotrexate resistance, suggests that the genetics of vincristine resistance will also yield to analysis.

Acknowledgments

The work performed in the authors' laboratory was supported in part by NIH grants CA-08748 and CA-24635 and by The Fairchild Foundation New Frontiers Fund.

References

1. D. J. Hutchison and F. A. Schmid, *in* "Drug Resistance and Selectivity: Biochemical and Cellular Basis" (E. Mihich, ed.), p. 73. Academic Press, New York, 1973.
2. H. E. Skipper, D. J. Hutchison, F. M. Schabel, Jr., L. H. Schmidt, A. Goldin, R. W. Brockman, J. M. Venditti, and I. Wodinsky, *Cancer Chemother. Rep.* **56,** 493 (1972).
3. H. Subak-Sharpe, *Exp. Cell Res.* **38,** 106 (1965).
4. K. T. Wong, S. Baron, H. B. Levy, and T. G. Ward, *Proc. Soc. Exp. Biol. Med.* **125,** 65 (1967).
5. D. Kessel, V. Botterill, and I. Wodinsky, *Cancer Res.* **28,** 938 (1968).
6. D. Kessel and I. Wodinsky, *Biochem. Pharmacol.* **17,** 161 (1968).
7. J. L. Biedler and H. Riehm, *Cancer Res.* **30,** 1174 (1970).
8. M. N. Goldstein, K. Hamm, and E. Amrod, *Science* **151,** 1555 (1966).
9. H. Riehm and J. L. Biedler, *Cancer Res.* **31,** 409 (1971).
10. K. Danø, *Cancer Chemother. Rep.* **56,** 701 (1972).
11. L. J. Wilkoff and E. A. Dulmadge, *J. Natl. Cancer Inst.* **61,** 1521 (1978).
12. A. A. Stavrovskaya, *Byull. Eksp. Biol. Med.* **76,** 112 (1973).
13. V. Ling and L. H. Thompson, *J. Cell. Physiol.* **83,** 103 (1974).
14. P. D. Minor and D. H. Roscoe, *J. Cell Sci.* **17,** 381 (1975).
15. N. T. Bech-Hansen, J. E. Till, and V. Ling, *J. Cell. Physiol.* **88,** 23 (1976).
16. C. D. Aldrich, *J. Natl. Cancer Inst.* **63,** 751 (1979).
17. R. Simard and R. Cassingena, *Cancer Res.* **29,** 1590 (1969).
18. Y. Langelier, R. Simard, and C. Brailovsky, *Differentiation* **2,** 261 (1974).
19. C. Cremisi, G. E. Sonnenshein, and P. Tournier, *Exp. Cell Res.* **89,** 89 (1974).
20. D. Kessel, *Proc. Int. Cancer Congr., 10th, 1970* p. 422 (1971).
21. H. Riehm and J. L. Biedler, *Cancer Res.* **32,** 1195 (1972).
22. R. H. F. Peterson, J. A. O'Neil, and J. L. Biedler, *J. Cell Biol.* **63,** 773 (1974).

23. J. L. Biedler, H. Riehm, R. H. F. Peterson, and B. A. Spengler, *J. Natl. Cancer Inst.* **55,** 671 (1975).
24. W. A. Bleyer, S. A. Frisby, and V. T. Oliverio, *Biochem. Pharmacol.* **24,** 633 (1975).
25. T. Skovsgaard, *Biochem. Pharmacol.* **27,** 1221 (1978).
26. D. Bowen and I. D. Goldman, *Cancer Res.* **35,** 3054 (1975).
27. H. Polet, *J. Pharmacol. Exp. Ther.* **192,** 270 (1975).
28. S. A. Carlsen, J. E. Till, and V. Ling, *Biochim. Biophys. Acta* **455,** 900 (1976).
29. M. Inaba and R. K. Johnson, *Cancer Res.* **37,** 4629 (1977).
30. M. Inaba and R. K. Johnson, *Biochem. Pharmacol.* **27,** 2123 (1978).
31. R. K. Johnson, M. P. Chitnis, N. M. Embrey, and E. B. Gregory, *Cancer Treat. Rep.* **62,** 1535 (1978).
32. M. Inaba, H. Kobayashi, Y. Sakurai, and R. K. Johnson, *Cancer Res.* **39,** 2200 (1979).
33. M. Inaba and Y. Sakurai, *Cancer Lett.* **8,** 111 (1979).
34. K. Danø, *Biochim. Biophys. Acta* **323,** 466 (1973).
35. T. Skovsgaard, *Cancer Res.* **38,** 1785 (1978).
36. T. Skovsgaard, *Cancer Res.* **38,** 4722 (1978).
37. Y. P. See, S. A. Carlsen, J. E. Till, and V. Ling, *Biochim. Biophys. Acta* **373,** 242 (1974).
38. S. A. Carlsen, J. E. Till, and V. Ling, *Biochim. Biophys. Acta* **467,** 238 (1977).
39. J. L. Biedler and R. H. F. Peterson, *Proc. Am. Assoc. Cancer Res.* **14,** 72 (1973).
40. J. Belehradek, Jr., J. L. Biedler, M. Thonier, and G. Barski, *Int. J. Cancer* **14,** 779 (1974).
41. R. E. Pollack, H. Green, and G. J. Todaro, *Proc. Natl. Acad. Sci. U.S.A.* **60,** 126 (1968).
42. Z. Rabinowitz and L. Sachs, *Nature (London)* **220,** 1203 (1968).
43. Z. Rabinowitz and L. Sachs, *Int. J. Cancer* **6,** 388 (1970).
44. J. R. Stephenson, R. K. Reynolds, and S. A. Aaronson, *J. Virol.* **11,** 218 (1973).
45. G. Marin and I. Macpherson, *J. Virol.* **3,** 146 (1969).
46. Z. Rabinowitz and L. Sachs, *Virology* **40,** 193 (1970).
47. M. Inbar, Z. Rabinowitz, and L. Sachs, *Int. J. Cancer* **4,** 690 (1969).
48. R. E. Pollack and M. M. Burger, *Proc. Natl. Acad. Sci. U.S.A.* **62,** 1074 (1969).
49. S. Mondal, M. J. Embleton, H. Marquardt, and C. Heidelberger, *Int. J. Cancer* **8,** 410 (1971).
50. S. Silagi and S. A. Bruce, *Proc. Natl. Acad. Sci. U.S.A.* **66,** 72 (1970).
51. S. Silagi, D. Beju, J. Wrathall, and E. de Harven, *Proc. Natl. Acad. Sci. U.S.A.* **69,** 3443 (1972).
52. M. Kitano, E. Mihich, and D. Pressman, *Cancer Res.* **32,** 181 (1972).
53. E. Bonmassar, A. Bonmassar, S. Vadlamudi, and A. Goldin, *Cancer Res.* **32,** 1446 (1972).
54. D. P. Hovchens, E. Bonmassar, M. R. Gaston, M. Kende, and A. Goldin, *Cancer Res.* **36,** 1347 (1976).
55. F. A. Schmid and D. J. Hutchison, *Cancer Res.* **33,** 2161 (1973).
56. A. Nicolin, A. Bini, P. Franco, and A. Goldin, *Cancer Chemother. Rep.* **58,** 325 (1974).
57. A. Nicolin, M. Cavalli, A. Missiroli, and A. Goldin, *Eur. J. Cancer* **13,** 235 (1977).
58. T. A. Calvelli, J. M. Gallo, D. J. Hutchison, E. de Harven, and J. L. Biedler, *Proc. Am. Assoc. Cancer Res.* **17,** 85 (1976).
59. T. A. Calvelli, E. de Harven, and D. J. Hutchison, *J. Cell Biol.* **70,** 379a (1976).
60. R. Wicker, M.-F. Bourali, H. G. Suarez, and R. Cassingena, *Int. J. Cancer* **10,** 632 (1972).
61. M. G. Blanchard, G. Barski, B. Léon, and D. Hémon, *Int. J. Cancer* **11,** 178 (1973).
62. I. Imbert, Y. Barra, and Y. Berebbi, *J. Cell Sci.* **18,** 67 (1975).
63. V. Ling, *Can. J. Genet. Cytol.* **17,** 503 (1975).
64. A. A. Stavrovskaya, T. V. Potapova, V. A. Rosenblat, and A. S. Serpinskaya, *Int. J. Cancer* **15,** 665 (1975).
65. L. Diamond, K. Kumagai, and J. L. Biedler, *In Vitro* **7,** 263 (1972).
66. D. Papahadjopoulos, G. Poste, W. J. Vail, and J. L. Biedler, *Cancer Res.* **36,** 2988 (1976).

67. J. S. Sobel, A. M. Albrecht, H. Riehm, and J. L. Biedler, *Cancer Res.* **31,** 297 (1971).
68. V. Ling and R. M. Baker, *Somatic Cell Genet.* **4,** 193 (1978).
69. G. L. Nicolson, *Biochim. Biophys. Acta* **458,** 1 (1976).
70. L. Warren, C. A. Buck, and G. P. Tuszynski, *Biochim. Biophys. Acta* **516,** 97 (1978).
71. A. Vaheri, *in* "Virus Transformed Cell Membranes" (C. Nicolau, ed.), p. 1. Academic Press, New York, 1978.
72. P. H. Atkinson and D. F. Summers, *J. Biol. Chem.* **246,** 5162 (1971).
73. U. K. Laemmli, *Nature (London)*, **227,** 680 (1970).
74. R. H. F. Peterson and J. L. Biedler, *J. Supramol. Struct.* **9,** 289 (1978).
75. D. Kessel and H. B. Bosmann, *Cancer Res.* **30,** 2695 (1970).
76. H. B. Bosmann, *Nature (London)* **233,** 566 (1971).
77. R. Juliano, V. Ling, and J. Graves, *J. Supramol. Struct.* **4,** 521 (1976).
78. R. L. Juliano and V. Ling, *Biochim. Biophys. Acta* **455,** 152 (1976).
79. W. T. Beck, T. J. Mueller, and L. R. Tanzer, *Cancer Res.* **39,** 2070 (1979).
80. J. R. Riordan and V. Ling, *J. Biol. Chem.* **254,** 12701 (1979).
81. M. E. Bramwell and H. Harris, *Proc. R. Soc. London, Ser. B* **201,** 87 (1978).
82. M. E. Bramwell and H. Harris, *Proc. R. Soc. London, Ser. B* **203,** 93 (1978).
83. K. Koyama, E. Nudelman, M. Fukuda, and S. Hakamori, *Cancer Res.* **39,** 3677 (1979).
84. S. Hakamori, *Biochim. Biophys. Acta* **417,** 55 (1975).
85. P. H. Fishman and R. O. Brady, *Science* **194,** 906 (1976).
86. R. O. Brady and P. H. Fishman, *Biochim. Biophys. Acta* **355,** 121 (1974).
87. C. L. Richardson, S. R. Baker, D. J. Morré, and T. W. Keenan, *Biochim. Biophys. Acta* **417,** 175 (1975).
88. R. H. F. Peterson, W. J. Beutler, and J. L. Biedler, *Biochem. Pharmacol.* **28,** 579 (1979).
89. K. Suzuki, *J. Neurochem.* **12,** 629 (1965).
90. G. Yogeeswaran, B. S. Stein, and H. Sebastian, *Cancer Res.* **38,** 1336 (1978).
91. G. Yogeeswaran, R. Sheinin, J. R. Wherret, and R. K. Murray, *J. Biol. Chem.* **247,** 5146 (1972).
92. P. T. Mora, *in* "Membrane Mediated Information" (P. W. Kent, ed.), Vol. 1, p. 64. Am. Elsevier, New York, 1974.
93. T. W. Keenan, E. Schmid, and W. W. Franke, *Lipids* **13,** 451 (1978).
94. V. N. Nigam, R. Lallier, and C. Brailovsky, *J. Cell Biol.* **58,** 307 (1973).
95. J. L. Biedler, A. M. Albrecht, and B. A. Spengler, *Genetics* **77,** s4 (1974).
96. J. L. Biedler and B. A. Spengler, *Science* **191,** 185 (1976).
97. F. W. Alt, R. E. Kellems, J. R. Bertino, and R. T. Schimke, *J. Biol. Chem.* **253,** 1357 (1978).
98. J. H. Nunberg, R. J. Kaufman, R. T. Schimke, G. Urlaub, and L. A. Chasin, *Proc. Natl. Acad. Sci. U.S.A.* **75,** 5553 (1978).
99. P. W. Melera, D. Wolgemuth, J. L. Biedler, and C. Hession, *J. Biol. Chem.* **255,** 319 (1980).
100. P. W. Melera, J. A. Lewis, J. L. Biedler, and C. Hession, *J. Biol. Chem.* **255,** 7024 (1980).
101. J. L. Biedler, A. M. Albrecht, and D. J. Hutchison, *Cancer Res.* **25,** 246 (1965).
102. B. J. Dolnick, R. J. Berenson, J. L. Bertino, R. J. Kaufman, J. H. Nunberg, and R. T. Schimke, *Proc. Am. Assoc. Cancer Res.* **20,** 150 (1979).
103. C. J. Bostock, E. M. Clark, N. G. L. Harding, P. M. Mounts, C. Tyler-Smith, V. van Heyningen, and P. M. B. Walker, *Chromosoma* **74,** 153 (1979).
104. S. Shanske, P. W. Melera, and J. L. Biedler, *J. Cell Biol.* **79,** 345a (1978).
105. J. L. Biedler, P. W. Melera, and B. A. Spengler, *Cancer Genet. Cytogenet.* **2,** 47 (1980).
106. J. L. Biedler and B. A. Spengler, *J. Natl. Cancer Inst.* **57,** 683 (1976).
107. J. L. Biedler and B. A. Spengler, *J. Cell Biol.* **70,** 117a (1976).
108. L. Wilson, *Ann. N.Y. Acad. Sci.* **253,** 213 (1975).
109. V. Ling, J. L. Aubin, A. Chase, and F. Sarangi, *Cell* **18,** 423 (1979).
110. G. M. Wahl, R. A. Padgett, and G. R. Stark, *J. Biol. Chem.* **254,** 8679 (1979).

23

Tubulin: A Target for Chemotherapeutic Agents

PETER B. SCHIFF AND SUSAN BAND HORWITZ

I. Microtubules

This chapter will review briefly the current literature on microtubules and small molecules that interact with the subunit of microtubules, tubulin. The molecular pharmacology of steganacin, an inhibitor of microtubule polymerization, and taxol, a promoter of microtubule polymerization, will be discussed in greater detail. The authors recommend other recent surveys of the microtubule literature (1–4).

Microtubules are an important part of the cytoskeleton of eukaryotic cells. They are an integral part of the mitotic spindle, eukaryotic flagella, and cilia and may contribute to the development and maintenance of cell shape. A relatively small class of drugs are capable of binding to tubulin. Such low-molecular-weight molecules have been useful tools in understanding the mechanism of microtubule polymerization *in vitro* and in cells, as well as in understanding cell

MOLECULAR ACTIONS AND TARGETS FOR CANCER CHEMOTHERAPEUTIC AGENTS

ISBN 0-12-619280-4

functions that may be mediated by microtubules. Some of these drugs are extremely useful in the therapy of specific diseases.

A. Structure, Biochemistry, and Polymerization

Microtubules have an outer diameter of approximately 250 Å, leaving a hollow core about 150 Å across, and vary in length from a fraction of a micrometer to several micrometers. They are made up of dimers composed of α and β subunits, each having a molecular weight of approximately 55,000. The heterodimer has a total molecular weight of 110,000 and a sedimentation coefficient of 6S. Guanine nucleotides have been found associated with brain tubulin (5). There are two nucleotide-binding sites per tubulin dimer; one exchanges rapidly with free GTP (the E site), and the other exchanges slowly or not at all with free GTP (the N site). Only the GTP at the E site is hydrolyzed during polymerization. It has been reported that there are single high-affinity binding sites for magnesium (6) and calcium (7) on the tubulin dimer.

Since the discovery of the conditions that support microtubule polymerization *in vitro* (8), an extensive literature has appeared characterizing the polymerization reaction. The most efficient polymerization occurs in organic buffers (pH 6.6–6.9) containing EGTA, magnesium, and GTP at 37°C. Microtubule polymerization is inhibited when tubulin preparations are sedimented at 230,000 *g* for 1.5 hours, conditions that remove structures larger than or equal to 36S but not most of the 6S tubulin (9). The loss of capacity for polymerization was shown to correlate with the removal of rings, oligomeric structures of tubulin dimers. It was proposed that microtubule polymerization *in vitro* required the presence of ring structures as nucleation centers.

Experimental data have been presented that support a nucleation condensation mechanism for microtubule polymerization *in vitro* (10–12). Oosawa and Kasai (13) first described this mechanism for the polymerization of actin. The mechanism predicts that the polymerization reaction consists of two steps; the first leads to formation of a nucleus and the second is helical polymer growth. Growth of the microtubule is favored over the formation of a nucleus, thus rendering the polymerization reaction cooperative. Timasheff (14) has pointed out three consequences of the process. First, there must exist a critical concentration C_c, below which tubulin is found only as tubulin dimers and linear tubulin oligomers. Second, all protein in excess of C_c is incorporated into microtubules. Third, C_c is related to the propagation equilibrium constant K_p^{app} as follows:

$$\text{Tubulin dimer} + \text{microtubule (length } n) \rightleftharpoons \text{microtubule (length } n + 1)$$

where $K_p^{app} = C_c^{-1}$. A measurement of C_c leads directly to the value of the apparent standard free energy (ΔG^0_{app}) of subunit addition to the cooperatively growing microtubule under the specific conditions of the experiment:

$$\Delta G^0_{\mathrm{app}} = -RT \ln K_{\mathrm{p}}^{\mathrm{app}} = -RT \ln C_{\mathrm{c}}^{-1}$$

For tubulin a C_c value of 0.2 mg/ml is required to achieve polymerization.

Repeated cycles of polymerization and depolymerization are used as a method to purify microtubules from brain extracts, although other methods have been described (see 2). The most common procedure was developed by Shelanski *et al.* (15). After two or three cycles of polymerization and depolymerization, this method yields tubulin that is approximately 85% pure. The remaining proteins are microtubule-associated proteins (MAPs) (16). These proteins copurify with tubulin with a constant stoichiometry and promote microtubule polymerization *in vitro*. Two of these proteins have been termed high-molecular-weight (HMW) proteins (MW $>$ 270,000) (17). Another class of MAPs, tau (MW $\sim$ 70,000), also has been studied extensively (18). The function of MAPs is not known, although they appear to be associated with microtubules in cells (19,20).

Microtubule assembly *in vitro* can be easily monitored by a variety of methods. The most common assay is measurement of the turbidity which develops during polymerization. Turbidity is relatively insensitive to the length of the microtubules formed and is mainly a function of the total mass of supramolecular structures present (10). Viscosity (21), sedimentation analysis (10), dark-field microscopy (22), and electron microscopy (23) have been used to quantitate assembly.

Many pathways have been proposed for the *in vitro* polymerization system (see 2). In general, these pathways can be summarized as follows (Figs. 1 and 2). Prior to the initiation of polymerization, tubulin exists as dimers and oligomeric rings. When initiation occurs, the rings uncoil or open to form short protofilaments; lateral and end-to-end association of the protofilament segments occurs. At the same time, tubulin dimers are incorporated into the protofilaments and their ribbonlike lateral aggregates. When the number of protofilaments reaches 13, the ribbon assumes the hollow cylindrical form of a microtubule. Additional dimers elongate the microtubule with one end growing at 3 times the rate of the opposite end (24,25). At steady state, a net polymerization and depolymerization reaction occurs at opposite ends of the microtubule (26). The exact mechanism of the microtubule polymerization reaction *in vitro* is not known, although it appears to consist of two distinct phases, nucleation and elongation (27).

There are two general classes of microtubules in cells: "labile" cytoplasmic microtubules and "stable" microtubules like those found in cilia and flagella (29,30). Stable microtubules are resistant to depolymerization by low temperatures and drugs, which normally block polymerization of microtubules *in vitro*. In living cells, centrioles, basal bodies, kinetochores, and possible other microtubule-organizing centers are thought to be involved in the spatial control of microtubule formation in cells (31,32). However, little is known about factors which may promote, stabilize, destabilize, or depolymerize microtubules in cells.

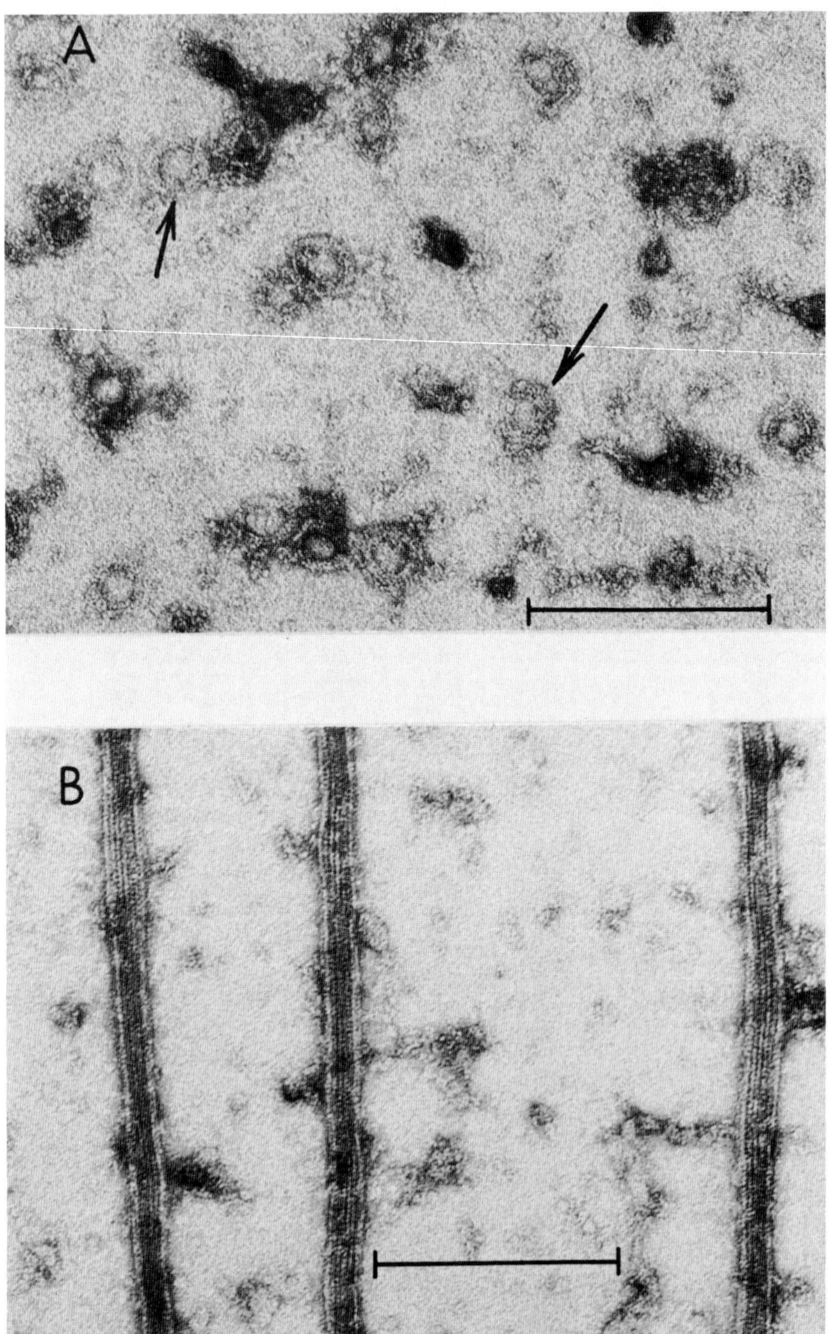

Fig. 1. (A) Electron micrograph of ring oligomeric forms of tubulin at 4°C prior to the initiation of microtubule polymerization *in vitro.* (B) Electron micrograph of microtubules. Structures were negatively stained with 2% uranyl acetate. Scale bar, 0.2 μm.

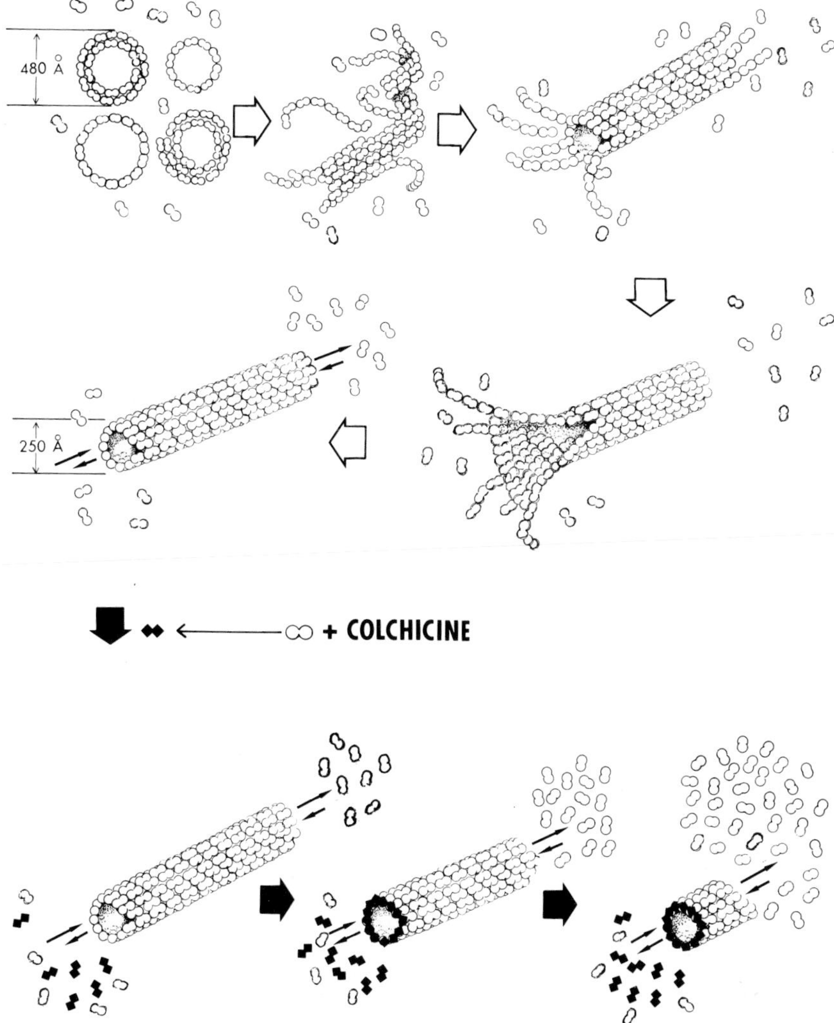

Fig. 2. Proposed pathway of microtubule polymerization *in vitro* (see 2) and the mechanism of substoichiometric poisoning at steady state by antimitotic agents [based on the work of Margolis and Wilson (26,28)]. Before polymerization is initiated, tubulin exists as oligomeric rings and free heterodimers. When polymerization takes place, a steady-state equilibrium is reached and opposite end net polymerization and net depolymerization occur. If an antimitotic drug (such as colchicine, podophyllotoxin, or vinblastine) is added to microtubules at steady-state equilibrium, the drug binds to the free tubulin dimer forming a drug-dimer complex which adds on to the net assembly ends of the microtubules and reduces further dimer additions. Disassembly continues at the opposite end of the "capped" microtubules.

Immunofluorescence microscopy, carried out with antibodies prepared against tubulin, has been used to study the microtubule cytoskeleton in individual cells in tissue culture (33–37). This technique has the advantage of being able to view large numbers of cells with a conventional fluorescence microscope. Interphase fibroblast cells present a characteristic display of cytoplasmic microtubules. The microtubules in these cells can be seen radiating outward from microtubule-organizing centers in the perinuclear region of the cell (Fig. 11A). It has been assumed that the organizing centers are associated with or include the centrioles. Microtubule-organizing structures are resistant to treatments which depolymerize cytoplasmic microtubules, i.e., colcemid and low temperature. There are usually one or two such structures per 3T3 fibroblast cell. When cells recover from colcemid or low temperature, microtubules polymerize from the organizing structures toward the plasma membrane in an ordered unidirectional manner. These experiments have demonstrated that the assembly of cytoplasmic microtubules in the cell is carefully orchestrated.

Many factors may be involved in regulating microtubule assembly in cells. Cyclic AMP (38) or GTP (39) may play a role in controlling microtubule polymerization in the cell. Posttranslational modifications of tubulin or MAPs could also be involved in the *in vivo* regulation of polymerization, and MAPs are thought to play a role in stabilizing microtubules (46,40,41). Calcium alone (8) or calcium and calcium-dependent regulator protein (calmodulin) (42) may also have a function in the depolymerization of microtubules in the cell.

B. Pharmacology

As mentioned in the introduction, many of the drugs that bind specifically to tubulin are useful in the therapy of specific diseases. Colchicine has been used for centuries in the treatment of acute gout, and vinblastine and vincristine are used individually or in combination with other drugs in the treatment of malignancies. However, these drugs are extremely toxic, probably because of their ability to disrupt microtubules and block cells in mitosis.

Colchicine (Fig. 3) is the microtubule-disrupting drug that has been studied most extensively. Synthesis of radioactive colchicine has made it possible to determine that the tubulin dimer has one high-affinity binding site with a binding constant of 2.3 μM (43–45). This site is probably blocked on the intact microtubule (46), although a limited number of sites on either of the two microtubule ends has not been ruled out.

Genetic and biochemical studies have been carried out to ascertain on which subunit of tubulin (α, β, or both) the colchicine-binding site is located. Tubulin isolated from *Aspergillus nidulans* that is resistant to benomyl, a competitive inhibitor of colchicine binding to tubulin (47,48), has been characterized by two-dimensional gel electrophoresis, copolymerization with porcine brain tubu-

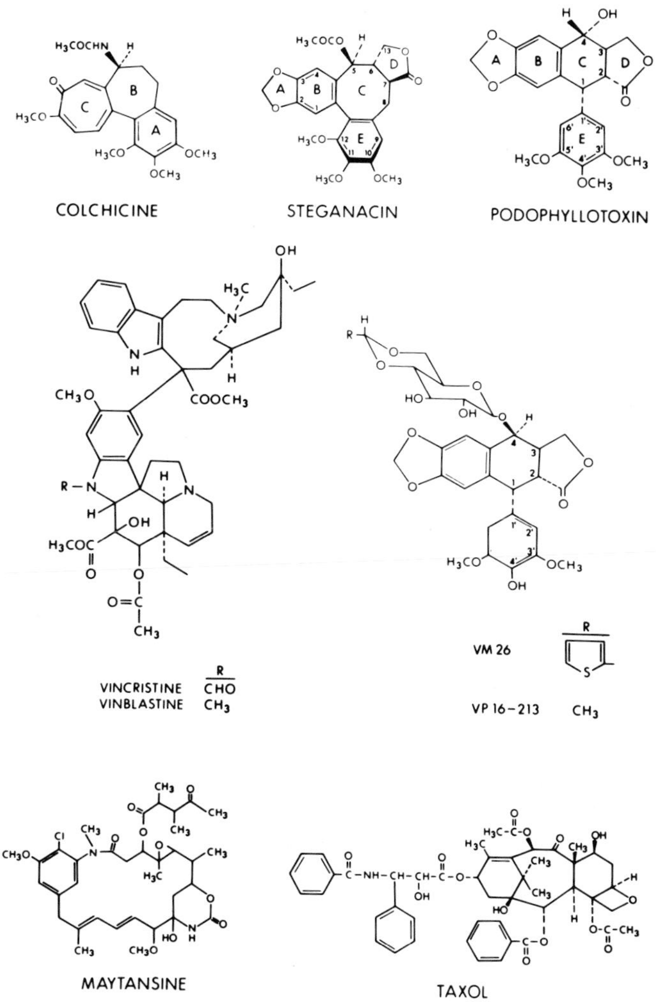

Fig. 3. Structural formulas of colchicine, steganacin, podophyllotoxin, vincristine, vinblastine, VM 26, VP 16-213, maytansine, and taxol.

lin, and peptide mapping (49). It has been concluded that the benomyl-binding site must be located on the β subunit, because of the variety of β-tubulins and the absence of abnormalities affecting α-tubulins seen in the benomyl-resistant mutants. Similar results have been obtained with Chinese hamster ovary cells resistant to colchicine (50). A photoaffinity labeled derivative of colchicine, bromocolchicine, has a high-affinity binding site on the α subunit of tubulin (51). This suggests that the colchicine and benomyl-binding site is located between the

α and β subunits, the benomyl part of the site on the β subunit and the colchicine part of the site near the α subunit.

It has been calculated that colchicine blocks cells in mitosis when less than 5% of the tubulin in cells is complexed with colchicine (52). Colchicine has also been shown to block microtubule polymerization *in vitro* in a substoichiometric manner (21). A mechanism has been proposed to explain this substoichiometric poisoning *in vitro* (28) (see Fig. 2). Colchicine first binds to the tubulin dimer, which then adds to the growing microtubule as a colchicine–dimer (CD) complex. Once this CD complex is added, further significant polymerization is inhibited. One CD complex per microtubule is sufficient to block further polymerization. Colchicine can also be thought of as a drug that increases the critical concentration of tubulin required for assembly, and microtubules containing CDs have been described (53). Recent studies using podophyllotoxin (Fig. 3), a competitive inhibitor of colchicine, indicate that at steady state the drug depresses the addition of dimers to the net polymerization end of the microtubule but does not alter the rate of depolymerization (26).

In addition to the effects of colchicine and podophyllotoxin on microtubule polymerization, at high concentrations these drugs inhibit nucleoside transport in cells (54). Lumicolchicine, a derivative of colchicine that does not inhibit cell replication or bind to tubulin (55,56), is a potent inhibitor of nucleoside transport (45). These data suggest that cellular receptors other than tubulin may exist for colchicine. Tubulin has also been found in cell membranes (57,58). Although the function of such tubulin is not known, it may be involved in the mobility of membrane surface constituents (59,60) and transport processes.

Podophyllotoxin has a mechanism of action similar to that of colchicine (55). A series of podophyllotoxin analogues have been studied with respect to their ability to inhibit (a) colchicine binding to tubulin (61), (b) microtubule assembly *in vitro,* and (c) nucleoside transport in HeLa cells (62,63). Two semisynthetic derivatives of podophyllotoxin, VP 16-213 and VM 26 (Fig. 3), do not inhibit microtubule polymerization *in vitro,* although they do inhibit nucleoside transport. VP 16-213 and VM 26 block cells in the late S–G_2 phase of the cell cycle (64). These two podophyllotoxin derivatives have demonstrated activity against a variety of human malignancies (65). Their antitumor activity may be related to the induction of single-strand breaks in cellular DNA (66). The 4′-hydroxy derivatives of podophyllotoxin have the ability to degrade cellular DNA and inhibit microtubule polymerization *in vitro*.

The vinca alkaloids vincristine and vinblastine (Fig. 3) have two binding sites that are distinct from the colchicine-binding site (67). Like the colchicine-binding site, the vinca alkaloid-binding sites are blocked on the intact microtubule. Vincristine and vinblastine inhibit microtubule polymerization by a substoichiometric mechanism similar to that of colchicine (Wilson, personal communication). At high drug concentrations, when both binding sites are occupied, tubulin crystals are formed (45,68). Maytansine (Fig. 3) inhibits microtubule polymerization *in vitro* and competitively inhibits vincristine binding to tubulin (69–71). However, its binding does not result in tubulin crystal formation (70).

II. Steganacin

The lactone steganacin was initially studied as an alcoholic extract from the wood and stems of *Steganotaenia araliacea* Hochst. This extract was active against P388 leukemia in mice (72), and a series of steganacin analogues were synthesized (73–75). Steganacin is structurally similar to both colchicine and podophyllotoxin (Fig. 3); all three molecules have a trimethoxybenzene ring. Steganacin arrests cell replication in mitosis and inhibits microtubule polymerization *in vitro* (76–78). The drug is a competitive inhibitor of colchicine binding to tubulin and inhibits the uptake of nucleosides by cells.

In our laboratory we have found that steganacin blocks HeLa cell replication in mitosis. The mitotic index of a 10 μM steganacin-treated suspension of HeLa cells (2×10^5 cells/ml) increased from 3 to 94% in 24 hours, but the cell number remained constant during the time course of the experiment. The cells were viable by the criterion of trypan blue exclusion.

Turbidity measurements and electron microscopy have been used to monitor the effects of steganacin on the microtubule assembly reaction. Figure 4A shows the results of turbidity experiments with two concentrations of steganacin. At 30 minutes, 0.39 μM steganacin inhibits polymerization by 36% and 3.9 μM by 86%. A log dose–response curve for the inhibition of microtubule assembly by steganacin is presented in Fig. 4B. Steganacin inhibits the yield of the polymerization reaction by 50% at a concentration of 1.5 μM. We have never observed inhibition greater than 90% with steganacin. The 10% residual turbidity observed at concentrations greater than 3.0 μM drug is most likely due to the small, protofilament-like structures seen with the electron microscope at 30 minutes.

Steganacin is a competitive inhibitor of [^{3}H]colchicine binding to purified tubulin. Double reciprocal plots of [^{3}H]colchicine binding to tubulin in the absence and presence of steganacin, vinblastine, and podophyllotoxin are given in Fig. 5. The apparent affinity (half-maximal binding) of [^{3}H]colchicine for tubulin was calculated to be 2.1 μM. Inhibition constants have been calculated for the three drugs (Table I). The inhibition constant (K_i) is assumed to be analogous to the dissociation constant for the drug (80). The inhibition constant for vinblastine, a noncompetitive inhibitor under these conditions (81), is 27.2 μM. Both steganacin and podophyllotoxin are competitive inhibitors of [^{3}H]colchicine binding to tubulin; steganacin has an inhibition constant of 3.1 μM and podophyllotoxin one of 1.5 μM (Table I). The inhibition constants for

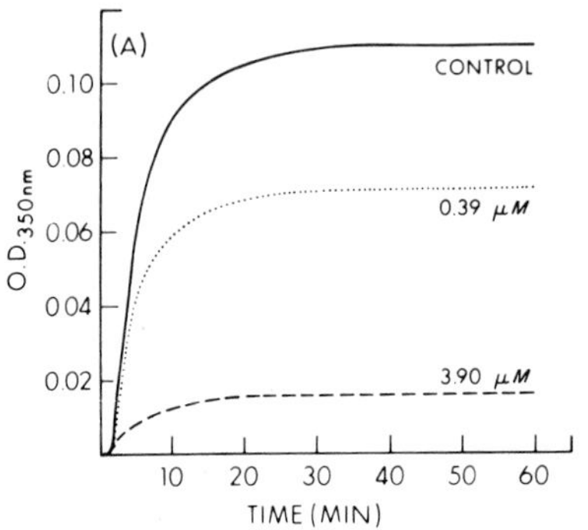

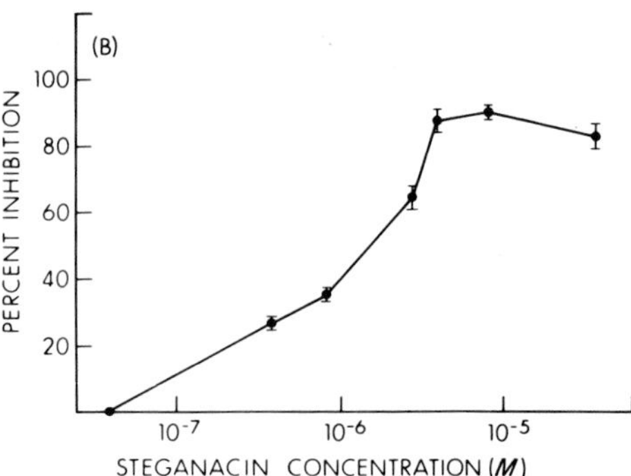

Fig. 4. Effect of steganacin on microtubule assembly *in vitro.* Chicken brain tubulin was prepared by two cycles of polymerization and depolymerization (15) and stored at -20°C in MES buffer (0.1 *M* MES, 1 m*M* EGTA, 0.5 m*M* $MgC1_2$, pH 6.6) containing 1 m*M* GTP and 4 *M* glycerol. Before each experiment, the tubulin was dialyzed for 3 hours at 4°C against 100 volumes of MES buffer and centrifuged at 120,000 *g* for 20 minutes at 4°C. Tubulin prepared by this procedure is approximately 85% pure as determined on 3-27% SDS- polyacrylamide gradient reducing slab gels (79). Microtubule polymerization was monitored by the method of Gaskin *et al.* (10). The cuvettes (1-cm path, 1 ml) containing 0.75 ml MES buffer, drug, and 1 m*M* GTP were kept at room temperature prior to the addition of 0.25 ml microtubule protein (1 mg) and shifting to 37°C. Turbidity measurements were made every 20 seconds at 350 nm on a Gilford spectrophotometer equipped with an automatic recorder and a thermostatically regulated sample chamber. Steganacin was dissolved in dimethyl sulfoxide at 10 m*M* and stored at -20°C. The final concentration of dimethyl sulfoxide (0.5%) had no detectable effect on the polymerization kinetics of tubulin. (A) Turbidity measurements in the absence and presence of 0.39 and 3.9 μ*M* steganacin. (B) Percent inhibition of microtubule polymerization at 30 minutes as a function of the concentration of steganacin. [From Schiff *et al.* (77), reproduced by permission of Academic Press.]

TABLE I

Relative Affinity of Steganacin, Vinblastine, and Podophyllotoxin for the Colchicine-Binding Site on Tubulin[a]

Inhibitor	K_i (μ*M*)
Steganacin	3.1
Vinblastine	27.2
Podophyllotoxin	1.5

[a] The apparent affinity of colchicine for tubulin under these conditions (see legend for Fig. 5) is 2.1 μ*M*.

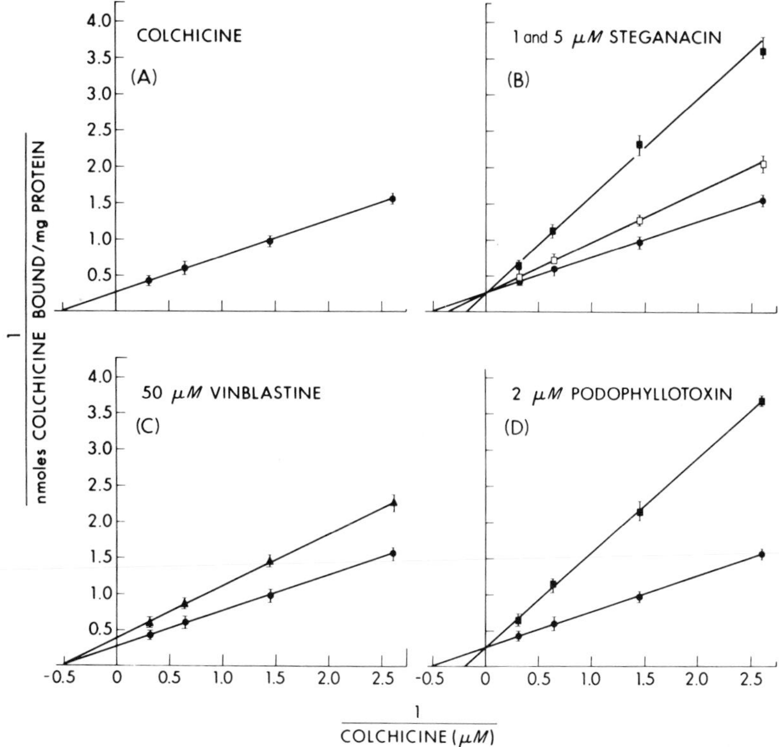

Fig. 5. Double reciprocal plots of drug-induced inhibition of [^{3}H]colchicine binding to purified chicken tubulin. The binding of [^{3}H]colchicine to tubulin was measured by a modification of the DEAE filter assay [5]. Tubulin (1 mg) in MES buffer was incubated for 1 hour at 37°C with 0.38, 0.75, 1.5, and 3 μM [^{3}H]colchicine (specific activity, 0.1 Ci/mmole) in a final volume of 1 ml. The reaction was stopped by the addition of 1 ml of 0.1 m*M* colchicine. The apparent affinity constants were computed from the least squares linear regression lines of the double reciprocal plots (see Table I). (A) Colchicine control reaction (●). (B) Steganacin, 1 μM (□) and 5 μM (■). (C) Vinblastine, 50 μM (▲). (D) Podophyllotoxin, 2 μM (■). [From Schiff *et al.*, (77), reproduced by permission of Academic Press.]

vinblastine and podophyllotoxin are in good agreement with those previously reported (see 1).

III. Taxol

A. *In Vitro* Studies

Taxol exhibits novel effects on the microtubule polymerization reaction *in vitro* (82); in contrast to steganacin, it enhances the rate, yield, and number of nucleations. In addition, taxol renders microtubules resistant to depolymerization by cold (4°C) and $CaCl_2$ (4 m*M*). The drug was first isolated from the plant *Taxus brevifolia* (83) and has shown significant activity against L1210, P388, and P1534 leukemia systems (84).

We have monitored microtubule polymerization in the presence of taxol by (a) an increase in turbidity at 350 nm as a function of time, (b) sedimentation, and (c) electron microscopy. Under our conditions, the control polymerization progress curve is sigmoid, but addition to 10 μM taxol gives hyperbolic kinetics (Fig. 6A). The control reaction, following a 3.5-minute lag time, progresses to 90% of its final turbidity value within approximately 15 minutes. The lag time is essentially eliminated when polymerization takes place in the presence of 10 μM taxol. The decrease in the lag time caused by taxol is a dose-dependent effect (Fig. 6B) and is independent of tubulin concentration. After the lag time, the control polymerization progress curve follows a single first-order exponential with a $t_{1/2}$ of 4.0 minutes (Fig. 6C). The taxol progress curve consists of two detectable phases: a rapid initial phase with a $t_{1/2}$ of 1.7 minutes and a slower

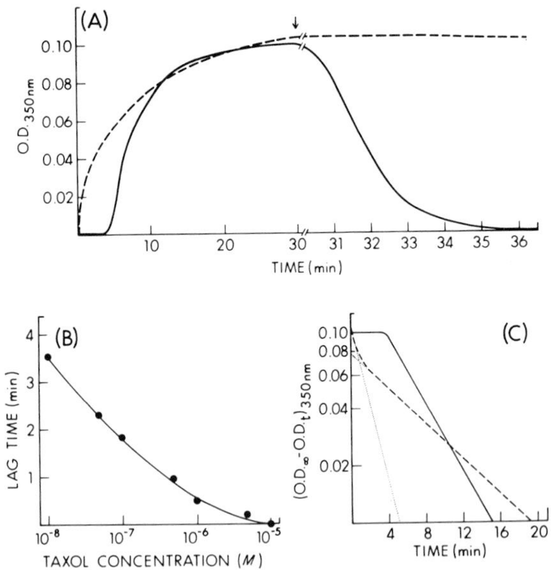

Fig. 6. Effect of taxol on the kinetics of calf brain microtubule polymerization and depolymerization. Polymerization conditions are as described in Fig. 4. (A) Control (—) and 10 μM taxol (———). The arrow (↓) indicates a shift in temperature from 37° to 8°C. (B) Lag time for the polymerization reaction plotted as a function of the concentration of taxol. (C) Analysis of the assembly progress curve as an exponential decay process. $O.D._{\infty}$ and $O.D._{t}$ are the equilibrium and time-dependent values, respectively, of the $O.D._{350\ nm}$. —, Control; ———, 10 μM taxol. (· · ·) extrapolations of the two kinetic phases of the taxol-treated reaction.

phase with a $t_{1/2}$ of 5.3 minutes. The rapid initial phase may result from increased nucleations, while the slower phase may represent elongation.

Ribbon structures and dimers are seen with the electron microscope at 30 seconds in reactions containing 10 μM taxol (Fig. 7); in the control there are only rings and tubulin dimers. The ribbon structures observed at 30 seconds with taxol are probably intermediates in assembly, as mainly microtubules are seen at 30 minutes.

Microtubules assembled in the presence of 10 μM taxol for 30 minutes are resistant to depolymerization by cold (4°C) (Fig. 6A). In the absence of taxol, the microtubules depolymerize and only the oligomeric tubulin rings and tubulin dimers are observed with the electron microscope 6 minutes after shifting the temperature from 37° to 8°C. Ribbon structures are observed when polymerization takes place at 4°C 30 minutes in the presence of 50 μM taxol. Microtubules assembled in the presence of 10 μM taxol are completely resistant to depolymerization by 4 mM $CaCl_2$ (82). Those assembled in the presence of 5 μM taxol are partially resistant to depolymerization by 4 mM $CaCl_2$. Dimers, rings, and microtubules are present 30 minutes after the addition of $CaCl_2$ to microtubules assembled in the presence of 5 μM taxol. Complete resistance to depolymerization occurs at a taxol concentration that is stoichiometric with the tubulin dimer concentration. Microtubule assembly will proceed in the presence of 4 mM $CaCl_2$ and 5 μM taxol.

Microtubules assembled in the absence of taxol become resistant to depolymerization by $CaCl_2$ after incubation with taxol (Fig. 8). Microtubules were polymerized at 37°C for 30 minutes and sedimented at 120,000 g for 30 minutes at 30°C. The sedimented microtubules were then resuspended in 1 ml of MES buffer with or without 10 μM taxol. After 4 minutes, 4 mM $CaCl_2$ was added to the resuspended samples. Continuous turbidity measurements and electron microscopy indicated that no microtubules were present in the non-drug-treated sample after the addition of the $CaCl_2$, whereas the taxol-treated microtubules were resistant to depolymerization by $CaCl_2$. Such experiments suggest that a taxol-binding site (or sites) is available on the intact microtubule.

Phosphocellulose-purified tubulin, which is free of MAPs (16,18), will polymerize in the presence of stoichiometric concentrations of taxol (P. B. Schiff and S. B. Horwitz, unpublished data). Normally, 1.5 mg/ml phosphocellulose-purified tubulin will not self-assemble, however, addition of 1–10 μM taxol will promote the assembly of such tubulin. These microtubules, when observed in the electron microscope at 30 minutes, tend to have more frayed ends than those assembled in the presence of MAPs plus taxol. Microtubules assembled from phosphocellulose-purified tubulin in the presence of taxol are resistant to depolymerization by $CaCl_2$.

Supernatant solutions remaining after sedimentation of tubulin at 230,000 g for 1.5 hours, conditions which will sediment proteins larger than approximately 36S, will not self-assemble (9). Taxol will promote the assembly of tubulin that

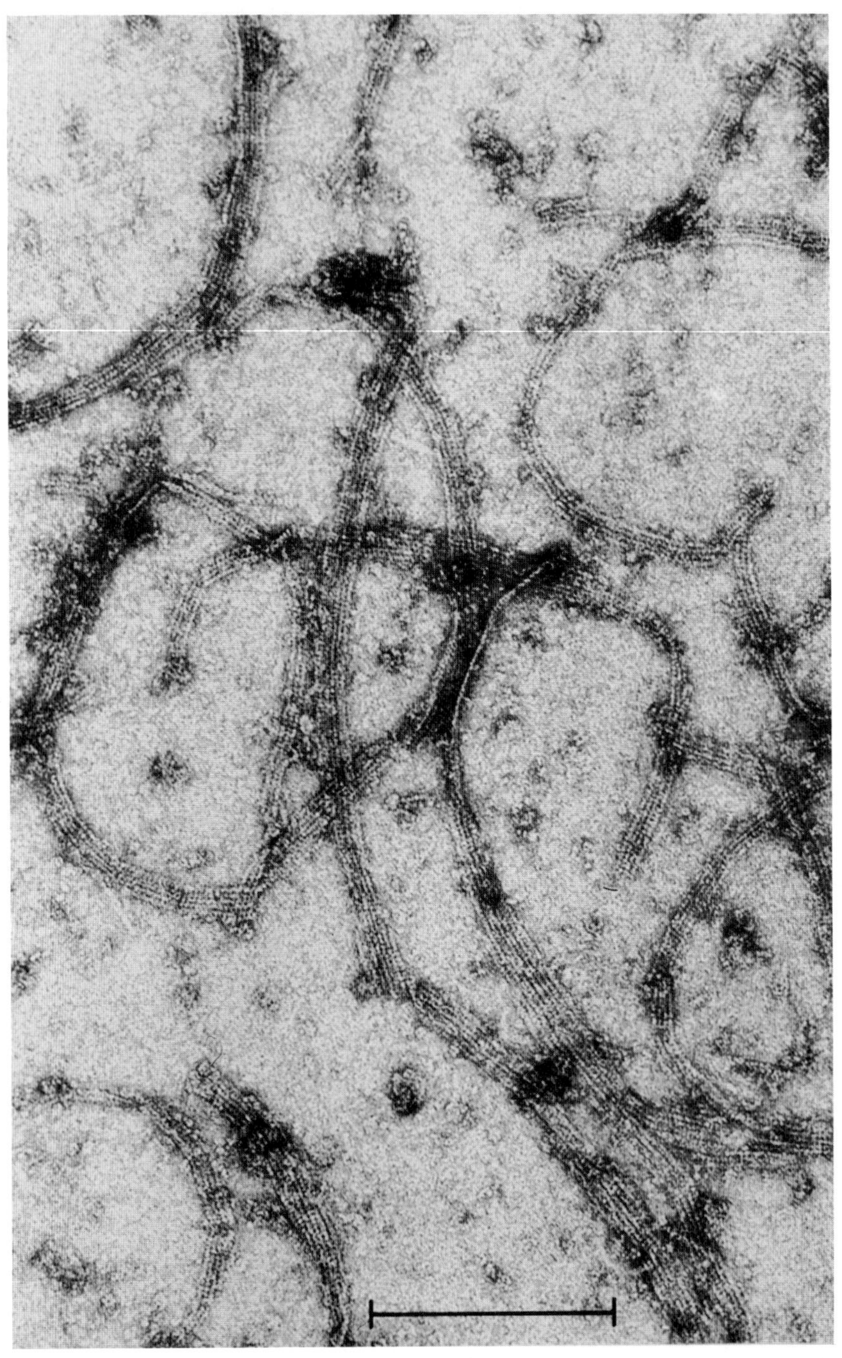

Fig. 7. Electron micrograph of ribbon structures observed at 30 seconds with 1 mg/ml tubulin and 10 μM taxol. Structures were negatively stained with uranyl acetate. Scale bar, 0.2 μm.

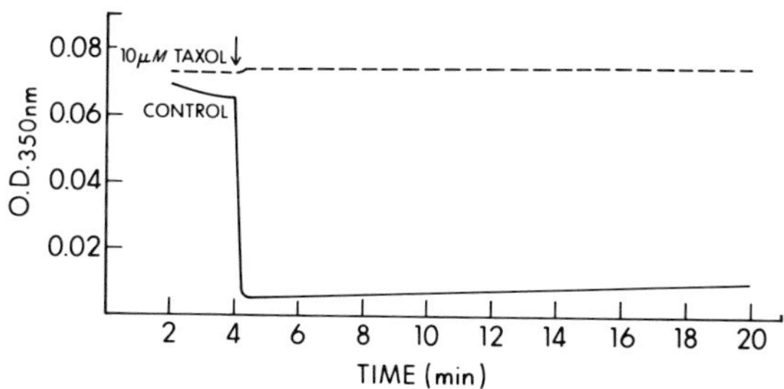

Fig. 8. Taxol confers calcium resistance to intact microtubules. Microtubules were polymerized for 30 minutes at 37°C and sedimented at 120,000 *g* for 30 minutes at 30°C. They were then resuspended in 1 ml of MES buffer in the absence (—) or presence (— — —) of 10 μM taxol (time 0). The arrow (↓) indicates the addition of 4 m*M* $CaCl_2$ at 4 minutes to the control and taxol-treated samples.

is depleted of 36S structures, as measured by turbidity and electron microscopy (P. B. Schiff and S. B. Horwitz, unpublished data). These microtubules have also been shown to be resistant to depolymerization by 4 m*M* $CaCl_2$.

Microtubules can be polymerized in the absence of added GTP and in the presence of taxol. When tubulin is charcoal-treated to remove GDP bound to be exchangeable site on the tubulin dimer (39), tubulin (0.8 mg/ml) will not self-assemble unless 1 m*M* GTP or taxol is added to the reaction mixture. Taxol (5 μM) decreases the lag time for the reaction in the absence of GTP. The microtubules assembled in the absence of GTP and in the presence of 5 μM taxol are resistant to depolymerization by 4 m*M* $CaCl_2$, and the addition of GTP does not reestablish calcium sensitivity. Taxol does not inhibit the hydrolysis of GTP or GDP under our polymerization conditions at 30 minutes.

Microtubules polymerized in the presence of taxol are, on the average, shorter than microtubules polymerized in the absence of the drug. Tubulin (1 mg/ml) was polymerized in the presence of various concentrations of taxol, and microtubule lengths determined at 30 minutes, at which time apparent equilibrium was reached. As the taxol concentration increased from 50 n*M* to 50 μM, the mean length of the microtubules decreased from 4.12 ± 2.21 to 1.49 ± 0.65 μm (Fig. 9A and B). The minimum microtubule length was reached at a taxol concentration that was approximately stoichiometric with the tubulin dimer concentration.

Taxol also shifts the equilibrium that exists between the tubulin dimer and the microtubule in favor of the microtubule (Fig. 9B). After assembly, the amount of microtubule protein in the 120,000-*g* pellets and supernatants was determined. In the absence of taxol, 0.57 mg of tubulin can be detected in the pellet. Like the effect of taxol concentration on the length of the microtubules, the concentration of taxol yielding a maximum amount of sedimented protein (0.78 mg) was approximately stoichiometric with the tubulin dimer. Up to 80% of the total protein in the drug-treated reaction is sedimented compared to 60% in the control

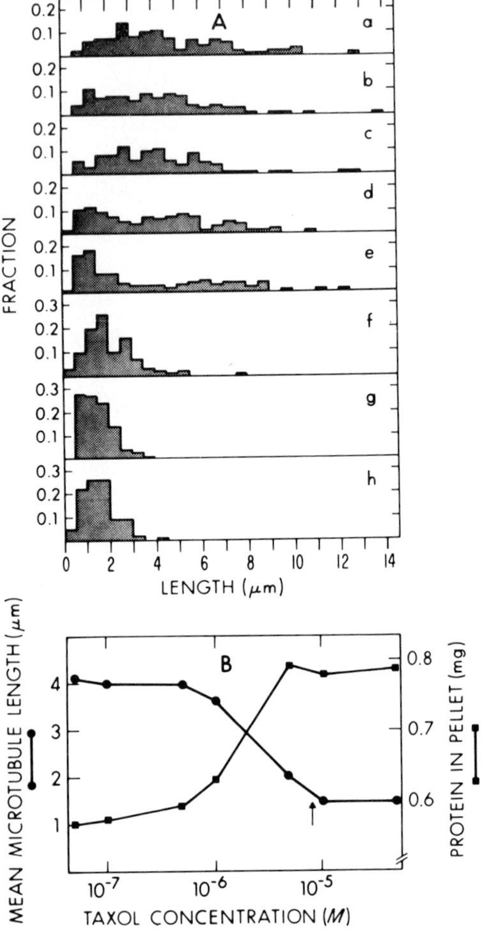

Fig. 9. Effect of taxol on microtubule length distribution and tubulin dimer–microtubule equilibrium. Microtubule lengths and the amount of tubulin sedimented were measured after 30 minutes at 37°C, when apparent equilibrium had been reached. Microtubule length measurements were made with a Numonics Graphics calculator, from electron micrographs printed at a magnification of 6000×. Statistical treatment of length measurements took into account microtubules with one end off the micrograph (27). A minimum of 150 microtubules were counted for each histogram. (A) Histograms show fraction of microtubules in each 0.5-μm-length range when polymerized from 1 mg/ml tubulin in the presence of taxol at concentrations of: a, 0; b, 0.05 *μM;* c, 0.1 *μM;* d, 0.5 *μM;* e, 1 *μM;* f, 5 *μM;* g, 10 *μM;* and h, 50 *μM* taxol. (B) Mean lengths of the microtubules (●) and amount of tubulin sedimented at 120,000 *g* (■) as a function of taxol concentration. The mean lengths (at each taxol concentration) were calculated to be: no taxol, 4.12 ± 2.21 μm; 0.05 *μM,* 4.10 ± 2.60 μm; 0.1 *μM,* 4.0 ± 2.28 μm; 0.5 *μM,* 3.89 ± 2.45 μm; 1.0 *μM,* 3.63 ± 3.01 μm; 5.0 *μM,* 2.0 ± 1.03 μm; 10 *μM,* 1.49 ± 0.65 μm; and 50 *μM,* 1.49 ± 0.73 μm. In the absence of taxol, 0.57 mg protein could be detected in the pellet. Each sedimentation point (■) represents the average of at least three experimental values that differ by less than 6%. The arrow (↑) indicates the corrected tubulin dimer concentration (7.7 *μM*).

reaction. A 1.5-fold increase in the yield of the polymerization reaction is attained at approximately 7.7 μM tubulin and taxol. When the polymerization products are analyzed by visualization of proteins with Coomassie blue on 3–27% sodium dodecyl sulfate (SDS) polyacrylamide gradient reducing slab gels (79), taxol does not appear to displace any of the MAPs that cosediment with microtubules when assembly takes place in the presence of 10 μM taxol and 1 mg/ml tubulin. If the average length of the microtubules and the mass of protein sedimented after polymerization in the presence of 10 μM taxol are taken into account, there is an approximate 3.8-fold increase in the number of microtubules in the drug-treated sample. Therefore, under these conditions, taxol causes a 3.8-fold increase in the number of nucleations.

Taxol decreases the critical concentration of microtubule protein required for microtubule assembly *in vitro* (Fig. 10). In the absence of drug (Fig. 10A), the critical concentration is 0.2 mg/ml (1.8 μM). In the presence of 5 μM taxol (Fig. 10B), the critical concentration decreases to $\leqslant$ 0.01 mg/ml (0.08 μM). The values for the apparent microtubule propagation equilibrium constant (K_p^{app}) and the apparent standard free energy (ΔG^0_{app}) on the addition of a tubulin dimer to a growing microtubule have been calculated (Table II). Turbidity at 30 minutes does not change appreciably as compared to the control, until the protein concentration is less than 0.25 mg/ml (Fig. 10A and B). Microtubules, tubulin hoops

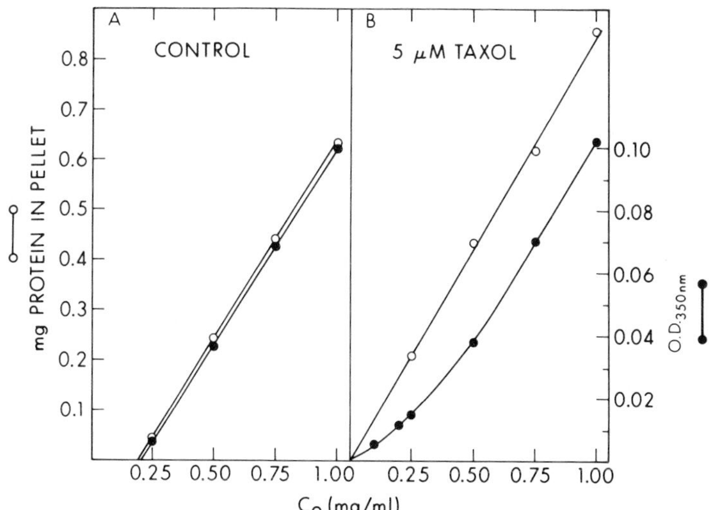

Fig. 10. Comparison of critical concentrations determined by sedimentation (120,000 *g* at 25°C for 30 minutes) of microtubules (○) and turbidity measurements (●) in the absence (A) and presence (B) of 5 μM taxol. C_0 is the total protein concentration. Determinations were made after a 30-minute incubation. [From Schiff *et al.* (82), reproduced by permission of Macmillan Journals.]

TABLE II

Effect of Taxol on the Apparent Microtubule Propagation Equilibrium Constant (K_p^{app})[a]

	C_c (mg/ml)	K_p^{app} (liters/mole)	ΔG^0_{app} (kcal/mole)
Control	0.20	5.7×10^5	-8.0
Taxol	$\leqslant 0.01$	$\geqslant 1.1 \times 10^7$	-10.0

[a] Standard assembly conditions in the absence and presence of 5 μM taxol. C_c is the critical concentration, and K_p^{app} is C_c^{-1}. The value of the apparent standard free energy (ΔG^0_{app}) is given by $\Delta G^0_{app} = -RT \ln K_p^{app}$.

(86) with less than 13 protofilaments, and ribbon structures were observed at 0.1 mg/ml tubulin in the presence of 5 μM taxol at 30 minutes, while the untreated reaction contained no structures (82). Such structures probably result from rapid and incomplete polymerization. At 1 mg/ml tubulin and 5 μM taxol, essentially no hoop or ribbon structures can be found at 30 minutes, only short microtubules.

B. Effects on Cell Structure and Function

Flow microfluorometry has been used to study the effect of taxol on the distribution of DNA in HeLa cells as a function of time. These experiments have demonstrated that cells treated with 0.25 μM taxol accumulate in the G_2 and M phases of the cell cycle. Approximately 70% of the taxol-treated cells were in mitosis at 20 hours (the nuclear membrane had disappeared and the DNA had condensed) as determined by electron microscopy (87).

Indirect immunofluorescence microscopy, using tubulin antiserum, has been used to determine whether taxol can convert labile cytoplasmic microtubules into stable microtubules like those found in cilia, flagella, and centrioles. Interphase fibroblast cells present a characteristic display of cytoplasmic microtubules (Figs. 11A and 12A). The microtubules in these cells radiate outward from the perinuclear region to the plasma membrane. Cells that have been treated for 22 hours with 10 μM taxol, a concentration of drug that completely inhibits fibroblast cell replication, display in addition to their cytoplasmic microtubules, "bundles" of microtubules that appear to radiate from a common site (or sites) which may be the microtubule-organizing centers (Figs. 11B and 12B). Small bundles of microtubules can be seen as early as 35 minutes after the addition of 10 μM taxol to the cells. Although it is difficult to rule out a redistribution of the microtubules in these cells, it is possible that these bundles represent new initiations that have occurred at the microtubule-organizing centers. Taxol-treated cells also have a microtubule-free zone between the distal ends of their mi-

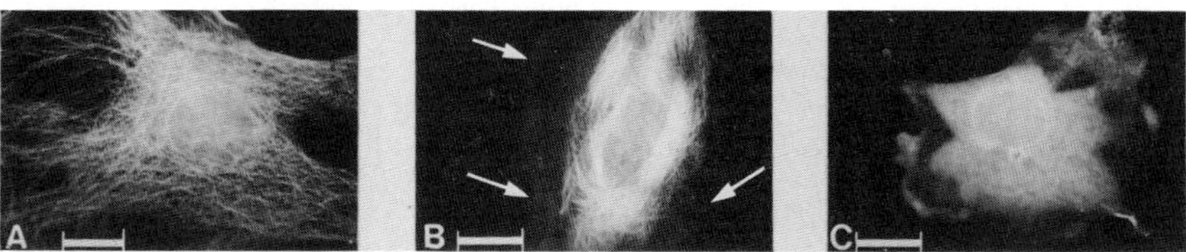

Fig. 11. Indirect immunofluorescence micrographs of BALB/c fibroblasts using tubulin antiserum. Fibroblast cells were grown on glass coverslips in Falcon culture dishes. Cells were allowed to attach to glass coverslips 24 hours prior to addition of the drugs. A technique for visualizing cytoplasmic microtubules in mammalian tissue cultures has been described (85). A Zeiss Photomicroscope III equipped with epifluorescence optics and a 63× oil-immersion objective lens was used to view the cells. Photographs were taken on Kodak Tri-X 35-mm film and developed in Diafine. (A) Control cell. (B) Cell exposed to 10 μM taxol for 22 hours. (C) Cell incubated with 10 μM steganacin for 22 hours. Arrows indicate the edge of the plasma membrane in the plane of focus. Scale bar, 20 μm.

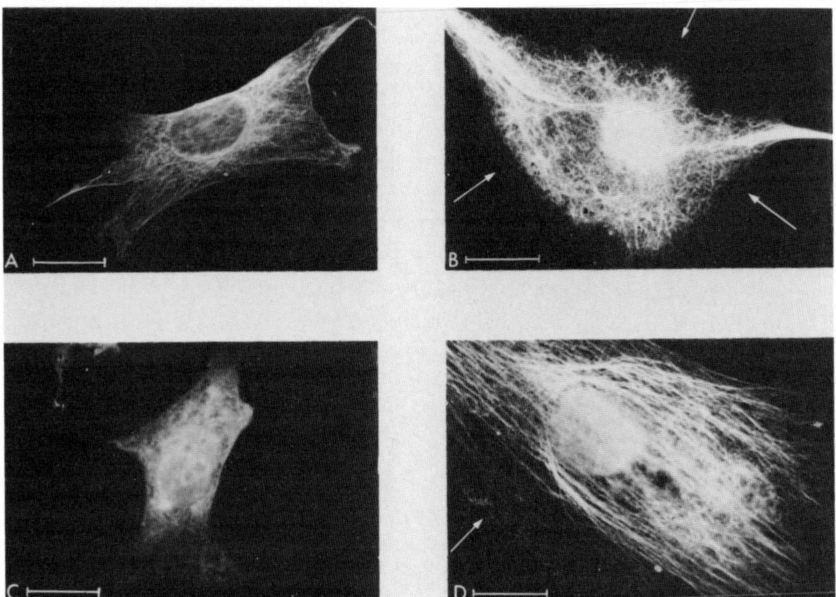

Fig. 12. Indirect immunofluorescence micrographs of BALB/c fibroblasts using tubulin antiserum. (A) Control cell. (B) Cell that has been in the presence of 10 μM taxol for 22 hours. (C) Cell that has been in the cold (4°C) for 16 hours. (D) Cell that has been incubated with 10 μM taxol for 22 hours and then shifted to 4°C for 16 hours. Arrows indicate the position of the plasma membrane in the plane of focus. Scale bar, 20 μm. [From Schiff and Horwitz (87), reproduced by permission of National Academy of Sciences U.S.A.]

crotubules and the plasma membrane. This zone may result from the cell preferentially initiating new microtubules at the microtubule-organizing centers, instead of elongating existing microtubules. In addition, the cell may not be able to depolymerize existing microtubules to provide additional dimers. The structure and distribution of the microtubules in taxol-treated cells have been confirmed by transmission electron microscopy.

Normally, cells that have been in the cold (4°C) for 16 hours lose their microtubules (Fig. 12C); however, cells incubated with 10 μM taxol for 22 hours at 37°C and then shifted to 4°C for 16 hours still display microtubules and bundles of microtubules (Fig. 12D). Cells treated with 10 μM taxol for 1 hour at 37°C also have cold-resistant cytoplasmic microtubule cytoskeletons. Fibroblasts incubated with 10 μM steganacin for 2 or 22 hours at 37°C do not display microtubules (Fig. 11C). However, fibroblasts pretreated with 10 μM taxol for 22 hours at 37°C and then treated with 10 μM steganacin for 2 hours continue to display microtubules.

Little is known about the biological machinery involved in cell migration. The microtubule cytoskeleton may play a role in migration by determining the polarity of a migrating cell (88). A model based on intrinsic microtubule behavior has been proposed to explain the orderly separation of chromosomes during mitosis (89). Colchicine and vinblastine, drugs that inhibit mitosis, also inhibit fibroblast and macrophage cell migration (90–92). However, these drug-treated cells are not utterly immobile. They are still able to produce mobile lamellipodia and filopodia. Ruffling of the plasma membranes becomes more evenly distributed around the cell perimeter of drug-treated cells instead of occurring mainly at the leading edge as in normal cells (93,94).

The effect of taxol and steganacin on 3T3 fibroblast cell migration behavior has been examined (87) using the phagokinetic track assay (95). When viewed at low magnification with dark-field microscopy at 24 hours, both taxol and steganacin completely inhibit cell migration at a concentration of 10 μM (Fig. 13A, C, and E). Control cultures produced numerous phagokinetic tracks of individual cells removing and ingesting gold particles in their paths. When drug-treated cells were viewed at higher magnification by phase-contrast microscopy, it was evident that they were able to clear and ingest gold particles from the area of attachment during the 24-hour experiment (Fig. 13 B, D, and F). Using time-lapse photography, we have shown that taxol-treated cells are able to produce mobile lamellipodia and filopodia. Thus the microtubule-free zone in a taxol-treated cell may also result from the cell extending lamellipodia beyond its stabilized microtubule cytoskeleton.

IV. Summary

The results described in the previous sections characterize the molecular pharmacology of two new drugs that interact with tubulin. Steganacin inhibits

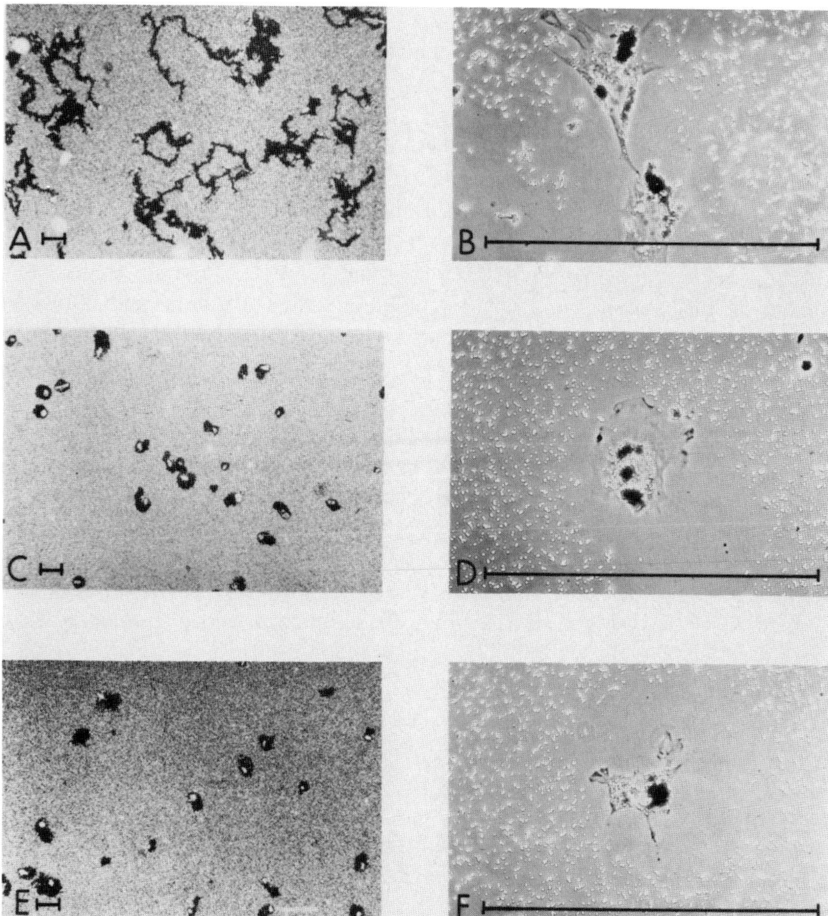

Fig. 13. Migration behavior of untreated, taxol-treated, and steganacin-treated Swiss 3T3 fibroblast cells. A technique for the visualization of phagokinetic tracks of individual cultured cells moving on a gold particle-coated substrate has been described (95). Cells (1000–2000 per dish) were seeded into drug-containing medium in 35 × 10mm tissue culture dishes at the start of the experiment. The phagokinetic tracks of the 3T3 cells were observed in dark-field illumination with a Zeiss Photomicroscope II, using a 25× objective lens at 24 hrs. (A) Control cells. (C) Taxol-treated (10 μM) cells. (E) Steganacin-treated (10 μM) cells. (B), (D), and (F) are phase-contrast micrographs of control, taxol-treated, and steganacin-treated cells, respectively, from the same experiment. Scale bar, 200 μm. [From Schiff and Horwitz (87), reproduced by permission of National Academy of Sciences U.S.A.]

microtubule polymerization *in vitro* and in cells. It poisons polymerization *in vitro* in a substoichiometric manner. Steganacin inhibits the yield of polymerization 50% at 1.5 μM, although the tubulin concentration is 7.4 μM. The mechanism of this poisoning is probably similar to that reported for colchicine (26,28), since steganacin is a competitive inhibitor of [^{3}H]colchicine binding to tubulin. The inhibition of microtubule assembly *in vitro* by steganacin most likely explains the drug's ability to block cells in mitosis. These properties may be responsible for the observed antitumor activity of the drug.

Taxol, a low-molecular-weight neutral drug, promotes the rate, extent, and number of nucleations in the *in vitro* polymerization of tubulin and stabilizes microtubules *in vitro* and in cells. Other workers have reported that microtubule assembly can be enhanced by MAPs (HMW proteins and tau proteins) (16,18,40,41,96), by basic proteins (97,98), and by polycations (98–101). Guanylyl-5′-methylene diphosphate (Gmp(CH_2)pp), an $\alpha\beta$ nonhydrolyzable analogue of GTP, has been shown to enhance microtubule polymerization and render microtubules resistant to depolymerization by 2 mM $CaCl_2$ (102). In addition, Gmp(CH_2)pp will promote the assembly of phosphocellulose-purified tubulin. Taxol, at stoichiometric concentrations, also promotes polymerization of MAP-free tubulin. It does not inhibit the hydrolysis of GTP or GDP in our preparations. Taxol promotes assembly of microtubules with substoichiometric concentrations of GTP at the E site on the tubulin dimer.

Taxol blocks cell replication in the G_2 and M phases of the cell cycle and stabilizes cytoplasmic microtubules. Like steganacin and other drugs that inhibit microtubule assembly, it inhibits the migration of mouse 3T3 fibroblast cells. However, taxol-treated cells do not lose their ability to produce mobile lamellipodia and filopodia. These experiments suggest that, in order to migrate, cells must be able to polymerize and depolymerize their cytoplasmic microtubules to differentiate between their front and back ends.

The inhibition of HeLa and fibroblast cell replication and the inability of fibroblasts to migrate in the presence of low concentrations of taxol could derive from cells being unable to depolymerize their microtubule cytoskeletons. This may represent a new mechanism of action for a chemotherapeutic agent and might explain the observed antitumor activity of taxol. A complete understanding of the action of taxol could lead to the development of new drugs with similar and modified activities. This drug should be a useful tool in studying the regulation of cellular functions, such as cell migration, that may be mediated by microtubules. Taxol could also provide a method for the isolation of intact cytoplasmic and spindle microtubules.

Finally, the presence of endogenous inhibitors of [^{3}H]colchicine binding to tubulin has been considered (103–105). Such factors may be important in the regulation of microtubule assembly and function in cells. There also may be endogenous molecules with activity like that of taxol; such molecules could be involved in the regulation of microtubule assembly and microtubule stability in cells.

Acknowledgment

Research that originated in the authors' laboratory was supported by an American Cancer Society Grant CH-86 and USPHS grants CA-15714 and CA-23187.

References

1. J. A. Snyder and J. R. McIntosh, *Annu. Rev. Biochem.* **45,** 699 (1976).
2. M. W. Kirschner, *Int. Rev. Cytol.* **54,** 1 (1978).
3. P. Dustin, *in* "Microtubules," Springer-Verlag, Berlin and New York, 1978.
4. K. Roberts, and J. S. Hyams (ed.) *Microtubules,* Academic Press, New York (1979).
5. R. C. Weisenberg, G. G. Borisy, and E. W. Taylor, *Biochemistry* **7,** 4466 (1968).
6. J. B. Olmsted, *Cold Spring Harbor Conf. Cell Proliferation* **3** (Book C), 1081 1976.
7. F. Solomon, *Biochemistry* **16,** 358 (1977).
8. R. C. Weisenberg, *Science* **177,** 1104 (1972).
9. G. G. Borisy and J. B. Olmsted, *Science* **177,** 1196 (1972).
10. F. Gaskin, C. R. Cantor, and M. L. Shelanski, *J. Mol. Biol.* **89,** 737 (1974).
11. G. G. Borisy, J. B. Olmsted, J. M. Marcum, and C. Allen, *Fed. Proc., Fed. Am. Soc. Exp. Biol.* **33,** 167 (1974).
12. J. C. Lee and S. N. Timasheff, *Biochemistry* **14,** 5183 (1975).
13. F. Oosawa and M. Kasai, *J. Mol. Biol.* **4,** 10 (1962).
14. S. N. Timasheff, *Trends Biochem. Sci.* **4,** 61 (1979).
15. M. L. Shelanski, F. Gaskin, and R. Cantor, *Proc. Natl. Acad. Sci. U.S.A.* **70,** 765 (1973).
16. R. D. Sloboda, W. L. Dentler, and J. L. Rosenbaum, *Biochemistry* **15,** 4497 (1976).
17. G. G. Borisy, J. M. Marcum, J. B. Olmsted, D. B. Murphy, and R. A. Johnson, *Ann. N.Y. Acad. Sci.* **253,** 107 (1975).
18. M. D. Weingarten, A. H. Lockwood, S. Y. Hwo, and M. W. Kirschner, *Proc. Natl. Acad. Sci. U.S.A.* **72,** 1858 (1975).
19. P. Sherline and K. Schiavone, *Science* **198,** 1038 (1977).
20. J. A. Connally, V. I. Kalnins, D. W. Cleveland, and M. W. Kirschner, *Proc. Natl. Acad. Sci. U.S.A.* **74,** 2437 (1977).
21. J. B. Olmsted and G. G. Borisy, *Biochemistry* **12,** 4282 (1973).
22. T. Miki-Noumura and R. Kamiya, *Expt. Cell Res.* **97,** 451 (1976).
23. M. W. Kirschner, L. S. Honig, and R. C. Williams, *J. Mol. Biol.* **99,** 263 (1975).
24. K. Summers and M. W. Kirschner, *J. Cell Biol.* **83,** 205 (1979).
25. L. G. Bergen and G. G. Borisy, *J. Cell Biol.* **84,** 141 (1980).
26. R. L. Margolis and L. Wilson, *Cell* **13,** 1 (1978).
27. K. A. Johnson and G. G. Borisy, *J. Mol. Biol.* **117,** 1 (1977).
28. R. L. Margolis and L. Wilson, *Proc. Natl. Acad. Sci. U.S.A.* **74,** 3466 (1977).
29. S. Inoué and H. Sato, *J. Gen. Physiol.* **50,** Suppl., 259 (1967).
30. L. Wilson, *Fed. Proc., Fed. Am. Soc. Exp. Biol.* **33,** 151 (1974).
31. K. Porter, *in* "Principles of Biomolecular Organization" (G. E. Wolstenholme and M. O'Connor, eds.), pp. 308–345. Little, Brown, Boston, Massachusetts, 1966.

32. J. Pickett-Heaps, *Cytobios* **1,** 257 (1969).
33. G. M. Fuller, B. R. Brinkley, and J. M. Broughter, *Science* **187,** 948 (1975).
34. K. Weber, R. Pollack, and T. Bibring, *Proc. Natl. Acad. Sci. U.S.A.* **72,** 459 (1975).
35. B. R. Brinkley, G. M. Fuller, and D. P. Highfield, *Proc. Natl. Acad. Sci. U.S.A.* **72,** 4981 (1975).
36. M. Osborn and K. Weber, *Proc. Natl. Acad. Sci. U.S.A.* **73,** 867 (1976).
37. B. M. Spiegelman, M. A. Lopata, and M. W. Kirschner, *Cell* **16,** 239 (1979).
38. K. R. Porter, T. T. Puck, A. W. Hsie, and D. Kelley, *Cell* **2,** 145 (1974).
39. S. M. Penningroth and M. W. Kirschner, *J. Mol. Biol.* **115,** 643 (1977).
40. M. D. Weingarten, M. S. Suter, D. R. Littman, and M. W. Kirschner, *Biochemistry* **13,** 5529 (1974).
41. D. B. Murphy and G. G. Borisy, *Proc. Natl. Acad. Sci. U.S.A.* **72,** 2696 (1975).
42. M. J. Welsh, J. R. Dedman, B. R. Brinkley, and A. R. Means, *Proc. Natl. Acad. Sci. U.S.A.* **75,** 1186 (1978).
43. G. G. Borisy and E. W. Taylor, *J. Cell Biol.* **34,** 535 (1967).
44. J. Bryan, *Biochemistry* **11,** 2611 (1972).
45. L. Wilson and J. Bryan, *Adv. Cell Mol. Biol.* **3,** 21 (1974).
46. L. Wilson and I. Meza, *J. Cell Biol.* **58,** 709 (1973).
47. J. Hoebeke, G. Van Nijen, and M. DeBrabander, *Biochem. Biophys. Res. Commun.* **69,** 319 (1976).
48. L. C. Davidse and W. Flach, *J. Cell Biol.* **72,** 174 (1977).
49. G. Sheir-Neiss, M. H. Lai, and N. R. Morris, *Cell* **15,** 639 (1978).
50. F. Cabral, M. E. Sobel, and M. M. Gottesman, *Cell* **20,** 29 (1980).
51. H. Schmitt and A. Daphine, *J. Mol. Biol.* **102,** 743 (1976).
52. E. W. Taylor, *J. Cell Biol.* **25,** 145 (1965).
53. H. Sternlicht and J. Ringel, *J. Biol. Chem.* **254,** 540 (1979).
54. S. B. Mizel and L. Wilson, *Biochemistry* **11,** 2573 (1972).
55. L. Wilson and M. Friedkin, *Biochemistry* **6,** 3126 (1967).
56. L. Wilson, *Biochemistry* **9,** 4999 (1970).
57. B. Bhattacharyya and J. Wolff, *J. Biol. Chem.* **250,** 7639 (1975).
58. B. Bhattacharyya and J. Wolff, *Nature (London)* **264,** 576 (1976).
59. T. E. Ukena and R. D. Berlin, *J. Exp. Med.* **136,** 1 (1972).
60. G. M. Edelman, I. Tahara, and J. L. Wang, *Proc. Natl. Acad. Sci. U.S.A.* **70,** 1442 (1973).
61. J. K. Kelleher, *Mol. Pharmacol.* **13,** 232 (1977).
62. J. D. Loike and S. B. Horwitz, *Biochemistry* **15,** 5435 (1976).
63. J. D. Loike, C. F. Brewer, H. Sternlicht, W. J. Gensler, and S. B. Horwitz, *Cancer Res.* **38,** 2688 (1978).
64. A. Krishan, K. Paika, and E. Frei, *J. Cell Biol.* **66,** 521 (1975).
65. M. Rozencweig, D. D. von Hoff, and J. E. Henney, *Cancer* **40,** 334 (1977).
66. J. D. Loike and S. B. Horwitz, *Biochemistry* **15,** 5443 (1976).
67. L. Wilson, *Ann. N.Y. Acad. Sci.* **253,** 213 (1975).
68. B. Bhattacharyya and J. Wolff, *Proc. Natl. Acad. Sci. U.S.A.* **73,** 2375 (1976).
69. S. Remillard, L. I. Rebhun, G. A. Howie, and S. M. Kupchan, *Science* **189,** 1002 (1975).
70. L. Rebhun, J. Nath, and S. Remillard, *Cold Spring Harbor Conf. Cell Proliferation* **3,** 1343 (1976).
71. F. Mandelbaum-Shavit, M. K. Wolpert-Defilippes, and D. G. Johns, *Biochem. Biophys. Res. Commun.* **72,** 47 (1976).
72. S. M. Kupchan, R. W. Britton, M. F. Ziegler, C. J. Gilmore, R. J. Restivo, and R. F. Bryan, *J. Am. Chem. Soc.* **95,** 1335 (1973).
73. A. S. Kende and L. S. Liebeskind, *J. Am. Chem. Soc.* **98,** 267 (1976).

74. A. S. Kende, L. S. Liebeskind, C. Kubiak, and R. Eisenberg, *J. Amer. Chem. Soc* **98,** 6389 (1976).
75. L. R. Hughes and R. A. Raphael, *Tetrahedron Lett.* **18,** 1543 (1976).
76. R. W. Wang, L. I. Rebhun, and M. S. Kupchan, *Cancer Res.* **37,** 3071 (1977).
77. P. B. Schiff, A. S. Kende, and S. B. Horwitz, *Biochem. Biophys. Res. Commun.* **85,** 737 (1978).
78. F. Zavala, D. Guenard, J. Robin, and E. Brown, *J. Med. Chem.* **23,** 546 (1980).
79. J. B. Swaney and K. S. Kuehl, *Biochim. Biophys. Acta* **446,** 561 (1976).
80. L. Wilson, J. R. Bamburg, S. B. Mizel, L. M. Grisham, and K. M. Creswell, *Fed. Proc., Fed. Am. Soc. Exp. Biol.* **33,** 158 (1974).
81. M. H. Zweig and C. F. Chignell, *Biochem. Pharmacol.* **22,** 2141 (1973).
82. P. B. Schiff, J. Fant, and S. B. Horwitz, *Nature (London)* **277,** 665 (1979).
83. M. C. Wani, H. L. Taylor, M. E. Wall, P. Coggon, and A. T. McPhail, *J. Am. Chem. Soc.* **93,** 2325 (1971).
84. M. E. Wall and M. C. Wani, *Annu. Rev. Pharmacol. Toxicol.* **17,** 117 (1977).
85. K. Weber, T. Bibring, and M. Osborn, *Exp. Cell Res.* **95,** 111 (1975).
86. E. Mandelkow, E. Mandelkow, N. Unwin, and C. Cohen, *Nature (London)* **265,** 655 (1977).
87. P. B. Schiff and S. B. Horwitz, *Proc. Natl. Acad. Sci. U.S.A.* **77,** 1561 (1980).
88. J. M. Vasiliev and I. M. Gelfand, *Int. Rev. Cytol.* **50,** 159 (1977).
89. R. L. Margolis, L. Wilson, and B. I. Kiefer, *Nature (London)* **272,** 450 (1978).
90. J. M. Vasiliev, I. M. Gelfand, L. V. Domnina, O. Y. Ivanova, S. G. Komm, and L. V. Olshevskaja, *J. Embryol. Exp. Morphol.* **24,** 625 (1970).
91. A. N. Bhisėy and J. J. Freed, *Exp. Cell Res.* **64,** 419 (1971).
92. M. H. Gail and C. W. Boone, *Exp. Cell Res.* **65,** 221 (1971).
93. M. Abercrombie, J. E. M. Heagsman, and S. M. Pegrum, *Exp. Cell Res.* **59,** 393 (1970).
94. M. Abercrombie, J. E. M. Heagsman, and S. M. Pegrum, *Exp. Cell Res.* **60,** 437 (1970).
95. G. Albrecht-Buehler, *Cell* **11,** 395 (1977).
96. A. Fellous, J. Francon, A. Lennon, and J. Nunez, *Eur. J. Biochem.* **78,** 167 (1977).
97. A. Levi, M. Cimino, D. Mercanti, J. S. Chen, and P. Calissano, *Biochim. Biophys. Acta* **399,** 50 (1975).
98. J. C. Lee, N. Tweedy, and S. N. Timasheff, *Biochemistry* **17,** 2783 (1978).
99. M. Jacobs, P. M. Bennett, and M. J. Dickens, *Nature (London)* **257,** 707 (1975).
100. O. Behnke, *Nature (London)* **257,** 709 (1975).
101. H. P. Erickson and W. A. Voter, *Proc. Natl. Acad. Sci. U.S.A.* **73,** 2813 (1976).
102. I. V. Sandoval, E. MacDonald, J. L. Jameson, and P. Cuatrecasas, *Proc. Natl. Acad. Sci. U.S.A.* **74,** 4881 (1977).
103. A. H. Lockwood, *Proc. Natl. Acad. Sci. U.S.A.* **76,** 1184 (1979).
104. J. Nunez, A. Fellous, J. Francon, and A. Lennon, *Proc. Natl. Acad. Sci. U.S.A.* **76,** 86 (1979).
105. P. Sherline, K. Schiavone, and S. Brocato, *Science* **205,** 593 (1979).

PART VII

Angiogenesis-Metastasis-Anticarcinogenesis-Differentiation

24

Angiogenesis Inhibitors

ROBERT LANGER AND JUDAH FOLKMAN

I. Angiogenesis as a Control Point in Tumor Growth

Most solid malignant tumors appear to have the property of inducing new capillaries from the host. This phenomenon has been called tumor angiogenesis. Accumulating evidence suggests that the growth of a solid tumor is bound to angiogenesis. Thus a successful tumor must continually induce new capillary blood vessels from the host, not only for maintenance of the original mass but also for further tumor growth (1).

We have previously advanced the hypothesis that, until a tumor nodule is penetrated by new capillaries, the limitations imposed by the diffusion of nutrients and oxygen prevent it from growing rapidly (2). The implication of this hypothesis is that, in the absence of angiogenesis, a tumor nodule might remain dormant or static at a few millimeters in diameter. For this reason, we propose

ISBN 0-12-619280-4

that "antiangiogenesis" might someday become a potential therapeutic approach (3).

Indirect support for this hypothesis has come from three lines of experimental evidence: (1) Tumor cells implanted in isolated perfused organs, where induction of new capillaries could not occur, grew to diameters of 0.5–1 mm and then became dormant (4). (2) Tumor implants in the anterior chamber of the rabbit eye remained avascular because new vessels could not reach them through the aqueous humor. These tumors never grew beyond 1 mm in diameter (5). (C) Tumor spheroids grown in soft agar medium that was continuously changed also reached a steady state of growth where generation of new cells and death of old cells became balanced. These spheroids ranged from 1 to 4 mm, with less than 1 million cells per spheroid (6).

However, there was previously no way to inhibit the vascularization of an implanted tumor directly and thus inhibit its growth. Most experimental tumors implanted subcutaneously in mice or rats induce new capillary growth rapidly and are penetrated by new vessels by the third or fourth day. Rapid tumor growth follows vascularization. The 3-day period before vascularization (the prevascular period) is too brief to measure the extent of tumor inhibition due to the absence of vascularization. A critical experiment to demonstrate that angiogenesis is a control point in tumor growth would require that the onset of vascularization be postponed or prevented by some type of angiogenesis inhibitor, and that subsequently an implanted tumor would stop growing as a small avascular tumor.

II. Inhibition of Tumor Angiogenesis Locally by Cartilage

We began to think that an angiogenesis inhibitor might be found in cartilage after learning about the work of Eisenstein *et al.* (7). In their experiment, pieces of cartilage were implanted in the chorioallantoic membrane of the chick embryo. It was found that cartilage could withstand invasion by vascular mesenchyme. They subsequently observed that, when cartilage was extracted with guanidine, it lost its resistance to invasion by the vascularized chorioallantoic membrane. They proposed that this ability of cartilage to resist invasion might be linked to protease inhibitors in the cartilage (8).

To test whether cartilage could continuously release some sort of angiogenesis inhibitor, we implanted V2 carcinoma in the cornea of the rabbit eye (9). The tumor implant was positioned at a distance of 2 mm from the normal vascular bed of the cornea. A 1-mm piece of cartilage from the scapula of a newborn rabbit was implanted between the tumor and the nearest vascular bed (Figs. 1 and 2). For control experiments, the cartilage was boiled or other tissues such as cornea or bone were implanted. New capillaries induced by the tumor grew across the cornea toward the tumor in eyes containing heat-killed cartilage (Fig. 3). In

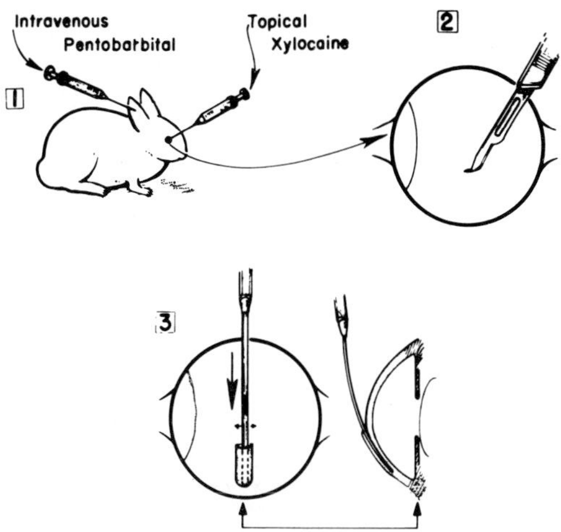

Fig. 1. Technique of corneal implantation. The rabbit is anesthetized with intravenous pentobarbital, and Xylocaine is applied topically to the cornea. An incision is made halfway through the thickness of the cornea, and an intrastromal pocket is made with a malleable iris spatula. The pocket ends approximately 1-2 mm from the limbus. Tumor fragments are inserted into the pocket.

contrast, when the cartilage implant was fresh, tumor-induced vessels growing toward it slowed and stopped their growth near the implant. In rabbits with a fresh cartilage implant, the majority of tumors did not become vascularized for periods of up to 3 months. In control rabbits, where the cartilage was inactivated, tumors became vascularized on schedule (i.e., at 10–15 days) and went on to become large, bulging tumor masses. In later studies, bovine cartilage produced

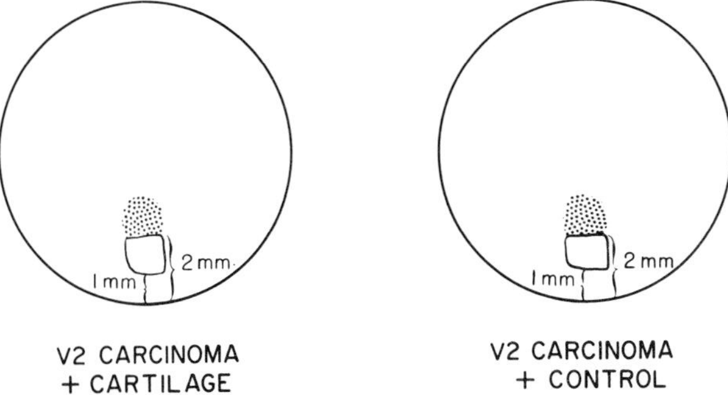

Fig. 2. Diagram of rabbit cornea. V2 carcinoma and neonatal rabbit cartilage are implanted together in a corneal pocket. As a control for neonatal cartilage, boiled cartilage or pieces of neonatal cornea are used. V2 carcinoma is implanted alone as another control. From Brem and Folkman (9), with permission of the publisher.

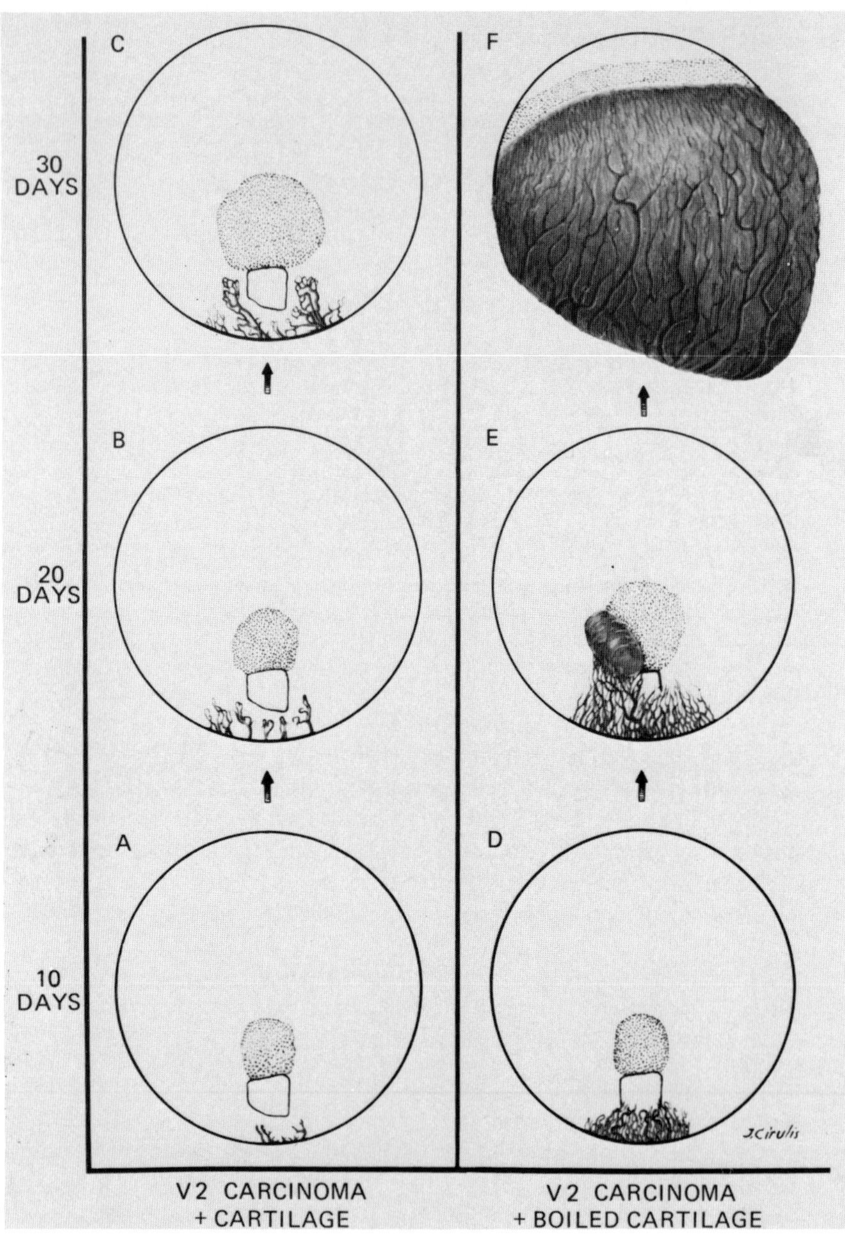

Fig. 3. V2 carcinoma implanted in rabbit corneas with active neonatal cartilage or with boiled cartilage. Scale drawings were made by tracing color photographs of the actual specimens. Vessels are inhibited from reaching the tumor when active cartilage is implanted with it (A–C). Cartilage inactivated by boiling is implanted with the tumor in (D). Vessels enter this tumor by day 15, and rapid tumor growth follows (E), leading to a large exophytic mass (F). A similar result (D–F) is obtained when the boiled cartilage is replaced by neonatal cornea or when the tumor is implanted alone. The diameter of the cornea is 12 mm. From Brem and Folkman (9).

the same effect. These studies implied that cartilage could release an angiogenesis inhibitor that was diffusible over short distances.

III. Isolation and Partial Purification of an Angiogenesis Inhibitor

Extracts of cartilage were then made by a variety of methods, including simple aqueous extraction, guanidine extraction, and Ringer's extraction, and were further purified using $(NH_4)_2SO_4$ precipitation and column chromatography. Most of the extracts caused severe inflammation. Only one turned out to have angiogenesis-inhibitory activity (10). This extract was made using 1 *M* guanidine extraction as suggested by Sorgente *et al.* (8), followed by trypsin-affinity chromatography (10). All extracts were dialyzed exhaustively against water at 4°C, passed through 0.45-μm Millipore filters, and lyophilized. Sterile technique was followed thereafter. It was difficult to assay these extracts in the cornea, because they rapidly diffused away from the site of implantation. This problem was solved by incorporating the cartilage extract into a sustained-release polymer that could be implanted as a 1-mm pellet in the cornea (11).

The sustained-release polymer permitted us to position a depot of cartilage extract in the cornea between a tumor and its vascular bed. These experiments confirmed the previous findings with cartilage implants, namely, that tumor-induced vessels could be stopped in their path of growth toward the tumor. A zone of inhibition appeared around the polymer implants containing the inhibitor. Comparative vessel growth rates are shown in Fig. 4.

IV. Control of Tumor Growth by Infusion of a Cartilage-Derived Angiogenesis Inhibitor

Before proceeding with further purification of the cartilage angiogenesis inhibitor, it was important to know if the soluble inhibitor could stop tumor-induced neovascularization if the material were given parenterally. Because of the scarcity of available material, the infusion of cartilage angiogenesis inhibitor was carried out in the following way.

A. V2 Carcinoma in Rabbits

A long-term indwelling catheter was placed in the right common carotid artery of rabbits using the system described by Conn and Langer (12) (Fig. 5). Ringer's solution was infused at the rate of 14.4 ml/day into rabbits weighing 4–5 lb. In this way, an inhibitor added to the Ringer's solution was delivered preferentially to the right eye, causing the left eye to receive inhibitor at a lower effective dose.

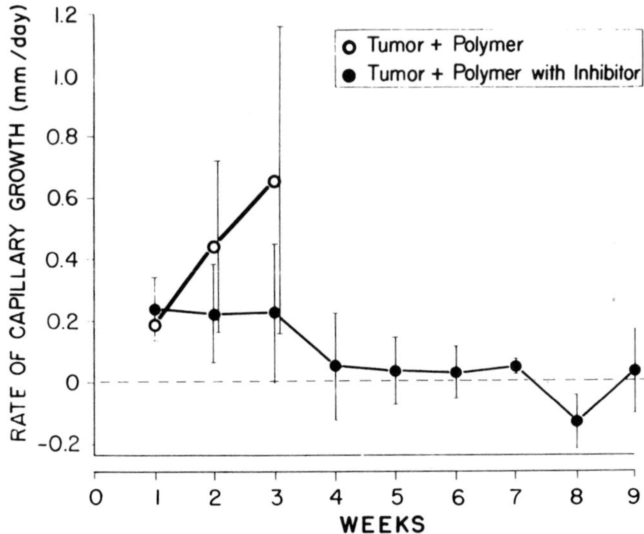

Fig. 4. Rate of capillary growth in 21 rabbit eyes with inhibitor and 16 controls. Rates were determined by weekly differences in the length of the longest vessels. Calculation of rates began at the onset of neovascularization, which occurred 5 ± 1 days after implantation for each of the 37 corneas. ○, Vessel growth rates in the absence of inhibitor; all rabbits were dead by the end of the third week. ●, Vessel growth rates when inhibitor was present; by the fourth week some vessels were regressing. From Langer *et al.* (10), with permission of the publisher.

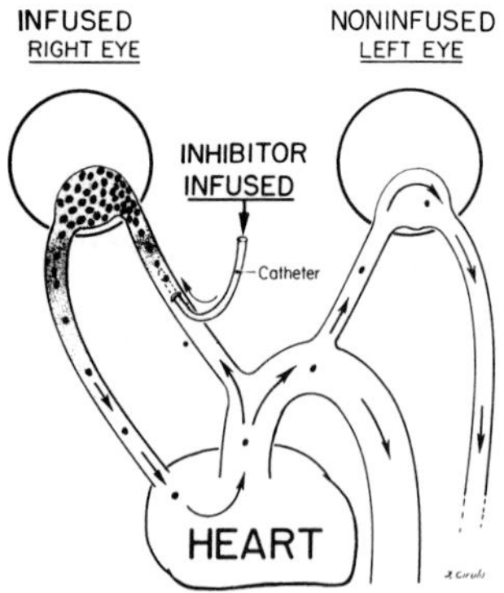

Fig. 5. Flow diagram of infusions through the right common carotid artery in rabbits and mice. Technetium pertechnate scans demonstrated that the concentration reaching the right eye was 15- to 60-fold times greater than that reaching the left eye. From Langer *et al.* (13), with permission of the publisher.

Therefore each rabbit received a high dose in the right eye and a low dose in the left eye, as proven by ^{199}Tc scanning. V2 carcinomas were implanted (1.5-mm pieces) in the rabbit cornea 1.0 mm central to the limbus, as described in Fig. 1. Rabbit corneas were examined daily with a Zeiss slit-lamp stereoscope at 6× and 16× magnification. Measurements of the lengths of new vessels were made to ±0.1 mm.

The angiogenesis inhibitor was prepared by using a scaled-up procedure of our earlier method (10). Cartilage was excised from fresh veal scapular bones, and connective tissue was removed. Cartilage slices (2.0 kg) were then extracted in 20 liter of 1.0 *M* guanidine–HCl and 0.02 *M* sodium malate buffer (pH 6) for 24 hours at 25°C. This solution was filtered and then concentrated to 500 ml in a Millipore ultrafiltration unit containing a PTGC cassette (nominal molecular weight limit 10,000). The retentate was dialyzed against water for 12 hours at 4°C and then desalted using the Millipore unit described above. The material was then lyophylized, subjected to trypsin–Sepharose affinity chromatography, and sterilized as described earlier.

V2 carcinoma was then implanted in both corneas of each rabbit. Three days after new blood vessels began to grow toward the tumor, infusion of the cartilage-derived inhibitor was begun in three rabbits (Fig. 6). The cartilage-derived inhibitor was infused at 1 mg/day and then increased to 3 mg/day as in Fig. 6. Controls consisted of 21 corneas infused with Ringer's solution, 4 with Trasylol, and 3 untreated eyes of the experimental animals. In the control animals, the mean corneal vessel growth rate was 0.32 mm/day (Ringer's), 0.35 mm/day (untreated eyes in the experimental group), and 0.46 mm/day (Trasylol) over the 6-day infusion period. In contrast, the average growth of vessels in the right corneas of animals receiving the cartilage-derived inhibitor was 0.01 mm/day.

The angiogenesis inhibitor affected the density of vessels, as well as their rate of growth. While all control corneas showed an increase in vessel number from approximately 4 to over 100 vessels per cornea during the 6-day infusion period, two of the three treated corneas showed no increase in vessel density. The third cornea showed only a small increase in vessel density and a 0.1-mm increase in length. Yet even this cornea was markedly less vascularized than the most mildly vascularized corneas of the controls (Fig. 7A and B).

The reason for infusing the rabbits at a slightly higher level of inhibitor (3 mg/day) was to determine if an increased dose would inhibit vascular growth in the contralateral eye. We did not observe any quantitative differences when comparisons with the controls were made.

All 28 controls developed large, bulging, vascularized tumors. In contrast, the tumors in the treated eyes grew much more slowly and did not become vascularized during the infusion. New vessels resumed growth toward the tumor implant once the inhibitor infusion was discontinued, although in some cases a

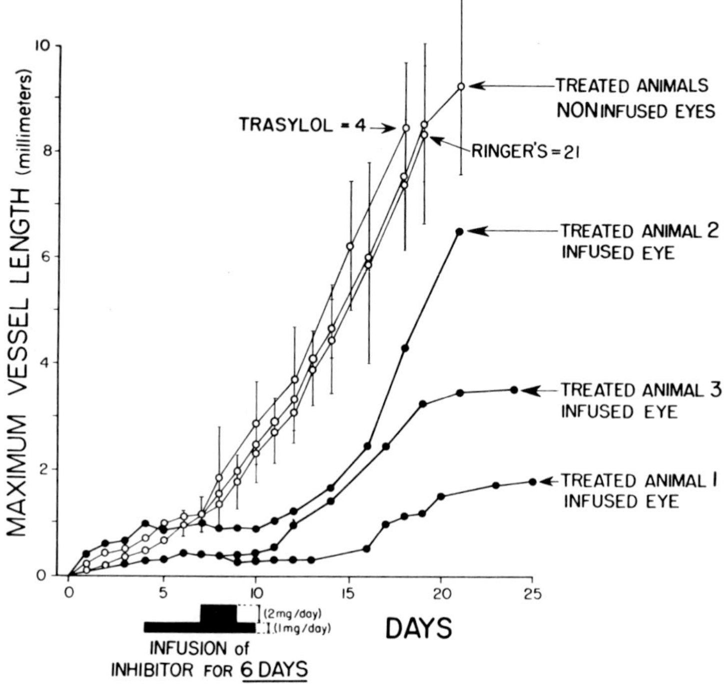

Fig. 6. Infusion of the inhibitor and control solutions through the right carotid artery in rabbits carrying V2 carcinoma in each cornea. Rabbits were sacrificed when tumors became large, protruding masses. The vessel length at this time averaged 9 mm. From Langer *et al.* (13), with permission of the publisher.

lag phase was observed (Fig. 6). When the vessels reached the edge of the tumor, tumor growth also resumed.

There were no toxic effects of the inhibitor infusion. Blood studies and histological studies on every organ showed no abnormality, with one exception, alkaline phophatase activity, which was below normal by a factor of 3 in the treated animals (13).

B. B16 Melanoma in Mice

In the rabbit experiments the tumor was separated from the host's vascular bed, and this permitted the daily measurement of vessel growth rate. However, in the clinical situation, most tumors are situated or arise in a previously existing vascular bed; thus tumor and host vasculature are not separated. Therefore we did a second set of experiments in which the tumor implant was placed contiguous to a vascular bed. Mouse melanoma (B16) was implanted directly in the dense capillary bed of the mouse conjunctiva. In this experimental design, tumor

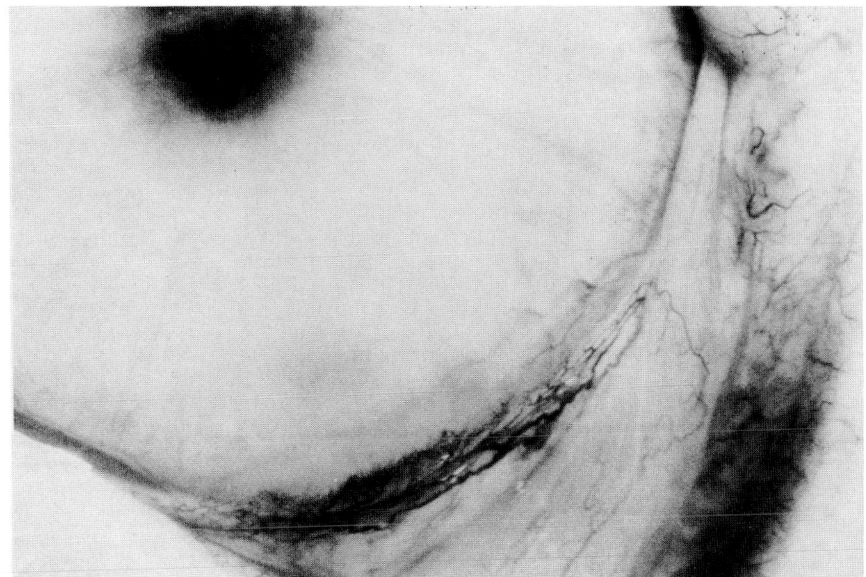
A

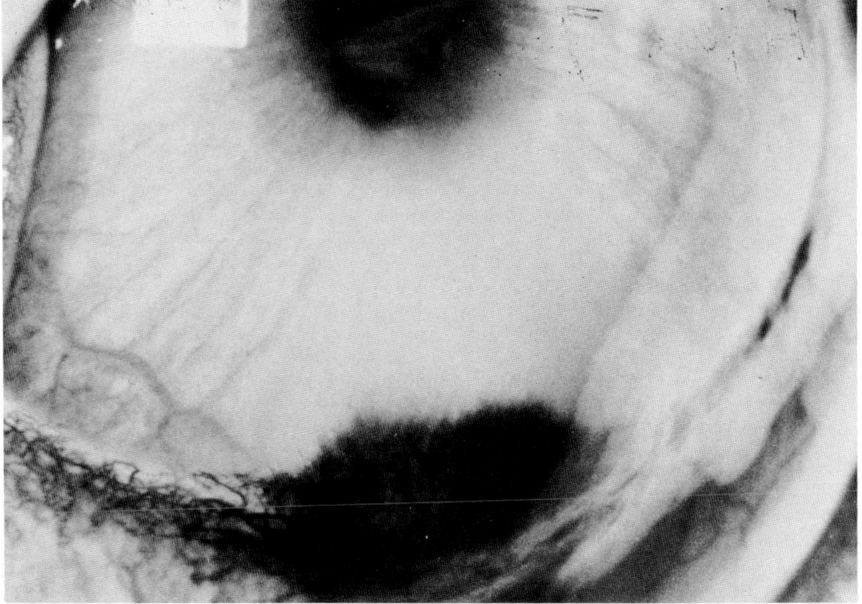
B

Fig. 7. Photographs of corneas in treated (A) and untreated (B) rabbits following the 6-day infusion period. Note the much larger, broader vascular front in the untreated cornea. Before the infusion started, the vessels in the untreated cornea were shorter and less dense than in the experimental cornea. From Langer *et al.* (13), with permission of the publisher.

growth was measured directly and the vascular response was determined histologically. It was not possible to measure the linear growth of vessels in this system.

Fragments of B16 melanoma (1.0 mm) were implanted in the conjunctival sac of C57BL/6J mice weighing 25–30 gm as described previously (13). A small silicone rubber catheter was placed in the right common carotid artery (Fig. 5) so that Ringer's solution could be infused at a rate of 0.96 ml/24 hours. Tumor measurements were made in anesthetized animals starting on day 5 after tumor implantation. The measurements were made with a Nikon stereomicroscope at 12× with an accuracy of ±0.1 mm and without knowledge of how the animals had been treated. The mice were sacrificed on day 7, and the tumors were excised and weighed. Twenty-four hours after implantation, little evidence of either the implant or of the procedure itself was evident. Between days 3 and 4, a small, flat, black plaque appeared in the area of the subconjunctiva pocket. The tumor cells grew rapidly into a three-dimensional mass. In untreated animals, focal hemorrhages occured on the tumor surface, and large, dilated vessels entered its base on days 5 and 6. This vascularization was not observed in treated animals. Measurement of tumor length was the only serial determination possible. Tumor width and height could not be accurately quantitated until after removal, because the vascularized tumors grew behind the orbital margin. The rate of tumor growth was similar in all the untreated animals. In noninfused mice, tumor length increased at a rate of 0.69 mm/day (Fig. 8). In mice infused with Ringer's solution, the rate was 0.64 mm/day. Tumors in mice infused with albumin or Trasylol grew at rates of 0.60 and 0.65 mm/day, respectively.

In contrast, tumors in the right eye of animals infused with the angiogenesis-inhibitor showed growth rates of only 0.06 mm/day. The left eyes of these animals served as internal controls with tumor growth rates similar to those of the other controls, i.e., 0.74 mm/day (Fig. 8). By day 7, the untreated tumors weighed an average of 7.6 mg and there was no statistically significant difference in tumor weight in any of the control groups. In contrast, the average tumor weight in the treated eyes was 0.18 mg, less than 2.5% of that of the controls (Figs. 9 and 10).

C. Histology

The histology of tumors in the untreated animals showed densely packed, healthy, pleomorphic tumor cells containing melanin in about half the cells of the tumor population. Within the densely packed tumor cells, there were prominent capillary blood vessels. The endothelial cell density in these vessels was higher than that in the flat endothelium in adjacent tissue not affected by the tumor. Animals treated with the angiogenesis inhibitor showed only a few viable melanin-producing cells which did not form a solid tumor mass but were scat-

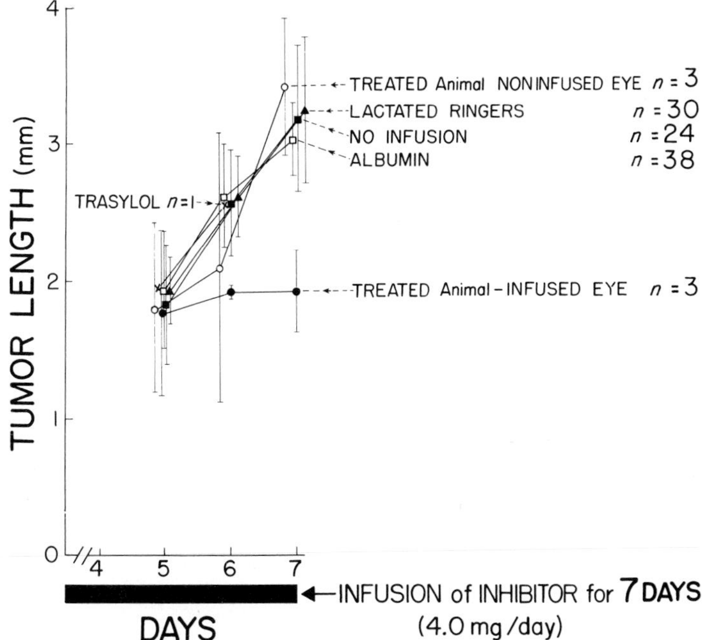

Fig. 8. Maximum tumor dimension of B16 melanoma implants in C57B1/6J mice in the subconjunctival space. From Langer *et al.* (13), with permission of the publisher.

tered as individual spindle cells within a loose edematous stroma. No new capillary proliferation was observed in the treated tumors, and adjacent vessels showed flat, quiescent endothelium. None of the treated mice showed any toxic effects from the infusion. Pathological surveys of all the major organs were normal. However, in two of the three treated animals, a widened femoral epiphyseal plate with increased numbers of chondrocytes was observed.

D. Cell Culture

B16 melanoma cells incubated with the angiogenesis inhibitor, Trasylol, or bovine serum albumin at concentrations of 1–1000 μg/ml grew at approximately the same rate as melanoma cells without the added compounds. At 4.0 mg/ml, all three solutions of inhibitor caused slight inhibition. Also, when V2 carcinoma was grown at 1.0 mg/ml, there was no reduction in growth rate compared to that of the controls. At 4.0 mg/ml the inhibitor caused a 10% reduction in growth rate of V2 carcinoma cells compared to that of the controls. These studies provided further evidence that the cartilage-derived angiogenesis inhibitor did not inhibit tumor cell growth directly but inhibited neovascularization and gave rise to an avascular tumor with restricted growth.

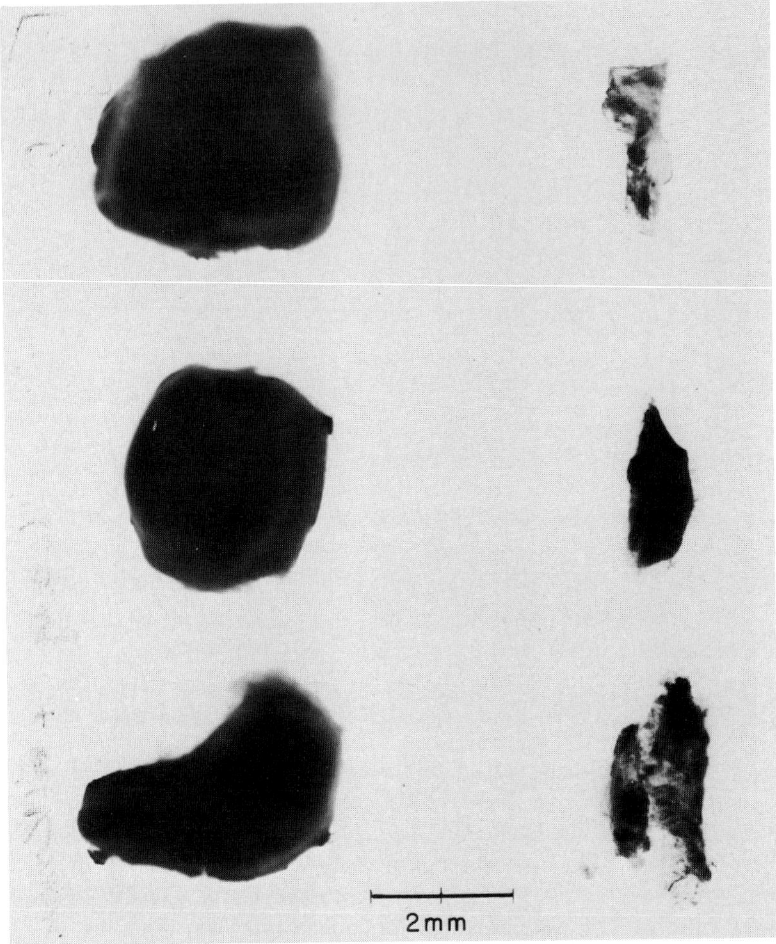

Fig. 9. Photographs of excised B16 melanoma implants. Untreated eye implants (left) and treated eye implants (right) at day 7.

E. Controls

To control for nonspecific inhibition due to infusion of protein in general, or antitrypsin activity in particular, other protein solutions were used including Trasylol, a bovine trypsin inhibitor. These infusions did not stop angiogenesis. To control for nonspecific inhibition of tumor growth due to "sickness" or debilitation of the animal, the left eye of all treated animals received the inhibitor, but at a substantially lower concentration than the right eye. If the animals were sick, tumor suppression would have occurred in the left eye as well as the right eye. In fact, all tumors in the left eye grew and became vascularized at the

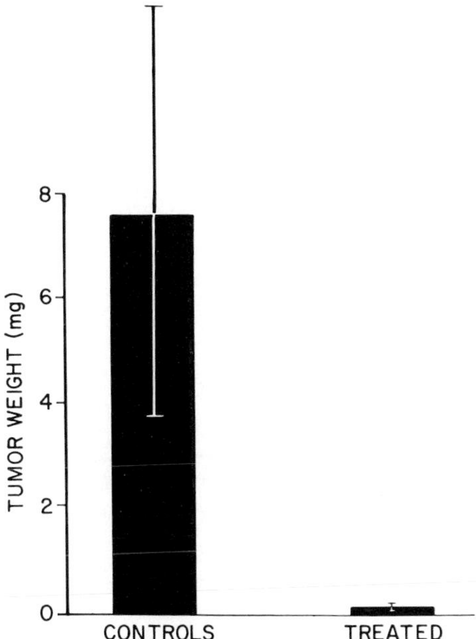

Fig. 10. Weights of excised untreated and treated B16 melanoma implants at day 7. The weights are for the 3 untreated tumors and all 15 controls (Ringer's, albumin, Trasylol, and the noninfused eyes of treated animals) run in the same series as the treated tumors. From Langer *et al.* (13), with permission of the publisher.

same rate as tumors in untreated eyes. To control for the possibility that the inhibited vessels might have stopped growing spontaneously or for some nonspecific reason, the pre- and postinfusion behavior of the tumors in the treated animals was studied carefully. While vessel growth essentially stopped in all eyes treated with the high dose of angiogenesis inhibitor, blood vessel growth always resumed after the angiogenesis inhibitor was discontinued. This result is further strengthened when considered against the experience of our laboratory with V2 carcinoma. In our experience over the past 9 years, V2 carcinoma has not regressed spontaneously in rabbit eyes.

V. Conclusions

These experiments show that an angiogenesis inhibitor can be isolated from cartilage. Its regional infusion will stop tumor vascularization and prevent subsequent tumor growth in two different species. The 41-fold inhibition of the growth of mouse melanoma further demonstrated that an aggressive solid tumor could be halted by an angiogenesis inhibitor, despite the fact that the tumor was implanted contiguous to a normal vascular bed. The angiogenesis inhibitor is a natural product of normal tissue, and it appears not to be toxic in any obvious way.

VI. Theoretical Considerations

The mechanism by which angiogenesis is inhibited by cartilage and its extracts is unknown. Nor do we know if such an angiogenesis inhibitor will be effective against a larger already vascularized tumor. The scarcity of the inhibitor precludes at this point the possibility of testing it on tumors at more advanced stages of growth and vascularization. However, work is underway to identify and purify the active molecule and, once characterized, the availability of the inhibitor may be increased. The point we wish to stress, however, is that this angiogenesis inhibitor derived from cartilage should be considered a prototype. It is possible that other angiogenesis inhibitors will be found or synthesized and that they may be even more potent. For example, an inhibitor of neovascularization has recently been isolated from the vitreous by Patz *et al.* (14). It also remains to be seen how a potent angiogenesis inhibitor would be used clinically, should one become available. One can speculate that infusion of an angiogenesis inhibitor might be carried out in patients a few days prior to excision of a primary tumor. Or, another speculation is that angiogenesis inhibitors may become important adjuncts in the treatment of brain tumors. Finally, in the more distant future it is possible that angiogenesis inhibitors will be used as a pretreatment in combination with chemotherapy or immunotherapy.

Whatever future direction is taken in this field, the present experiments provide strong support for the concept of antiangiogenesis (3) and suggest that control of tumor growth may be possible through control of neovascularization.

Acknowledgment

This work was supported by USPHS grant CA-14019 from the National Cancer Institute, and by a grant to Harvard University from the Monsanto Company. The polymer studies were also supported by a gift from the Alza Corporation. We thank Ms. Vicki Elms for typing the manuscript for this chapter.

References

1. J. Folkman and R. S. Cotran, *Int. Rev. Exp. Pathol.* **16,** 207 (1976).
2. J. Folkman, *Adv. Cancer Res.* **19,** 331 (1974).
3. J. Folkman, *Ann. Surg.* **175,** 409 (1972).

4. J. Folkman, P. Cole, and S. Zimmerman, *Ann. Surg.* **164,** 491 (1966).
5. M. A. Gimbrone, Jr., S. B. Leapman, R. S. Cotran, and J. Folkman, *J. Natl. Cancer Inst.* **50,** 219 (1973).
6. J. Folkman and M. Hochberg, *J. Exp. Med.* **138,** 745 (1973).
7. R. Eisenstein, N. Sorgente, L. W. Soble, A. Miller, and K. E. Kuettner, *Am. J. Pathol.* **73,** 765 (1973).
8. N. Sorgente, K. E. Kuettner, L. W. Soble, and R. Eisenstein, *Lab. Invest.* **32,** 217 (1975).
9. H. Brem and J. Folkman, *J. Exp. Med.* **141,** 427 (1975).
10. R. Langer, H. Brem, K. Falterman, M. Klein, and J. Folkman, *Science* **193,** 70 (1976).
11. R. Langer and J. Folkman, *Nature* (*London*) **263,** 797 (1976).
12. H. Conn and R. Langer, *Lab. Anim. Sci.* **28,** 598 (1978).
13. R. Langer, H. Conn, J. Vacanti, C. Haudenschild, and J. Folkman, *Proc. Natl. Acad. Sci. U.S.A.* **77,** 4331 (1980).
14. A. Patz, S. Brem, D. Finkelstein, C-H. Chen, G. Lutty, A. Bennett, W. R. Coughlin, and J. Gardner, *Trans. Am. Acad. Ophthalmol. Otolaryngol.* **85,** 626 (1978).

25

Effects of β-All-*Trans*-Retinoic Acid on the Growth and Implantation Properties of Metastatic B16 Melanoma Cell Lines

REUBEN LOTAN AND GARTH L. NICOLSON

I. Introduction

Retinoids (vitamin A analogues; see Fig. 1) are well recognized for their ability to suppress the effects of carcinogens both *in vitro* and *in vivo* [for reviews, see references 1–4]. In addition to their anticarcinogenesis properties, they inhibit the growth of malignant cells [reviewed in Lotan (4)]; however, the potential use of retinoids as antitumor agents is still being explored. Several studies have shown that retinoids alone (5–11) or in combination with X-irradiation (12), cyclophosphamide and 1,3-bis(2-chloroethyl)- 1-nitrosourea (13), 5-fluorouracil and cobalt-60 radiation (14,15), or *Mycobacterium bovis* (strain BCG) (16) exhibit antitumor activities, while other studies with different

MOLECULAR ACTIONS AND TARGETS FOR CANCER CHEMOTHERAPEUTIC AGENTS

ISBN 0-12-619280-4

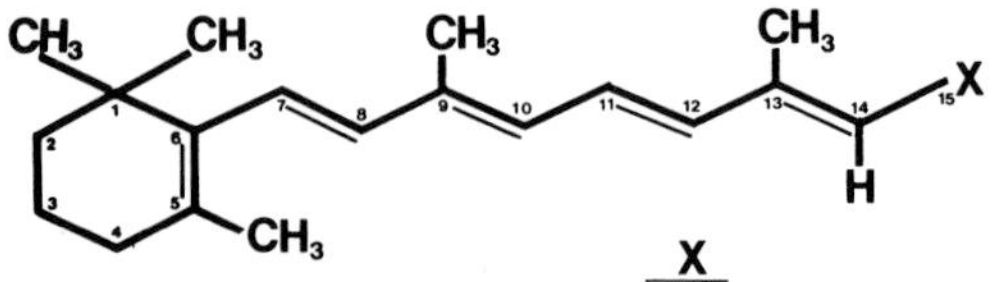

	X
Retinol	CH_2OH
Retinoic acid	COOH
Retinyl acetate	CH_2OCOCH_3

Fig. 1. Chemical structure of some retinoids.

tumor systems have failed to detect significant inhibitory effects of retinoids on malignant cells (17).

The results of recent investigations in our laboratory have demonstrated the potential use of retinoids for inhibition of tumor growth in a number of systems. First, we have shown that the proliferation of numerous transformed and tumor cell lines of rodent or human origin can be inhibited by retinoids in culture (18–21) and, second, we have found that retinoids stimulate host antitumor cell-mediated immune responses (22). Thus, with certain tumors, retinoids can be expected to inhibit cell proliferation directly and/or act indirectly to destroy tumor cells via augmentation of host antitumor immune responses. A recent report on the ability of retinoids to reduce the efficiency of colony formation of freshly prepared human melanoma cells in soft agar has led to the initiation of clinical trials using retinoids in selected patients with malignant melanoma (23).

We are utilizing the murine B16 melanoma system to evaluate the potential of using conventional cytotoxic drugs, as well as retinoids, as antimetastatic agents (24). Cell lines are available in the B16 system that show enhanced colonization of lung (25), brain (26), or ovary (27) in C57BL/6 mice. In addition, some of the *in vivo*-selected B16 lines have been selected further *in vitro* for resistance to killing by immune syngeneic populations to obtain lymphocyte-resistant sublines (28). The selections for tumor cell subpopulations with differing properties were successful in part because the parent B16 melanoma is a heterogeneous cell population that contains clones with widely different metastatic phenotypes (29,30). Heterogeneity in the metastatic properties of preexistent cells in the unselected B16 tumor has been demonstrated by *in vitro* cloning experiments where clones of quite dissimilar metastatic potential have been obtained (31). Other studies have shown that, in addition to B16 melanoma, other quite different tumors such as murine sarcoma (32), mammary carcinoma (33), and fibrosarcoma (34,35) contain rare, highly metastatic subpopulations.

II. Retinoid Inhibition of B16 Melanoma Cell Growth

Our previous studies examined the effects of β-all-*trans*-retinoic acid or retinyl acetate on the growth of a B16 melanoma subline (B16-F1) of low lung

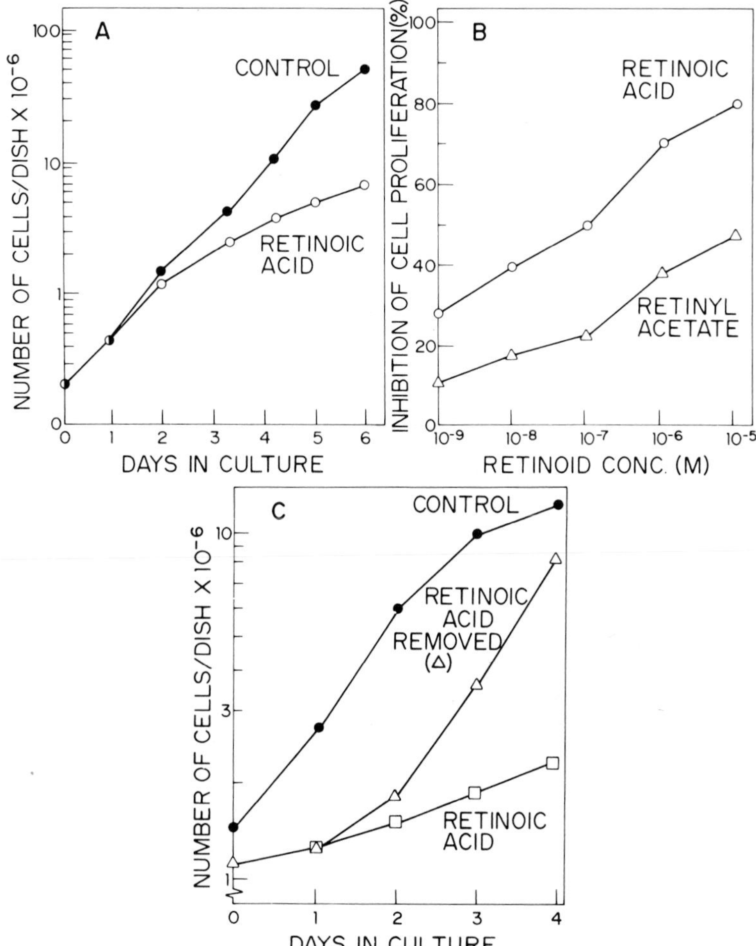

Fig. 2. Time course (A), dose-response (B), and reversibility (C) of retinoid-induced growth inhibition of mouse B16-F1 cells *in vitro.* (A) Cells (2×10^5/dish) were plated in 150-mm dishes in 30 ml growth medium containing 0.1% ethanol (●) or retinoic acid (10^{-5} *M*) added in ethanol (○). Medium was changed on alternate days, and cultures were harvested at the indicated times and the cell number determined. (B) Cells (2×10^5/dish) were cultured as in (A) in the absence or in the presence of the indicated concentrations of retinoids. On day 6, the cells were counted and percent inhibition of growth was calculated according to the equation $1 - (R/C) \times 100$, where R and C are the numbers of cells in retinoic acid-treated and untreated cultures, respectively. (C) Cells were plated in 100-mm dishes in 10 ml medium at 4×10^3 cells/dish in control medium and at 3×10^4 cells/dish in medium containing 10^{-5} *M* retinoic acid. Medium was changed on alternate days and from day 6 on control cultures (●) and half of the retinoic acid-treated cultures (Δ) were refed medium without retinoic acid, whereas the other half of the retinoic acid-treated cultures (□) were refed medium containing retinoic acid. Cultures were harvested every 24 hours thereafter, and the cell number determined.

colonization potential (18,19). These experiments revealed that retinoid-mediated inhibition of B16-F1 cell proliferation *in vitro* was time-dependent (Fig. 2A), dose- and drug-dependent (Fig. 2B), and reversible (Fig. 2C). Growth inhibition was apparent only after 2 days of treatment (Fig. 2A) and was not related to cell density in culture. Retinoid inhibition of B16-F1 proliferation was effective in sparse cultures (Fig. 3); therefore it does not represent restoration of density-dependent growth control of the melanoma cultures. Nor does it represent cytotoxicity of retinoic acid as the cause of growth inhibition, because cell viabilities were similar in treated and control cell cultures (19) and there were no differences in the cytoplasmic contents of the lysosomal enzymes, acid phosphatase and aryl sulfatase (19), indicating that inhibition was not the result of a sublethal release of lysosomal enzymes. In addition, the lysosomal stabilizers hydrocortisone and cortisone failed to prevent the inhibitory effects of retinoic acid on the growth of cells. Further studies failed to detect any change in cyclic AMP (cAMP) levels in retinoic acid-treated cells as compared to controls, suggesting that growth inhibition was not the result of elevated cAMP which has been implicated in reducing the growth rate of B16 melanoma (36). The main effect of retinoic acid on B16-F1 cells is a reduction in the growth rate to about half that of untreated control cells (Fig. 2A). This is not due to a loss of plating ability, because plating efficiencies are not affected by retinoic acid concentrations as high as 10^{-5} *M*.

Treatment of B16-F1 cells with 10^{-5} *M* retinoic acid causes characteristic morphological changes. In retinoic acid-treated cultures cells exhibit an enhanced tendency to grow in clumps (Fig. 3B), a phenomenon that only occurs in

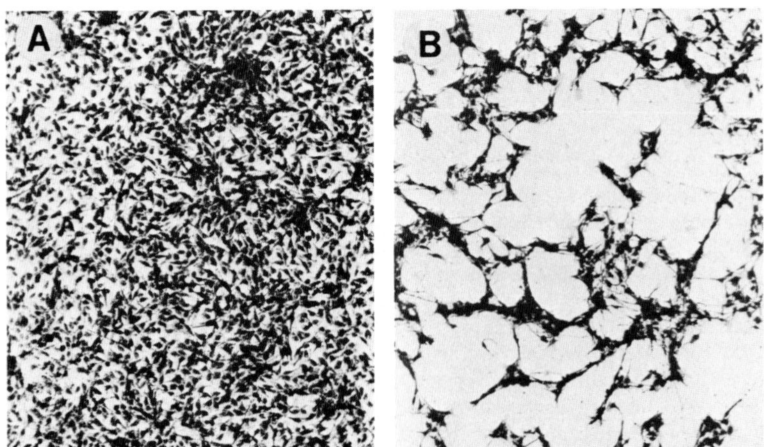

Fig. 3. Photomicrographs of B16-F1 melanoma cells plated at 3×10^4 cells/35-mm tissue culture dishes in the absence (A) or presence (B) of 10^{-5} *M* retinoic acid and cultured for 5 days. Cells were fixed and stained with Diff-Quick, Harleco (Gibbstown, N.J.). ×70.

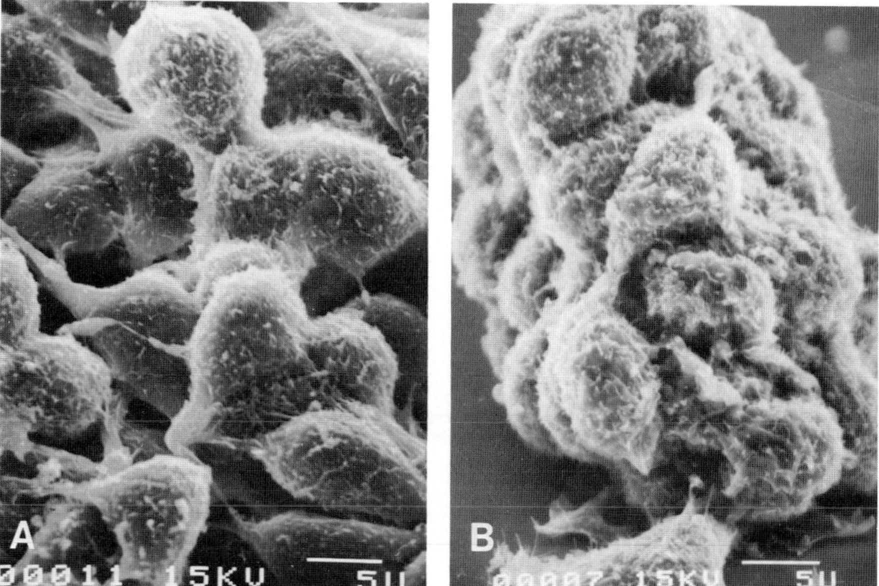

Fig. 4. Scanning electron micrographs of B16-F1 melanoma cells cultured as in Fig. 2 in the absence (A) or presence (B) of 10^{-5} *M* retinoic acid. Bars equal 5 μm.

untreated cultures of B16-F1 cells that have reached confluency (Fig. 3A). Examination of control (Fig. 4A) and retinoic acid-treated (Fig. 4B) cell cultures by scanning electron microscopy reveals the enhanced degree of intercellular interactions among the retinoic acid-treated cells and the apparent presence of more membrane ruffles, as compared to untreated cells.

The B16 clones and selected cell lines also varied in their melanin content (Table I). Lines B16-O10 and B16-F10$^{Lr\text{-}6}$ produced negligible amounts of melanin and appeared amelanotic; line B16-B10n and parental clone 12 produced small but significant amounts of melanin, whereas all the other clones and cell lines produced large amounts of melanin. There was no relationship between melanin production and the biological properties of the clones and lines or their ability to be growth-inhibited by retinoic acid (Table I).

III. Heterogeneity in Retinoid Inhibition of B16 Variant Lines

Previous studies on the effects of anticancer drugs on tumor cells have found that various cell lines derived from the same tumor differ widely in drug susceptibility (33,38,39). Therefore we examined the ability of retinoic acid to inhibit proliferation of the parental B16 melanoma line, as well as clones derived from

TABLE I

Properties of Clones and Variant Cell Lines of Metastatic B16 Melanoma and Their

B16 melanoma line	Source and reference	Metastatic potential	Organ colonization preference
Parental	Subcutaneous C57BL/6 tumor established in culture (25)	Moderate	Lung > lymph node > ovary > liver > kidney
Clone 12	*In vitro* cloning of the parental B16 line (31)	Low	Lung
Clone 15		Low	Lung > lymph node
Clone 9		High	Lung >> lymph node > brain
Clone 14		High	Lung >> ovary
F1	Parental B16 selected once *in vivo* for lung colonization (25)	Moderate	Lung > Lymph node > brain > ovary
F10	Parental B16 selected 10 times *in vivo* for lung colonization (25)	High	Lung
$F10^{Lr-6}$	B16-F10 selected for resistance to lymphocyte-mediated cytotoxicity *in vitro* (28)	Low	Lung
B10n	B16-F1 selected 10 times *in vivo* for brain colonization (26)	Moderate	Brain > > lung
O10	B16-F1 selected 10 times *in vivo* for ovary colonization (27)	High	Ovary > lung

this line, and variant cell lines of varying metastatic and organ colonization potential selected *in vivo* (Table I). Retinoic acid reduced the growth rates of all B16 cell lines and clones tested without affecting their respective plating efficiencies; however, there was a dramatic difference in the extent of growth inhibition among the various B16 lines and clones. Parental B16, parental clone 14, and line B16-F1 were especially sensitive to retinoic acid, and their growth rates were inhibited approximately 85–90% after 5 days in media containing 10^{-5} *M* retinoic acid. Parental clone 12 and line B16-B10n were moderately inhibited in 10^{-5} *M* retinoic acid after 5 days, while the other parental clones and the lines selected *in vivo* were more resistant to the effects of the drug (Table I).

Response to the Growth-Inhibitory Effect of Retinoic Acid

Doubling time in culture (hours)[a]	Melanin content (A_{400nm}/ 5 × 10^6 cells)[b]	Growth inhibition by 10^{-5} *M* retinoic acid (%)[c]	Approximate concentration required for 50% growth inhibition (μ*M*)[d]
14-16	0.39 ± 0.03	88 ± 4	0.01
13-14	0.15 ± 0.02	62 ± 3	0.3
14-15	0.41 ± 0.03	40 ± 2	>10.0
14-15	0.37 ± 0.04	51 ± 3	1.0
14-15	0.53 ± 0.03	85 ± 3	0.06
14-16	0.35 ± 0.03	89 ± 4	0.01
14-16	0.66 ± 0.04	42 ± 4	>10.0
14-15	<0.05	54 ± 3	1.0
17-18	0.09 ± 0.02	75 ± 3	0.07
17-19	<0.05	48 ± 2	10.0

[a] Determined after following the growth of the cell lines from an inoculum of 5 × 10^4 cells per dish to confluence (1-2 × 10^7 cells/10-cm dish) during 5 days with medium changes on alternate days.

[b] Melanin was assayed according to the method of Whittaker (37).

[c] Calculated as in Fig. 1.

[d] Determined graphically from the curves in Fig. 4.

To further characterize the differences in the sensitivities of the various cell lines to retinoic acid, their growth in the presence of decreasing concentrations of the drug was studied. In all the cell lines and clones, cell growth inhibition by retinoic acid was concentration-dependent, and even at very low concentrations growth of some of the lines were dramatically inhibited (Fig. 5). Nonetheless,

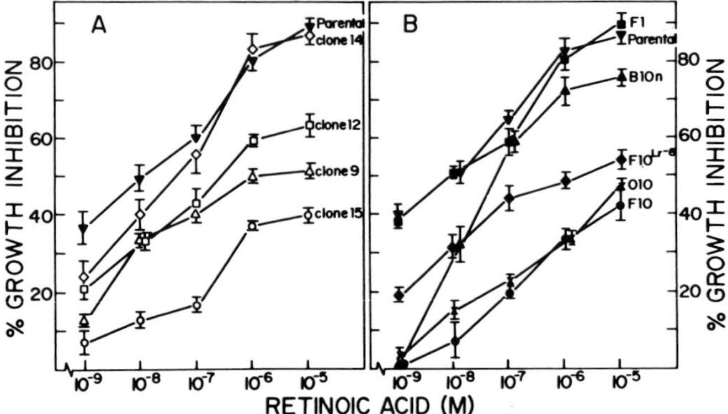

Fig. 5. Dose-response relationship of retinoic acid-induced growth inhibition of B16 melanoma parental cell line and its clones (A) and of cell variants selected *in vivo* (B). The cells were plated at 5 × 10^4 cells/dish in 100-mm diameter dishes in the absence or presence of the indicated retinoic acid concentrations and cultured for 6 days. Percent growth inhibition was determined as in Fig. 2 (21).

there were certain cell lines that were relatively unaffected. At the lowest retinoic acid concentration tested (10^{-9} *M*), where the growth of the parental B16 line and of B16-F1 was still inhibited by nearly 40%, the growth of parental clones 12 and 14 and B16-F10^{Lr-6} was inhibited by about 25%, and parental clones 9 and 15 and sublines B16-O10, B16-B10n, and B16-F10 were not significantly inhibited. The dose–response relationship for retinoic acid was quite linear for the cell lines and clones, except for line B16-B10n, which was completely insensitive to retinoic acid at 10^{-9} *M* but was sensitive at high drug concentrations (Fig. 5B). Comparison of the concentrations of retinoic acid required for 50% growth inhibition (ID_{50}) of the various cell lines (Table I) indicates that differences in the drug sensitivities of the B16 cell lines were greater than the twofold values obtained when absolute percent growth inhibition was compared at most concentrations. Parental B16 line and B16-F1 had an ID_{50} of approximately 10^{-8} *M*, whereas the corresponding values for parental clone 14, B16-B10n, parental clone 12, B16-F10^{Lr-6}, parental clone 9, and B16-O10 were 6 × 10^{-8}, 7 × 10^{-8}, 3 × 10^{-7}, 10^{-6}, 10^{-6}, and 10^{-5} *M*, respectively, and parental clone 15 and line B16-F10 were not inhibited 50% at 10^{-5} *M* retinoic acid (Fig. 5 and Table I). By this criterion the difference between the most sensitive lines and clones and the most resistant is about 1000 times. The sensitivities of the various lines and clones to retinoic acid-mediated growth inhibition was a stable characteristic, since inhibition did not change by more than 10% after continuous weekly subculture in the presence of 10^{-5} *M* retinoic acid for 3 months (21).

We have also studied the effect of retinoic acid on the growth of individual colonies of B16-F1 cells, because the heterogeneity observed in the response to retinoic acid of the various B16 clones and cell lines was greater than expected from cells originating from a sensitive population. To test whether this heterogeneity existed in subpopulations of an uncloned cell line, we examined the effect of retinoic acid on the proliferation of cells within individual randomly selected colonies of B16-F1 (21). Table II shows that there was a direct correlation between the inhibitory effect of retinoic acid on the proliferation of cells in the whole B16-F1 population and in individual colonies. Comparison of the average number (and the range) of cells per colony in cultures exposed to retinoic acid for 4 or 5 days with that of untreated control cultures demonstrated that most colonies consisted of cells sensitive to retinoic acid. We also noted the presence of a few less sensitive cell subpopulations in the B16-F1 colonies.

IV. Retinoid Inhibition of B16 Melanoma *in Vivo* Implantation

The various clones and lines of B16 melanoma used in our studies were all sensitive to retinoic acid at high concentrations which are pharmacologically achievable (40). Therefore our results do not denegate the potential use of retinoids as antitumor agents. In fact, retinoids have been used *in vivo* to inhibit the growth of transplantable rodent tumors (6–8), and recent reports suggest that they may be useful as adjuvants to chemotherapy (13–15), radiotherapy (12), or immunotherapy (16). The last-mentioned possibility is interesting, since we have found that retinoids can stimulate host immune systems (22).

As a prelude to studies on the effects of retinoids on the *in vivo* growth of B16 melanoma and metastatic colonization of specific organs via blood-borne arrest and survival, we have determined the effect of retinoic acid pretreatment on the ability of B16-F1 cells to implant, survive, and grow in the lungs after intravenous inoculation into syngeneic hosts. Our experiments indicate that retinoic acid treatment (10^{-5} *M* for 5 days) will significantly ($P < 0.001$) depress the lung implantation and survival characteristics of B16-F1 cells if care is taken to disaggregate nonspecific clumps of retinoid-treated cells before injection (Table III). Although there are several possible explanations for these results, we are investigating the following possibilities. The most likely is that retinoids modify cell surface properties of B16 melanoma cells so that they improperly interact with vascular endothelial cells in the microcirculation and fail to become implanted. Studies on the kinetic distributions of B16 melanoma and their pulmonary arrest (41) with or without retinoid pretreatment, as well as examination of the effect of retinoic acid on the interaction of melanoma cells with endothelial cell monolayers (42), should test this possibility. Retinoids are known to affect the synthesis and display of cell surface components such as glycoproteins and glycosaminoglycans (reviewed in Lotan [4]), and in preliminary experiments (R. Lotan and G. L. Nicolson, unpublished observations) we have found that retinoic

TABLE II

Inhibitory Effects of Retinoic Acid on Population and Colony Growth of B16-F1 Melanoma Cultures

Days in culture	Number of cells per dish ($\times 10^{-5}$)[a]		Inhibition of population growth (%)[b]	Number of cells per colony and range[c]		Inhibition of colony growth (%)[b]
	Control	Retinoic acid		Control	Retinoic acid	
1	1.6 ± 0.09	1.7 ± 0.11	0	3.2 ± 1.2 (1–6)	3.3 ± 1.2 (1–6)	0
2	3.9 ± 0.15	3.8 ± 0.23	0	7.0 ± 1.7 (4–12)	6.8 ± 1.9 (4–12)	0
3	11.2 ± 1.1	7.8 ± 0.3	30.4	15.6 ± 2.1 (8–22)	11.2 ± 2.2 (8–16)	28.2
4	32.5 ± 1.9	11.7 ± 1.2	64.0	43.6 ± 13.2 (20–66)	16.8 ± 3.0 (8–20)	61.5
5	88.6 ± 3.1	12.2 ± 0.9	86.2	103.5 ± 20.7 (61–138)	18.7 ± 3.5 (12–56)	81.9

[a] B16-F1 cells were plated at 1×10^5 cells per dish in a series of 10-cm diameter dishes in 10 ml growth medium in the absence or presence of 10^{-5} *M* retinoic acid. At 24-hour intervals thereafter, duplicate cultures were removed from the incubation media and the total number of cells per dish determined. The values represent the average ± SEM of duplicate cultures. Similar results were obtained in several independent experiments.

[b] Percent growth inhibition was calculated as $100 - (R/C) \times 100$, where R and C are the numbers of cells per dish (or per colony) in retinoic acid-treated and control cultures, respectively.

[c] Cells from the same culture of B16-F1 were plated at 10^2, 10^3, or 10^4 cells per dish in a series of 6-cm diameter dishes with 5 ml growth medium in the absence or presence of 10^{-5} *M* retinoic acid. At 24-hour intervals thereafter, duplicate cultures at the different cell densities were removed from incubation, the cells fixed and stained (Diff-Quik, Harelco, Gibbstown, N.J.), and the number of cells per colony determined. The values are the mean ± SEM and range of cells per colony in 50 individuals colonies in each duplicate culture.

TABLE III

Effect of Pretreatment of B16 Melanoma Cells with Retinoic Acid on Their Lung Implantation Potential

Cells[a]	Number of lung colonies per mouse[b]	Range
Untreated	34 ± 14	18–65
Retinoic acid-treated	7 ± 4	3–15

[a] B16-F1 cells were cultured for 5 days in the absence (untreated) or presence of 10^{-5} *M* retinoic acid. The cells were detached by brief trypsinization, suspended as a single-cell suspension, and passed through a no. 53 Nitex nylon screen to remove a few aggregates.

[b] Mice were injected in the tail vein with 10^5 untreated or retinoic acid-treated cells. After 2 weeks, they were sacrificed and their lungs removed for scoring pigmented tumor colonies under a dissecting microscope. The values are the mean ± SD and the range of results obtained with 10 mice per group ($p < 0.001$).

acid modifies B16-F1 cell surface components accessible to lactoperoxidase-catalyzed iodination (43). Retinoic acid is also known to modify cell membrane fluidity (44), which could result in an alteration in cellular deformability during microcirculatory passage. Other possibilities include altered cell–cell interactions with circulating host cells such as platelets (45) and lymphocytes (46), as well as abnormalities in cellular interactions with endothelial basement membrane (42) after arrest of retinoid-treated cells. Surface changes in retinoid-treated B16 cells could also alter their immunogenicity, resulting in diminished survival after implantation in the pulmonary microcirculation. These explanations and others are currently under investigation along with experiments designed to test the usefulness of retinoids alone or in combination with other drugs to inhibit tumor metastasis.

V. Summary

In vitro cloning techniques and sequential *in vivo* selection procedures have been used to obtain variant sublines of murine B16 melanoma with differing metastatic potentials and organ preferences for colonization in syngeneic hosts. Retinoids such as β-all-*trans*-retinoic acid inhibited cell proliferation of these B16 sublines and clones *in vitro,* and the retinoic acid-mediated inhibition was time-, drug-, and dose-dependent, and reversible. Retinoic acid caused characteristic morphological changes in B16 cell cultures, such as an enhanced tendency to grow in cell clumps, and scanning electron microscopy revealed more membrane ruffles on drug-treated cells. When the sensitivities of various B16 clones and sublines to retinoic acid-induced growth inhibition were examined in culture, there was considerable heterogeneity in the extent of drug-mediated inhibition. The parental B16 line and line B16-F1, selected once for lung colonization, were much more sensitive to retinoic acid (up to 1000 times) than the sublines selected 10 times *in vivo* for organ preference of metastatic colonization. Moreover, clones obtained from the parental B16 line also showed variability in retinoic acid sensitivity to growth inhibition. When the effect of retinoic acid treatment on the pulmonary implantation and survival of B16-F1 cells was examined after intravenous injection of drug-treated and control cells into syngeneic hosts, the drug-treated cells formed significantly fewer experimental pulmonary metastases. The significance of these findings in the development of retinoid therapy for malignant melanoma was discussed.

Acknowledgments

We thank D. Lotan and A. Brodginski for excellent assistance. These studies were supported by USPHS grants RO1-CA-22823 and RO1-CA-28867 and contract NO1-CB-74153 from the National Cancer Institute. Dr. Lotan was a Lievre Senior Fellow of the American Cancer Society, Inc.

References

1. M. B. Sporn, *Nutr. Rev.* **35,** 65 (1977).
2. H. Mayer, W. Bollag, R. Hänni, and R. Rüegg, *Experientia* **34,** 1106 (1978).
3. M. B. Sporn and D. L. Newton, *Fed. Proc., Fed. Am. Soc. Exp. Biol.* **38,** 2528 (1979).
4. R. Lotan, *Biochim. Biophys. Acta Rev. Cancer* **605,** 33 (1980).
5. W. Bollag, *Eur. J. Cancer* **10,** 731 (1974).
6. G. Rettura, A. Schittek, M. Hardy, S. M. Levenson, A. Demetriou, and E. Seifter, *J. Natl. Cancer Inst.* **54,** 1489 (1975).
7. E. L. Felix, B. Loyd, and M. H. Cohen, *Science* **189,** 886 (1975).
8. P. W. Trown, M. J. Buck, and R. Hansen, *Cancer Treat. Rep* **60,** 1647 (1976).
9. M. Micksche, C. Cerni, O. Kokron, R. Titscher, and H. Wrba, *Oncology* **34,** 234 (1977).
10. G. S. Kistler and H. J. Peter, *Schweiz. Med. Wochenschr.* **109,** 847 (1979).
11. G. L. Peck, T. G. Olsen, D. Butkus, M. Pandya, J. Arnaud-Battandier, R. Yoder, and W. R. Levis, *Proc. Am. Assoc. Cancer Res.* **20,** 56 (1979).
12. D. Brandes, J. O. Rundell, and H. Ueda, *J. Natl. Cancer Inst.* **52,** 945 (1974).
13. M. H. Cohen and P. P. Carbone, *J. Natl. Cancer Inst.* **48,** 921 (1972).
14. S. Komiyama, I. Hiroto, S. Ryu, T. Nakashima, M. Kuwano, and H. Endo, *Oncology* **35,** 253 (1978).
15. M. Kurka, C. E. Orfanos, and H. Pullmann, *Hautarzt* **29,** 313 (1978).
16. T. Kurata and M. Micksche, *Oncology* **34,** 212 (1977).
17. W. Bollag, *Cancer Chemother. Rep.* **55,** 53 (1971).
18. R. Lotan and G. L. Nicolson, *J. Natl. Cancer Inst.* **59,** 1717 (1977).
19. R. Lotan, G. Giotta, E. Nork, and G. L. Nicolson, *J. Natl. Cancer Inst.* **60,** 1035 (1978).
20. R. Lotan, *Cancer Res.* **39,** 1014 (1979).
21. R. Lotan and G. L. Nicolson, *Cancer Res.* **39,** 4767 (1979).

22. R. Lotan and G. Dennert, *Cancer Res.* **39,** 55 (1979).
23. F. L. Meyskens and S. E. Salmon, *Cancer Res.* **39,** 4055 (1979).
24. G. L. Nicolson, R. Lotan, and A. Rios, *Cancer Chemother. Rep.,* (in press).
25. I. J. Fidler, *Nature (London), New Biol.* **242,** 148 (1973).
26. K. W. Brunson, G. Beattie, and G. L. Nicolson, *Nature (London)* **272,** 543 (1978).
27. K. W. Brunson and G. L. Nicolson, *J. Supramol. Struct.,* **11,** 517 (1979).
28. I. J. Fidler and C. Bucana, *Cancer Res.* **37,** 3945 (1977).
29. G. L. Nicolson, *BioScience* **28,** 441 (1978).
30. I. J. Fidler, D. M. Gersten, and I. R. Hart, *Adv. Cancer Res.* **28,** 149 (1978).
31. I. J. Fidler and M. L. Kripke, *Science* **197,** 893 (1977).
32. G. L. Nicolson, K. W. Brunson, and I. J. Fidler, *Cancer Res.* **38,** 4105 (1978).
33. G. H. Heppner, D. L. Dexter, T. DeNucci, F. R. Miller, and P. Calabresi, *Cancer Res.* **38,** 3758 (1978).
34. H. Suzuki, H. R. Withers, and M. W. Koehler, *Cancer Res.* **38,** 3349 (1978).
35. M. L. Kripke, E. Gruys, and I. J. Fidler, *Cancer Res.* **38,** 2962 (1978).
36. J. W. Kreider, D. R. Wade, M. Rosenthal, and T. Densley, *J. Natl. Cancer Inst.* **54,** 1457 (1975).
37. J. R. Whittaker, *Dev. Biol.* **8,** 99 (1963).
38. S. C. Barranco, D. H. W. Ho, B. Derwinko, M. M. Romsdahl, and R. M. Humphrey, *Cancer Res.* **32,** 2733 (1972).
39. S. C. Barranco, B. R. Haenelt, and E. L. Gee, *Cancer Res.* **38,** 656 (1978).
40. C. A. Frolik, T. E. Tavela, G. L. Peck, and M. B. Sporn, *Anal. Biochem.* **86,** 743 (1978).
41. I. J. Fidler, and G. L. Nicolson, *J. Natl. Cancer Inst.* **57,** 1199 (1976).
42. R. H. Kramer and G. L. Nicolson, *Proc. Natl. Acad. Sci. U.S.A.* **76,** 5705 (1979).
43. G. L. Nicolson, C. R. Birdwell, K. W. Brunson, J. C. Robbins, G. Beattie, and I. J. Fidler, *in* "Cell and Tissue Interactions" (J. Lash and M. M. Burger, eds.), p. 225, Raven Press, New York, 1977).
44. R. G. Meeks and R. F. Chen, *Fed. ;Proc., Fed. Am. Soc. Exp. Biol.* **38,** 540 (1979).
45. G. J. Gasic, T. B. Gasic, N. Galanti, T. Johnson, and S. Murphy, *Int. J. Cancer* **11,** 704 (1973).
46. I. J. Fidler, *Cancer Res.* **35,** 218 (1975).

26

Retinoids and Suppression of the Effects of Polypeptide Transforming Factors—A New Molecular Approach to Chemoprevention of Cancer

MICHAEL B. SPORN, DIANNE L. NEWTON, ANITA B. ROBERTS, JOSEPH E. DE LARCO, AND GEORGE J. TODARO

I. Introduction

We have recently described a new biological approach to the chemoprevention of cancer and have reviewed the use of retinoids (the set of molecules comprised of vitamin A and its synthetic analogues) for this purpose (1,2). It is by now well established that retinoids have the following important properties with respect to

ISBN 0-12-619280-4

chemoprevention of cancer: (1) They suppress malignant transformation *in vitro,* whether it is caused by chemical carcinogens (3), ionizing radiation (4), or transforming peptides from virally transformed cells (5); (2) they are potent inhibitors of the tumor-promoting effects of phorbol esters (6–11); and (3) they are effective agents for the prevention of cancer in experimental animals, particularly for prevention of carcinoma of the bladder (12–15), breast (16–18), and skin (19,20). The ability of retinoids to enhance the differentiation of both premalignant (21) and malignant (22) cells is yet another one of their important properties of relevance to cancer prevention. Since our reviews have considered the above phenomena at some length, we will not discuss further details in this chapter.

Instead we shall attempt to deal with the difficult question of the molecular mechanisms whereby retinoids exert their chemopreventive effects, since this approach will provide additional information for their more effective use. Furthermore, understanding the molecular action of retinoids should help to define molecular targets for the development of new chemopreventive or chemotherapeutic agents. We shall stress the importance of the interaction of retinoids with transforming polypeptide growth factors, and the potential significance of these factors as molecular targets for future development of new chemopreventive agents. We will develop the concept that retinoids and transforming growth factors represent antagonistic biological forces and that each can be used as an investigative tool to dissect out the biological role of the other. Since carcinogenesis may be considered a distorted version of embryogenesis (23), certain answers to some of the critical problems in carcinogenesis may lie in the study of embryological mechanisms. Particularly useful will be the study of pairs of molecules which can be shown to have significant biological effects in studies on both carcinogenesis (malignant transformation) and embryogenesis (cellular differentiation), and which can be shown to have antagonistic effects with respect to each other in both systems. Basic to this approach is an attempt to understand the problem of the evolutionary and functional origins of both retinoids and transforming polypeptide growth factors, since this knowledge should then help to define the appropriate development of a specific new molecular pharmacology.

II. Retinoids and Normal Cell Differentiation

Although it has been known for more than 50 years that retinoids play a fundamental, essential role in controlling normal epithelial cell differentiation throughout the body (24), the basic mechanism of this phenomenon has remained obscure. Moreover, the physiological role, if any, of retinoids in controlling growth and differentiation of cells derived from mesoderm and mesenchyme has also remained unclear. Retinoids are undoubtedly an ancient family of regulatory molecules. Their progenitors, carotenoids, are widely distributed in various species, including very primitive organisms such as bacteria and algae, in which they are believed to have a protective effect against the damaging effects of visible light, particularly photosensitized oxidation (25,26). The biosynthesis of tetraterpenoid (C_{40}) carotenoids from the classic terpene precursors mevalonic acid and isopentenyl pyrophosphate has been demonstrated in many species of both primitive and higher plants, as well as in microorganisms (27), but has not been shown to occur in animals. However, the C_{40} carotenoid molecule can be centrally cleaved in animals to form two C_{20} retinoid molecules (28), and this cleavage is the principal source of the biologically useful retinoid molecules animals obtain from plants.

The phenomenon of mucociliary differentiation of cells, which is one of the classic effects of retinoids that has been studied in mammalian and avian organisms over the past 50 years (24,29,30), is an important mechanism in as primitive an animal as the protochordate *Amphioxus*. In the case of *Amphioxus,* the mucus-secreting and ciliated cells that line the pharynx are involved in the direct intake and capture of food and the conveying of this food to the intestine (31). In mammals, a mucociliary mechanism still is retained in the epithelial lining of the trachea and bronchi (pharyngeal derivatives during embryogenesis), but in this case the mucociliary action is used to capture undesirable particulate material, such as bacteria and dust, and to convey this material out of the body, thus keeping the airway clean and sterile. Retinoids have even been found in a variety of invertebrate species (32), including lobsters and shrimps, as well as in simple molluscs (33). Even though a great deal is known about the overall biology of retinoids and normal cell differentiation (32), elucidation of the molecular basis of control of cellular differentiation has been difficult. However, study of a pathological process may provide a useful tool for understanding a normal one. In the case of retinoids, study of the mechanism of malignant transformation of normal cells by viruses, chemicals, or radiation is already proving to be an important tool for investigating molecular action.

III. Malignant Transformation of Cells and the Role of Polypeptide Transforming Factors

When normal cells are exposed to specific viruses, chemicals, or radiation, *permanent, genetic* transformation of clones of cells may result, as has been shown in many classic experiments. However, the mechanism of transformation, particularly after exposure to chemicals and radiation, has been difficult to study because of the prolonged delay between exposure and measurable transformation. The recent identification, isolation, and characterization of transforming polypeptide growth factors derived from murine cells transformed by Moloney sarcoma virus (MSV) has now provided a new way to study *reversible, phenotypic* transformation of cells (34). These polypeptides are direct reversible effectors of cell transformation. When applied to nontransformed cells, they rapidly cause phenotypic properties characteristic of the transformed state, particularly anchorage-independent growth in soft agar, as well as morphological changes and altered growth pattern in monolayer culture. The property of anchorage-independent growth has been closely correlated with expression of the malignant phenotype (35,36). In parallel experiments, using new methods for extraction of tumor tissue, we have recently shown that transforming activity is also found in extracts of sarcomas from chickens that have been inoculated with Rous sarcoma virus, as well as in extracts of sarcomas induced by inoculation of mice with MSV-transformed fibroblasts (37). Furthermore, transforming activity has recently been found in extracts of epithelial cancers, derived from chemically transformed rat tracheal epithelial cells (38). Thus it appears that factors capable of conferring the property of anchorage-independent growth on normal cells (which ordinarily will not grow in soft agar) can be found in a variety of malignant cells, of both mesenchymal and epithelial origin, from several different species of animals.

We may thus postulate the existence of a class of substances, which we shall call transforming growth factors, characterized by their ability to cause final expression of the malignant phenotype. The molecular and biological properties of these transforming growth factors appear to be clearly different from those of the protein which results from transcription and translation of the *src* gene in the avian sarcoma system (39). Elsewhere, we have suggested that a transforming growth factor, such as sarcoma growth factor (SGF), may be regarded as an ultimate carcinogen, in that it is responsible for the phenotypic changes which confer the properties of malignancy on a transformed cell (2).

IV. Sarcoma Growth Factor and Its Inhibition by Retinoids

Although transforming activity (as defined by enhancement of the growth of normal cells in soft agar and alteration of cellular morphology) has recently been detected in a variety of malignant cells, only one transforming growth factor, namely, SGF, from murine 3T3 cells transformed by MSV, has been well characterized up to the present time (34). This factor is a heat-stable, acid-stable polypeptide with a molecular weight of approximately 12,000; it is sensitive to the reducing agent dithiothreitol and presumably contains disulfide bonds. The transforming effects of low concentrations of SGF on normal cells can be blocked by retinoids. When normal rat kidney fibroblasts were treated simultaneously with SGF and nanogram levels of retinoids (retinoic acid, retinyl acetate, retinyl methyl ether, or retinylidene dimedone at $1.0–2.0 \times 10^{-8}$ *M*), the transforming effects of SGF were suppressed (5). As shown in Table I, retinyl acetate (1.9×10^{-8} *M*) inhibited the ability of SGF to release normal fibroblasts from density-dependent inhibition of growth. Normal fibroblasts treated with SGF alone formed multiple layers and crisscrossed each other in a random fashion resembling MSV-transformed cells, while cells treated with both SGF and retinyl acetate did not have a disordered growth pattern and did not have increased saturation density in monolayer culture. Furthermore, as shown in Table II, all four retinoids were effective in diminishing the ability of SGF to induce the growth of normal rat fibroblasts in soft agar. The cell system used in these assays (a clone of rat kidney fibroblasts) has a very low background of growth in soft agar in the absence of SGF and is extremely sensitive to the addition of SGF. Retinoids markedly suppressed the effect of SGF; the few colonies that formed in the presence of both SGF and retinoids were smaller and contained fewer cells than those treated with SGF alone. In both sets of experiments described in Tables I and II, the effect of the retinoids was clearly not a cytotoxic one, since they inhibited neither normal rat fibroblastic cell growth in monolayer nor the ability of rat or mouse cells which had been permanently transformed by murine sarcoma virus to form colonies in soft agar.

TABLE I

Effect of Sarcoma Growth Factor and Retinyl Acetate on the Final Cell Density of Rat Fibroblast Cell Cultures[a]

Treatment	Cells per plate ($\times 10^{-6}$)	
	Experiment 1	Experiment 2
Untreated control	1.2	1.0
Plus retinyl acetate (1.9×10^{-8} *M*)	1.3	1.1
SGF-treated (10 μg/ml)	3.6	2.6
Plus retinyl acetate (1.9×10^{-8} *M*)	1.4	0.9
Plus DMSO (1:1000)	3.3	2.5

[a] Reprinted, with permission, from *Nature* (5).

[b] A subclone (536-7) of a normal rat fibroblast cell clone, NRK 49F, susceptible to the growth-stimulating effect of SGF, was seeded at 2×10^5 cells per plate in 60-mm plastic Petri dishes. The cells were treated at the time of inoculation and refed with medium (Dulbecco's modified medium with 1% fetal calf serum) containing the additions shown every third day. Cell counts were made 10 days after seeding. The SGF came from conditioned medium of MSV-transformed mouse NIH/3T3 cells. Retinyl acetate was dissolved in dimethyl sulfoxide (DMSO). The final concentration of DMSO in all experiments was 0.1%. Neither retinyl acetate nor DMSO alone showed any effect on the growth, final cell density, or cloning efficiency of normal rat fibroblasts at the concentrations used.

TABLE II

Effect of Sarcoma Growth Factor and Various Retinoids on the Colony-Forming Ability of Rat Fibroblasts Plated in Soft Agar[a]

Treatment[b]	Colonies per plate[c]		
	Experiment 1	Experiment 2	Experiment 3
Untreated controls	0	0	0
Plus retinyl acetate, (1.9×10^{-8} *M*)	0	0	0
Plus retinoic acid, (2.0×10^{-8} *M*)	NT	0	NT
Plus retinylidene dimedone, (1.5×10^{-8} *M*)	NT	NT	0
Plus retinyl methyl ether, (2.0×10^{-8} *M*)	NT	NT	0
SGF-treated (10 μg/ml)	44.5	39.0	49.5
Plus retinyl acetate, (1.9×10^{-8} *M*)	2.5	1.5	8.0
Plus retinoic acid, (2.0×10^{-8} *M*)	NT	3.2	NT
Plus retinylidene dimedone, (1.5×10^{-8} *M*)	NT	NT	0.5
Plus retinyl methyl ether, (2.0×10^{-8} *M*)	NT	NT	14.5

[a] Reprinted, with permission, from *Nature* (5).

[b] On day 0, 1×10^5 rat fibroblast cells, clone 536-7, were treated in monolayer cultures using Dulbecco's modified medium with 1% fetal calf serum as described in Table I, footnote *b.* On day 2, they were seeded at 1×10^4 cells per plate in 0.3% soft agar containing the additions shown. All cells not treated with SGF (whether treated with retinoid or not) remained as single cells with occasional (<10%) small colonies of 2–4 cells. Colonies with greater than 20 cells after 2 weeks in agar were scored as positive.

[c] NT, Not tested.

V. Physiological Role of Transforming Growth Factors

In Section I we suggested that understanding the evolutionary and functional origins of both retinoids and transforming growth factors is important in defining their roles in both carcinogenesis and embryogenesis. With respect to SGF, the function of enhancing the development of malignancy has no obvious evolutionary advantage, suggesting a more benign, unknown, physiological function. The exact molecular specification of this putative normal function will be important if we wish to achieve the most effective control of the aberrant functions of transforming growth factors associated with transformation and carcinogenesis.

Transforming growth factors are thus molecules in search of a normal physiological function. In attempting to define this function experimentally, the oncogene hypothesis (40,41) provides a useful conceptual framework. This hypothesis essentially states that carcinogenesis results from the inappropriate expression, in adult life, of cellular genes (coding for transforming proteins) that were required for normal embryological development. The nucleotide sequence coding for SGF may be one such gene, since SGF is involved in expression of the malignant phenotype.

How, then, may one experimentally test the proposition that transforming growth factors are required for normal embryological development? Several new direct approaches to this question have very recently been started in our laboratories. A conceptually simple approach is to determine if addition of exogenous SGF (derived from malignant cells) to an early explanted rodent or chick embryo will enhance the differentiation, growth, or morphogenesis of any embryonic tissue; this makes the assumption that the early embryo is not fully saturated with respect to the ability of receptors to respond to exogenous SGF. Another direct approach is to attempt to isolate and characterize SGF-like molecules from early embryos and then to attempt to define the physiological role of such endogenous polypeptides. A third direct approach is to make an antibody (or a peptide antagonist) to SGF (or a similar transforming growth factor) and to determine the effect of such an antagonist on embryogenesis; one might expect to find some specific teratogenic effect if SGF is critically involved in embryogenesis. This last approach was used successfully to determine the specific role of the polypeptide nerve growth factor in development of the sympathetic nervous system; treatment of young mice with antibody to nerve growth factor resulted in an "immunosympathectomy" (42).

Although all the above approaches are being pursued in our laboratories, definitive answers will not come easily. Could there be other clues from information that already exists which might implicate transforming growth factors in the process of normal embryological development? Just as we earlier suggested that study of a pathological process (namely, malignant transformation and the role of SGF as a direct effector of this process) might help to elucidate the role of retinoids in normal cell differentiation, we will again attempt to use a pathological process to elucidate the role of transforming growth factors in normal embryological differentiation. If, as we showed earlier, retinoids and SGF represent antagonistic mechanisms, then one should be able to utilize a *selective, specific* pathological process induced by retinoids as a probe for the normal physiological role of SGF. In this case we will deal with the classic embryological experiments which have used retinoids as selective, specific teratogens, and we will now briefly summarize this literature, with particular emphasis on mechanism.

VI. Retinoids as Selective Teratogens

Marked teratogenic effects of high doses of retinol and/or retinyl esters, administered to pregnant female rats, were first reported more than 25 years ago (43). Similar teratogenic effects were soon reported in other species of mammals (44), and the types of malformations that occurred were found to depend on the age of the embryo at the time the mother was treated (45). In rat and mouse embryos, treatment on days 8 and 9 of gestation with retinol and/or retinyl esters led to a variety of malformations. Craniofacial abnormalities were striking, particularly malformation of various parts of the cartilaginous and bony facial and oral skeleton, including abnormalities of the mandible, maxilla, and palate, as well as absence of the external ear (46). Subsequently, administration of retinoic acid was found to produce a similar series of embryonic malformations; retinoic acid is considerably more potent than retinyl acetate (47). With retinoic acid, too, the types of embryonic malformations were dependent on the time at which the mother received a single dose; the interesting observation was made that retinoic acid could produce a given malformation well before there was any morphologically identifiable precursor (anlage) of the structure destined to be affected (48). It is important to note that retinoids are unique among experimental teratogens in their specific ability to produce some of the classic craniofacial abnormalities (46).

It has been difficult to approach the question of the mechanism of teratogenesis by administration of retinoids to pregnant animals, since one cannot be certain whether the effects of the retinoids are mediated by a direct action on the embryo or by an indirect action on the mother. In spite of these limitations of interpretation, the important observation was made some time ago that administration of high doses of retinol (as retinyl ester) to pregnant animals caused a significant lessening of the formation of cephalic mesenchyme in the embryos (49); this observation has been further expanded with *in vitro* studies, as will be described below.

The recent development of defined systems for isolated explant culture of both mammalian and avian embryos (in which essentially normal development takes place over a brief period *in vitro*) has allowed investigation of the mechanism of teratogenesis by retinoids (50,51). Direct effects of retinol on cell migration and differentiation in cultured 8-day (primitive streak) rat embryos were first reported by Morriss and Steele (52), who noted that retinol (1.7×10^{-6} *M*) caused neural folds to remain flat and widely open and reduced the formation of cephalic mesenchyme in a manner previously observed in embryos that had been exposed to retinol *in utero* (49,53). Further *in vitro* studies (54) on 9-day (neural plate) rat embryos have shown that retinoic acid (1.7×10^{-6} *M*) prevents the formation of pharyngeal arches; these structures are derived from cephalic mesenchyme and provide the morphological precursors of the mandible and maxilla. In addition, retinoic acid also causes a striking inhibition of formation of the yolk sac circulation (54), which is also derived from mesenchymal elements. Thus retinoids have been shown to have a potent direct effect *in vitro* on the differentiation of structures derived from mesenchyme; moreover, these *in vitro* effects provide a reasonable explanation for some of the teratogenic effects seen *in vivo*.

The cellular mechanism of teratogenesis induced by retinoids has been investigated in several *in vitro* studies. It has been shown that retinoids can inhibit the migration of primitive mesenchymal cells, either within the embryo itself (55) or when such cells are cultured in a Petri dish (56) or on glass coverslips (57). Of particular note is the ability of retinol to prevent the migration of cranial neural crest cells to the first pharyngeal arch (55), although an effect on proliferation of neural crest cells may also be involved. Facial development in vertebrate embryos requires migration of mesenchymal cells, derived from the neural crest, into the pharyngeal arches (58); the distance these cells migrate *in vivo* is very great. These observations may account in part for the classic facial malformations described earlier. In addition to these effects on cell migration, direct inhibitory effects of retinoic acid on cell proliferation and differentiation have also been reported in cultured embryos at concentrations as low as 1.7×10^{-7} *M* (54).

If one is looking for a molecular mechanism to explain the above teratogenic effects of retinoids, an inhibitory effect on embryonic growth factors resembling SGF is a possibility. One obviously cannot prove this with a deductive argument. However, given the data that retinoids inhibit the proliferative and transforming effects of SGF in a cell transformation system, it is entirely plausible to suggest that a similar interaction might occur in an embryonic system. Particularly intriguing are the effects of retinoids on cell migration. During normal early embryonic development, massive cell movements are a very prominent feature, and the suggestion that the normal trophoblast is an invasive tissue, resembling malignant tissue, is a very old one (59,60). Thus, although many polypeptide factors have now been described which promote cell proliferation and growth, one must also look for a molecular definition of invasiveness in a transforming growth factor. The ability of transformed cells to undergo marked cell movement and migration, rather than their mere ability to proliferate and grow, might be more closely correlated with their invasive potential. In the case of the early embryo, there is clearly a normal, physiological need for hormonelike factors which can markedly enhance cell movement, proliferation, and growth; based on the experimental data dealing with both transformation and teratogenesis, it seems reasonable to postulate that SGF may be such a factor.

Retinoids and SGF thus appear to be intimately linked to each other with respect to their mechanism of action. Each can be used as a probe to study the mechanism of action of the other. We have shown data from one defined experimental situation (phenotypic transformation) in which retinoids can block the proliferative and transforming action of SGF. The converse situation, in which SGF is used to block the teratogenic action of retinoids on a developing embryo, has yet to be demonstrated but is experimentally testable. Hamster tracheal organ culture (30) and mouse teratocarcinoma cell culture (22) represent two other systems in which potential and antagonism between retinoids and SGF may be experimentally tested.

VII. Need for Development of New Pharmacological Agents to Inhibit Transforming Growth Factors

If, as we stated earlier, transforming growth factors are ultimate carcinogens (i.e., if they are direct effectors which confer the properties of malignancy on a transformed cell), then they should be ideal molecular targets for pharmacological agents which can be used for chemoprevention of cancer. Indeed, it is reasonable to attribute some part of the capacity of retinoids for cancer prevention to their ability to antagonize the activity of hormones involved in cell proliferation. A striking example of this is seen (Figs. 1–3) in the antiproliferative effect of both retinyl acetate and 4-hydroxyphenyl retinamide on the development of mammary epithelium in the rat (18). The complex role of the peptide hormones insulin and prolactin, as well as steroid hormones, in enhancing proliferation in mammary epithelium has been the subject of numerous studies (61). In addition to their antiproliferative effect on mammary epithelium, both retinyl acetate and 4-hydroxyphenyl retinamide are also effective agents for inhibiting the development of mammary cancer in the rat (18). However, although retinoids have been used very efficiently in a variety of experimental situations for prevention of carcinoma of the bladder (12–15), breast (16–18), and skin (19,20), they undoubtedly do not represent the ultimate preventive agent, since they do not effectively inhibit tumorigenesis when a very high level of carcinogenic exposure occurs. Similarly, when strong transforming viruses such as MSV or simian virus 40 (SV40) were used to effect genotypic transformation of either mouse 3T3 cells or rat fibroblasts, retinoids were found to be ineffective in blocking either the initiation or maintenance of transformation (5).

A more direct approach to control of the ultimate carcinogen, namely, competitive inhibition of the action of transforming growth factors, is therefore an attractive possibility. As these polypeptide factors are isolated, purified, and eventually sequenced, it should be possible to develop synthetic peptide antagonists as has been done with several other hormonal polypeptides (62–65). The comparative biochemistry of transforming factors isolated from different tumor types and different species of animals will be an important guide to the design of appropriate antagonistic peptides. Beyond synthetic peptide an-

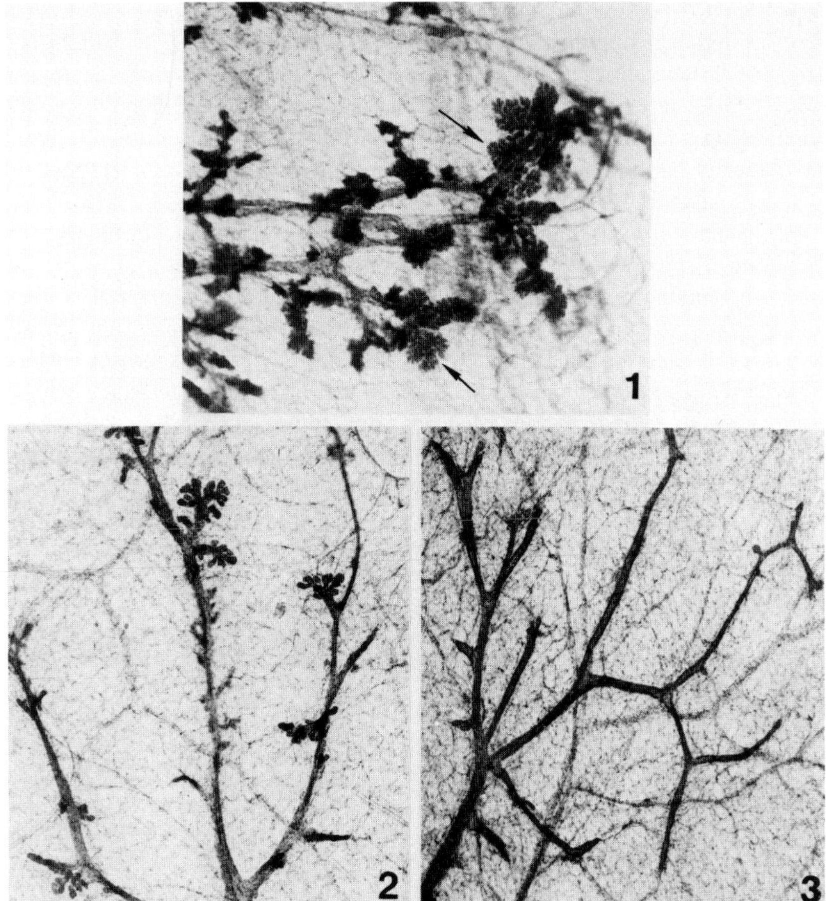

Figs. 1–3. Representative areas of mammary gland whole mounts from virgin female rats fed special diets from age 2 months to 8 months. Reprinted, with permission, from *Cancer Research* (18).

Fig. 1. Control diet. Note the marked end bud proliferation (arrows). Alum carmine. ×40.

Fig. 2. Retinyl acetate (328 mg/kg of diet). A marked decrease in end bud proliferation is noted. Compare to Fig. 1. Alum carmine. ×40.

Fig. 3. 4-Hydroxyphenyl retinamide (782 mg/kg of diet). An almost total absence of end bud proliferation is noted. Compare to Fig. 1. Alum carmine. ×40.

tagonists, it is possible that screening of natural products, such as alkaloids or peptides derived from fermentation, will yield useful agonists and antagonists in a manner similar to the relationships among morphine, morphine analogues, enkephalins, and endorphins (66,67). The development of simple competitive binding assays should facilitate such screening. The partial success that retinoids have already had in chemoprevention should provide some optimism that this new approach will be useful.

We have not discussed the possible use of antagonists to transforming growth factors in the chemotherapy of invasive disease. It is not yet known to what extent the continued expression of these factors, produced by tumor cells themselves, is required for the maintenance of malignant cell behavior, but presumably this is necessary. Thus it is quite conceivable that the new approach we have outlined will also have some use in the therapy of invasive or metastatic disease. Some of the recent reports that low doses of retinoids can control the differentiation or proliferation of both rodent (22,68,69) and human (70,71) malignant cells suggest that the use of antagonists of transforming growth factors might also be of some interest in this area.

Acknowledgments

We thank Ellen C. Friedman for expert assistance in preparing the manuscript for this chapter, and Peter J. Becci and Richard C. Moon for Figs. 1–3.

References

1. M. B. Sporn, N. M. Dunlop, D. L. Newton, and J. M. Smith, *Fed. Proc., Fed. Am. Soc. Exp. Biol.* **35,** 1332 (1976).
2. M. B. Sporn and D. L. Newton, *Fed. Proc., Fed. Am. Soc. Exp. Biol.* **38,** 2528 (1979).
3. R. L. Merriman and J. S. Bertram, *Cancer Res.* **39,** 1661 (1979).
4. L. Harisiadis, R. C. Miller, E. J. Hall, and C. Borek, *Nature (London)* **274,** 486 (1978).
5. G. J. Todaro, J. E. De Larco, and M. B. Sporn, *Nature (London)* **276,** 272 (1978).
6. W. Bollag, *Eur. J. Cancer* **8,** 689 (1972).
7. A. K. Verma and R. K. Boutwell, *Cancer Res.* **37,** 2196 (1977).
8. A. K. Verma, H. M. Rice, B. G. Shapas, and R. K. Boutwell, *Cancer Res.* **38,** 793 (1978).
9. A. K. Verma, B. G. Shapas, H. M. Rice, and R. K. Boutwell, *Cancer Res.* **39,** 419 (1979).
10. T. W. Kensler and G. C. Mueller, *Cancer Res.* **38,** 771 (1978).
11. T. W. Kensler, A. K. Verma, R. K. Boutwell, and G. C. Mueller, *Cancer Res.* **38,** 2896 (1978).
12. M. B. Sporn, R. A. Squire, C. C. Brown, J. M. Smith, M. L. Wenk, and S. Springer, *Science* **195,** 487 (1977).
13. R. A. Squire, M. B. Sporn, C. C. Brown, J. M. Smith, M. L. Wenk, and S. Springer, *Cancer Res.* **37,** 2930 (1977).
14. C. J. Grubbs, R. C. Moon, R. A. Squire, G. M. Farrow, S. F. Stinson, D. G. Goodman, C. C. Brown, and M. B. Sporn, *Science* **198,** 743 (1977).

15. P. J. Becci, H. J. Thompson, C. J. Grubbs, R. A. Squire, C. C. Brown, M. B. Sporn, and R. C. Moon, *Cancer Res.* **38,** 4463 (1978).
16. C. J. Grubbs, R. C. Moon, M. B. Sporn, and D. L. Newton, *Cancer Res.* **37,** 599 (1977).
17. R. C. Moon, C. J. Grubbs, M. B. Sporn, and D. G. Goodman, *Nature* (*London*) **269,** 620 (1977).
18. R. C. Moon, H. J. Thompson, P. J. Becci, C. J. Grubbs, R. J. Gander, D. L. Newton, J. M. Smith, S. L. Phillips, W. R. Henderson, L. T. Mullen, C. C. Brown, and M. B. Sporn, *Cancer Res.* **39,** 1339 (1979).
19. W. Bollag, *Experientia* **28,** 1219 (1972).
20. H. Mayer, W. Bollag, R. Hänni, and R. Rüegg, *Experientia* **34,** 1105 (1978).
21. I. Lasnitzki, *Br. J. Cancer* **9,** 434 (1955).
22. S. Strickland and V. Mahdavi, *Cell* **15,** 393 (1978).
23. G. B. Pierce, R. Shikes, and L. M. Fink, "Cancer—A Problem of Developmental Biology," p. 27. Prentice-Hall, Englewood Cliffs, New Jersey, 1978.
24. S. B. Wolbach and P. R. Howe, *J. Exp. Med.* **42,** 753 (1925).
25. R. Y. Stanier, *Harvey Lect.* **54,** 219 (1960).
26. N. I. Krinsky, *in* "Carotenoids" (O. Isler, ed.), p. 669. Birkhaeuser, Basel, 1971.
27. T. W. Goodwin, *in* "Carotenoids" (O. Isler, ed.), p. 577. Birkhaeuser, Basel, 1971.
28. D. S. Goodman, H. S. Huang, and T. Shiratori, *J. Biol. Chem.* **241,** 1929 (1966).
29. H. B. Fell, *Proc. R. Soc. London, Ser. B* **157,** 242 (1957).
30. M. B. Sporn, N. M. Dunlop, D. L. Newton, and W. R. Henderson, *Nature* (*London*) **263,** 110 (1976).
31. A. S. Romer and T. S. Parsons, "The Vertebrate Body," p. 18. Saunders, Philadelphia, Pennsylvania, 1977.
32. T. Moore, "Vitamin A." Elsevier, Amsterdam, 1957.
33. L. R. Fisher, S. K. Kon, and S. Y. Thompson, *J. Mar. Biol. Assoc.* **35,** 41 (1956).
34. J. E. De Larco and G. J. Todaro, *Proc. Natl. Acad. Sci. U.S.A.* **75,** 4001 (1978).
35. S. Shin, V. H. Freedman, R. Risser, and R. Pollack, *Proc. Natl. Acad. Sci. U.S.A.* **72,** 4435 (1975).
36. P. Kahn and S. Shin, *J. Cell Biol.* **82,** 1 (1979).
37. A. B. Roberts, L. C. Lamb, D. L. Newton, M. B. Sporn, J. E. De Larco, and G. J. Todaro, *Proc. Natl. Acad. Sci. U.S.A.* **77,** 3494 (1980).
38. A. C. Marchok, A. B. Roberts, M. B. Sporn, J. E. De Larco, and G. J. Todaro, unpublished experiments.
39. M. S. Collett and R. L. Erikson, *Proc. Natl. Acad. Sci. U.S.A.* **75,** 2021 (1978).
40. R. J. Huebner and G. J. Todaro, *Proc. Natl. Acad. Sci. U.S.A.* **64,** 1087 (1969).
41. G. J. Todaro and R. J. Huebner, *Proc. Natl. Acad. Sci. U.S.A.* **69,** 1009 (1972).
42. R. Levi-Montalcini and S. Cohen, *Ann. N.Y. Acad. Sci.* **85,** 324 (1960).
43. S. Q. Cohlan, *Pediatrics* **13,** 556 (1954).
44. A. Giroud and M. Martinet, *C. R. Seances Soc. Biol. Ses Fil.* **153,** 201 (1959).
45. A. Giroud and M. Martinet, *Arch. Anat. Microsc. Morphol. Exp.* **45,** 77 (1956).
46. H. Kalter and J. Wárkány, *Am. J. Pathol.* **38,** 1 (1961).
47. D. M. Kochhar, *Acta Pathol. Microbiol. Scand.* **70,** 398 (1967).
48. R. E. Shenefelt, *Teratology* **5,** 103 (1972).
49. M. Marin-Padilla, *J. Embryol. Exp. Morphol.* **15,** 261 (1966).
50. D. A. T. New, "The Culture of Vertebrate Embryos." Academic Press, New York, 1966.
51. D. A. T. New, P. T. Coppola, and D. L. Cockroft, *J. Embryol. Exp. Morphol.* **36,** 133 (1976).
52. G. M. Morriss and C. E. Steele, *J. Embryol. Exp. Morphol.* **32,** 505 (1974).
53. G. M. Morriss, *J. Anat.* **113,** 241 (1972).
54. G. M. Morriss and C. E. Steele, *Teratology* **15,** 109 (1977).

55. J. R. Hassell, J. H. Greenberg, and M. C. Johnston, *J. Embryol. Exp. Morphol.* **39,** 267 (1977).
56. T. E. Kwasigroch and D. M. Kochhar, *Exp. Cell Res.* **95,** 269 (1975).
57. G. M. Morriss, *in* "New Approaches to the Evaluation of Abnormal Embryonic Development" (D. Neubert and H. J. Merker, eds.), p. 678. Thieme, Stuttgart, 1976.
58. M. C. Johnston, *Anat. Rec.* **156,** 143 (1966).
59. W. B. Bell, *Lancet* **209,** 1003 (1925).
60. B. G. Böving, *Ann. N.Y. Acad. Sci.* **80,** 21 (1959).
61. Y. J. Topper and C. S. Freeman, *Physiol. Rev.* **60,** 1049 (1980).
62. P. Newmark, *Nature* (*London*) **280,** 637 (1979).
63. J. E. Mahaffey, M. Rosenblatt, G. L. Shepard, and J. T. Potts, Jr., *J. Biol. Chem.* **254,** 6496 (1979).
64. D. H. Coy, I. Mezo, E. Pedroza, M. V. Nekola, A. V. Schally, W. Murphy, and C. A. Meyers, "Miles Symposium on Peptide Hormones." Raven, New York (in press).
65. H. D. Niall and G. W. Tregear, *N. Engl. J. Med.* **301,** 940 (1979).
66. W. A. Klee, *Adv. Protein Chem.* **33,** 243 (1979).
67. C. Zioudrou, R. A. Streaty, and W. A. Klee, *J. Biol. Chem.* **254,** 2446 (1979).
68. R. Lotan, G. Giotta, E. Nork, and G. L. Nicolson, *J. Natl. Cancer Inst.* **60,** 1035 (1978).
69. L. D. Dion, J. E. Blalock, and G. E. Gifford, *Exp. Cell Res.* **117,** 15 (1978).
70. R. Lotan, *Cancer Res.* **39,** 1014 (1979).
71. F. L. Meyskens, Jr. and S. E. Salmon, *Cancer Res.* **39,** 4055 (1979).

27

New Human Hematopoietic Cell Systems for the Study of Growth, Differentiation, and Involved Factors: Some Therapeutic Implications

ROBERT C. GALLO AND FRANCIS W. RUSCETTI

MOLECULAR ACTIONS AND TARGETS FOR CANCER CHEMOTHERAPEUTIC AGENTS

ISBN 0-12-619280-4

I. Introduction

Growth of human blood cells *in vitro* has generally been limited to growth on solid surfaces, e.g., colonies on soft agar. The exception to this was the growth of Epstein–Barr virus (EBV)-positive B lymphoblasts which can occasionally be established as cell lines from human blood by apparent spontaneous transformation. We sought to grow other types of human blood cells in long-term liquid suspension. It was and still is our opinion that long-term liquid suspension tissue culture provides major advantages over colony growth for biochemical, immunological, and virological studies.

In this chapter we will summarize some new systems developed in our laboratory over the past few years that allow the long-term growth of specific human blood cells in liquid suspension cultures. The use of these systems for the study of regulation of blood cell growth and differentiation will also be described. Finally, because of the objectives of this volume we will try, whenever possible, to show how some of these systems may be useful to the development of new approaches to treatment of hematopoietic neoplasias.

II. Factor-Dependent Long-Term Growth of Normal Human T Lymphocytes in Liquid Suspension Culture

A. Discovery of T-Cell Growth Factor and a Description of the System

Several years ago, we found that the media in which human lymphocytes were incubated and treated with phytohemagglutinin (PHA) released active growth factors. The first one identified was colony-stimulating activity (CSA) (1). When this so-called lymphocyte-conditioned medium (Ly-CM) was concentrated, added to normal blood cells, and incubated in standard liquid suspension culture, we obtained growth of lymphoblasts. We assumed that this was growth of B lymphoblasts and initially did not give this observation its due attention. Subsequent studies indicated that these lymphoid cultures consisted entirely of thymus-derived lymphocytes, i.e., T cells (2,3). Successful cultures were started from human bone marrow, peripheral blood, and spleen. Cultures were continuously maintained for more than 1 year with a 5- to 10-fold increase in cell number every 3–4 days. These cells could be distinguished from permanently transformed lymphoblastoid cell lines by their (1) dependence for growth upon the continuous presence of a protein factor(s) in Ly-CM, (2) lack of detectable EBV, and (3) exhibition of immunological reactivities not associated with transformed lymphoblastoid cells.

The morphological and functional characteristics of these cultured cells were characteristic of mature T lymphocytes (Table I) as assayed by methods described in the literature (4,5). The cells were positive by the sheep red blood cell or "E" rosette test for T cells and did not contain detectable levels of terminal deoxynucleotidyltransferase, an enzyme marker for immature T cells (6,7). The cells were functionally mature, since they responded to mitogens such as concanavalin A (Con A) and released lymphokines. Finally, as another test of T-cell-specific function, they responded to, but were unable to stimulate, allogeneic cells in one-way mixed leukocyte cultures.

The population of growing cells appeared to be purely T cells, since there were no markers for other types of leukocytes. For example, histochemical and functional tests for myeloid and monocytic cells were negative. Similarly, surface

TABLE I

Characteristics of Cultured Human T Cells

		Peripheral blood		
Assay	Cultured cells	T cells	B cells	Myeloid or monocyte
Sheep erythrocyte E receptor[a]	+	+	−	−
Surface immunoglobulin[b]	−	−	+	+
Epstein-Barr viral antigen[b]	−	−	+	−
Myeloid histochemical stains[c]	−	−	−	+
Monocyte-specific tests[c]	−	−	−	+
Mitogen response (Con A)[a]	+	+	−	−
Mixed lymphocyte culture				
Stimulator[b]	−	−	+	±
Responder[a]	+	+	−	−
Cytolysis[a]	+	+	−	−

[a] Functional and morphological characteristics of peripheral blood T cells (4,5).

[b] Functional and morphological characteristics of peripheral blood B cells (4,5).

[c] Functional and cytochemical tests specific for myeloid and/or monocytoid cells, such as phagocytosis, peroxidase, chloroacetate esterase, and nonspecific esterase, were all carried out by standard techniques.

markers for B lymphoblastoid cells were not detectable, including tests for surface immunoglobulin, EBV receptors, and B-cell-specific complement receptors. On the other hand, the surface markers associated with T cells were quite heterogeneous. Some cells were negative for Fc receptors, while some were positive for Fc receptors for IgG or for IgM, and still others had non-B-cell complement receptors. More homogeneous T-cell strains, as judged by surface markers, were developed by initiation of cloned strains from single cells (F. Ruscetti and R. Gallo, unpublished observations).

The methods we have developed for culturing human T cells is as follows. After erythrocytes are removed, the cells (5×10^5/ml) are suspended in RPMI-1640 medium containing 20% heat-inactivated fetal calf serum (FCS) and 20% Ly-CM. The cells reach their saturation density (at approximately a 10-fold increase) every 4–5 days and are refed and split to the original cell density. We prepared Ly-CM by culturing mononuclear leukocytes from single or multiple donors at 10^6 cells/ml in RPMI-1640 containing 5% autologous serum and 1% PHA. As stated before, Ly-CM, in addition to T-cell growth factor (TCGF) contained CSA and a variety of lymphokines.

The human T-lymphocyte culture system can be used for at least four different general purposes: (1) studies on growth promotion and regulation of a specific cell type involving factor–cell receptor interactions; (2) studies on various aspects of cell-mediated immunity; (3) studies on this subset of hematopoietic cells for the presence of viral information and for the interaction of viruses with these cells; and (4) development of cytotoxic T cells in large numbers specifically directed against tumor cells carrying recognizable specific antigens, i.e., in immunotherapy.

B. Properties of Purified Human T-Cell Growth Factor

Starting with human Ly-CM pooled from numerous healthy blood donors, we recently purified human TCGF by using a sequence of ion-exchange chromatography, gel filtration, and isoelectric focusing (8). The characteristics of the purified TCGF are listed in Table II. The molecular weight as estimated by gel filtration is about 23,000. This factor is trypsin-sensitive, is RNase- and DNase-resistant, does not adhere to various lectins, and after purification is very labile unless stored in the presence of albumin or polyethylene glycol. Purified TCGF does *not initiate* blastogenesis of peripheral blood lymphocytes, *but it is a selective mitogen for T lymphocytes that have already been activated (blast-"transformed") after earlier exposure to a lectin or antigen.*

Human TCGF will exert its effect over a broad range of species. We have found that it has mitogenic activity for activated T lymphocytes derived from other primates as well as rodents (9). In contrast, it appears very specific for the

TABLE II

Some Characteristics of Purified Human T-Cell Growth Factor

Nature of molecule	Protein
Size	13,000 daltons*
pI	6.8
Glycosyl moiety	None detected
Target cell	Activated T lymphocyte
Mode of action	Unknown
Cell of origin	Probably activated T lymphocyte
Stability	Very labile unless stored in albumin or polyethylene glycol

*As estimated by gel filtration SDS PAGE shows a doublet of approximately 12,000 daltons.

kind of cell it affects. Thus TCGF has no detectable effect on fibroblasts, B lymphocytes, myeloid cells, or nonactivated T lymphocytes.

C. Schematic Model for the Mechanism of Action of T-Cell Growth Factor

As stated above, purified TCGF has no detectable effect on "resting" peripheral blood lymphocytes. Moreover, early results indicate that peripheral blood cells do not contain receptors for this factor. These assays are carried out by incubating blood cells with TCGF and showing that the activity can be quantitatively recovered in the medium. In contrast, when peripheral blood lymphocytes are blast-transformed (activated) with PHA or antigen and TCGF subsequently added, the TCGF is no longer found in the supernatant fraction, and the activated T lymphocytes are induced to proliferate continually as long as TCGF is supplied. Although proof of receptor presence will depend on chemical isolation of receptors and on binding studies with labeled, purified TCGF, these results clearly and strongly suggest that in normal situations receptors for TCGF are either newly synthesized or newly exposed only after T lymphocytes are antigen-activated. These results led us to propose the mechanism shown in Fig. 1.

The fundamental observations on growing T lymphocytes in long-term suspension culture dependent on a factor called TCGF have been confirmed in many laboratories during the past few years (10–17). The results have been extended to include rat and murine cells (10–12). Moreover, some groups have used concentrates of crude Ly-CM to generate cytotoxic T cells (13–16), a subject we have explored using purified TCGF as described below. Others have used crude Ly-CM to study the role of these cultured cells in helper–suppressor assays (17).

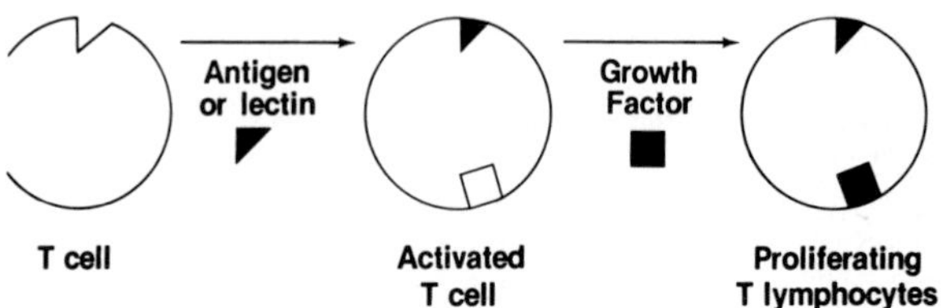

Fig. 1. Proposed mechanism of action of T-lymphocyte growth factor.

D. Therapeutic Implications of the System

There are two possibilities we wish to discuss here concerning the potential use of this system in the therapy of human neoplasias. The first of these is based upon immunotherapy. There is abundant evidence that some tumor cells contain surface antigens which can elicit immune stimulation of T cells *in vitro*. It is therefore possible that, after mixing malignant cells with autologous normal lymphocytes obtained when a patient is in remission, the remission normal T cells activated by exposure to the autologous malignant cells can be propagated in culture with TCGF and that some of these T cells will include cytotoxic T cells. The cytotoxic T cells in turn could be used to kill the tumor cells *in vivo*. Using the TCGF present in crude Ly-CM, Zarling and Bach (16) have recently reported some success with a few samples, although the length of time the normal cytotoxic cells were grown was rather limited and the effector cell/target cell ratio was high. We have performed similar experiments with a larger number of patients and with purified TCGF (18). In summary, we activated remission normal T cells from six patients with acute myeloblastic leukemia by initially coculturing normal lymphocytes with autologous leukemic myeloblasts. After activation, the lymphocytes were treated with TCGF and then expanded in culture with TCGF continuously added. The leukemic myeloblasts died out, and the cultures consisted only of T lymphocytes. The cultured T lymphocytes were assayed for cytotoxicity against different targets by the ^{15}Cr release assay. The T lymphocytes have maintained cytotoxic activity for their autologous leukemic cells for over 6 months. Cytotoxicity has ranged from 15 to 50% (18). The effector cell/target cell ratio is still high (50:1, or at best 25:1), precluding a practical clinical adaptation of the system at this time. However, by various manipulations it may be possible to reduce this ratio substantially. If this can be achieved, then in our opinion clinical trials based on these studies would be merited.

A second approach is based upon inhibiting TCGF activity in T cell neoplasias, e.g., by antibodies to TCGF. This assumes that in some or all cases of T-cell neoplasias TCGF is an important aspect of the abnormal proliferation. Some evidence for this is described below.

III. Growth of Neoplastic T Cells

A. Growth Dependent on T-Cell Growth Factor

We have noted above that TCGF activity on normal cells depends upon previous activation of normal T cells by an antigen or mitogenic lectin such as PHA. We have suggested that normally only activated T cells have receptors for TCGF. In contrast, when we added TCGF to neoplastic T cells the cells grew without prior antigen activation. This result was obtained with Sezary cells. Similar results have also been obtained in an acute T-cell leukemia (B. Poiesz *et al.*, in press). These findings indicate that human neoplastic T cells have TCGF receptors, suggesting prior *in vivo* antigen activation.

B. T-Cell Growth Factor-Independent Growth

Preliminary results indicate that some neoplastic human T cells stimulated by TCGF eventually become TCGF-independent and in these cases may continuously release TCGF. This leads us to propose that a "driving force" for continued growth of some human neoplastic T cells may involve abnormal TCGF production. These results also suggest that the cell of origin of TCGF may normally be the very T cell which responds to it.

IV. Long-Term Factor-Dependent Growth of Human Myeloid (Granulocytic) Leukemic Leukocytes in Liquid Suspension Culture

We reported previously that conditioned medium (CM) from some early-passage whole human embryo cultures (WHE-CM) could stimulate extended growth and differentiation of myeloid cells in suspension culture (19–21). Briefly, we prepared CM from monolayer cells by allowing the cells to grow to confluency in culture flasks, changing to fresh media containing 10% FCS and harvesting the CM 48 hours later. The effect of WHE-CM on cell growth was tested essentially in the same manner as described for Ly-CM. One particular embryonic cell strain (WHE-1) was a much more potent source of CM than the other cultures tested. This CM stimulated the logarithmic growth of peripheral blood cells from patients with myelogenous leukemia. The cell cultures had to be refed and diluted to a low cell density weekly for growth to continue. Leukocyte growth remained dependent upon the CM, even after 300 days in culture. The most remarkable property of WHE-1 CM was its specificity. Logarithmic growth of peripheral blood leukocytes was stimulated from 16 successive cases of myelogenous leukemias, whereas there was no effect on the number of leukocytes from blood or marrow of normal donors or patients with lymphatic leukemia. In addition, the CM could not support clonal growth of myeloid cells in agar. The differentials of the cells growing in cultures varied from case to case. All contained a subpopulation of blast cells, which presumably accounted for the self-renewal capability of these cultures. Some cultures contained the whole spectrum of myeloid and monocytoid cells, including mature neutrophils, eosinophils, and basophils. Histochemical stains and functional tests certified the dominant myeloid nature of the cells. Even after 4 months in culture, the majority of the cells stained with peroxidase, Sudan black B, and chloroacetate esterase, substances specific for the myeloid series of leukocytes. These cells also were able to phagocytize latex particles, a function of mature granulocytes. Two of the cultures had chromosome markers, indicating the proliferation *in vitro* of leukemic myeloid cells. However, only a portion of the metaphases had the marker chromosome, indicating either the growth of different clones of leukemic cells or a mixture of normal and leukemic cells.

We also tested a variety of other human cultured cells for myeloid stimulatory activity, but only rare samples yielded detectable activity. All were from embryonic tissues and included two embryo cultures from first-trimester abortuses, a fibroblast culture of fetal thymic origin, three amnionic fluid cell cultures, and a fetal lung fibroblast culture (Section V). Positive results were achieved with one source of whole human embryo and amnionic fluid, but they were less potent than the original WHE-1, only a portion of the leukocyte specimens responded, and the magnitude and duration of cell proliferation were more limited. In most, the cells in culture developed a declining growth fraction and a longer doubling time after a few weeks. This was usually coincident with an increasing degree of differentation into mature neutrophils.

The release of active CM was restricted in every case, including WHE-1, to early-passage, unfrozen, cellular material. This has severely limited our ability to purify and characterize these factors. Nevertheless, the results indicated that leukemic myeloid cells could be grown in suspension culture and that many human leukemic cells could be stimulated to mature into nondividing granulocytes. They also suggested that cell membranes of myeloid leukemia cells may preferentially recognize fetal growth and differentiation-promoting factors.

V. Factor-Independent Growth: The HL-60 Promyelocytic Leukemic Cell Line

A. Development of the HL-60 Line

As noted above, previous experiments in our laboratory indicated that continuous growth in suspension culture of human myeloid leukemic cells could be maintained using CM from certain whole human embryo cultures (19–21). These cultures remained factor-dependent with one exception. HL-60 cells, obtained by leukophoresis from the peripheral blood of a patient with acute promyelocytic leukemia, were incubated in standard medium supplemented with media conditioned by various human embryonic (first-trimester) fibroblast cultures (22). Growth initially occurred only in flasks containing CM from a human embryonic lung culture. However, unlike our previous experience with growing myeloid leukemic cells, growth of HL-60 cells soon became independent of this CM and continuous proliferation of these cells occurred in standard medium supplemented with fetal calf serum alone (22). It is intriguing to speculate that these cells, once dependent on an exogenous factor for *in vitro* growth, now produce such a factor endogenously. Recently, continuous proliferation of HL-60 cells in standard medium supplemented only with insulin and transferrin has been achieved (T. R. Breitman *et al.*, unpublished results). This may make it easier to test such a hypothesis.

B. Characteristics of HL-60 Cells

1. *Leukemic Phenotype*

Cell lines derived from patients with myeloid leukemia frequently consist of B lymphoblasts containing the EBV genome, which probably arise from contaminating B lymphocytes and not from the patient's leukemic cells. In contrast, cultured HL-60 cells are truly representative of the patient's leukemic cells. Striking morphological and histochemical similarities exist between the patient's fresh leukemic cells and the cultured HL-60 cells. Moreover, the major karyotypic changes in the patient's fresh bone marrow (deleted chromosomes 5 and 8 and an abnormal E-group chromosome) are present in metaphases of cultured HL-60 cells. These cells also show other malignant characteristics, including tumorigenicity in nude mice (myeloid tumors, i.e., chloromas) and spontaneous colony formation in soft agar. The HL-60 cells were repeatedly negative for EBV by the nuclear antigen test (EBNA), and we found no evidence of replicating type-C oncornavirus in these cells (23).

2. *Myeloid Features*

HL-60 cells show a firm commitment to differentiation along myeloid-granulocytic lines. The cultured cells resemble promyelocytes with large, round nuclei, each containing two to four nucleoli and dispersed nuclear chromatin (Fig. 2). The cytoplasm is basophilic and has prominent azurophilic granules. Virtually 100% of the cells are histochemically positive for myeloid-specific chloroacetate esterase, myeloperoxidase, and Sudan black (22). In addition, HL-60 cells package and release lysozyme and β-glucuronidase (24). The cells display Fc receptors but lack Ia antigen (23).

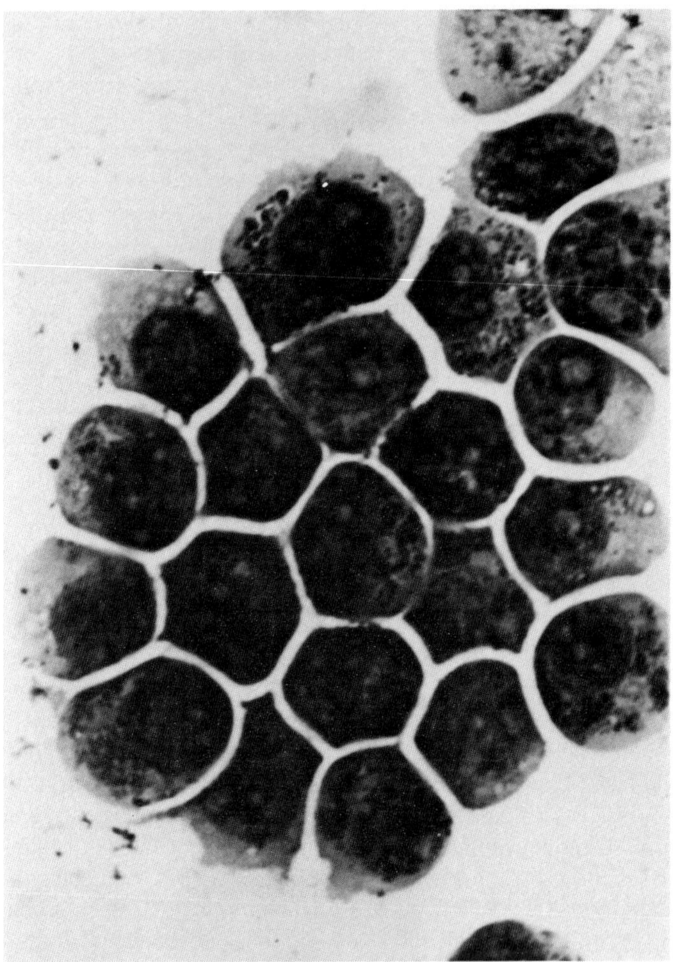

Fig. 2. Wright-Giemsa stain of HL-60 cells. ×1000.

The distinct morphological and histochemical myeloid characteristics make the HL-60 culture unique among human leukemic cell lines. A number of cell lines have been developed with leukemic characteristics of B cells, T cells, or null cells (25,26), but none of these have the morphological or histochemical characteristics of HL-60 cells. In addition, the KG-1 cell line, recently derived from a patient with erythroleukemia (27), initially displayed a positive myeloperoxidase reaction in approximately 20% of the cells, but this reaction was gradually reduced to near zero with serial passage of the culture (D. Golde, personal communication). In contrast, virtually 100% of the HL-60 cells have remained peroxidase-positive after more than 100 passages over a 2-year period.

C. Terminal Differentiation of HL-60 Cells

1. *Spontaneous*

A small percentage of HL-60 cells (up to 10–12% in early passages and about 2–7% in later passages) spontaneously differentiate past promyelocytes into more mature myeloid cells, including myelocytes, metamyelocytes, and banded and segmented neutrophils. This spontaneous terminal differentiation is analogous to that seen in cultured Friend mouse erythroleukemia cells which consist predominantly of erythroblasts, a small percentage of which spontaneously differentiate into more mature erythroid cells producing hemoglobin.

2. *Induction by Dimethyl Sulfoxide*

Dimethy sulfoxide (DMSO), which markedly enhances Friend cell erythroid differentiation (28), similarly increases the percent of mature myeloid cells in the HL-60 culture (Fig. 3) (29).

3. *Comparison of Uninduced and Induced HL-60 Cells*

Unlike uninduced HL-60 cells, DMSO-treated cells display functional characteristics of mature granulocytes. These include the ability to phagocytose and kill microorganisms (29), the capacity to respond to chemoattractants (29), development of complement receptors (29), increased hexose monophosphate shunt activity (24), increased capacity to release packaged enzymes including β-glucuronidase, lysozyme, and peroxidase (24,29), and the capacity to generate superoxide anion ($0^{-}{}_{2}$) and reduce NBT dye. However, at least two characteristics of normal mature granulocytes are not found in DMSO-treated HL-60 cells: leukocyte alkaline phosphatase (LAP), as determined histochemically, and lactoferrin. LAP is also commonly absent in the granulocytes of chronic-phase CML. Its physiological leukemia relevance is unknown. Lactoferrin, found in mature granulocytes, may play a role in inhibiting the release of CSA from certain producer cells (30). It is interesting to speculate that the absence of lactoferrin from a patient's mature granulocytes could thus lead to an excess production of CSA, resulting in granulocytic hyperplasia with subsequent leukemia. The characteristics of uninduced and DMSO-induced HL-60 cells are summarized in Table III.

The ability of mature, DMSO-treated HL-60 cells to reduce NBT dye is of practical importance in assessing HL-60 response to various inducing agents. In a reaction mediated by superoxide, NBT, a water-soluble dye, is converted to insoluble intracellular blue formazan by phagocytizing or phorbol myristate acetate (TPA)-treated neutrophils (31,32). The percent of HL-60 cells reducing this dye closely parallels the percent of morphologically mature cells in the culture (33). Moreover, NBT reduction is one of the earliest differentiation markers expressed in maturing HL-60 cells (33). Thus this test is a sensitive, easily quantitated differentiation marker which eliminates observer subjectivity as-

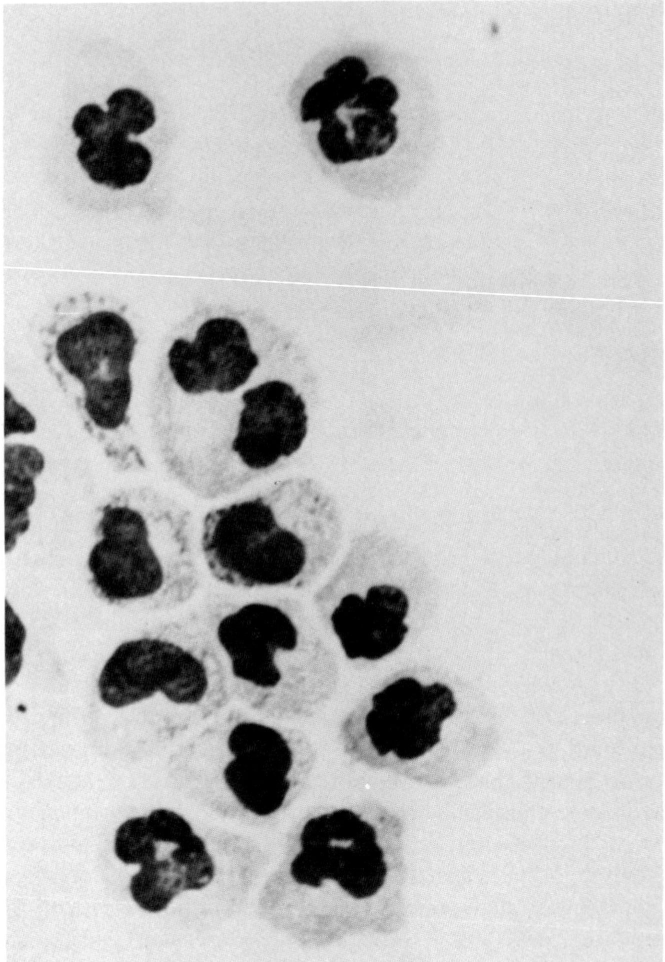

Fig. 3. HL-60 cells after a 6-day incubation in 1.2% DMSO. ×1000.

sociated with morphological assessment alone. As such, it is similar to the benzidine stain of Friend cells in providing an easily reproducible technique for assessing HL-60 response to a large number of potential differentiation-inducing compounds.

4. *Comparative Effect of Various Chemicals*

Although DMSO was the first compound reported to induce differentiation in Friend cells (28) and has been the most extensively studied inducing agent, a wide variety of other compounds similarly induce differentiation in both Friend

TABLE III

Characteristics of Uninduced and Induced HL-60 Cells

Characteristic	Uninduced HL-60 cells	DMSO-induced HL-60 cells
Morphology	Promyelocytes	Granulocytes
Histochemistry	Specific myeloid	Specific myeloid
Karyotype	Aneuploid ($N = 45$)	Aneuploid ($N = 45$)
Growth		
DNA synthesis	+	−
Proliferation in suspension	+	−
Colony formation in soft agar	+	−
Tumorigenicity in nude mice	+	−
Functional		
Chemotaxis	−	+
Phagocytosis	−	+
NBT reduction	−	+
Bactericidal activity	−	+
Fc receptors	+	+
Complement receptors	−	+
Leukocyte alkaline phosphatase	−	−
Lactoferrin	−	−

cells (34,35) and HL-60 cells (29). These include a group of polar-planer compounds, including DMSO (29), and a more recently synthesized compound, hexamethylene bisacetamide (HMBA) (29,36). The optimal molar concentrations of the polar inducers in the HL-60 system are 40–60% less than the concentrations used in Friend cells, but the relative potency of these compounds in inducing differentation is strikingly similar in both systems (29,34). The concentrations which induce maximum differentiation are only slightly below concentrations which produce nonspecific cytotoxicity. Compounds other than DMSO which are active in inducing differentiation at similar concentrations in both Friend cells and HL-60 cells include butyric acid, hypoxanthine, and actinomycin D (37). Some compounds, including hemin, ouabain, and prostaglandin E_1, induce Friend cell differentiation but have no effect on HL-60 cell differentiation (37). However, all compounds presently known to induce HL-60 cell differentiation also induce analogous differentiation in Friend cells. The mechanism of action of these inducing agents is presently unknown, but the marked similarity in behavior of HL-60 cells and Friend cells in the presence of these compounds suggests that similar molecular mechanisms are involved in the induction of differentiation of these human myeloid and murine erythroid leukemic cells.

D. Development of Special Clones

1. *Superinducible*

Clones of Friend cells resistant to the inducing action of DMSO and other compounds have been previously described (38,39). Since at least 10–15% of uncloned HL-60 cells retain the immature promyelocytic phenotype even after prolonged incubation in optimal concentrations of DMSO, we felt that it would be relatively simple to clone these HL-60 cells apparently resistant to DMSO induction. the HL-60 cells were cloned in semisolid medium as previously described (29), and the resultant clones treated with DMSO. Over 100 clones were analyzed, all of which developed increased differentiation with DMSO treatment. Some of these clones are hyperinducible and display both spontaneous and DMSO-induced differentiation significantly higher than the parent line (Table IV). It is surprising that uninducible clones have not been obtained in this manner. It may be that the cloning technique used (picking colonies from methylcellulose) in some way selects for HL-60 cells that are firmly committed to granulocytic differentiation.

2. *Partially Resistant to Differentiation Induction*

In order to develop clones resistant to differentiation induction, the HL-60 parent cells were incubated in gradually increasing concentrations of DMSO and dimethylformamide, a particularly potent HL-60 inducer (29). After at least a 7-day incubation, the viable cells remaining were harvested, cultured, and then resuspended in medium containing a slightly higher concentration of inducer. After several such procedures the cells were cloned and assessed for differentiation capacity. Clones incubated with dimethylformamide showed the most marked resistance to DMSO induction (Table IV). Moreover, the cells displayed little if any spontaneous differentiation. Nevertheless, even in these relatively resistant clones there was still significant differentiation (20–25%) after DMSO treatment. Thus, clones of HL-60 cells absolutely resistant to inducing agent are presently not available.

E. Response to Colony-Stimulating Activity

Friend mouse erythroleukemic cells do not show any response to erythropoietin, one of the *in vivo* regulators of normal erythropoiesis (40). In contrast, the HL-60 myeloid cell line develops a definite response to various sources of CSA which may be an *in vivo* regulator of normal granulopoiesis. This response is most clearly demonstrated in semisolid medium. HL-60 cells plated in methylcellulose in the presence of various sources of CSA display a 5- to 30-fold increase in colony-forming efficiency when compared to cells plated without CSA (20). Moreover, colonies stimulated by CSA are significantly

TABLE IV

Dimethyl Sulfoxide-Induced Differentiation of Various Clones of HL-60 Cells

HL-60 cell type	DMSO concentration (%)	Mature myeloid cells (%)[a]	NBT reduction (%)
Parent	None	4	5
	0.8	25	28
	1.0	50	55
	1.2	79	83
	1.5	Dead	Dead
Clone A (none)[b]	None	12	15
	0.8	53	60
	1.0	82	85
	1.2	98	99
	1.5	Dead	Dead
Clone B (1.6% DMSO)	None	3	3
	0.8	21	23
	1.0	53	48
	1.2	79	76
	1.5	Dead	Dead
Clone C (110 m*M* DMF)[c]	None	<1	<1
	0.8	4	6
	1.0	5	7
	1.2	18	24
	1.4	24	22
	1.6	Dead	Dead

[a] Morphologically mature myelocytes, metamyelocytes, and banded and segmented neutrophils.

[b] The figures in parentheses refer to the highest concentration of inducing agent the HL-60 parent cells were incubated in before cloning in methylcellulose.

[c] DMF, Dimethylformamide.

larger than those arising spontaneously. This effect is most clearly demonstrated in early passages of HL-60 cells when the spontaneous colony formation (i.e., without CSA) is less than in later passages. Morphological assessment of Wright–Giemsa-stained cells picked from individual colonies stimulated by CSA reveals that most (>80%) of these colonies still consist of immature promyelocytes. This is in contrast to normal bone marrow where colonies stimulated by CSA consist predominantly of mature granulocytes or macrophages. Thus, in semisolid medium, CSA enhances cloning efficiency and proliferation but not differentiation of HL-60 cells.

This factor also exerts an effect on HL-60 cells in suspension culture. When these cells are incubated with 10–20% CM containing CSA, a slight enhancement of proliferation is noted. Moreover, after 5–7 days, the cells become morphologically altered; thus cytoplasmic granules become less prominent, the nucleus/cytoplasm ratio decreases, and the nuclear chromatin condenses slightly. Similar, more extensive studies of CSA effects on HL-60 cells have been performed by L. Sachs and his colleagues, and they believe that the effect of CSA (or MGI as they call it) is to induce conversion of HL-60 promyelocytes to macrophages (see L. Sachs elsewhere in this book).

In our laboratory, these cells no longer are myeloperoxidase-positive but become positive for nonspecific esterase, which is characteristic of monocytes and macrophages. However, these cells exhibit few if any functional characteristics commonly associated with monocytes and macrophages (41), such as a response to chemoattractants, phagocytosis, complement receptors, CSA production, and NBT reduction. The significance of these CSA-treated HL-60 cells, in our opinion, therefore is not completely clear.

The distinct, reproducible response of HL-60 cells to CSA suggests that these cells possess a receptor for this growth-promoting factor. In this respect, HL-60 cells resemble the KG-1 cell line which also shows increased cloning efficiency in semisolid medium in the presence of CSA. The existence of these cell lines thus provides a unique opportunity for assessing CSA–receptor interaction and for isolating the specific receptor for this particular growth promoter. Moreover, compared to the previous use of human bone marrow, these cell lines should provide a more available and more reproducible assay system for human CSA. However, these studies could be hampered by the apparent molecular heterogeneity of human CSA and the difficulty of purifying this molecule(s) in sufficient quantity (42–44).

F. Effect of Glucocorticoids

Glucocorticoids, particularly dexamethasone, exert markedly diverse effects on certain murine leukemic cells. The differentiative response of Friend cells to DMSO and other inducing agents is blocked in the presence of dexamethasone (45,46). In contrast, dexamethasone directly induces varying degrees of differentiation in murine myeloid leukemic cells (47,48). Incubation of HL-60 cells in concentrations as high as 10^{-5} M dexamethasone results in no change in cell viability, proliferation, or differentiation. Moreover, at this concentration, response to differentiation-inducing agents is similar to the response of cells in the absence of dexamethasone. Thus, unlike murine leukemia cells, glucocorticoids neither induce nor block differentiation of HL-60 cells. However, these compounds may still exert some important effect on HL-60 cells, since a reduction in the number of Fc receptor sites on the HL-60 membrane after incubation with glucocorticoids has been recently reported (49), and confirmed in our laboratory (A. Ganguly, R. Gallo, and I. Witz, unpublished results).

G. Effect of Phorbol Myristate Acetate

Tumor promoters are a group of closely related membrane-active compounds which, though not carcinogens themselves, promote tumor formation *in vivo* in the mouse two-stage carcinogenesis system (50,51). The most potent and widely studied of these compounds is phorbol myristate acetate (TPA). This compound blocks both spontaneous and DMSO-induced differentiation in certain clones of Friend erythroleukemia cells (52,53). Moreover, differentiation in various other cultured cells is blocked by TPA (54–56). These findings have led to the hypothesis that tumor promoters exert their effect by similarly blocking terminal differentiation *in vivo* and allowing unrestricted growth of more immature cells (57).

In contrast to its effect on other cell systems, TPA does not block differentiation of HL-60 but rather induces distinct phenotypic changes in these cells (58,59). These include increased adherence to plastic substrate, degranulation, and release of lysozyme, inhibition of cell division, activation of intracellular enzymes, and increased ingestion of latex particles. These results have been interpreted in different ways: TPA induces differentiation of HL-60 cells into terminally differentiated granulocytes (58), or TPA induces HL-60 cells to differentiate into macrophages (59). We think that one reason for this confusion is that the well-documented effects of TPA on normal myeloid cells have been insufficiently considered. This compound is routinely used to mimic the membrane changes that occur with phagocytosis, resulting in distinct metabolic changes in normal myeloid cells (60–63). These include degranulation and release of lysozyme and activation of certain membrane and intracellular enzymes, resulting in the production of superoxide anion and H_2O_2, increased hexose monophosphate shunt activity, and increased cellular chemiluminescence. Since HL-60 cells have such distinct myeloid characteristics, it is likely that TPA exerts effects on this cell line similar to those it exerts on normal myeloid cells. Thus the differentiation of HL-60 cells induced by TPA in our opinion is most likely a result of stimulation of their cell membranes resulting in degranulation and activation of membrane-associated and intracellular enzymes normally activated during and after phagocytosis. The marked difference in response of Friend cells and HL-60 cells to TPA suggests that significant membrane differences exist in these erythroid and myeloid cells.

H. Possible Use of HL-60 Cells as Test Indicators for Certain Antileukemic Compounds

In view of the fact that frank leukemic cells can sometimes be induced to differentiate terminally into nondividing and functional normal-appearing cells, it seems prudent to consider the possibility that some antileukemic compounds might work this way and/or that new compounds might be developed with this as its major effect rather than cell killing. Sachs has already suggested this from data he and his colleagues have obtained in mouse myeloid leukemias (see L. Sachs elsewhere in this book). Obviously, the HL-60 system provides an ideal choice to test this. Here we present some data for known antileukemic agents. As shown in Tables V–VII, compounds such as daunorubicin and actinomycin D have differentiation-promoting activity. These results have been obtained by S. Collins in our group in collaboration with A. Bodner and R. Ting of Biotech

TABLE V

Effect of Miscellaneous Cell Differentiation Inducers on Differentiation of HL-60 Cells[a]

Compound	Concentration (mM)	Viable cell count ($\times 10^{-5}$/ml)	Mature myeloid cells (%)[b]	NBT reduction (%)
None		22	8	7
DMSO	180	11	75	80
HMBA	3	9	95	97
Dexamethasone	0.1	22	7	10
	0.01	23	6	8
	0.001	23	7	10
Hemin	1	4.4	5	7
	0.5	10	6	6
	0.1	20	5	6
Prostaglandin E_1	0.1	Dead		
	0.01	3.8	9	7
	0.001	12	10	12
Ouabain	4×10^{-5}	Dead		
	3×10^{-5}	2	4	3
	2×10^{-5}	10	6	5
	10^{-5}	20	6	6
Hypoxanthine	5	4.2	86	90
	3	11	76	74
	1	25	16	19
6-Thioguanine	6×10^{-3}	Dead		
	3×10^{-3}	7.6	49	45
	1.5×10^{-3}	10.7	35	35
6-Mercaptopurine	0.5	Dead		
	0.25	0.4	NT	NT
	0.10	4.0	27	25
	0.05	7.0	12	10

[a] HL-60 cells were seeded at 2.5×10^5/ml in the indicated concentration of inducing agent and incubated under standard conditions. After 6 days, the cultured cells were assessed for viability, morphological, and functional (NBT reduction) differentiation. NT, Not tested; HMBA, hexamethylene bis(acetamide).

[b] Myelocytes, metamyelocytes, and banded and segmented neutrophils.

TABLE VI

Effect of Standard Chemotherapeutic Agents on Induction of Differentiation of HL-60 Cells

Compound	Concentration (μg/ml)	Cell count ($\times 10^{-5}$/ml)	Mature myeloid cells (%)[a]
None		21	8
Adriamycin	0.02	6.4	23
	0.01	16	14
	0.005	20	9
Daunorubicin	0.01	2.4	35
	0.005	8.8	19
	0.00125	21.2	15
Arabinosylcytosine	0.1	4.2	15
	0.05	8.2	15
	0.025	12.2	11
Vincristine	0.005	8.8	18
	0.0025	18.4	12
	0.00125	20.2	8
Hydroxyurea	8	5.0	13
	4	11.6	8

[a] Myelocytes, metamyelocytes, and banded and segmented neutrophils. HL-60 cells were seeded at 2.5×10^5/ml in growth media containing the indicated concentration of drug. After 6 days of incubation, morphological assessment of Wright-Giemsa-stained cytospin preparations was performed.

TABLE VII

Effect of Actinomycin D on Growth and Differentiation of HL-60 Cells[a]

Concentration (ng/ml)	Viable cells ($\times 10^{-5}$/ml)	Mature myeloid cells (%)[b]	NBT reduction (%)
None	23	8	8
2.5	8.0	40	44
2.5[c]	5.8	52	56
5.0	4.5	62	66
5.0[c]	3.5	89	93
7.5	Dead		

[a] HL-60 cells were seeded at 2.5×10^5/ml in growth media containing the indicated concentrations of actinomycin D. After 6 days of incubation, the cells were assessed for viability, morphological, and functional differentiation.

[b] Myelocytes, metamyelocytes, and banded and segmented neutrophils.

[c] Media changed on day 4 of a 6-day incubation and replaced with fresh media containing actinomycin D.

Research Laboratories. On the other hand, it should be stressed that, when *fresh* human leukemic cells are evaluated in this way, most show no differentiation induction. It seems to us then that at the present time the best use of this system with the objective of obtaining better treatment of these diseases is to determine (1) the mechanism of differentiation induction in HL-60 cells, and (2) why some cells respond and others do not.

I. Summary and Future Objectives with HL-60 Cells

HL-60 human myeloid leukemic cells share with Friend mouse erythroid leukemic cells the capacity to be induced to differentiate terminally by various polar-planar compounds, as well as by butyric acid, hypoxanthine, and actinomycin D. These compounds are active in both systems at similar concentrations. However, HL-60 cells differ markedly from Friend cells in their response to glucocorticoids and to the tumor-promoting phorbol esters. In addition, Friend cells do not respond to erythropoietin, while HL-60 cells display a distinct phenotypic response to CSA (a possible granulopoietin). Therefore, despite karyotypic abnormalities, HL-60 cells contain the genetic information for coding for most of the characteristics of normal functionally mature granulocytes. Why then was this information not expressed in the leukemic patient from whom these cells were derived? What is the cause and nature of the blockage in normal differentiation found in this particular patient and in other patients with leukemia, as well as in Friend erythroleukemic cells? The similarity in response of Friend cells and HL-60 cells to various inducing agents which somehow overcome this blockage in differentiation suggests that the molecular basis of this blockage is similar in both systems. Friend disease itself is induced by a type-C oncornavirus, and most Friend cell lines produce replicating virus. We could not detect a replicating type-C virus in HL-60 cells by standard techniques, but this does not necessarily rule out a viral etiology for the blockage in differentiation of HL-60 cells, since in most *in vitro* systems specific viral sequences rather than whole replicating virus are what is necessary for transformation. It is of interest in this respect that recent experiments in our laboratory suggest that immunoglobulins eluted from human leukemic cells react with certain type-C viral proteins (notably, reverse transcriptases purified from some mammalian type-C viruses) (64), and that these immunoglobulins bind preferentially to HL-60 cell membranes.

Friend erythroleukemic cells have been useful in elucidating some of the molecular events associated with normal erythropoiesis (65). Such studies have concentrated on the well-characterized mRNA coding for globin, the major differentiation product of erythroid cells. Similar studies theoretically could be done with differentiating HL-60 cells to outline the molecular events associated with normal myeloid differentiation. These studies are hampered by the extensive functional complexity of differentiating myeloid cells and by the present lack of knowledge of specific proteins and mRNAs associated with these multiple functional characteristics. We are presently analyzing cytoplasmic RNA from HL-60 cells to determine whether new mRNA sequences accumulate as the HL-60 cells differentiate into functionally mature cells.

It is presently unclear whether the differentiation-inducing agents active in both Friend and HL-60 cells have their primary site of action at the cell membrane or at nuclear chromatin. A histone-related polypeptide (HP) has been recently detected among the acid-extractable chromosomal proteins of HL-60 cells (66). It is related to histone H2a and is apparently a cleavage product of H2a. Differentiation of HL-60 cells induced by DMSO is accompanied by increased cleavage of HP from H2a. Whether the increased HP level directly leads to alteration of the transcription pattern of HL-60 genes, leading to terminal differentiation, or is merely another expression of the more differentiated phenotype is as yet undetermined. It is of interest that different levels of histone H2a are also found in particular clones of Friend cells having different capacities to differentiate (66). Isolation and purification of HP, together with its quantitation in other cells and cell lines at various stages of differentation should provide more clues in elucidating its potential role in the regulation of differentiation.

References

1. J. Prival, M. Paran, R. C. Gallo, and A. M. Wu, *J. Natl. Cancer Inst.* **53,** 1583 (1974).
2. D. A. Morgan, F. W. Ruscetti, and R. C. Gallo, *Science* **193,** 1007 (1976).
3. F. W. Ruscetti, D. A. Morgan, and R. C. Gallo, *J. Immunol.* **119,** 131 (1977).
4. M. Jondal, H. Wigzell, and F. Aiuti, *Transplant. Rev.* **16,** 63 (1973).
5. E. M. Shevach, E. S. Jaffe, and I. Green, *Transplant. Rev.* **16,** 3 (1973).
6. F. J. Bollum, *in* "The Enzymes" (P. D. Boyer, ed.), 3rd ed., Vol. 10, p. 145. Academic Press, New York, 1974.
7. P. S. Sarin, P. N. Anderson, and R. C. Gallo, *Blood* **47,** 11 (1976).
8. J. Mier and R. Gallo, *Proc. Natl. Acad. Sci.* (*U.S.*) **77,** 6134 (1980).
9. F. Ruscetti, J. Mier, and R. Gallo, unpublished observations.
10. S. Gillis, M. Ferm, W. Ou, and K. Smith, *J. Immunol.* **120,** 2027 (1978).
11. S. Rosenberg, P. Spiess, and S. Schwarz, *J. Immunol.* **121,** 1946 (1978).
12. J. T. Kurnick, K. Gronvik, A. Kimura, J. Lindblom, V. T. Skoog, O. Sjöberg, and H. Wigzell, *J. Immunol.* **122,** 1255 (1979).
13. S. Kasakura, *J. Immunol.* **118,** 43 (1977).
14. P. Baker, S. Gillis, M. Ferm, and K. Smith, *J. Immunol.* **121,** 2168 (1978).
15. J. L. Strausser and S. A. Rosenberg, *J. Immunol.* **121,** 1491 (1978).
16. J. Zarling and F. Bach, *Nature* (*London*) **280,** 685 (1979).
17. R. Raca, G. Bonnard, and R. Herberman, *J. Immunol.* **123,** 246 (1979).
18. A. Jurjus, J. Mier, A. Ridgeway, G. Bonnard, R. Herberman, I. Witz, and R. Gallo, unpublished observations.
19. R. E. Gallagher, S. Z. Salahuddin, W. T. Hall, K. B. McCredie, and R. C. Gallo, *Proc. Natl. Acad. Sci. U.S.A.* **72,** 4137 (1975).
20. R. C. Gallo, F. Ruscetti, S. Collins, and R. Gallagher, *in* "Hematopoietic Cell Differentiation"

(D. W. Golde, M. J. Cline, D. Metcalf, and C. F. Fox, eds.), p. 335 Academic Press, New York, 1978.
21. R. C. Gallo, F. Ruscetti, and R. E. Gallagher, *Cold Spring Harbor Conf. Cell Proliferation* **5,** 671 (1978).
22. S. J. Collins, R. C. Gallo, and R. E. Gallagher, *Nature* (*London*) **270,** 347 (1977).
23. R. Gallagher, S. Collins, J. Trujillo, K. McCredie, M. Ahearn, S. Tsai, R. Metzgar, G. Aulakh, R. Ting, F. Ruscetti, and R. C. Gallo, *Blood* **54,** (1979).
24. P. Newburger, M. Chovaniec, J. Greenberg, and H. Cohen, *J. Cell Biol.* **82,** 315 (1979).
25. C. B. Lozzio and B. B. Lozzio, *Blood* **45,** 321 (1975).
26. K. Nilsson and J. Pontén, *Int. J. Cancer* **15,** 321 (1975).
27. H. P. Koeffler and D. W. Golde, *Science* **200,** 1153 (1978).
28. C. Friend, W. Scher, J. G. Holland, and T. Soto, *Proc. Natl. Acad. Sci. U.S.A.* **68,** 378 (1971).
29. S. H. Collins, F. W. Ruscetti, R. E. Gallagher, and R. C. Gallo, *Proc. Natl. Acad. Sci. U.S.A.* **75,** 2458 (1978).
30. H. E. Broxmeyer, A. Smithyman, R. R. Eger, P. A. Meyers, and M. DeSousa, *J. Exp. Med.* **148,** 1052 (1978).
31. A. W. Segal, *Lancet* **2,** 1248 (1974).
32. R. L. Baehner, L. Boxer, and J. David, *Blood* **48,** 309 (1976).
33. S. J. Collins, F. W. Ruscetti, R. E. Gallagher, and R. C. Gallo, *J. Exp. Med.* **149,** 969 (1979).
34. M. Tanaka, J. Levy, M. Terada, R. Breslow, R. Rifkind, and P. Marks, *Proc. Natl. Acad. Sci. U.S.A.* **72,** 1003 (1975).
35. H. P. Preisler and G. Lyman, *Cell Differ.* **4,** 179 (1975).
36. R. Reuben, R. Wife, R. Breslow, R. Rifkind, and P. Marks, *Proc. Natl. Acad. Sci. U.S.A.* **73,** 862 (1976).
37. S. Collins, A. Bodner, R. Ting, and R. C. Gallo, *Int. J. Cancer* **25,** 213 (1980).
38. Y. Ohta, M. Tamara, M. Terada, O. Miller, A. Bank, P. Marks, and R. Rifkind, *Proc. Natl. Acad. Sci. U.S.A.* **73,** 1232 (1976).
39. H. D. Preisler, G. Christoff, and R. Taylor, *Blood* **47,** 363 (1976).
40. N. Kluge, G. Gaedicke, G. Steinheider, S. Dube, and W. Ostertag, *Exp. Cell Res.* **88,** 257 (1974).
41. M. Territo and M. Cline, *J. Immunol.* **118,** 187 (1977).
42. G. B. Price, J. S. Senn, E. M. McCulloch, and J. E. Till, *Biochem. J.* **148,** 209 (1975).
43. A. W. Burgess, E. M. A. Wilson, and D. Metcalf, *Blood* **49,** 573 (1977).
44. K. Motoyoshi, F. Takaku, H. Mizoguchi, and Y. Miura, *Blood* **52,** 1012 (1978).
45. W. Scher, D. Tsui, S. Sassa, P. Price, A. Gabelman, and C. Friend, *Proc. Natl. Acad. Sci. U.S.A.* **75,** 3851 (1978).
46. S. C. Lo, R. Aft, J. Ross, and G. C. Mueller, *Cell* **15,** 447 (1978).
47. J. Lotem and L. Sachs, *Int. J. Cancer* **15,** 731 (1975).
48. Y. Honma, T. Kasukabe, J. Okabe, and M. Hozumi, *Gann* **68,** 241 (1977).
49. G. R. Crabtree, A. Munck, and K. Smith, *Nature* (*London*) **279,** 338 (1979).
50. I. Berenblum, *Prog. Exp. Tumor Res.* **11,** 21 (1969).
51. B. L. Van Durren and A. Sibak, *Cancer Res.* **28,** 2349 (1968).
52. G. Rovera, T. G. O'Brien, and L. Diamond, *Proc. Natl. Acad. Sci. U.S.A.* **74,** 2894 (1977).
53. H. Yamasaki, E. Fibach, V. Nudel, I. B. Weinstein, R. A. Rifkind, and P. A. Marks, *Proc. Natl. Acad. Sci. U.S.A.* **74,** 3451 (1977).
54. R. Cohen, M. Racifici, N. Rubinstein, J. Biehl, and H. Holtzer, *Nature* (*London*) **266,** 538 (1977).
55. L. Diamond, T. G. O'Brien, and G. Rovera, *Nature* (*London*) **269,** 247 (1977).
56. D. N. Ishii, E. Fibach, H. Yamasaki, and I. B. Weinstein, *Science* **200,** 556 (1978).
57. A. M. Raick, *Cancer Res.* **34,** 2915 (1974).

58. E. Huberman and M. F. Callahan, *Proc. Natl. Acad. Sci. U.S.A.* **76,** 1293 (1979).
59. G. Rovera, D. Santoli, and C. Damsky, *Proc. Natl. Acad. Sci. U.S.A.* **76,** 2779 (1979).
60. R. D. Estensen, J. G. White, and B. Holmes, *Nature* (*London*) **248,** 347 (1974).
61. I. M. Goldstein, S. T. Hoffstein, and G. Weissman, *J. Cell Biol.* **66,** 647 (1975).
62. J. E. Repine, J. G. White, C. C. Clawson, and B. Holmes, *J. Lab. Clin. Med.* **83,** 911 (1974).
63. L. R. De Chatelet, P. S. Shirley, and R. B. Johnston, *Blood* **47,** 545 (1976).
64. P. C. Jacquemin, C. Saxinger, and R. C. Gallo, *Nature* (*London*) **276,** 230 (1978).
65. P. A. Marks and R. A. Rifkind, *Annu. Rev. Biochem.* **47,** 419 (1978).
66. T. Pantazis, P. Sarin, and R. C. Gallo, unpublished observations.

28

Induction of Normal Differentiation in Malignant Cells as an Approach to Cancer Therapy

LEO SACHS

I. Introduction

Evidence has been obtained in various cell systems that malignant cells have not lost the genes for the normal control of growth and differentiation (1,2). Normal response to the physiological factors that control growth and differentiation appears to be due to a balance between genes for the expression (E) and suppression (S) of these properties (1–6). Normal genes present in malignant cells can be activated in two ways. If they are suppressed in the malignant cells because of an excess of S genes, they can be activated by segregation of the chromosomes that carry S genes either without cell hybridization (1,3,4–6) or after cell hybridization (7,8). If, however, they are normal genes in malignant cells which are not involved in the origin of the malignant state, they can be

ISBN 0-12-619280-4

activated by the normal physiological inducer without the necessity for chromosome segregation (2). The activation of normal growth control in sarcomas seems to belong to the first category (1,4,5), and the activation of normal differentiation in myeloid leukemic cells to the second (1,2). Both the activation of normal growth control in sarcomas due to chromosome segregation (1,4,5) and the activation of normal differentiation in myeloid leukemia which produces mature macrophages and granulocytes (1,2) result in the formation of cells that are no longer malignant. The expression of normal properties in the progeny of teratoma cells (9) could be due to either of these mechanisms.

Normal growth control could thus be induced therapeutically in malignant cells either by inducing the appropriate chromosome segregation in tumors belonging to the first category (1) or by using the appropriate inducer to activate the normal genes in tumors belonging to the second category (2). In tumors belonging to the second category, I have developed this approach with myeloid leukemia and would therefore like to discuss our studies with this type of leukemia.

II. Normal Differentiation of Myeloid Leukemia by the Physiological Macrophage and Granulocyte Inducer

My approach was originally based on *in vitro* studies on the differentiation of different types of white blood cells (1,2,10–16), including our identification (13–15) of a normal regulatory protein that we now call macrophage and granulocyte inducer (MGI) (17), and our development of an *in vitro* colony-forming assay for this protein with mouse (10,13–15) and human (18) cells (Fig. 1). We have shown that this protein is required for the viability, growth, and differentiation of normal macrophages and granulocytes (2). The discovery of MGI has made it possible to examine whether leukemic cells can still be induced to differentiate by this normal protein regulator. These experiments have shown that there is one type of myeloid leukemia cell, which we call $MGI^{+}D^{+}$, that can be induced by purified MGI (17,19,20) to differentiate normally to mature cells via the normal sequence of cell differentiation (2,21–23). This type of leukemic cell has been identified in different strains of mice (21,24) and in humans (18,25), and normal differentiation in these cells can be induced *in vitro* (2,25) (Figs. 2 and 3) and *in vivo* (20) (Fig. 4). differentiation *in vivo* can be enhanced by injecting MGI or grafting MGI-producing cells and seems to be regulated by cells involved in the immune response (20). Like normal mature macrophages and granulocytes, the mature cells induced from these leukemic cells are no longer malignant *in vivo* and no longer multiply *in vitro* (2). The protein regulator (13–15) called MGI has also been referred to by other names. After we had identified it we first called it *mashran gm* (26), and it has also been referred to as colony-stimulating factor (27) and colony-stimulating activity (28).

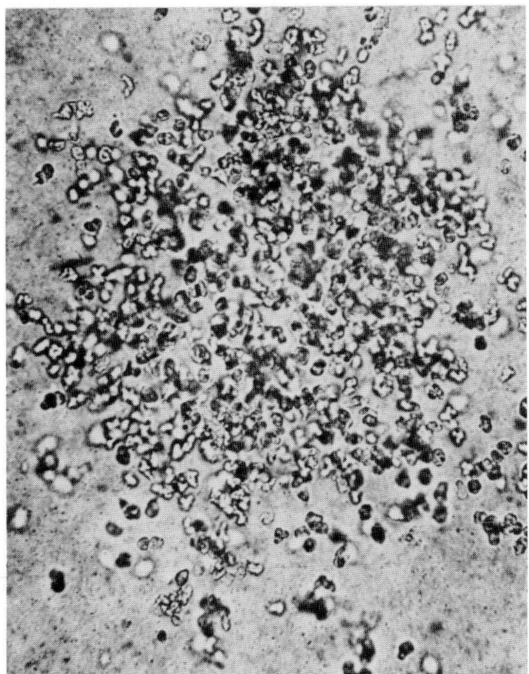

Fig. 1. Granulocyte colony induced *in vitro* from normal human bone marrow myeloid precursor cells by MGI (18).

III. Origin and Further Development of Myeloid Leukemia

Our experiments have shown that undifferentiated $MGI^{+}D^{+}$ leukemic cells are malignant, not because they cannot be induced to differentiate by normal regulatory protein MGI but because, unlike normal myeloid precursor cells, they no longer require MGI for cell viability and growth (2). The leukemic cells can therefore continue to multiply in the absence of MGI. These results have shown that leukemia can originate from the loss of a requirement of a normal regulatory protein for viability and growth in cells that can still be induced to differentiate normally by the normal protein regulator (2). This origin of leukemia is genetic and is associated with a chromosome change (6).

Experiments with different clones of myeloid leukemic cells have then shown that there can be further stages in the development of leukemia. The genetic change which allows leukemic cells to grow in the absence of MGI but still to differentiate normally, can then be followed by other genetic changes that can produce different blocks in differentiation (2,21,23,29). The isolation and study of such cell mutants has also made it possible to develop an experimental system that has been used to dissect genetically the controls that

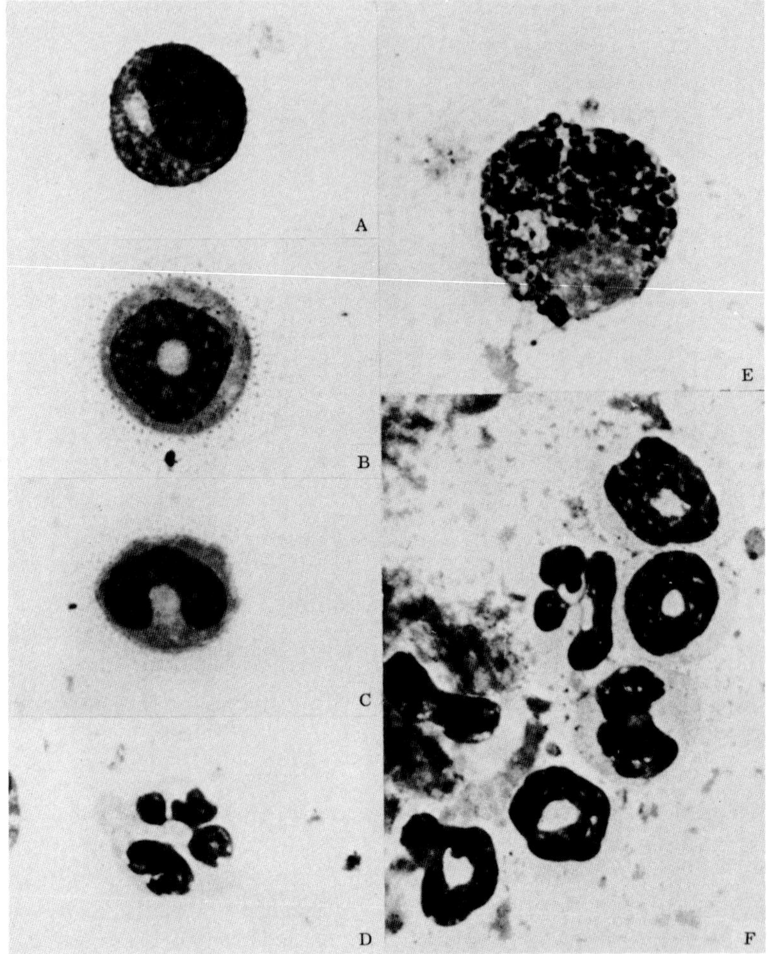

Fig. 2. *In vitro* differentiation of MGI^+D^+ mouse myeloid leukemia cells to macrophages and granulocytes by MGI. (A) Blast cell; (B-D) stages in differentiation to mature granulocytes; (E) macrophages; (F) group of granulocytes in different stages of differentiation (2).

regulate induction of a variety of internal and external differentiation-associated markers that are switched on by the normal regulatory protein during differentiation to mature macrophages and granulocytes (2,22,23).

IV. Cell Competence for Normal Differentiation

Experiments with leukemic cell clones with different degrees of competence for the induction of normal differentiation by MGI have shown that differences in

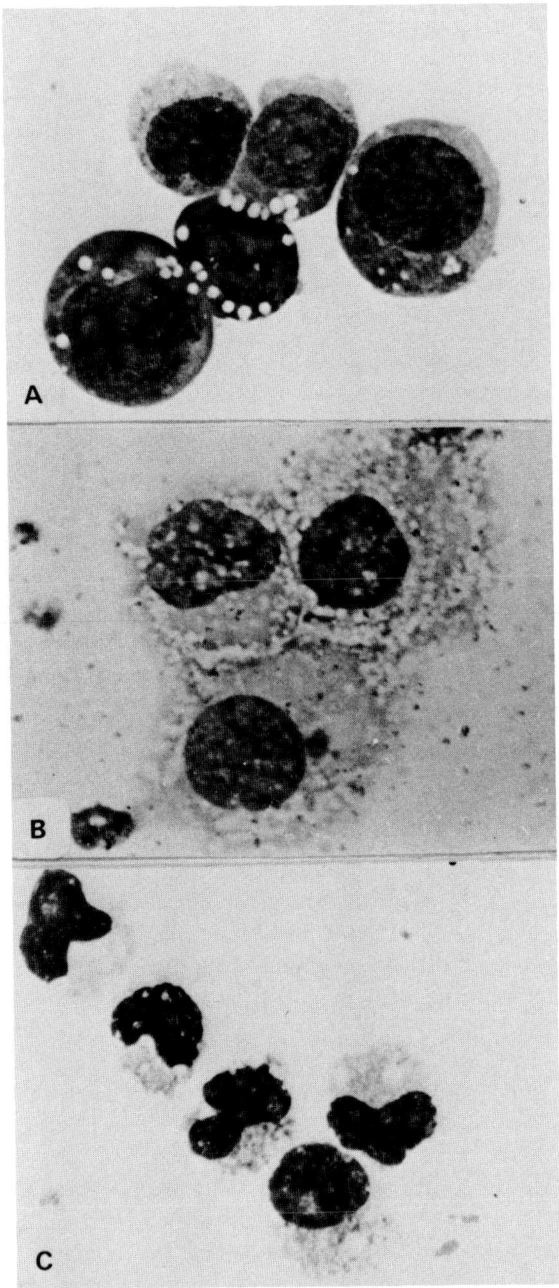

Fig. 3. *In vitro* differentiation of $MGI^{+}D^{+}$ human myeloid leukemia cells to macrophages and granulocytes. (A) Blast cells; (B) macrophages induced by MGI; (C) granulocytes induced by actinomycin D.

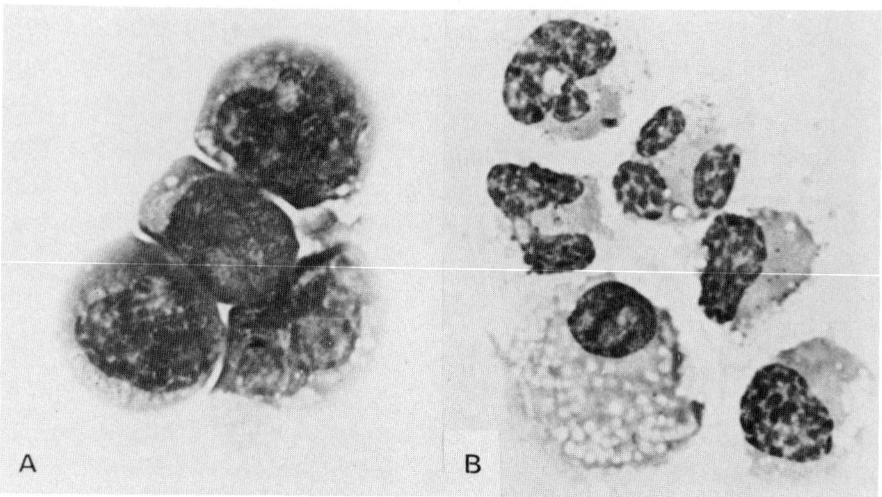

Fig. 4. *In vivo* differentiation of MGI^+D^+ mouse myeloid leukemic cells. (A) Blast cells in mice pretreated 1 day before cell implantation with cyclophosphamide; (B) cells in different stages of differentiation in normal mice: metamyelocyte (top), two mature granulocytes (center), macrophage (bottom left), two myelocytes (bottom right) (20).

competence are associated with specific membrane changes, including the mobility of certain surface receptors (1,22), the ability for hormone desensitization (30), and the production of type-C RNA viruses (29). The association between the mobility of certain surface receptors, as measured by cap formation, and the ability to respond to a differentiation inducer may be useful as an aid in the clinical diagnosis of various diseases (31,32). Genes for the expression and genes for the suppression of cell competence have been identified on two different chromosomes in the mouse, chromosomes 2 and 12, and it has been found that inducibility for differentiation by MGI is controlled by the balance between these genes (6).

Studies with various compounds other than MGI, including those used in the present forms of cytotoxic cancer therapy, have shown that some of the stages of differentiation can be induced in appropriate clones of myeloid leukemic cells by various steroids, certain surface-acting compounds, and some compounds that interact with DNA (Table I) (2,21,25,33). The use of appropriate cell mutants has shown that there can be different cellular sites for different compounds and that some compounds can act in mutant cells at differentiation sites no longer susceptible to the normal regulator MGI (2). There are also compounds that can induce cell susceptibility to MGI in mutants that are not induced to differentiate by adding only MGI (25). In certain cases, this activation of some stages of differentiation in leukemic cells appears to be due to inhibition of the formation

TABLE I

Inducers and Noninducers for Normal Differentiation-Associated Properties in MGI^+D^+ Myeloid Leukemic Cells[a]

Type of compound	Inducers	Noninducers
Peptide hormones	MGI	Erythropoietin, nerve growth factor, insulin, ubiquitin, thymopoietin, interferon
Steroids	Dexamethasone, prednisolone, hydrocortisone, estradiol	Progesterone, testosterone, epitestosterone, androstenedione, cortisone
Lectins	Concanavalin A, phytohemagglutinin, pokeweed mitogen	
Polycyclic hydrocarbons	Benzo(*a*)pyrene, dimethylbenz(*a*)anthracene	Benz(*a*)anthracene, dibenz (*a,c*) anthracene, dibenz (*a,h*) anthracene, phenanthrene
Other compounds	Lipopolysaccharide, lipid A, mitomycin C, dimethyl sulfoxide, arabinosylcytosine, hydroxyurea, thymidine, 5-iododeoxyuridine, 5-bromodeoxyuridine, nitrosoguanidine, actinomycin D, adriamycin, daunorubicin, X-irradiation, 12-*O*-tetradecanoylphorbol-13-acetate	Colchicine, vinblastine, sodium butyrate, cycloheximide, dibutyryl cyclic AMP, dibutyryl cyclic GMP, cordycepin, deoxyglucose, ouabain, ionophore 23187

[a] The different inducers were not all active on the same clone and did not all induce the same differentiation-associated properties (2).

of repressors of the differentiation process (2). It has also been found that some surface-acting compounds can induce differentiation in clones with the appropriate genotype by inducing in cells that differentiate the ability to produce the differentiation-inducing protein MGI (25,34) (Fig. 5).

V. Autoregulation of Differentiation Inducers

This induction of MGI production in cells that can be differentiated by MGI (25,34) has shown that induction of differentiation by a normal regulatory protein may not necessarily be dependent upon interaction between different types of cells but can be controlled by autoregulation. The induction, in cells that differentiate, of regulatory proteins like MGI that can induce specific cell differentiation may be a more general mechanism for the induction of differentiation by different inducers in various types of cells (2,34). Our finding of another protein inducer, the T-cell inducer (TCI) (35,36) that can induce the formation of normal T-cell colonies and can be produced by T cells (35) lends further support to the possibly important role of autoregulation in the control of normal cell growth and differentiation. Mouse erythroleukemic cells cannot be induced to differentiate by the normal erythroid-inducing protein erythropoietin but can be induced for some stages of differentiation by nonphysiological compounds such as dimethyl sulfoxide (37) and other surface-acting compounds (38). It will be of

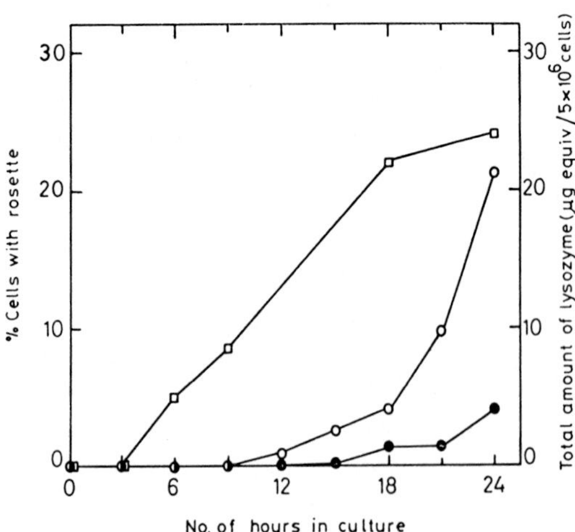

Fig. 5. Induction of MGI activity (□), Fc (○), and C3 rosettes (●) after treatment of MGI^+D^+ mouse myeloid leukemic cells *in vitro* with lipopolysaccharide. The presence of MGI activity in the medium of the treated cells was tested by the ability of the conditioned medium to induce lysozyme in a MGI^+D^+ clone that was resistant to lipopolysaccharide (34).

interest to determine if this involves the induction of a specific normal erythroid differentiation-inducing protein in leukemic cells.

VI. Therapeutic and Diagnostic Possibilities

Our results suggest novel forms of therapy for leukemia (1,2,20), which may be applicable to other diseases. The finding of myeloid leukemic cells that can be induced to differentiate normally by MGI indicates that MGI injection, grafting of MGI-producing cells (20), or stimulation of the *in vivo* production of MGI induces normal differentiation of these leukemic cells. This would be a form of tumor therapy not based on the search for cytotoxic agents that selectively kill tumor cells. The membrane differences among cells which differ in their competence to be induced to differentiate by MGI (1,2,16,22,30) may be useful predictive markers of the response to MGI *in vivo*. MGI^+D^+ leukemic cells can be induced to MGI to require again this protein for cell viability and growth (2). This suggests that induction of differentiation of leukemic cells to this stage, followed by the withdrawal of MGI, may also result in the loss of viability and growth of the induced MGI^+D^+ leukemic cells *in vivo*. Injection or *in vivo* stimulation of MGI may also be useful for treatment of nonmalignant granulocyte diseases (2,18).

Our results can also help to explain the response of some but not all patients to chemical and irradiation cytotoxic therapy. The chemicals and irradiation used in the present forms of cytotoxic therapy can induce some stages of differentiation in clones of myeloid leukemic cells with the appropriate genotype, and clonal differences in inducibility for normal differentiation-associated properties are not necessarily associated with differences in the response of these clones to the cytotoxic effect of these compounds (2). Some clones can be induced for properties such as Fc and C3 receptors, phagocytosis, and other macrophage-like properties, and such cells can be expected to behave differently in the body in their response to a variety of factors, including antibodies, than cells without these properties. The *in vivo* growth of leukemic cells with the appropriate genotype may thus be controlled by the therapeutic agents used, not only because of their cytotoxic effect but also because they induce these differentiation-associated properties. Differences in competence to be induced by these agents may thus explain differences in response to therapy in different individuals. The possible induction of MGI by these compounds may also play a role in the therapeutic effect observed with these compounds *in vivo* (2). Although treatment with dibutyryl cyclic AMP did not seem to induce differentiation in the myeloid leukemic clones tested, treatment with this compound has induced changes in the growth of some other types of tumor cells (39–42).

The results obtained with these leukemic cells therefore suggest possible new forms of therapy based on the use of a normal regulatory protein such as MGI to induce normal differentiation in malignant myeloid cells and a more rapid recovery of the normal cell population after the present forms of therapy. They also suggest the use of other compounds that can induce the normal regulatory protein, affect mutant malignant cells at differentiation sites no longer susceptible to the normal regulator (2), or induce the susceptibility of mutant cells to MGI (25). The finding of another regulatory protein such as TCI which acts on T lymphocytes (35,36) suggests that this approach may also be of value in cases of lymphoid leukemia. The induction of normal differentiation in malignant cells may be generally applicable as an approach to cancer therapy, and it is advisable that screening tests for compounds that act in this way on different types of tumor cells be widely introduced.

References

1. L. Sachs, *Harvy Lect.* **68,** 1 (1974).
2. L. Sachs, *Nature (London)* **274,** 535 (1978).
3. Z. Rabinowitz and L. Sachs, *Nature (London)* **225,** 136 (1970).
4. T. Yamamoto, Z. Rabinowitz, and L. Sachs, *Nature (London), New Biol.* **243,** 247 (1973).
5. N. Bloch-Shtacher and L. Sachs, *J. Cell. Physiol.* **87,** 89 (1976).
6. J. Azumi and L. Sachs, *Proc. Natl. Acad. Sci. U.S.A.* **74,** 253 (1977).
7. F. Wiener, G. Klein, and H. Harris, *J. Cell Sci.* **16,** 189 (1974).
8. N. R. Ringertz and R. E. Savage, "Cell Hybrids." Academic Press, New York, 1976.
9. B. Mintz and K. Illmensee, *Proc. Natl. Acad. Sci. U.S.A.* **72,** 3585 (1975).
10. H. Ginsburg and L. Sachs, *J. Natl. Cancer Inst.* **31,** 1 (1963).
11. L. Sachs, *in* "New Perspectives in Biology," ed. M. Sela p. 246. Elsevier, Amsterdam, 1964.
12. H. Ginsburg and L. Sachs, *J. Cell. Comp. Physiol.* **66,** 199 (1965).
13. D. H. Pluznik and L. Sachs, *J. Cell. Comp. Physiol.* **66,** 319 (1965).
14. D. H. Pluznik and L. Sachs, *Exp. Cell Res.* **43,** 553 (1966).
15. Y. Ichikawa, D. H. Pluznik, and L. Sachs, *Proc. Natl. Acad. Sci. U.S.A.* **56,** 488 (1966).
16. L. Sachs, *Isr. J. Med. Sci.* **13,** 654 (1977).
17. T. Landau and L. Sachs, *Proc. Natl. Acad. Sci. U.S.A.* **68,** 2540 (1971).
18. M. Paran, L. Sachs, Y. Barak, and P. Resnitzky, *Proc. Natl. Acad. Sci. U.S.A.* **67,** 1542 (1970).
19. E. Fibach, T. Landau, and L. Sachs, *Nature (London)* **237,** 276 (1972).
20. J. Lotem and L. Sachs, *Proc. Natl. Acad. Sci. U.S.A.* **75,** 3781 (1978).
21. J. Lotem and L. Sachs, *Proc. Natl. Acad. Sci. U.S.A.* **71,** 3507 (1974).
22. J. Lotem and L. Sachs, *Proc. Natl. Acad. Sci. U.S.A.* **74,** 5554 (1977).
23. B. Hoffman-Liebermann and L. Sachs, *Cell* **14,** 825 (1978).
24. Y. Ichikawa, *J. Cell. Physiol.* **74,** 223 (1969).
25. J. Lotem and L. Sachs, *Proc. Natl, Acad. Sci. U.S.A.* **76,** 5158 (1979).
26. Y. Ichikawa, D. H. Pluznik, and L. Sachs, *Proc. Natl. Acad. Sci. U.S.A.* **58,** 1480 (1967).
27. D. Metcalf, *J. Cell. Physiol.* **74,** 323 (1969).
28. P. E. Austin, E. A. McCulloch, and J. E. Till, *J. Cell. Physiol.* **77,** 121 (1971).
29. D. Liebermann and L. Sachs, *Cell* **15,** 823 (1978).
30. R. Simantov and L. Sachs, *Proc. Natl. Acad. Sci. U.S.A.* **75,** 1805 (1978).

31. U. Mintz and L. Sachs, *Proc. Natl. Acad. Sci. U.S.A.* **72,** 2428 (1975).
32. U. Mintz and L. Sachs, *Int. J. Cancer* **19,** 345 (1977).
33. S. J. Collins, F. W. Ruscetti, R. E. Gallagher, and R. C. Gallo, *Proc. Natl. Acad, Sci. U.S.A.* **75,** 2458 (1978).
34. B. Weiss and L. Sachs, *Proc. Natl. Acad. Sci. U.S.A.* **75,** 1374 (1978).
35. E. Gerassi and L. Sachs, *J. Immunol.* **121,** 2547 (1978).
36. D. Douer and L. Sachs, *J. Immunol.* **122,** 2473 (1979).
37. C. Friend, W. Sher, J. G. Holland, and T. Sato, *Proc. Natl. Acad. Sci. U.S.A.* **68,** 378 (1971).
38. R. C. Reuben, R. L. Wife, R. Breslow, R. Rifkind, and P. A. Marks, *Proc. Natl. Acad. Sci. U.S.A.* **73,** 862 (1976).
39. A. W. Hsie and T. T. Puck, *Proc. Natl. Acad. Sci. U.S.A.* **68,** 358 (1971).
40. K. N. Prasad and A. Vernadakis, *Exp. Cell Res.* **70,** 27 (1972).
41. R. Simantov and L. Sachs, *Europ. J. Biochem.* **30,** 123 (1972).
42. T. T. Puck, *Proc. Natl. Acad. Sci. U.S.A.* **74,** 4491 (1977).

Index

E

F